Pocket Guide to Medical-Surgical Nursing

Mosby's

POCKET GUIDE SERIES

Medical-Surgical Nursing

Second Edition

Pamela L. Swearingen, RN
Special Projects Editor

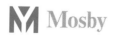 Mosby

St. Louis Baltimore Boston Carlsbad Chicago Naples New York
Philadelphia Portland London Madrid Mexico City Singapore
Sydney Tokyo Toronto Wiesbaden

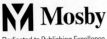

Mosby
Dedicated to Publishing Excellence

A Times Mirror Company

Editor: Robin Carter
Developmental Editor: Jeanne Allison
Project Manager: Mark Spann
Production Editor: Melissa Martin
Designer: David Zielinski
Manufacturing Supervisor: Betty Richmond

Printed in the United States of America
Composition by The Clarinda Company
Printing/binding by R.R. Donnelley & Sons Company

Mosby–Year Book, Inc.
11830 Westline Industrial Drive
St. Louis, Missouri 63146

Library of Congress Cataloging in Publication Data
Medical-surgical nursing / Pamela L. Swearingen, special projects editor.—2nd ed.
     p.   cm.—(Mosby's pocket guide series)
    Rev. ed. of: Pocket guide to medical-surgical nursing. c1992.
    Includes bibliographical references and index.
    ISBN 0-8151-8692-4
    1. Nursing—Handbooks, manuals, etc. 2. Surgical nursing--Handbooks, manuals, etc. I. Swearingen, Pamela L. II. Pocket guide to medical-surgical nursing. III. Series.
    [DNLM: 1. Nursing—methods—handbooks. 2. Surgical Nursing--handbooks. 3. Nursing Diagnosis—handbooks. WY 49 M489 1995]
RT51.S97 1995
610.73—dc20
DNLM/DLC
for Library of Congress
                          95-42113
                          CIP

96 97 98 99 00 / 9 8 7 6 5 4 3 2 1

Preface

Using a convenient-size format, *Mosby's Pocket Guide to Medical-Surgical Nursing*, second edition, offers nurses quick, easy access to information on over 170 medical-surgical disorders. Written and reviewed by expert nurses, this pocket guide was designed to be a clinical companion to medical-surgical textbooks and will help staff and student nurses plan and evaluate care of the adult medical-surgical patient. Its goal of being a portable, practical clinical reference has been met by both its size and its content, which in turn enhance its usefulness in the clinical setting. Focusing on NANDA-approved nursing diagnoses, this pocket guide includes the most important interventions for each of the most common medical-surgical disorders. The outcome criteria are explicit, positive statements that facilitate evaluation of care. In addition, generic information that applies to many of the specific disorders in the book, including physical and psychosocial nursing diagnoses and interventions for preoperative and postoperative patients, patients on prolonged bed rest, patients with cancer and other life-disrupting illnesses, and the elderly, is presented for reference in succinct, unified discussions in the appendixes.

Readers familiar with *Manual of Medical-Surgical Nursing Care: Nursing Interventions and Collaborative Management*, third edition (1994), may recognize many of the same nursing diagnoses and interventions in this pocket guide. Nursing diagnoses and interventions from the manual have been updated for the pocket guide and enhanced with information from the manual's other sections, including the pathophysiology, assessment, diagnostic testing, and collaborative management discussions. We suggest that readers who want more information than was possible to include in this more portable guide refer to the manual for greater detail and specific background information.

Finally, a word about the medical-surgical disorders that were selected: we chose those that either are commonly seen as primary admission diagnoses or are seen frequently as secondary diagnoses in hospitalized patients. To reduce the number of pages and ensure a portable, pocket-size reference, we did not include specific discussions of pediatrics, critical care, mental health, or other specialized areas.

Mosby's Pocket Guide to Medical-Surgical Nursing was designed to help students and staff nurses apply nursing diagnoses in the "real world" of the acute care hospital. Our reviewers believe that it achieves this objective; however, the ultimate judgment rests with the nurses who read and use the pocket guide on a daily basis. We welcome your comments on how we might enhance its usefulness in future editions.

Pamela L Swearingen

Contributors

Lolita Adrien, RN, MS, CETN
Clinical Nurse Specialist, Enterostomal Therapy
John Muir Medical Center
Walnut Creek, California

Linda S. Baas, RN, PhD, CCRN
Assistant Professor
University of Cincinnati, College of Nursing and Health
Cincinnati, Ohio

Marianne S. Baird, RN, MN, CCRN
Clinical Specialist, Critical Care
St. Joseph's Hospital of Atlanta
Atlanta, Georgia

Kathryn Schroeder Clark, RN, BSN, CCRN
Clinical Services Facilitator/Staff Nurse
Indiana University Hospitals
Indianapolis, Indiana

Mary E. Cooley, RN, CRNP, MSN, OCN
Oncology Clinical Specialist/Adult Nurse Practitioner
Philadelphia Veterans Affairs Medical Center
Philadelphia, Pennsylvania

Patricia Hall, RN, PhD
Clinical Nurse Specialist, Cardiac Services
Kennestone Hospital
Marietta, Georgia

Mima M. Horne, RN, MS, CDE
Diabetes Clinical Nurse Specialist
New Hanover Regional Medical Center
Adjunct Lecturer
University of North Carolina–Wilmington

Cheri A. Howard, RN, MSN
Unit Director
Indiana University Hospitals
Indianapolis, Indiana

Marguerite M. Jackson, RN, MS, CIC, FAAN
Administrative Director
Medical Center Epidemiology Unit
Assistant Clinical Professor
Community and Family Medicine
University of California–San Diego

Patricia E.R. Jansen, RN, MSN, CS
Geriatric Clinical Nurse Specialist
Consultant
San Jose, California

Janet Hicks Keen, RN, MS, CCRN, CEN
Staff Nurse, Level II, Emergency Department
St. Joseph's Hospital of Atlanta
Atlanta, Georgia
Clinical Instructor
Gordon College
Barnsville, Georgia

LCDR Kenneth Miller, RN, PhD, FAAN
Director, Clinical Nursing Research
National Naval Medical Center (US Navy)
Bethesda, Maryland

Dennis G. Ross, RN, PhD, MAE
Professor of Nursing
Castleton State College
Castleton, Vermont

Barbara Tueller Steuble, RN, MS
Education Coordinator
Sutter Amador Hospital
Jackson, California

Nancy A. Stotts, RN, MN, EdD
Associate Professor
Department of Physiological Nursing
University of California–San Francisco

Carol Monlux Swift, RN, BSN
Clinical Nurse III, Critical Care Unit
El Camino Hospital
Mountain View, California

Diane Wind Wardell, RN,C, PhD
Associate Professor
University of Texas Health Science Center at Houston

Karen S. Webber, RN, MN
Assistant Professor, School of Nursing
Memorial University of Newfoundland
St. John's, Newfoundland, Canada

Contents

Respiratory Disorders

SECTION ONE: ACUTE RESPIRATORY DISORDERS

Atelectasis

NURSING DIAGNOSES AND INTERVENTIONS

PATIENTS WITH ATELECTASIS

Impaired gas exchange related to altered oxygen supply or alveolar hypoventilation secondary to ventilation/perfusion mismatch occurring as a result of alveolar collapse

Desired outcomes: After intervention/treatment, patient has adequate gas exchange, as evidenced by normal skin color and orientation to time, place, and person. At a minimum of 24 h before hospital discharge, patient's ABG results are normal: Pa_{O_2} $\geq$80 mm Hg, pH 7.35-7.45, Pa_{CO_2} <45 mm Hg (or ABG results consistent with patient's baseline parameters).

1. Auscultate breath sounds at least q2-4h. Report any decrease in breath sounds or an increase in adventitious breath sounds.
2. Monitor patient for signs and symptoms of hypoxia: restlessness, agitation, changes in LOC, cyanosis. Report significant changes to physician.
3. Maintain a patent airway and ensure removal of secretions at least q2h; suction as indicated or prescribed.
4. Position patient for comfort and to promote optimal gas exchange (usually semi-Fowler's position).
5. Monitor serial ABG values. Be alert for decreasing Pa_{O_2} or increasing Pa_{CO_2}, both of which can signal impending respiratory compromise.

PATIENTS AT RISK FOR ATELECTASIS

Ineffective breathing pattern related to decreased lung expansion secondary to inactivity or omission of deep breathing

Desired outcome: Patient demonstrates deep breathing and effective coughing at least qh and is eupneic (RR 12-20 breaths/min with normal depth and pattern) at all other times.

1. Auscultate breath sounds at least q4h and during hyperinflation therapy. Report any decrease in breath sounds or presence of/increase in adventitious breath sounds.
2. Instruct patient in the use of hyperinflation device. Ensure that patient inhales slowly and deeply 2× normal tidal volume and holds the breath at least 5 sec at the end of inspiration. Ten breaths per hour is recommended to maintain adequate alveolar inflation. Deep breathing expands the alveoli, and coughing mobilizes and clears secretions. Monitor patient's progress and document in nurses' notes.
3. Administer analgesics as prescribed to reduce pain, since this may facilitate patient's coughing and deep-breathing exercises.
4. Encourage activity as prescribed to help mobilize secretions and promote effective airway clearance.

PATIENT-FAMILY TEACHING AND DISCHARGE PLANNING

Give patient and significant others verbal and written instructions about the following:
1. Use of hyperinflation device if patient is to continue this therapy at home. Conduct a predischarge check of patient's technique, and document assessment in progress notes.
2. Importance of maintaining activity level as prescribed to promote optimal lung expansion, mobilize secretions, and promote effective airway clearance.
3. Medications, including drug name, purpose, dosage, schedule, precautions, drug/drug and food/drug interactions, and potential side effects.
4. Precipitating factors in the development of atelectasis.
5. Importance of notifying physician if signs and symptoms recur.
6. Importance of medical follow-up; review date and time of next appointment.

Pneumonia

NURSING DIAGNOSES AND INTERVENTIONS

PATIENTS WITH PNEUMONIA

Impaired gas exchange related to altered oxygen supply and alveolar capillary membrane changes secondary to inflammatory process in the lungs

Desired outcomes: After intervention/treatment, patient has adequate gas exchange, as evidenced by RR 12-20 breaths/min with normal depth and pattern, and absence of signs and symptoms of respiratory distress. At a minimum of 24 h before hospital discharge, patient's Pao_2 is ≥80 mm Hg, $Paco_2$ is 35-45 mm Hg, and pH is 7.35-7.45 (or values consistent with patient's baseline).
1. Observe for signs and symptoms of respiratory distress: restlessness, anxiety, SOB, tachypnea, use of accessory muscles of respiration. Remember that cyanosis of the lips and nail beds may be a late indicator of hypoxia.

2. Monitor and document VS q2-4h. Be alert for a rising temperature and other changes in VS that may indicate infection (e.g., increased HR, increased RR).
3. Auscultate breath sounds q2-4h. Monitor for decreased or adventitious sounds (e.g., crackles or wheezes).
4. Monitor ABG results. A decreasing Pao_2 often indicates a need for oxygen therapy.
5. Position patient for comfort (usually semi-Fowler's position) to promote diaphragmatic descent, maximize inhalation, and decrease WOB. In patients with unilateral pneumonia, positioning on the unaffected side (i.e., "good side down") will promote ventilation/perfusion matching.
6. Deliver oxygen as prescribed; monitor FIo_2 to ensure that oxygen is within prescribed concentrations. Be aware that patients with chronic obstructive pulmonary disease (COPD) may not tolerate oxygen at a delivery of >2 L/min, which can suppress the centrally mediated respiratory drive in individuals with chronic CO_2 retention.
7. Provide periods of rest between care activities to decrease oxygen demand.

Ineffective airway clearance related to presence of tracheobronchial secretions secondary to infection or related to pain and fatigue secondary to lung consolidation

Desired outcomes: Patient demonstrates effective cough. After intervention, patient's airway is free of adventitious breath sounds.

1. Maintain a patent airway, and ensure that secretions are removed at least q2h. Suction as indicated or prescribed. Auscultate breath sounds q2-4h, and report changes in the patient's ability to clear pulmonary secretions.
2. Inspect sputum for quantity, color, and consistency; document findings. As patient's condition worsens, sputum can change in color from clear→white→yellow→green.
3. Ensure that patient performs deep breathing with coughing exercises at least q2h. Assist patient into position of comfort, usually semi-Fowler's position, to facilitate effectiveness and ease of these exercises.
4. Assess need for hyperinflation therapy (i.e., inability to take deep breaths). Report complications of hyperinflation therapy to physician: hyperventilation, gastric distention, headache, hypotension, signs and symptoms of pneumothorax (SOB, sharp chest pain, dyspnea, cough).
5. Teach patient to splint chest with pillow or crossed arms when coughing to reduce pain.
6. Ensure that patient gets prescribed chest physiotherapy. Document patient's response to treatment.
7. Assist patient with position changes q2h to help mobilize secretions. If patient is ambulatory, encourage ambulation to patient's tolerance.

Fluid volume deficit related to increased insensible loss secondary to tachypnea, fever, or diaphoresis

Desired outcome: At a minimum of 24 h before hospital discharge, patient is normovolemic, as evidenced by urine output ≥30

ml/h with specific gravity 1.010-1.030, stable weight, HR and BP within patient's normal limits, CVP >2 mm Hg (5 cm H_2O), moist mucous membranes, and normal skin turgor.

1. Monitor I&O. Consider insensible losses if patient is diaphoretic and tachypneic. Be alert for urinary output <30 ml/h.
2. Weigh patient daily, at the same time of day and on the same scale; record weight. Report weight decreases of 1-1.5 kg/day.
3. Encourage fluid intake (at least 2-3 L/day in unrestricted patient) to ensure adequate hydration.
4. Maintain IV fluid therapy as prescribed.
5. Promote oral hygiene, including lip and tongue care to moisten dried tissues and mucous membranes.

Altered nutrition: Less than body requirements related to anorexia

Desired outcome: At a minimum of 24 h before hospital discharge, patient has adequate nutrition, as evidenced by stable weight, balanced or positive nitrogen state, and serum albumin 3.5-5.5 g/dl.

1. Provide small, frequent feedings of nutritious foods that are easy to consume. Monitor and record amount of nutrients consumed.
2. Request dietetic consultation so that patient can discuss food likes and dislikes.
3. Ask physician to prescribe dietary supplements if patient is unable to consume adequate diet.
4. Discuss with patient and significant others the importance of good nutrition in the treatment of pneumonia.
5. For other interventions, see "Providing Nutritional Support," p. 378.

PATIENTS AT RISK FOR DEVELOPING PNEUMONIA

Risk for infection (nosocomial pneumonia) related to inadequate primary defenses (e.g., decreased ciliary action), invasive procedures (e.g., intubation), and/or chronic disease

Desired outcome: Patient is free of infection, as evidenced by normothermia, WBC count ≤11,000/μl, and sputum clear to whitish in color.

1. Perform good handwashing technique before and after contact with patient (even though gloves were worn).
2. Identify presurgical candidate who is at increased risk for nosocomial pneumonia because of the following: older adult (>70 yr), obesity, COPD, history of smoking, abnormal pulmonary function tests (especially decreased forced expiratory flow rate), intubation, upper abdominal/thoracic surgery.
3. Provide preoperative teaching, explaining and demonstrating the following pulmonary exercises, which will be used postoperatively to prevent respiratory infection: deep breathing, coughing, turning in bed, ambulation, use of hyperinflation device. Make sure patient verbalizes knowledge of exercises and their rationale and *returns* demonstrations appropriately. Encourage individuals who smoke to discontinue smoking, especially during preoperative and postoperative periods.
4. Control pain, which interferes with lung expansion, by administering analgesics 30 min before deep-breathing exercises. Support

(splint) surgical wound with hands or pillows placed firmly across site of incision.

5. Identify patients who are at increased risk for aspiration: depressed LOC, dysphagia, nasogastric (NG) tube in place. Maintain HOB at 30-degree elevation, and turn patient onto side rather than back. When patient receives enteral alimentation, recommend continuous rather than bolus feedings.

6. Recognize risk factors for patients with tracheostomy: underlying lung disease or other serious illness, increased colonization of oropharynx or trachea by aerobic gram-negative bacteria, greater access of bacteria to lower respiratory tract, cross-contamination due to manipulation of tracheostomy tube.

7. Use "no touch" technique or wear sterile gloves on both hands until tracheostomy wound has healed or formed granulation tissue around tube.

8. Suction prn rather than on a routine basis because frequent suctioning increases risk of trauma and cross-contamination.

9. Use sterile catheter for each suctioning procedure and sterile solutions if secretions are tenacious and catheter flushing is necessary. Consider use of closed suction system to further minimize risk of contamination.

10. Always wear gloves on both hands to suction.

11. Recognize the following ways in which nebulizer reservoirs can contaminate patient: introduction of nonsterile fluids or air, manipulation of nebulizer cup, backflow of condensate from delivery tubing into reservoir or into patient when tubing is manipulated.
   - Use only sterile fluids, and dispense them aseptically.
   - Replace (rather than replenish) solutions and equipment at frequent intervals. For example, empty reservoir completely and refill with sterile solution q8-24h, according to agency protocol.
   - Change breathing circuits q48h or according to agency policy; if used for multiple patients, replace breathing circuit with sterilized or disinfected breathing circuit between patients.
   - Fill fluid reservoirs immediately before use (not far in advance).
   - Discard any fluid that has condensed in tubing; do not allow it to drain back into reservoir or patient.

PATIENT-FAMILY TEACHING AND DISCHARGE PLANNING

Give patient and significant others verbal and written information about the following:

1. Techniques that promote gas exchange and minimize stasis of secretions: deep breathing, coughing, use of hyperinflation device, increasing activity level as appropriate for patient's medical condition, percussion and postural drainage as necessary.

2. Medications, including drug name, purpose, dosage, schedule, precautions, drug/drug and food/drug interactions, and potential side effects, particularly of antibiotics (see p. 317).

3. Signs and symptoms of pneumonia and the importance of reporting them promptly to health professional should they recur. Teach patient's significant others that changes in sensorium may be the only indicator of pneumonia if patient is elderly.
4. Importance of preventing fatigue by pacing activities and allowing for frequent rest periods.
5. Importance of avoiding exposure to individuals known to have flu or colds. Recommend that patient get annual flu and pneumococcal vaccinations.
6. Minimizing factors that can cause reinfection: close living conditions, poor nutrition, poorly ventilated living quarters or work environment.

Pleural Effusion

NURSING DIAGNOSES AND INTERVENTIONS

Ineffective breathing pattern related to decreased lung expansion secondary to fluid accumulation in the pleural space
Desired outcome: After intervention, patient's breathing pattern moves toward eupnea.
1. Auscultate breath sounds q2-4h, monitoring for decreasing breath sounds or pleural friction rub.
2. Ensure patency of chest drainage system (see guidelines, p. 10, in "Pneumothorax/Hemothorax").
3. Position patient for maximum chest expansion, generally semi-Fowler's position.
4. If hyperinflation therapy is prescribed, instruct patient in its use. Reinforce teaching, and document patient's progress.
5. For patients with gross pleural effusion, provide the following instructions for apical expansion breathing exercises:
   - Sit upright.
   - Position fingers just below the clavicles.
   - Inhale and attempt to push upper chest wall against the pressure of the fingers.
   - Hold breath for a few seconds, and then exhale passively.
When performed at frequent intervals, this exercise will help expand the involved lung tissues, minimize flattening of the upper chest, and mobilize secretions.

Also see "Pneumonia" for **Impaired gas exchange,** p. 2, and **Altered nutrition,** p. 4. See "Pneumothorax/Hemothorax" for **Pain,** p. 11.

PATIENT-FAMILY TEACHING
AND DISCHARGE PLANNING

Give patient and significant others verbal and written instructions about the following:
1. Importance of quitting smoking. Provide patient with resources related to "stop smoking" programs.

2. Signs of respiratory distress (restlessness, agitation, changes in behavior, complaints of SOB or dyspnea) and the importance of notifying physician if these signs occur.
3. Use of equipment at home: hyperinflation device, nebulizer, oxygen.
4. Medications, including drug name, purpose, dosage, schedule, precautions, drug/drug and food/drug interactions, and potential side effects.

Pulmonary Embolus

NURSING DIAGNOSES AND INTERVENTIONS

Impaired gas exchange related to altered oxygen supply secondary to ventilation/perfusion mismatch

Desired outcomes: After intervention/treatment, patient exhibits adequate gas exchange and ventilatory function, as evidenced by RR 12-20 breaths/min with normal pattern and depth (eupnea) and orientation to time, place, and person. At a minimum of 24 h before hospital discharge, patient has $Pao_2 \geq 80$ mm Hg, $Paco_2$ 35-45 mm Hg, and pH 7.35-7.45 (or values consistent with patient's baseline parameters).

1. Monitor patient for signs and symptoms of increasing respiratory distress: RR increased from baseline, increasing dyspnea, anxiety, restlessness, confusion, cyanosis.
2. Position patient for comfort and optimal gas exchange. Ensure that area of lung affected by embolus is not dependent when patient is in lateral decubitus position. Elevate HOB 30 degrees to improve ventilation.
3. Avoid positioning patient with knees bent (i.e., gatching the bed), because this impedes venous return from the legs and can increase the risk of pulmonary embolus (PE).
4. Reduce metabolic demands for oxygen by limiting or pacing patient's activities and procedures.
5. Ensure that patient performs deep-breathing and coughing exercises q2h.
6. Ensure delivery of prescribed concentrations of oxygen.
7. Monitor serial ABG values, assessing for desired response to treatment. Report lack of response to treatment or worsening ABG values.

Altered protection related to risk of prolonged bleeding or hemorrhage secondary to anticoagulation therapy

Desired outcome: Patient is free of frank or occult bleeding; body secretions/excretions test negative for blood.

1. Monitor VS for indicators of profuse bleeding or hemorrhage resulting from anticoagulant therapy: hypotension, tachycardia, tachypnea.
2. At least once a shift, check stool, urine, sputum, and vomitus for occult blood, using agency-approved method for testing.
3. At least once a shift, inspect wounds, oral mucous membranes, any entry site of an invasive procedure, and nares for evidence of bleeding.

4. At least once per shift, inspect torso and extremities for petechiae or ecchymoses.
5. To prevent hematoma formation, do not give an IM injection unless it is unavoidable.
6. Apply pressure to all venipuncture or arterial puncture sites until bleeding stops completely.
7. Ensure easy access to antidotes for prescribed treatment.
   - *Protamine sulfate:* 1 mg counteracts 100 U of heparin. Usually, the initial dose is 50 mg.
   - *Vitamin K:* 20 mg given SC to counteract the effects of oral anticoagulants.
   - *ε-Aminocaproic acid* (e.g., Amicar): Administered *via* slow IV infusion of 5 g; reverses the fibrinolytic condition related to thrombolytic therapy.
8. If patient is undergoing heparin therapy, monitor serial PTT (desired range is 1½-2½ × control). If patient is undergoing warfarin (Coumadin) therapy, monitor serial PT (desired range is 1¼-1½ × control). Report values outside desired range.
9. To prevent negative interactions with anticoagulants or thrombolytic therapy, establish compatibility of all drugs before administering them.
   - *Heparin:* Digitalis, tetracyclines, nicotine, and antihistamines decrease the effect of heparin therapy. Consult pharmacist about compatibility before infusing other IV drugs through heparin IV line.
   - *Warfarin sodium:* Numerous drugs can decrease or increase the response to treatment with warfarin. Consult pharmacist to obtain specific information about patient's medication profile.
   - *Thrombolytic therapy (e.g., streptokinase, urokinase):* No specific drug interactions are noted. However, consult pharmacist before infusing any other medication through the same IV line.
10. Because aspirin and nonsteroidal antiinflammatory drugs (NSAIDs), such as ibuprofen, are platelet-aggregation inhibitors and can prolong bleeding, avoid use of *any* drug that contains these medications.
11. Discuss with patient and significant others the importance of promptly reporting bleeding from any source.
12. Explain to patient the need to use sponge-tipped applicators and mouthwash for oral care to minimize the risk of gum bleeding. Instruct patient to shave with an electric razor rather than a straight or safety razor.
13. If patient is restless and combative, provide a safe environment: Pad side rails, restrain patient as necessary to prevent falls, and use extreme care when moving patient to avoid bumping extremities into side rails.

Knowledge deficit: Oral anticoagulant therapy, potential side effects, and foods and medications to avoid during therapy

Desired outcome: Within the 24 h before hospital discharge, patient verbalizes knowledge of prescribed anticoagulant drug, potential side effects, and foods and medications to avoid while undergoing oral anticoagulant therapy.

1. Determine patient's knowledge of oral anticoagulant therapy. As appropriate, discuss the drug name, purpose, dosage, schedule, precautions, drug/drug and food/drug interactions, and side effects.
2. Inform patient of potential side effects/complications of anticoagulant therapy: easy bruising; prolonged bleeding from cuts; spontaneous nosebleeds; black, tarry stools; blood in urine and sputum.
3. Discuss with patient the importance of laboratory testing and follow-up visits with physician.
4. Explain the importance of informing all health care providers (e.g., dentists and other physicians) that patient is taking anticoagulants. Suggest that patient wear a Medic-Alert tag or other means of informing health care providers about the anticoagulant therapy.
5. Teach patient about foods high in vitamin K (e.g., fish, bananas, dark green vegetables, tomatoes, and cauliflower), which can interfere with anticoagulation.
6. Caution patient that a soft-bristled, rather than hard-bristled, toothbrush and an electric razor rather than a straight or safety razor should be used during anticoagulant therapy to minimize the risk of injury that could cause bleeding.
7. Instruct patient to consult physician before taking OTC or prescribed drugs that were used before anticoagulant therapy was begun. Aspirin, cimetidine, and trimethaphan are among the many drugs that enhance the response to warfarin. Drugs that decrease the response include antacids, diuretics, oral contraceptives, and barbiturates, among others.

Also, if appropriate, see Appendix One, "Caring for Preoperative and Postoperative Patients," p. 395, and "Caring for Patients on Prolonged Bed Rest," p. 413.

PATIENT-FAMILY TEACHING
AND DISCHARGE PLANNING

Give patient and significant others verbal and written instructions about the following:
1. Risk factors related to the development of thrombi and embolization and preventive measures to reduce the risk.
2. Signs and symptoms of *thrombophlebitis:* swelling of the calf, tenderness or warmth in the involved area, possible pain in affected calf when ankle is flexed, slight fever, distention of veins in affected leg. Also, signs and symptoms of *pulmonary embolism:* sudden onset of dyspnea and anxiety, nonproductive cough, palpitations, nausea, syncope.
3. Purpose of and procedure for putting on antiembolism hose. Explain that patient should put them on in the morning before getting out of bed.
4. Importance of preventing impairment of venous return from the lower extremities by avoiding prolonged sitting, crossing legs, and constrictive clothing.

N O T E :   Rehabilitation and family teaching concepts for fat emboli are nonspecific.

Pneumothorax/Hemothorax

NURSING DIAGNOSES AND INTERVENTIONS

Impaired gas exchange related to altered oxygen supply secondary to ventilation/perfusion mismatch

Desired outcomes: After treatment/intervention, patient exhibits adequate gas exchange and ventilatory function, as evidenced by RR $\leq$20 breaths/min with normal depth and pattern (eupnea) and orientation to time, place, and person. At a minimum of 24 h before hospital discharge, patient's ABG values are as follows: Pao_2 $\geq$80 mm Hg and $Paco_2$ 35-45 mm Hg (or values within patient's acceptable baseline parameters).

1. Monitor serial ABG results to detect decreasing Pao_2 and increasing $Paco_2$, which can signal impending respiratory compromise. Report significant findings to physician.
2. Observe for indicators of hypoxia: increased restlessness, anxiety, changes in mental status. Cyanosis may be a late sign.
3. Assess patient's VS and breath sounds q2-4h (patient will require checks q15min after thoracotomy until stable) for signs of respiratory distress: increased RR, diminished or absent movement of chest wall on affected side, paradoxic movement of chest wall, increased WOB, use of accessory muscles of respiration, complaints of increased dyspnea, cyanosis. Evaluate HR and BP for indications of shock (i.e., tachycardia and hypotension).
4. Position patient to allow for full expansion of unaffected lung. Semi-Fowler's position usually provides comfort and allows adequate expansion of chest wall and descent of diaphragm.
5. Change patient's position q2h to promote drainage and lung reexpansion and to facilitate alveolar perfusion.
6. Encourage patient to take deep breaths, providing analgesia necessary to reduce discomfort during deep-breathing exercises. Deep breathing promotes full lung expansion and may reduce the risk of atelectasis. Coughing facilitates mobilization of tracheobronchial secretions, if present.
7. Deliver and monitor oxygen as indicated.

Ineffective breathing pattern (or risk for same) related to decreased lung expansion secondary to malfunction of chest drainage system

Desired outcome: After intervention, patient becomes eupneic.

1. Monitor patient at frequent intervals (q2-4h, as appropriate) to assess breathing pattern while chest drainage system is in place. Auscultate breath sounds and report a decrease; be alert for and report signs of respiratory distress: restlessness, anxiety, changes in mental status.
2. Assess and maintain the closed chest-drainage system.
   - Tape all connections, and secure chest tube to thorax with tape.
   - Ensure that there are no kinks in the tubing, and that the bed and equipment are not compressing any component of the system.

- Eliminate all dependent loops in the tubing, because they may impede removal of air and fluid from the pleural space.
- Maintain fluid in underwater-seal chamber, and suction chamber at appropriate levels.

3. Be aware that the suction apparatus does not regulate the amount of suction applied to the closed chest-drainage system. The amount of suction is determined by the water level in the suction control chamber. Minimal bubbling in this chamber is acceptable and desirable. **Note:** Suction aids in the reexpansion of the lung, but removing suction for short periods of time, such as for transporting, is not detrimental and will not disrupt the closed chest-drainage system.

4. Follow institution's policy about chest tube stripping. Be aware that this mechanism for maintaining tube patency is controversial and has been associated with creating high negative pressures in the pleural space, which can damage fragile lung tissue. Tube stripping may be indicated when bloody drainage or clots are visible in the tubing. Squeezing alternately hand over hand along the drainage tube may generate sufficient pressure to move fluid along the tube.

5. Be aware that fluctuations in the long tube of the underwater-seal chamber are characteristic of a patent chest tube. Fluctuations stop when either the lung has reexpanded or a kink or obstruction is present in the chest tube.
   - Bubbling in the underwater-seal chamber occurs on expiration and is a sign that air is leaving the pleural space.
   - Continuous bubbling in the underwater-seal chamber may be a signal that air is leaking into the drainage system. Locate and seal the leak, if possible.

6. Keep necessary emergency supplies at bedside: petrolatum gauze pad to apply over insertion site if the chest tube becomes dislodged, and sterile water in which to submerge chest tube if it becomes disconnected from the underwater-seal system. *Never* clamp a chest tube without a specific directive from the physician, inasmuch as clamping may lead to tension pneumothorax because air in the pleural space can no longer escape.

Pain related to impaired pleural integrity, inflammation, or presence of a chest tube

Desired outcome: Within 30-60 min of intervention, patient's subjective perception of pain decreases, as documented by a pain scale.

1. At frequent intervals, assess patient's degree of discomfort. Devise a pain scale with patient (e.g., rating pain from 0 [no pain] to 10 [worst pain]). Medicate with analgesics as prescribed, using pain scale to evaluate and document medication's effectiveness.

2. Premedicate patient 30 min before initiating coughing, exercising, or repositioning.

3. Teach patient to splint affected side when coughing, moving, or repositioning.

4. Schedule activities to provide for 90-min periods of undisturbed rest, which may raise patient's pain threshold.

5. Stabilize chest tube to reduce pull or drag on latex connector tubing. Tape chest tube securely to thorax.

6. For additional interventions, see Appendix One, p. 396.

See "Abdominal Trauma" for **Fluid volume deficit,** p. 265. Also see psychosocial nursing diagnoses and interventions in Appendix One, "Caring for Patients with Cancer and Other Life-Disrupting Illnesses," p. 450.

PATIENT-FAMILY TEACHING AND DISCHARGE PLANNING

Give patient and significant others verbal and written instructions about the following:

1. Purpose of chest tube placement and maintenance.
2. Potential for recurrence of spontaneous pneumothorax (average interval between occurrences is 2-3 yr). Explain the importance of seeking medical care immediately if symptoms recur (Table 1-1).
3. Medications, including drug name, purpose, dosage, schedule, precautions, drug/drug and food/drug interactions, and potential side effects.

Pulmonary Tuberculosis

NURSING DIAGNOSES AND INTERVENTIONS

Knowledge deficit: Spread of tuberculosis (TB) and procedure for AFB isolation

Desired outcome: After instruction, patient and significant others verbalize how TB is spread and measures necessary to prevent spread of the disease.

1. Teach patient about TB and the mechanism by which it is spread.
2. Explain isolation to patient and significant others. Post a notice of isolation/airborne precautions on patient's room door.
3. Explain to staff and visitors the importance of wearing high-efficiency masks, including proper fit and use. Provide masks at doorway or other convenient place.
4. Teach patient the importance of covering mouth and nose with tissue when sneezing or coughing and of disposing of used tissue in container suitable for biohazardous waste disposal.
5. Stress the importance of good handwashing technique to reduce the risk of ingesting the organism.

PATIENT-FAMILY TEACHING AND DISCHARGE PLANNING

Give patient and significant others verbal and written information about the following:

1. Importance of good handwashing technique.
2. Antituberculosis medications, including drug name, purpose, dosage, schedule, precautions, drug/drug and food/drug interactions, and potential side effects. Remind patient that medications are to be taken uninterruptedly for the prescribed period.
3. Importance of periodic reculturing of sputum.

Table 1-1   Assessment of patient with pneumothorax or hemothorax

	Spontaneous or Traumatic Pneumothorax		Tension Pneumothorax	Hemothorax
	Closed	Open		
Signs and Symptoms	SOB, cough, chest tightness, chest pain	SOB, sharp chest pain	Dyspnea, chest pain	Dyspnea, chest pain
Physical Assessment	Tachypnea, decreased thoracic movement, cyanosis, subcutaneous emphysema, hyperresonance over affected area, diminished breath sounds, paradoxic movement of chest wall (may signal flail chest), change in mental status	Agitation, restlessness, tachypnea, cyanosis, presence of chest wound, hyperresonance over affected area, sucking sound on inspiration, diminished breath sounds, change in mental status	Anxiety, tachycardia, cyanosis, jugular vein distention, tracheal deviation toward unaffected side, absent breath sounds on affected side, distant heart sounds, hypotension, change in mental status	Tachypnea, pallor, cyanosis, dullness over affected side, tachycardia, hypotension, diminished or absent breath sounds, change in mental status

SECTION TWO: ACUTE RESPIRATORY FAILURE

NURSING DIAGNOSES AND INTERVENTIONS

See "Pneumonia" for **Impaired gas exchange**, p. 2, and **Fluid volume deficit**, p. 3.

Also see "Atelectasis," p. 1, "Pleural Effusion," p. 6, "Pulmonary Embolus," p. 7, "Pneumothorax/Hemothorax," p. 10, "Asthma," p. 15, "Chronic Bronchitis," p. 16, "Emphysema," p. 18, "Pulmonary Fibrosis," p. 20, "Pulmonary Edema," p. 49, "Guillain-Barré Syndrome," p. 20, and "Multiple Sclerosis," p. 113, because these disorders may be precursors to acute respiratory failure.

For psychosocial nursing diagnoses and interventions, see Appendix One, "Caring for Patients with Cancer and Other Life-Disrupting Illnesses," p. 450.

PATIENT-FAMILY TEACHING AND DISCHARGE PLANNING

Acute respiratory failure (ARF) is symptomatically treated during the patient's hospitalization. Discharge planning and teaching should be di-

Table 1-2   Disease processes leading to the development of respiratory failure

Impaired Alveolar Ventilation	Ventilation or Perfusion Disturbances
Chronic obstructive pulmonary disease (emphysema, bronchitis, asthma, cystic fibrosis)	Pulmonary emboli
	Atelectasis
	Pneumonia
Restrictive pulmonary disease (interstitial fibrosis, pleural effusion, pneumothorax, kyphoscoliosis, obesity, diaphragmatic paralysis)	Emphysema
	Chronic bronchitis
	Bronchiolitis
	Adult respiratory distress syndrome
Neuromuscular defects (Guillain-Barré syndrome, myasthenia gravis, multiple sclerosis, muscular dystrophy)	**Diffusion Disturbances**
	Pulmonary/interstitial fibrosis
	Pulmonary edema
Depression of respiratory control centers (drug-induced cerebral infarction, inappropriate use of high-dose O_2 therapy)	Adult respiratory distress syndrome
	Anatomic loss of functioning lung tissue (tumor pneumonectomy)

From Howard C. In Swearingen PL, Keen JH: *Manual of critical care nursing: nursing interventions and collaborative management,* ed 3, St Louis, 1995, Mosby.

rected at educating the patient and significant others about the underlying pathophysiology and specific treatment for that process. See sections in this chapter that relate specifically to the underlying disease process contributing to the development of ARF. See Table 1-2 for more information.

SECTION THREE: CHRONIC OBSTRUCTIVE PULMONARY DISEASE

Asthma

NURSING DIAGNOSES AND INTERVENTIONS

Impaired gas exchange related to altered oxygen supply secondary to decreased alveolar ventilation as a result of narrowed airways
Desired outcomes: After treatment/intervention, patient has adequate gas exchange, as evidenced by RR 12-20 breaths/min. Before hospital discharge, patient's ABG values are as follows: Pao_2 $\geq$80 mm Hg, $Paco_2$ 35-45 mm Hg, and pH 7.35-7.45 (or values consistent with patient's baseline).

1. Observe for signs and symptoms of hypoxia: agitation, restlessness, changes in LOC. Remember that cyanosis of the lips and nail beds is a late indicator of hypoxia.
2. Position patient for comfort and to promote optimal gas exchange. Usually this is accomplished using high Fowler's position, with the patient leaning forward and elbows propped on the over-the-bed table to promote maximal chest expansion. Record patient's response to positioning.
3. Auscultate breath sounds q2-4h. Monitor for decreased or adventitious sounds (e.g., crackles or wheezes).
4. Monitor ABG results. Be alert for decreasing Pao_2 and increasing $Paco_2$, which can signal respiratory compromise.
5. Deliver and monitor O_2 as prescribed.

See "Chronic Bronchitis" for **Ineffective airway clearance,** p. 16.
See "Emphysema" for **Ineffective breathing pattern,** p. 18.
For anxiety, see Appendix One, p. 451. For other nursing diagnoses related to psychosocial interventions, see Appendix One, "Caring for Patients with Cancer and Other Life-Disrupting illnesses," p. 450.

PATIENT-FAMILY TEACHING AND DISCHARGE PLANNING

Give patient and significant others verbal and written instructions about the following:

1. Irritants that can precipitate an attack, and the importance of removing these irritants from patient's environment.
2. Signs and symptoms of pulmonary infection (increased cough, increasing sputum production, change in color of sputum from clear white to yellow-green, fever) or bronchial irritation (dry, hacking cough).
3. Medications, including drug name, purpose, dosage, schedule, precautions, drug/drug and food/drug interactions, and potential side effects. In addition, teach patient the proper use of metered-dose inhalers, documenting accurate return of demonstration before hospital discharge. Remind patient that OTC inhalers contain medications that can interfere with the prescribed therapy. Instruct patient to contact physician before taking any OTC medications.
4. Importance of avoiding contact with infectious individuals, especially those with respiratory infections. Encourage patient to get yearly flu and pneumococcal vaccinations.
5. Importance of follow-up care. Confirm date and time of next appointment.

Chronic Bronchitis

NURSING DIAGNOSES AND INTERVENTIONS

Ineffective airway clearance related to decreased energy, which results in ineffective cough, or related to presence of increased tracheobronchial secretions

Desired outcome: After intervention, patient coughs appropriately and has effective airway clearance, as evidenced by absence of adventitious breath sounds.

1. Auscultate breath sounds q2-4h and after coughing. Be alert for and report changes in adventitious breath sounds.
2. Teach patient the "double cough" technique:
   - Sit upright with upper body flexed forward slightly.
   - Take two to three breaths, and exhale passively.
   - Inhale again, but only to the mid-inspiratory point.
   - Exhale by coughing quickly two or three times.

This technique prevents collapse of small airways, which can occur with forceful coughing.

3. Administer chest physiotherapy as prescribed to mobilize secretions.

Altered nutrition: Less than body requirements, related to decreased intake secondary to fatigue and anorexia

Desired outcome: For at least the 24 h before hospital discharge, patient has adequate nutrition, as evidenced by stable weight, positive nitrogen (N) state on N studies, and serum albumin 3.5-5.5 μg/dl.

Table 1-3   Guidelines on calorie sources for patients with COPD

Foods High in Fat	Foods to Avoid
Whole milk	Cakes
Cream	Cookies
Evaporated milk	Jams
Cream soups	Pastries
Custards	Sugar-concentrated snacks
Cheese	
Salad and cooking oils	
Margarine	
Mayonnaise	
Nuts	
Meat	
Poultry	
Fish	

1. Monitor patient's food and fluid intake. If indicated, obtain dietary consultation for calorie counts.
2. Provide diet in small, frequent meals that are nutritious and easy to consume.
3. Request a dietetic consultation so that patient can discuss food likes and dislikes.
4. Unless otherwise indicated, provide calories more from unsaturated fat sources (Table 1-3) than from carbohydrate sources. During the process of carbohydrate metabolism, the body uses O_2 and produces CO_2, which is dissipated by the lungs. A patient with chronic obstructive pulmonary disease (COPD) takes in less O_2 and retains CO_2. A high-fat diet minimizes this problem because fat generates the least amount of CO_2 for a given amount of O_2 used, whereas carbohydrates generate the most.
5. Discuss with patient and significant others the importance of good nutrition in the treatment of chronic bronchitis.

Also see "Asthma" for **Impaired gas exchange,** p. 15.
See "Emphysema" for **Ineffective breathing pattern,** p. 18, and **Activity intolerance,** p. 19.
See "Heart Failure" for **Fluid volume excess,** p. 34.
In addition, see Appendix One, p. 451, for **Anxiety.**

PATIENT-FAMILY TEACHING AND DISCHARGE PLANNING

Give patient and significant others verbal and written instructions about the following:
1. Use of home O_2, including instructions for when to use it, importance of not increasing prescribed flow rate, precautions, and community resources for O_2 replacement when necessary.

Table 1-4   Foods high in sodium

Bouillon
Celery
Cheeses
Dried fruits
Frozen, canned, or packaged foods
Monosodium glutamate (MSG)
Mustard
Olives
Pickles
Preserved meat
Salad dressings and prepared sauces
Sauerkraut
Snack foods (e.g., crackers, chips, pretzels)
Soy sauce

2. Medications, including drug name, purpose, dosage, schedule, precautions, drug/drug and food/drug interactions, and potential side effects.
3. Signs and symptoms of congestive heart failure (CHF) that necessitate medical attention: increased dyspnea; fatigue; increased coughing; changes in the amount, color, or consistency of sputum; swelling of the ankles and legs; fever; sudden weight gain. Patients with COPD often have right-sided heart failure secondary to cardiac effects of the disease. For more information, see "Heart Failure," p. 34.
4. Avoiding individuals known to be infectious, especially those with upper respiratory infections.
5. Review of sodium-restricted diet (Table 1-4) and other dietary considerations, as indicated.
6. Importance of pacing activity level to conserve energy.
7. Importance of yearly flu and pneumococcal vaccinations.
8. Follow-up appointment with physician; confirm date and time of next appointment.
9. Introduction to local chapter of American Lung Association activities and pulmonary rehabilitation programs. Physical training programs may improve ventilation and cardiac muscle function, which may compensate for irreversible lung disease.

Emphysema

NURSING DIAGNOSES AND INTERVENTIONS

Ineffective breathing pattern related to decreased lung expansion secondary to chronic air flow limitations
Desired outcome: After treatment/intervention, patient's breathing pattern improves, as evidenced by reduction in or absence of dyspnea and movement toward a state of eupnea.

1. Assess patient's respiratory status q2-4h, being alert for indicators of respiratory distress: agitation, restlessness, decreased LOC, use of accessory muscles of respiration. Auscultate breath sounds; report a decrease in breath sounds or an increase in adventitious breath sounds.

2. Instruct patient in the use of pursed-lip breathing (which provides internal stability to the airways and may prevent airway collapse during expiration):
   - Sit upright with hands on thighs or lean forward with elbows propped on the over-the-bed table.
   - Inhale slowly through the nose with the mouth closed.
   - Form lips in an O shape as though whistling.
   - Exhale slowly through pursed lips. Exhalation should take twice as long as inhalation (e.g., count to five on inhalation; count to 10 on exhalation).

   Record patient's response to breathing technique.

3. Administer bronchodilator therapy as prescribed. Monitor patient for side effects, including tachycardia and dysrhythmias.

4. Monitor patient's response to prescribed O_2 therapy. Be aware that high concentrations of O_2 can depress the respiratory drive in individuals with chronic CO_2 retention.

5. Monitor serial ABG values. Patients with chronic CO_2 retention may have chronically compensated respiratory acidosis with a low-normal pH (7.35-7.38) and a $Paco_2$ >45 mm Hg.

Activity intolerance related to imbalance between oxygen supply and demand secondary to inefficient work of breathing

Desired outcome: Patient reports decreasing dyspnea during activity or exercise and rates his or her perceived exertion at ≤3 on a 0-10 scale.

1. Maintain prescribed activity levels, and explain rationale to patient.

2. Monitor patient's respiratory response to activity. Activity intolerance is indicated by excessively increased respiratory rate (e.g., >10 breaths/min over baseline) and depth, dyspnea, and use of accessory muscles of respiration. Ask patient to rate perceived exertion (see p. 413 for a description). If activity intolerance is noted, instruct patient to stop the activity and rest.

3. Organize care so that periods of activity are interspersed with periods of at least 90 min of undisturbed rest.

4. Assist patient with active ROM exercises to build stamina and prevent complications of decreased mobility. For more information, see **Risk for activity intolerance** in Appendix One, "Caring for Patients on Prolonged Bed Rest," p. 13.

See "Asthma" for **Impaired gas exchange,** p. 15.

See "Chronic Bronchitis" for **Ineffective airway clearance,** p. 16, and **Altered nutrition:** Less than body requirements, p. 16.

Also see psychosocial nursing diagnoses and interventions in Appendix One, "Caring for Patients with Cancer and Other Life-Disrupting Illnesses," p. 450.

PATIENT-FAMILY TEACHING AND DISCHARGE PLANNING

See "Chronic Bronchitis," p. 17.

SECTION FOUR: RESTRICTIVE PULMONARY DISORDERS

Pulmonary Fibrosis

NURSING DIAGNOSES AND INTERVENTIONS

Ineffective breathing pattern related to decreased lung expansion secondary to fibrotic condition in the lungs

Desired outcomes: After treatment/intervention, patient verbalizes a subjective relief of dyspnea; patient moves toward a state of eupnea.

1. Assess respiratory status q2-4h. Auscultate breath sounds and report increasing crackles or other adventitious sounds.
2. Monitor patient's serial ABG values for decreasing Pao_2 and be alert for early signs of hypoxia (restlessness, anxiety, dyspnea), especially with activity.
3. Assist patient in identifying ways to conserve energy during daily activities (e.g., planning frequent rest periods before and after activities as needed, stopping the activity and resting if dyspnea increases, and waiting for 1 h after eating before engaging in activities, because digestion draws blood and hence O_2 away from the muscles). As indicated, arrange for a consultation with occupational therapist or physical therapist.
4. Deliver O_2 as prescribed. Remember that the Pao_2 may be normal at rest but may decrease with exercise. The patient may require supplemental O_2 with activity.

Knowledge deficit: Side effects of corticosteroids

Desired outcome: Within the 24 h before hospital discharge, patient verbalizes knowledge of the side effects of corticosteroids and the importance of reporting them promptly to staff or physician should they occur.

1. Corticosteroids are potent medications that have potentially serious side effects and are used to suppress the immune system. Alert patient taking corticosteroids to the potential for the following, depending on dosage and duration of therapy: poor resistance to infection, increasing BP, mental changes, hyperglycemia, capillary fragility, and gastrointestinal (GI) bleeding. Stress the importance of avoiding individuals known to have infections. If the patient has been undergoing corticosteroid therapy for a prolonged period, sodium and water retention, hypokalemia, and indicators similar to Cushing's syndrome can occur, as manifested by edema, buffalo

hump, hirsutism, moon face, skin striae and thinning, weight gain, peptic ulcer, headache, nervousness, insomnia, and metabolic acidosis, in addition to the initial indicators described previously.

See "Chronic Bronchitis" for **Altered nutrition:** Less than body requirements, p. 16.

Also see psychosocial nursing diagnoses in Appendix One, "Caring for Patients with Cancer and Other Life-Disrupting Illnesses," p. 450.

PATIENT-FAMILY TEACHING
AND DISCHARGE PLANNING

Give patient and significant others verbal and written instructions about the following:

1. Importance of pacing activities to tolerance and avoiding strenuous exercises that would increase cardiac and respiratory symptoms.
2. Medications, including drug name, purpose, dosage, schedule, precautions, drug/drug and food/drug interactions, and potential side effects. It is likely that the patient will take corticosteroids while at home. Provide instructions accordingly to ensure that patient takes the correct amount, particularly during the period in which the medication will be tapered.
3. Use of O_2 and the necessary precautions if it is to be used at home.
4. Avoiding exposure to individuals known to have pulmonary infections. Recommend annual flu and pneumococcal vaccinations.
5. Date and time of follow-up visit.

SECTION FIVE: BRONCHOGENIC CARCINOMA

NURSING DIAGNOSES AND INTERVENTIONS

Pain related to biologic and physiologic agents secondary to compression of nerves by the tumor
Desired outcome: Within 30-60 min of intervention, patient's subjective perception of pain decreases, as documented by a pain scale.

1. Assess and document the following: location, description, onset, duration, and factors that precipitate and alleviate patient's pain. Devise a pain scale with patient (e.g., rating pain from 0 [no pain] to 10 [worst pain]).
2. Offer prescribed analgesics. Encourage patient to ask for pain medication before pain becomes severe. If patient has more than one analgesic, confer with patient about which would be more beneficial for pain relief. Document the amount of pain relief obtained, using the pain scale.
3. Position patient for comfort.

4. Encourage patient to use relaxation techniques (deep breathing, imagery, meditation, biofeedback) and diversional activities (television, books, radio, crafts). For a description of an effective relaxation technique, see "Coronary Artery Disease" for **Health-seeking behaviors:** p. 27.
5. For other effective pain interventions, see Appendix One, "Caring for Preoperative and Postoperative Patients," **Pain or Chronic pain,** p. 396.

See "Pulmonary Fibrosis" for **Ineffective breathing pattern,** p. 20.
Also see Appendix One, "Caring for Preoperative and Postoperative Patients," p. 395, and "Caring for Patients with Cancer and Other Life-Disrupting Illnesses," p. 423.

PATIENT-FAMILY TEACHING
AND DISCHARGE PLANNING

Give patient and significant others verbal and written instructions about the following:
1. Signs and symptoms of respiratory complications that may necessitate medical attention: increased dyspnea, agitation, cyanosis.
2. If surgery was performed, the indicators of wound infection: redness at wound site, local warmth, purulent drainage, pain, fever.
3. Medications, including drug name, purpose, dosage, schedule, precautions, drug/drug and food/drug interactions, and potential side effects.
4. Operation of all equipment that will be used at home, including O_2.
5. Need for follow-up care with physician; confirm date and time of next appointment.
6. Local American Cancer Society and American Lung Society programs. Provide available literature.

Cardiovascular Disorders

2

SECTION ONE: DEGENERATIVE CARDIOVASCULAR DISORDERS

Pulmonary Hypertension

NURSING DIAGNOSES AND INTERVENTIONS

Impaired gas exchange related to altered blood flow secondary to pulmonary capillary constriction

Desired outcome: Within the 24 h before hospital discharge, patient has improved gas exchange, as evidenced by O_2 saturation >90% and Pao_2 ≥80 mm Hg.

1. Monitor O_2 saturation *via* bedside monitor; be alert for values <90%.
2. Monitor ABG results for evidence of hypoventilation: decreased Pao_2, increased $Paco_2$, and decreased pH; and for hyperventilation: low $Paco_2$ and high pH.
3. Auscultate lung fields q4-8h to assess lung sounds. Note adventitious sounds, which can occur with fluid extravasation.
4. Assess respiratory rate, pattern, and depth; chest excursion; and use of accessory muscles of respiration q4h.
5. Observe for and document cyanosis or skin color change, which can occur with decreased gas exchange.
6. Teach patient to take slow, deep breaths to enhance gas exchange.
7. Help patient into Fowler's position, if possible, to reduce WOB and maximize chest excursion.
8. Administer prescribed low-flow O_2 as indicated.

Activity intolerance related to generalized weakness and imbalance between oxygen supply and demand secondary to right and left ventricular failure

Desired outcome: By a minimum of 24 h before hospital discharge, patient rates perceived exertion at ≤3 on a 0-10 scale and exhibits cardiac tolerance to activity, as evidenced by RR ≤20 breaths/min, HR ≤20 bpm over resting HR, and systolic BP within 20 mm Hg of resting range.

1. Monitor patient for evidence of activity intolerance, and ask him or her to rate perceived exertion (see Appendix One, p. 413, for a description).

2. Observe for and document any changes in VS. Monitor BP at least q4h. Report drops >10-20 mm Hg, which can signal decompensation of the cardiac muscle. Also be alert for other signs of left ventricular failure: dyspnea, SOB, crackles.

3. Measure and document I&O and weight, reporting any steady gains or losses. Be alert for other signs of right ventricular failure: peripheral edema, both pedal and sacral; ascites; distended neck veins; and increased CVP (>12 cm H_2O).

4. Administer diuretics, vasodilators, and calcium channel blockers as prescribed.

5. Provide periods of undisturbed rest; limit visitors as appropriate.

6. Keep frequently used items within patient's reach so that exertion can be avoided as much as possible.

7. Assist patient with maintaining prescribed activity level and progress as tolerated. If activity intolerance is observed, stop the activity and have patient rest.

8. Assist patient with ROM exercises at frequent intervals. To help prevent complications caused by immobility, plan progressive ambulation and exercise based on patient's tolerance and prescribed activity restrictions (see Appendix One, "Caring for Patients on Prolonged Bed Rest," **Risk for activity intolerance,** p. 413, and **Risk for disuse syndrome,** p. 416).

Knowledge deficit: Disease process and treatment

Desired outcome: Within the 24 h before hospital discharge, patient and significant others verbalize knowledge of the disease, its treatment, and measures that promote wellness.

1. Assess patient's level of knowledge of the disease process and its treatment.

2. Discuss the purposes of the medications: to ease the work load of the heart (vasodilators); to "relax" the heart (calcium antagonists); and to prevent fluid accumulation (diuretics).

3. Support patient in dealing with the concept of having a chronic disease.

4. If the cause of pulmonary hypertension is known, reinforce explanations of the disease process, treatment, and need for changing lifestyle, if appropriate.

5. Explain the value of relaxation techniques: tapes, soothing music, meditation, biofeedback. See "Coronary Artery Disease," **Health-seeking behaviors:** Relaxation technique effective for stress reduction, p. 27.

6. If patient smokes, explain that smoking increases the work load of the heart by causing vasoconstriction. Provide materials that explain the benefits of quitting smoking, such as pamphlets prepared by the American Heart Association.

7. Confer with physician about type of exercise program that will benefit patient; provide patient teaching as indicated.

8. If appropriate, involve dietitian to help patient with planning low-sodium meals.

See "Heart Failure" for **Fluid volume excess,** p. 34, **Knowledge deficit:** Precautions and side effects of diuretic therapy, p. 35, and **Knowledge deficit:** Precautions and side effects of vasodilators, p. 36.

Also see psychosocial nursing diagnoses in Appendix One, "Caring for Patients with Cancer and Other Life-Disrupting Illnesses," p. 450.

PATIENT-FAMILY TEACHING AND DISCHARGE PLANNING

Give patient and significant others verbal and written information about the following:

1. Indicators that require medical attention: decreased exercise tolerance, increasing SOB or dyspnea, swelling of ankles and legs, steady weight gain.
2. Medications, including drug name, purpose, dosage, schedule, precautions, drug/drug and food/drug interactions, and potential side effects.

Coronary Artery Disease

NURSING DIAGNOSES AND INTERVENTIONS

Pain (angina) related to decreased oxygen supply to the myocardium
Desired outcomes: Within 30 min of onset of pain, patient's subjective perception of angina decreases, as documented by a pain scale. Objective indicators, such as grimacing and diaphoresis, are absent.

1. Assess location, character, and severity of pain. Record severity on a subjective scale from 0 (no pain) to 10 (worst pain). Also record the number of nitroglycerin (NTG) tablets needed to relieve each episode, the factor or event that precipitated the pain, and alleviating factors. Document angina relief obtained, using pain scale.
2. Keep sublingual NTG within patient's reach, and explain that it is to be taken as soon as angina begins, repeating q5min × 3 if necessary.
3. Stay with patient and provide reassurance during periods of angina. If indicated, request that visitors leave the room.
4. Monitor HR and BP during episodes of chest pain. Be alert for and report irregularities in HR and changes in systolic BP >20 mm Hg from baseline.
5. Monitor for headache and hypotension after administering NTG. Keep patient recumbent during angina and NTG administration.
6. Administer O_2 as prescribed to increase O_2 supply to myocardium.
7. Emphasize to patient the importance of immediately reporting angina to health care team.
8. Instruct patient to avoid activities and factors that are known to cause stress and that may precipitate angina.
9. Discuss the value of relaxation techniques: tapes, soothing music, biofeedback, meditation, yoga. See **Health-seeking behaviors** diagnosis.
10. Administer beta-blockers and calcium channel blockers as prescribed to reduce cardiac work load and O_2 demand.

11. Administer long-acting and/or topical nitrates to reduce O_2 demand and the likelihood of angina.

Activity intolerance related to generalized weakness and imbalance between oxygen supply and demand secondary to tissue ischemia (MI)

Desired outcome: During activity, patient rates perceived exertion at ≤3 on a 0-10 scale and exhibits cardiac tolerance to activity, as evidenced by RR ≤20 breaths/min, HR ≤120 bpm (or within 20 bpm of resting HR), systolic BP within 20 mm Hg of patient's resting systolic BP, and absence of chest pain or new dysrhythmias.

1. Observe for and report increasing frequency of angina, angina that occurs at rest, angina that is not relieved by NTG, or decreased exercise tolerance without angina. See Table 2-1 for classification of angina.
2. Assess patient's response to activity. Be alert for chest pain, increase in HR (>20 bpm), change in systolic BP (20 mm Hg over or under resting BP), excessive fatigue, and SOB. Ask patient to rate perceived exertion (see p. 413 for details).
3. Help patient recognize and limit activities that increase O_2 demands, such as exercise and anxiety.
4. Maintain O_2 as prescribed for angina episodes.
5. Have patient perform ROM exercises, depending on tolerance and prescribed activity limitations. Because cardiac intolerance to activity can be aggravated by prolonged bed rest, consult physician about in-bed exercises and activities that patient can perform as his or her condition improves. Examples are found in Appendix One, "Caring for Patients on Prolonged Bed Rest," **Risk for activity intolerance,** p. 413, and **Risk for disuse syndrome,** p. 416.

Altered nutrition: More than body requirements of calories, sodium, or fats

Desired outcome: Within the 24 h before hospital discharge, patient demonstrates knowledge of healthy dietary regimen by planning a 3-day menu that includes and excludes appropriate foods.

Table 2-1   Classification of angina

Stable angina: Pattern of frequency, duration, and severity stable over several months.

Unstable angina: Pattern of frequency, duration, and severity changed or increased; associated with decreased exercise or exertion. This broad category includes:

- Wellens syndrome: Unstable angina usually associated with left arterial descending (LAD) lesions
- Rest angina
- New-onset angina
- Preinfarction (also called crescendo): Unstable angina with progression to MI possible (this term sometimes is used interchangeably with *unstable angina*)

Prinzmetal's angina (also called **variant angina**): Often occurs at rest (unrelated to exercise) or during sleep; usually caused by coronary artery spasm

1. If patient is over ideal body weight, explain that a low-calorie diet is necessary.
2. Teach patient how to reduce dietary intake of saturated (animal) fats and increase intake of polyunsaturated (vegetable oil) fats. See Table 2-2.
3. Teach patient to limit dietary intake of cholesterol to <300 mg/day (see Table 2-3).
4. Teach patient to limit dietary intake of refined/processed sugar.
5. Teach patient to limit dietary intake of sodium chloride (NaCl) to <4 g/day (mild restriction) (see Table 1-4, p. 18, for a list of high-sodium foods to avoid).
6. Encourage patient to eat fresh fruits, natural carbohydrates, fish, poultry, legumes, fresh vegetables, and grains for a healthy, balanced diet.

Health-seeking behaviors: Relaxation technique effective for stress reduction

Desired outcome: Patient reports subjective relief of stress after using relaxation technique.

1. Discuss with patient the importance of relaxation for reducing SNS tone, energy requirements, and O_2 consumption.
2. Many techniques use breathing, concentration, or imagery to promote relaxation and reduce energy requirements. The following is an example of a technique that can be used easily by anyone. Speaking slowly and softly, give patient these guidelines:
   - Find a comfortable position. Close your eyes.
   - Relax all your muscles. First, concentrate on your toes. Relax your toes. Now move to your feet. Relax the muscles of your feet. Continue with each muscle group, moving up your body, until finally you reach your facial muscles. Concentrate on your facial muscles and relax them.
   - Now breathe through your nose. Concentrate on feeling the air move in and out. As you exhale, say the word *one* silently to

Table 2-2   Guidelines for a diet low in saturated fat

Foods to Avoid	Foods to Choose
Red meat, especially when highly "marbled"; salami, sausages, bacon	Lean cuts of meat, fresh fish, poultry with skin removed before cooking, grilled meats
Whole milk, whipping cream	Low-fat or skim milk
Tropical oils (coconut, palm oils; cocoa butter)	Monosaturated cooking oils (e.g., olive or canola oil)
Candy	Fresh fruit, vegetables
Sweet rolls, donuts	Whole grain breads, cereals
Ice cream	Nonfat yogurt, sherbet
Salad dressings	Vinegar, lemon juice
Peanut butter, peanuts, hot dogs, potato chips	Unbuttered popcorn
Butter	Margarine (safflower oil listed as the first ingredient)

Table 2-3   Guidelines for a low-cholesterol diet

Foods to Avoid	Foods to Choose
Egg yolks (no more than three per week)	Egg whites, cholesterol-free egg substitutes
Foods made with many egg yolks (e.g., sponge cakes)	Lean, well-trimmed meats (minimize servings of beef, lamb, and pork)
Fatty cuts of meat, fat on meats	Fish (except shellfish), chicken and turkey (without the skin)
Skin on chicken and turkey	
Luncheon meats or cold cuts	
Sausage, frankfurters	Dried peas and beans as meat substitutes
Shellfish (e.g., lobster, shrimp, crab)	
Whole milk, cream, whole milk cheese	Nonfat (skim) or low-fat (2%) milk
Ice cream	Partially skim milk cheeses
Commercially prepared foods with hydrogenated shortening (saturated fat)	Ice milk and sherbet
	Polyunsaturated oils for cooking and food preparation: corn, safflower, cottonseed, sesame, and sunflower
Coconut and palm oils and products made with them (e.g., cream substitutes)	
Butter, lard, hydrogenated shortening	Margarines that list one of the above oils as their first ingredient
Fried meats and vegetables	Foods prepared "from scratch" with the above suggested oils
Seasonings containing large amounts of sugar and saturated fats	Meats (in acceptable quantity) and vegetables prepared by broiling, steaming, or baking (never frying)
Sauces and gravies	
Salad dressings containing cream, cheeses, or mayonnaise	Spices, herbs, lemon juice, wine, flavored wine vinegars

yourself. Again, continue feeling the air move in and out of your lungs. Continue for approximately 20 min.

- Try to clear your mind of worries; be passive. Let relaxation occur. If distractions appear, gently push them away. Continue breathing through your nose, repeating *one* silently.
- After approximately 20 min, slowly begin to allow yourself to become aware of your surroundings. Keep your eyes closed for a few moments.
- Open your eyes.

3. Encourage patient to practice this technique 2-3 ×/day or whenever feeling stressed or tense. Acknowledge that this technique may feel strange at first but that it becomes easier and more effective with practice.

4. Explain that baroque music, played softly, helps many individuals achieve an even greater state of relaxation.

Knowledge deficit: Precautions and side effects of nitrates

Desired outcome: Within the 24 h before hospital discharge, patient verbalizes understanding of the precautions and side effects of the prescribed medication.

1. Instruct patient to report to physician or staff a headache associated with NTG because the physician may alter the dose.
2. Teach patient to assume a recumbent position if a headache occurs. Explain that the vasodilatation effect of the drug causes a drop in BP, which can result in orthostatic hypotension and transient headache.

Knowledge deficit: Precautions and side effects of beta-blockers

Desired outcome: Within the 24 h before hospital discharge, patient verbalizes understanding of the precautions and side effects of beta-blockers.

1. Instruct patient to be alert for depression, fatigue, dizziness, erythematous rash, respiratory distress, and sexual dysfunction, which can occur as side effects of beta-blockers. Explain the importance of notifying the physician promptly if these side effects occur.
2. Explain that weight gain and peripheral and sacral edema can occur as side effects of beta-blockers. Teach patient how to assess for edema, and the importance of reporting signs and symptoms promptly if they occur.
3. Explain that BP and HR are assessed before administration of beta-blockers because the drug can cause hypotension and excessive slowing of the heart.
4. Caution patient not to omit or abruptly stop taking beta-blockers because this can result in rebound angina or even MI.

Knowledge deficit: Disease process and life-style implications of coronary artery disease (CAD)

Desired outcome: Within the 24 h before hospital discharge, patient verbalizes knowledge of the disease process of CAD and the concomitant life-style implications.

1. Teach patient about CAD, including the pathophysiologic processes of cardiac ischemia, angina, and infarction.
2. Assist patient with identifying risk factors for CAD and risk-factor modification:
   - Diet low in cholesterol and saturated fat
   - Quitting smoking
   - Regular activity/exercise programs
3. Discuss symptoms that require medical attention, such as chest pain that is not relieved by NTG.
4. Discuss guidelines for sexual activity: resting before intercourse, finding a comfortable position, taking prophylactic NTG, postponing intercourse for 1-1½ h after a heavy meal.
5. Discuss medical procedures, such as cardiac catheterization, and surgical procedures, such as percutaneous transluminal coronary angioplasty and coronary artery bypass graft, if appropriate.

PATIENT-FAMILY TEACHING
AND DISCHARGE PLANNING

Give patient and significant others verbal and written information about the following:

1. Medications, including drug name, purpose, dosage, schedule, precautions, drug/drug and food/drug interactions, and potential side effects. Discuss the potential for headache and dizziness after NTG administration. Caution patient about using NTG more often than prescribed and about notifying physician if 3 tablets do not relieve angina.

2. Importance of reducing intake of caffeine, which causes vasoconstriction and increases HR.

3. Dietary changes: low saturated fat (see Table 2-2), low sodium (see Table 1-4, p. 18, which discusses high-sodium foods that should be avoided), low cholesterol (see Table 2-3), and the need for weight loss if appropriate.

4. Pulse monitoring: how to self-measure pulse, including parameters for target heart rates and limits.

5. Prescribed exercise program and the importance of maintaining a regular exercise schedule. Remind patient of the need to measure pulse, to stop if pain occurs, and to stay within prescribed exercise limits. See Table 2-4 for a progressive, at-home walking program. Caution patient not to exercise during extremes of weather (hot or cold), which can place an additional strain on the heart.

6. Indicators that require medical attention: progression to unstable angina, loss of consciousness, decreased exercise tolerance, unrelieved pain, angina that is not relieved by NTG, increasing occurrence of angina, or the need to increase the number of NTG tablets to relieve angina.

7. Quitting smoking; refer patient to a "stop smoking" program, as appropriate.

8. Importance of involvement and support of significant others in patient's life-style changes.

9. Importance of getting BP checked at regular intervals (at least once a month if the patient is hypertensive).

Table 2-4   Guidelines for a progressive at-home walking program

Week	Distance	Time
1	100-200 ft	2 ×/day
2	200-400 ft	2 ×/day
3	¼ mi	8-10 min
4	½ mi	15 min
5	1 mi	30 min
6	1¾ mi	30 min
7	2 mi	40 min

10. Importance of avoiding strenuous activity for at least 1 h after meals to avoid excessive O_2 demands.
11. Importance of reporting to health care provider any change in pattern or frequency of angina.
12. Sexual activity guidelines:
    ■ Rest is beneficial before sexual activity.
    ■ Medications such as NTG may be taken prophylactically if pain occurs with activity.
    ■ Postpone sexual activity for 1-1½ h after a meal.

Myocardial Infarction

NURSING DIAGNOSES AND INTERVENTIONS

Pain related to ischemia and infarction of myocardial tissue
Desired outcomes: Within 30 min of onset, patient's subjective perception of pain decreases, as documented by a pain scale. Objective indicators, such as grimacing and diaphoresis, are absent.
1. Assess location, character, duration, and intensity of pain, using a pain scale of 0 (no pain) to 10 (worst pain). Assess associated symptoms, such as nausea and diaphoresis.
2. Assess and document BP and HR with episodes of pain. BP and HR may increase because of sympathetic stimulation or decrease because of ischemia and decreased cardiac function.
3. Administer prescribed pain medications (usually morphine sulfate); document quality of relief obtained, using pain scale, and time the interval from administration to expressed relief.
4. Provide reassurance during episodes of pain; stay with patient if possible.
5. Observe for and report side effects of pain medications: hypotension, slowed RR, difficulty with urination.
6. Administer O_2 as prescribed, usually 2-4 L/min per nasal cannula.
7. Prepare to transport patient to CCU.

Decreased cardiac output related to negative inotropic changes (decreased cardiac contractility) secondary to ischemia and infarction
Desired outcome: Within 1 h of treatment/intervention, patient has adequate cardiac output, as evidenced by systolic BP ≥90 mm Hg, HR ≤100 bpm, urinary output ≥30 ml/h, RR 12-20 breaths/min with normal depth and pattern (eupnea), absence of crackles, and edema ≤1+ on a 0-4+ scale.
1. Assess for and document the following as indicators of decreased cardiac output: restlessness and/or change in LOC, extra heart sounds (e.g., S_3), systolic BP <90 mm Hg, and HR >100 bpm.
2. Observe for and report any indicators of fluid accumulation in the lungs: dyspnea, crackles, SOB.
3. Be alert for and report decreasing urine output (particularly <30 ml/h) and increasing specific gravity (>1.030).
4. Assess for peripheral (sacral, pedal) edema.
5. Maintain IV infusion as prescribed. Usually fluids are monitored closely to prevent failure and circulatory overload.

6. As prescribed, administer medications such as beta-blockers and vasodilators to reduce cardiac work load and prevent a decrease in cardiac output.
7. Prepare patient for possible transfer to CCU.

Activity intolerance related to imbalance between oxygen supply and demand secondary to diminished strength of cardiac contraction and decreased cardiac output

Desired outcome: During exercise/activity, patient rates perceived exertion at ≤3 on a 0-10 scale and exhibits cardiac tolerance to activity, as evidenced by systolic BP within 20 mm Hg of resting systolic BP, RR ≤20 breaths/min, and HR ≤120 bpm (or ≤20 bpm over resting HR).

1. Monitor patient for signs of activity intolerance, and ask patient to rate perceived exertion (see **Risk for activity intolerance** in Appendix One, "Caring for Patients on Prolonged Bed Rest," p. 413, for details).
2. Observe for and report any symptoms of decreased cardiac output or cardiac failure: decreasing BP, cold extremities, oliguria, decreased peripheral pulses, increased HR.
3. Monitor I&O and be alert to urinary output <30 ml/h. Auscultate lung fields q2h for crackles, which can occur with fluid retention and cardiac failure.
4. Palpate peripheral pulses at frequent intervals. Be alert for irregularities and decreased amplitude, which can signal cardiac failure.
5. Administer O_2 and medications as prescribed.
6. During acute periods of decreased cardiac output and as prescribed, support patient in maintaining bed rest by keeping personal articles within reach, providing a calm and quiet atmosphere, and limiting visitors to ensure periods of undisturbed rest.
7. Assist patient to commode when bathroom privileges are allowed.
8. Assist patient with passive or assistive ROM exercises as determined by activity tolerance and activity limitations. Consult physician about type and amount of in-bed exercises patient can perform as his or her condition improves. Examples of in-bed exercises are found in Appendix One, "Caring for Patients on Prolonged Bed Rest," **Risk for activity intolerance,** p. 413; and **Risk for disuse syndrome,** p. 416. Also, discuss with physician patient's participation in an exercise program after hospital discharge.
9. As appropriate, teach patient self-measurement of HR for gauging exercise tolerance.
10. Make sure patient has undisturbed rest periods of ≥90 min. Plan activities accordingly.

Impaired gas exchange related to alveolar capillary membrane changes secondary to fluid accumulation in the lungs

Desired outcome: Within 30 min of treatment/intervention, patient has adequate gas exchange, as evidenced by a state of eupnea. For a minimum of 24 h before hospital discharge, patient's Pao_2 is ≥80 mm Hg, $Paco_2$ is 35-45 mm Hg, and O_2 saturation is ≥95%.

1. Assess ABG levels and be alert for evidence of hypoxemia (decreased Pao_2), decreased O_2 saturation, or hyperventilation (decreased $Paco_2$).

2. Auscultate lung fields q2h for crackles, which occur with fluid accumulation.
3. Monitor for sudden changes in respiratory pattern (increased dyspnea or reduced RR), which can occur with an extension of infarction and decreased cardiac output; report immediately if they occur.
4. Monitor BP. In the absence of marked hypotension, place patient in semi-Fowler's position to ease dyspnea.
5. Administer O_2 as prescribed. Deliver O_2 with humidity to help prevent drying effects on oral and nasal mucosa.
6. Administer prescribed analgesics (usually morphine sulfate) to reduce cardiac work load by vasodilatation and ease respiratory effort.

See "Coronary Artery Disease" for **Health-seeking behaviors:** Relaxation technique effective for stress reduction, p. 27, and **Knowledge deficit:** Disease process and life-style implications of coronary artery disease (CAD), p. 29.

Also see Appendix One, "Caring for Preoperative and Postoperative Patients," p. 395, and psychosocial nursing diagnoses and interventions in "Caring for Patients with Cancer and Other Life-Disrupting Illnesses," p. 450.

PATIENT-FAMILY TEACHING
AND DISCHARGE PLANNING

Give patient and significant others verbal and written information about the following:

1. Process of MI and extent of patient's injury.
2. Indicators that require immediate medical attention: unrelieved pain, decreased activity tolerance, sudden onset of SOB, weight gain.
3. Medications, including drug name, purpose, dosage, schedule, precautions, drug/drug and food/drug interactions, and potential side effects. Provide instructions for taking prophylactic NTG before activities, such as sexual activity.
4. Exercise program specific to patient's condition. Guidelines for walking are provided in Table 2-4. Caution patient to start slowly, walk 3-5 ×/wk, warm up and cool down with stretching exercises, avoid overexertion, stop when tired, and notify physician of any change in exercise tolerance.
5. Importance of avoiding overexertion and getting rest when tired.
6. Resumption of sexual activity as directed, usually after 2-4 wk, but this varies with each patient.
7. Diet regimen as prescribed. For descriptions of appropriate diets, see Table 1-4, p. 18 (high-sodium foods to avoid); Table 2-2 (low fat); and Table 2-3 (low cholesterol).
8. Quitting smoking; refer patient to programs that specialize in this process.
9. Phone number and address of the local branch of the American Heart Association, local heart rehabilitation programs, family physician, and primary nurse.

Cardiovascular

10. Referral to stress management programs, if appropriate. See "Coronary Artery Disease" for **Health-seeking behaviors:** Relaxation technique effective for stress reduction, p. 27.

Heart Failure

NURSING DIAGNOSES AND INTERVENTIONS

Activity intolerance related to generalized weakness and imbalance between oxygen supply and demand secondary to decreased strength of cardiac contraction

Desired outcome: During activity/exercise, patient rates perceived exertion at ≤3 on a 0-10 scale and exhibits cardiac tolerance to activity, as evidenced by RR ≤20 breaths/min with normal depth and pattern (eupnea), HR ≤120 bpm (or within 20 bpm of resting HR), systolic BP within 20 mm Hg of resting systolic BP, and absence of chest pain or new dysrhythmias.

1. Monitor HR, BP, and RR during periods of activity. Note signs of activity intolerance: HR >120 bpm, RR >20 breaths/min, and systolic BP >20 mm Hg from resting range. Ask patient to rate perceived exertion (see Appendix One, p. 413, for a description).
2. Monitor VS q2h or as necessary, and report decreasing BP, increasing HR, or increasing RR, which can occur with worsening failure related to sympathetic nervous system discharge and fluid retention.
3. Administer vasodilators and other cardiac drugs, such as digitalis, as prescribed.
4. If symptoms worsen, discuss with patient the need for activity limitations. Assist patient with ADLs to prevent SOB, and plan nursing care and limit visitors to allow periods of undisturbed rest.
5. Discuss ways to decrease activities at home (e.g., not climbing stairs).
6. If appropriate, refer patient to an occupational therapist to learn how to conserve energy so that ADLs can be performed with a minimum of exertion.
7. Assist patient with passive or assistive ROM exercises, depending on activity tolerance and prescribed activity limitations. Because cardiac intolerance to activity can be aggravated by prolonged bed rest, consult physician about type and amount of in-bed exercises that can be initiated as patient's condition improves. For details, see Appendix One, "Caring for Patients on Prolonged Bed Rest," **Risk for activity intolerance,** p. 413, and **Risk for disuse syndrome,** p. 416.

Fluid volume excess related to compromised regulatory mechanisms secondary to decreased cardiac output

Desired outcome: For a minimum of 24 h before hospital discharge, patient is normovolemic, as evidenced by urinary output ≥30 ml/h, balanced I&O, stable weight (or weight loss attributable to fluid loss), edema ≤1+ on a 0-4+ scale, HR ≤100 bpm, and absence of crackles.

1. Auscultate lung fields at least q8h; report crackles, which occur with fluid volume excess and heart failure.

2. Monitor and document I&O at least q8h. Report imbalances, including urinary output <30 ml/h, which can occur with decreased renal blood flow.

3. Monitor weight daily, and report unusual gains. Be alert for pitting edema. To assess for this condition, apply firm pressure to edematous area with a finger. If indentation remains after finger has been removed, pitting edema is present.

4. Auscultate heart sounds; be alert for S_3 gallop, an early sign of heart failure.

5. Administer diuretics as prescribed. Observe for indicators of decreased effective circulating volume: hypotension, decreased CVP (<5 cm H_2O), tachycardia. Monitor potassium (K^+) levels, and consult physician about levels <3.5 mEq/L.

6. If appropriate, teach patient the importance of reducing intake of sodium (or table salt). See Table 1-4, p. 18, for a list of foods high in sodium.

7. If fluids are restricted, help relieve patient's thirst by offering ice chips or popsicles. Record amount of intake on I&O record.

Knowledge deficit: Precautions and side effects of diuretic therapy

Desired outcome: Within the 24 h before hospital discharge, patient verbalizes knowledge of the precautions and side effects of diuretic therapy.

1. Depending on type of diuretic used, teach patient to report signs and symptoms of the following:
   - *Hypokalemia:* Anorexia, irregular pulse, nausea, apathy, muscle cramps.
   - *Hyperkalemia:* Muscle weakness, hyporeflexia, and irregular HR, which can occur with potassium-sparing diuretics.
   - *Hyponatremia:* Fatigue, weakness, and edema (owing to fluid extravasation).

2. For patients undergoing long-term diuretic therapy, explain the importance of follow-up monitoring of blood levels of sodium (Na^+) and potassium (K^+).

3. As appropriate, instruct patient to use care when rising from a sitting or recumbent position to prevent injury from orthostatic hypotension.

Knowledge deficit: Precautions and side effects of digitalis therapy

Desired outcome: Within the 24 h before hospital discharge, patient verbalizes understanding of the precautions and side effects associated with digitalis therapy.

1. Teach patient the technique and importance of assessing HR before taking digitalis. Explain that he or she should obtain HR parameters from the physician, but that digitalis usually is withheld when HR is <60 bpm if the usual HR before digitalis administration is greater. Teach patient to notify physician if he or she has omitted a dose because of the low HR.

2. Explain that serum K^+ levels are monitored routinely because low levels can potentiate digitalis toxicity.

3. Explain that the apical HR and peripheral pulses are assessed for irregularity, which is a sign of digitalis toxicity.

4. Teach patient to be alert for other indicators of digitalis toxicity: nausea, vomiting, anorexia, diarrhea, blurred vision, yellow haze vision, mental confusion. Explain the importance of reporting signs and symptoms promptly to physician or staff if they occur.

Knowledge deficit: Precautions and side effects of vasodilators

Desired outcome: Within the 24 h before hospital discharge, patient verbalizes knowledge of the precautions and side effects associated with vasodilators.

1. Explain that a headache can occur after administration of a vasodilator and that lying down will help alleviate the pain.
2. Teach the importance of assessment for weight gain and signs of peripheral or sacral edema, any of which can occur as side effects of vasodilator therapy.
3. Instruct patient to alert physician to side effects of this therapy.

See "Coronary Artery Disease" for **Altered nutrition,** p. 26, and **Knowledge deficit:** Precautions and side effects of beta-blockers, p. 29. See "Myocardial Infarction" for **Impaired gas exchange,** p. 32.

Also see Appendix One, "Caring for Patients on Prolonged Bed Rest," p. 395, and psychosocial nursing diagnoses in "Caring for Patients with Cancer and Other Life-Disrupting Illnesses," p. 450.

PATIENT-FAMILY TEACHING AND DISCHARGE PLANNING

Give patient and significant others verbal and written information about the following:

1. Medications, including drug name, purpose, dosage, schedule, precautions, drug/drug and food/drug interactions, and potential side effects. Stress the importance of taking medications regularly and of not discontinuing them without consulting physician. Teach patient and significant others how to measure HR for digitalis therapy.
2. Diet: Advise patient that sodium restriction may be lessened as cardiac function improves. Assist patient with diet planning, or refer to a nutrition specialist if major dietary changes are necessary. Foods high in sodium that should be avoided are listed in Table 1-4, p. 18.
3. Signs and symptoms that require medical attention: irregular pulse, bradycardia, unusual SOB, increased orthopnea, decreased exercise tolerance, unusual or steady weight gain.
4. Importance of quitting smoking, which causes vasoconstriction and increases cardiac work load. As appropriate, refer patient to "stop smoking" programs.
5. Importance of limiting exertional activities at home (e.g., minimize bending and lifting and avoid stair climbing). Stress, though, the importance of a progressive increase in activity.
6. Emergency telephone numbers to call if needed.
7. Importance of follow-up care: confirm date and time of next medical appointment.

SECTION TWO: VALVULAR HEART DISORDERS

Mitral Stenosis

NURSING DIAGNOSES AND INTERVENTIONS

Decreased cardiac output related to decreased preload secondary to decreased ventricular filling

Desired outcomes: By a minimum of the 24 h before hospital discharge, patient has adequate cardiac output, as evidenced by urine output ≥30 ml/h; systolic BP within 20 mm Hg of baseline systolic BP; HR 60-100 bpm with regular rhythm; pedal pulse amplitude >2+ on a 0-4+ scale; extremities warm and normal in color; and orientation to time, place, and person. For at least the 48 h before hospital discharge, patient is free of new dysrhythmias.

1. Monitor BP and HR q4h unless patient is unstable. Report changes such as irregular heart rhythm, HR <60 bpm or >100 bpm, or systolic BP >20 mm Hg over or under baseline.
2. Monitor urine output, noting amount <30 ml/h for 2 h.
3. Assess pedal pulses and color and temperature of extremities, along with other assessment factors. Be alert for pulse amplitude ≤2+ and extremities that are cool, pale, and mottled.
4. Administer inotropic drugs as prescribed to increase cardiac contractility.
5. Consult physician about significant findings.

Activity intolerance related to generalized weakness and imbalance between oxygen supply and demand secondary to decreased left ventricular filling

Desired outcome: By a minimum of the 24 h before hospital discharge, patient rates perceived exertion at ≤3 on a 0-10 scale and exhibits cardiac tolerance to activity, as evidenced by HR ≤20 bpm over resting HR, systolic BP within 20 mm Hg of resting systolic BP, and RR ≤20 breaths/min with normal depth and pattern (eupnea).

1. Monitor VS with patient activity, and report significant decrease or increase in BP (≥20 mm Hg). Be alert for indicators of activity intolerance: SOB, dyspnea, fatigue. Ask patient about perceived exertion (see description, p. 413).
2. Assess for orthostatic changes in BP that occur when patient moves from supine to standing position.
3. Assess peripheral pulses, capillary refill, and temperature and color of extremities as indicators of cardiac output.
4. Provide rest periods at frequent intervals, especially between care activities.
5. Confer with physician about in-bed exercises that can be incorporated into patient's routine as his or her condition improves. Ex-

amples are found in Appendix One, **Risk for activity intolerance,** p. 413, and **Risk for disuse syndrome,** p. 416. Increase ambulation progressively and to patient's tolerance.

Fluid volume excess related to compromised regulatory mechanisms secondary to right-sided heart failure

Desired outcome: Within 24 h of treatment, patient is normovolemic, as evidenced by CVP 5-12 cm H_2O, balanced I&O, stable weight, urine output $\geq$30 ml/h, edema $\leq$1+ on a 0-4+ scale, flattened neck veins, and lungs clear on auscultation.

1. Observe for and report the following indicators of right-sided heart failure: increasing CVP (>12 cm H_2O), peripheral edema, dyspnea, hepatic enlargement on palpation, jugular vein distention.
2. Monitor I&O, and administer fluids only as prescribed to ensure that patient maintains adequate volume without overload. Weigh patient daily, and report significant I&O imbalance.
3. If fluids are limited, offer ice chips and popsicles to help patient control thirst. Record amount of intake.
4. As prescribed, administer inotropic drugs, such as digitalis, to increase the strength of cardiac contraction.
5. Administer diuretics as prescribed to reduce volume load.

Risk for infection (with concomitant endocarditis) related to tissue destruction and increased exposure secondary to lodging of bacteria in the malfunctioning valve

Desired outcome: Patient is free of infection, as evidenced by normothermia, WBC count $\leq$11,000/μl, and HR $\leq$100 bpm.

1. Maintain aseptic technique for all invasive procedures.
2. Monitor temperature q4h, and report significant increases.
3. Be alert for rising HR, which can signal an infection.
4. Administer prescribed antibiotics on time.
5. Maintain hydration as prescribed, through oral and IV fluids, making sure patient has adequate volume without overload.

Knowledge deficit: Disease process and treatment/management

Desired outcome: Within the 24 h before hospital discharge, patient verbalizes knowledge of valvular disorder, its treatment/management, and the potential for developing endocarditis.

1. Discuss patient's disorder and associated physiologic effects and symptoms. Describe treatment options, including commissurotomy, percutaneous balloon valvuloplasty, and valve surgery.
2. Assess patient's knowledge of the potential for endocarditis. As indicated, explain how endocarditis affects the heart and its valves and why individuals with valvular disorders are predisposed to developing this disorder.
3. Teach patient the following indicators of endocarditis: temperature increases, malaise, anorexia, tachycardia, pallor. Explain the importance of reporting symptoms early.
4. Teach patient the indicators of frequently encountered infections (e.g., URI, UTI, and wound infection). For a description, see "Care of the Renal Transplant Recipient," p. 86, and Table 2-5. Stress the importance of reporting symptoms promptly should they occur, since a systemic infection can lead to endocarditis.

Table 2-5   Infectious processes requiring medical intervention

Upper respiratory infection	Fever, chills, cough productive of sputum, crackles, rhonchi, dyspnea, inflamed pharynx, sore throat
Urinary tract infection	Burning or pain with urination, cloudy or malodorous urine, fever, chills, tachycardia, diaphoresis, nausea, vomiting, abdominal pain
Systemic sepsis	Fever, chills, tachycardia, diaphoresis, nausea, vomiting, hypothermia, flushed skin, hypotension
Localized (IV sites)	Erythema, swelling, purulent drainage, warmth

5. Discuss the importance of antibiotic prophylaxis before and after any major or minor surgical procedures.

PATIENTS UNDERGOING CARDIAC CATHETERIZATION

Knowledge deficit: Catheterization procedure and postcatheterization regimen

Desired outcome: Before procedure, patient verbalizes knowledge of cardiac catheterization and postcatheterization regimen.

1. Assess patient's knowledge about catheterization procedure. As appropriate, reinforce physician's explanation of procedure and answer any questions or concerns of patient and significant others. If possible, arrange for an orientation visit to catheterization laboratory before procedure.
2. Before cardiac catheterization, have patient practice techniques that will be used during catheterization (e.g., Valsalva maneuver, coughing, deep breathing).
3. Explain that bed rest will be required after the procedure and that VS, circulation, and the insertion site will be checked at frequent intervals to ensure integrity. In addition, explain that sandbags may be used over the insertion site, and that flexing of the insertion site (arm or groin) is contraindicated to prevent bleeding.
4. Stress the importance of promptly reporting signs and symptoms of hemorrhage, hematoma formation, or embolization.

Altered cardiopulmonary, peripheral, and cerebral tissue perfusion related to interrupted arterial flow secondary to the catheterization procedure

Desired outcome: Within 1 h after procedure, patient has adequate perfusion, as evidenced by HR regular and within 20 bpm of baseline HR; apical/radial pulse equality; BP within 20 mm Hg of baseline BP; peripheral pulse amplitude >2+ on a 0-4+ scale; warmth and normal color in extremities; and orientation to time, place, and person.

1. Monitor BP q15min until stable on three successive checks, q2h for the next 12 h, and q4h thereafter. If the systolic pressure drops 20 mm Hg below previous recordings, lower HOB and consult physi-

cian. **Note:** If insertion site was the antecubital space, measure BP in unaffected arm.

2. Be alert for and report indicators of decreased perfusion: cool extremities, decreased amplitude of peripheral pulses, cyanosis, decreased LOC, SOB.
3. Monitor patient's HR, and consult physician if dysrhythmias occur. If patient is not on a cardiac monitor, auscultate apical and radial pulses with every BP check, and report irregularities or apical/radial discrepancies.
4. If femoral artery was the insertion site, maintain HOB at a 30-degree elevation to prevent acute hip joint flexion.

Risk for fluid volume deficit related to hemorrhage or hematoma formation due to arterial puncture and/or osmotic diuresis owing to the dye

Desired outcomes: Patient remains normovolemic, as evidenced by HR ≤100 bpm; BP ≥90/60 mm Hg (or within 20 mm Hg of baseline range); and orientation to time, place, and person. Dressing is dry, and puncture site shows no swelling.

1. Be alert for indicators of shock or hemorrhage: decreased BP, increased HR, decreasing LOC.
2. Inspect dressing on groin or antecubital space for frank bleeding or hematoma formation (fluctuating swelling).
3. Monitor peripheral perfusion, and be alert for decreased amplitude or absence of distal pulses, delayed capillary refill, coolness of extremities, and pallor, which can signal embolization or hemorrhagic shock.
4. To minimize the risk of bleeding, caution patient about flexing elbow or hip for 6-8 h, or as prescribed.
5. If bleeding occurs, maintain pressure at insertion site as prescribed. Typically this is done with a pressure dressing or a 2½- to 5-lb sandbag.

Altered peripheral (involved limb) tissue perfusion (or risk for same) related to interrupted arterial flow secondary to embolization

Desired outcome: Patient has adequate perfusion in involved limb, as evidenced by peripheral pulse amplitude >2+ on a 0-4+ scale; normal color, sensation, and temperature; and brisk capillary refill (<2 sec).

1. Assess peripheral perfusion by palpating peripheral pulses q15min for 30 min, then q30min for 1 h, then qh for 2 h or per protocol.
2. Monitor for and report any indicators of embolization in the involved limb: faintness or absence of pulse, coolness of extremity, mottling, decreased capillary refill, cyanosis, complaints of numbness, tingling, and pain at insertion site. Instruct patient to report any of these indicators promptly.
3. If there is *no* evidence of an embolus or thrombus formation, instruct patient to move fingers or toes and rotate wrist or ankle to promote circulation.
4. Ensure that patient maintains bed rest for 4-6 h, or as prescribed.

Altered renal tissue perfusion (or risk for same) related to interrupted blood flow secondary to decreased cardiac output or reaction to contrast dye

Desired outcome: Patient has adequate renal perfusion, as evidenced by urinary output ≥30 ml/h, good skin turgor, and moist mucous membranes.

1. Because contrast dye for cardiac catheterization may cause osmotic diuresis, monitor for indicators of dehydration: poor skin turgor, dry mucous membranes, high urine specific gravity.
2. Monitor I&O. Consult physician if urinary output is <30 ml/h despite adequate intake.
3. If urinary output is insufficient despite adequate intake, restrict fluids. Be alert for and report indicators of fluid overload: crackles on auscultation of lung fields, distended neck veins, SOB. Consult physician about significant findings.
4. If patient does not exhibit signs of cardiac or renal failure, encourage daily intake of 2-3 L of fluids, or as prescribed, to flush contrast dye out of the system.

See "Pulmonary Embolus" for **Altered protection** related to risk of prolonged bleeding or hemorrhage secondary to anticoagulant therapy, p. 7. See "Heart Failure" for **Knowledge deficit:** Precautions and side effects of diuretic therapy, p. 35, and **Knowledge deficit:** Precautions and side effects of digitalis therapy, p. 35.

Also see Appendix One, "Caring for Preoperative and Postoperative Patients," p. 395.

PATIENT-FAMILY TEACHING AND DISCHARGE PLANNING

Give patient and significant others verbal and written information about the following:

1. Medications, including drug name, purpose, dosage, schedule, precautions, drug/drug and food/drug interactions, and potential side effects.
2. Gradually increasing exercise, avoiding heavy lifting (>10 lb), and incorporating rest periods.
3. Name and phone number of a resource person (e.g., physician, primary nurse) should questions arise after discharge from the hospital.
4. Referral to a cardiac rehabilitation program if appropriate.
5. Resumption of sexual activity as directed by physician.
6. Indicators that require immediate medical attention: decreased exercise tolerance, signs of infection, SOB, bleeding.
7. Importance of consulting physician before using OTC medications, especially aspirin products for individuals taking oral anticoagulants (aspirin can affect coagulation times).
8. Importance of follow-up care; confirm date and time of next medical appointment.

Mitral Regurgitation

NURSING DIAGNOSES AND INTERVENTIONS

Activity intolerance related to generalized weakness and imbalance between oxygen supply and demand secondary to decreased cardiac output with valvular regurgitation

Desired outcome: By a minimum of 24 h before hospital discharge, patient rates perceived exertion at ≤3 on a 0-10 scale and exhibits cardiac tolerance to activity, as evidenced by HR ≤20 bpm over resting HR, systolic BP within 20 mm Hg of resting systolic BP, and RR ≤20 breaths/min with normal depth and pattern (eupnea).

1. Assess patient's VS during activities, being alert for HR >20 bpm over resting HR, systolic BP >20 mm Hg over or under resting systolic BP, and RR >20 breaths/min. Ask patient to rate perceived exertion (see p. 413 for description).
2. Provide frequent rest periods, especially between care activities.
3. As necessary, assist patient with ADLs to avoid SOB.
4. Discuss ways to decrease energy output at home.
5. Progressively increase ambulation to patient's tolerance. Be alert for dyspnea, fatigue, and SOB with activity. Modify or restrict activities as indicated. See **Risk for activity intolerance,** p. 413, and **Risk for disuse syndrome,** p. 416, in Appendix One.

See "Pulmonary Embolus" for **Altered protection** related to risk of prolonged bleeding or hemorrhage secondary to anticoagulant therapy, p. 7.

See "Coronary Artery Disease" for **Knowledge deficit:** Precautions and side effects of beta-blockers, p. 29.

See "Heart Failure" for **Fluid volume excess,** p. 34, **Knowledge deficit:** Precautions and side effects of diuretic therapy, p. 35, **Knowledge deficit:** Precautions and side effects of digitalis therapy, p. 35, **Knowledge deficit:** Precautions and side effects of vasodilators, p. 36.

See "Mitral Stenosis" for **Decreased cardiac output,** p. 37, **Risk for infection** (with concomitant endocarditis), p. 38, and **Knowledge deficit:** Disease process and treatment/management, p. 38.

Also see "Cardiac Surgery," p. 53, and Appendix One, "Caring for Preoperative and Postoperative Patients," p. 395.

PATIENT-FAMILY TEACHING AND DISCHARGE PLANNING

See "Heart Failure," p. 36, and "Cardiac Surgery," p. 55, depending on patient's clinical course.

Aortic Stenosis

NURSING DIAGNOSES AND INTERVENTIONS

See "Pulmonary Embolus" for **Altered protection** related to risk of prolonged bleeding or hemorrhage secondary to anticoagulant therapy, p. 7.

See "Coronary Artery Disease" for **Knowledge deficit:** Precautions and side effects of beta-blockers, p. 29.

See "Heart Failure" for **Fluid volume excess,** p. 34, **Knowledge deficit:** Precautions and side effects of diuretic therapy, p. 35, **Knowledge deficit:** Precautions and side effects of digitalis therapy, p. 35, and **Knowledge deficit:** Precautions and side effects of vasodilators, p. 36.

See "Mitral Stenosis" for **Decreased cardiac output,** p. 37, **Activity intolerance,** p. 37, **Risk for infection** (with concomitant endocarditis), p. 38, and **Knowledge deficit:** Disease process and treatments/management, p. 38.

As appropriate, see "Mitral Stenosis," p. 37, "Cardiac Surgery," p. 53, and Appendix One, "Caring for Preoperative and Postoperative Patients," p. 395.

Aortic Regurgitation

NURSING DIAGNOSES AND INTERVENTIONS

See "Pulmonary Embolus" for **Altered protection** related to risk of prolonged bleeding or hemorrhage secondary to anticoagulant therapy, p. 7.

See "Coronary Artery Disease" for **Knowledge deficit:** Precautions and side effects of beta-blockers, p. 29.

See "Heart Failure" for **Fluid volume excess,** p. 34, **Knowledge deficit:** Precautions and side effects of diuretic therapy, p. 35, **Knowledge deficit:** Precautions and side effects of digitalis therapy, p. 35, and **Knowledge deficit:** Precautions and side effects of vasodilators, p. 36.

See "Mitral Stenosis" for **Risk for infection** (with concomitant endocarditis), p. 38, and **Knowledge deficit:** Disease process and treatments/management, p. 38.

As appropriate, see "Mitral Stenosis," p. 37, "Cardiac Surgery," p. 53, and Appendix One, "Caring for Preoperative and Postoperative Patients," p. 395.

PATIENT-FAMILY TEACHING AND DISCHARGE PLANNING

See "Heart Failure," p. 36, and "Cardiac Surgery," p. 55, depending on patient's clinical course.

Cardiovascular

SECTION THREE: CARDIOVASCULAR CONDITIONS SECONDARY TO OTHER DISEASE PROCESSES

Cardiac and Noncardiac Shock (Circulatory Failure)

NURSING DIAGNOSES AND INTERVENTIONS

Altered peripheral, cardiopulmonary, cerebral, and renal tissue perfusion related to decreased circulating blood volume

Desired outcome: Within 1 h of treatment, patient has adequate perfusion, as evidenced by peripheral pulse amplitude >2+ on a 0-4+ scale; brisk capillary refill (<2 sec); BP within patient's normal range; CVP ≥5 cm H_2O; HR regular and ≤100 bpm; orientation to time, place, and person; and urine output ≥30 ml/h.

1. Assess and document peripheral perfusion status. Report significant findings: coolness and pallor of the extremities, decreased amplitude of pulses, delayed capillary refill.
2. Monitor BP at frequent intervals; be alert for readings more than 20 mm Hg below patient's normal range or to other indicators of hypotension: dizziness, altered mentation, decreased urinary output.
3. If hypotension is present, place patient in a supine position to promote venous return. Remember that BP must be ≥80/60 mm Hg for adequate coronary and renal artery perfusion.
4. Monitor CVP (if line is inserted) to determine adequacy of venous return and blood volume; 5-10 cm H_2O usually is considered an adequate range. Values near zero can indicate hypovolemia, especially when associated with decreased urinary output, vasoconstriction, and increased HR, which are found with hypovolemia.
5. Observe for indicators of decreased cerebral perfusion: restlessness, confusion, decreased LOC. If positive indicators are present, protect patient from injury by raising side rails and placing bed in lowest position. Reorient patient as indicated.
6. Monitor for indicators of decreased coronary artery perfusion: chest pain, irregular HR.
7. Monitor urinary output qh. Consult physician if it is <30 ml/h despite adequate intake. Check weight daily for evidence of gain.
8. Monitor laboratory results for elevated BUN (>20 mg/dl) and creatinine (>1.5 mg/dl); report increases.
9. Monitor serum electrolyte values for evidence of imbalances, particularly sodium (Na^+) (>147 mEq/L) and potassium (K^+) (>5 mEq/L). Be alert for signs of hyperkalemia: muscle weakness, hy-

poreflexia, irregular HR. Also monitor for signs of hypernatremia: fluid retention, edema.

10. Administer fluids as prescribed to increase vascular volume. The type and amount of fluid depend on the type of shock and the patient's clinical situation. See Table 2-6 for a description of clinical signs associated with different types of shock.
    - *Cardiogenic shock:* Fluids probably are limited to prevent overload, yet dehydration must be avoided to ensure support of vascular space and cardiac muscle.
    - *Hypovolemic shock:* Amount lost is replaced. As much as 1,000 ml/h of Ringer's solution may be administered if volume loss is severe. Most often this includes blood replacement.
    - *Septic shock:* Ringer's solution, plasma, and blood are administered.
11. Prepare for transfer of patient to ICU if appropriate.

Impaired gas exchange related to altered oxygen supply secondary to decreased respiratory muscle function occurring with altered metabolism

Desired outcome: Within 1 h of intervention, patient has adequate gas exchange, as evidenced by O_2 saturation $\geq$95%; Pao_2 $\geq$80 mm Hg; $Paco_2$ $\leq$45 mm Hg; pH $\geq$7.35; eupnea; and orientation to time, place, and person.

1. Monitor ABG results. Be alert for and report hypoxemia (decreased O_2 saturation, decreased Pao_2), hypercapnia (increased $Paco_2$), and acidosis (decreased pH, increased $Paco_2$). Report significant findings.
2. Monitor respirations q30 min; note and report tachypnea or dyspnea. Be alert for restlessness, irritability, and confusion, which are indicators of hypoxia.
3. Teach patient to breathe slowly and deeply to promote oxygenation.
4. Ensure that patient has a patent airway; suction secretions as needed to assist with gas exchange.
5. Administer O_2 as prescribed.

Also see psychosocial nursing diagnoses and interventions in Appendix One, "Caring for Patients with Cancer and Other Life-Disrupting Illnesses," p. 450.

PATIENT-FAMILY TEACHING AND DISCHARGE PLANNING

See patient's primary diagnosis.

Dysrhythmias and Conduction Disturbances

NURSING DIAGNOSES AND INTERVENTIONS

Decreased cardiac output related to altered rate, rhythm, or conduction or negative inotropic changes secondary to cardiac disease

Table 2-6   Systemic clinical signs of shock

	Cardiogenic	Septic	Hypovolemic	Neurogenic	Anaphylactic
Cardiovascular	↓ BP ↑ HR ↓ Pulses	*Early:* ↑ BP ↑ Pulses *Late:* ↓ BP ↓ Pulses	↓ BP ↑ HR Flat neck veins	*Early:* vasodilatation, ↑ BP	↓ BP ↑ HR ↓ Pulses
Respiratory	Dyspnea, crackles	*Early:* ↑ RR *Late:* ↓ RR, crackles	Lungs clear	Lungs clear	Dyspnea to air hunger; wheezes and complete obstruction
Neurologic	Confusion, lethargy, drowsiness	↓ LOC	↓ LOC	Normal or ↓ LOC	↓ LOC
Renal	↓ Urinary output	↓ Urinary output	↓ Urinary output	Normal or ↓ urinary output	↓ Urinary output
Cutaneous	Cool skin	*Early:* warm *Late:* cool	Cool skin	Warm (due to vasodilatation)	Urticaria, angioedema

Desired outcome: Within 1 h of treatment/intervention, patient has adequate cardiac output, as evidenced by BP ≥90/60 mm Hg, HR 60-100 bpm, and normal sinus rhythm on ECG.

1. Monitor patient's heart rhythm continuously; note BP and symptoms if dysrhythmias occur or become more frequent.
2. If symptoms of reduced cardiac output occur, prepare to transfer patient to CCU.
3. Document dysrhythmias with rhythm strip. Use a 12-lead ECG as necessary to identify dysrhythmia.
4. Monitor patient's laboratory data, particularly electrolyte and digoxin levels. Serum potassium (K^+) levels <3.5 mEq/L or >5 mEq/L can cause dysrhythmias.
5. Administer antidysrhythmic agents as prescribed; note patient's response to therapy.
6. Provide O_2 as prescribed. O_2 may be beneficial if dysrhythmias are related to ischemia.
7. Maintain a quiet environment, and administer pain medications promptly. Both stress and pain can increase sympathetic tone and cause dysrhythmias.
8. If life-threatening dysrhythmias occur, initiate emergency procedures and cardiopulmonary resuscitation (as indicated).
9. When dysrhythmias occur, stay with patient; provide support and reassurance while performing assessments and administering treatment.

Knowledge deficit: Mechanism by which dysrhythmias occur and life-style implications

Desired outcome: Within the 24 h before hospital discharge, patient and significant others verbalize knowledge of causes of dysrhythmias and implications for life-style modification.

1. Discuss causal mechanisms for dysrhythmias, including resulting symptoms. Use a heart model or diagrams as necessary.
2. Teach the signs and symptoms of dysrhythmias that require medical attention: unrelieved and prolonged palpitations, chest pain, SOB, rapid pulse (>150 bpm), dizziness, syncope. Teach patient and significant others how to check pulse rate for a full minute.
3. Teach patient and significant others about medications that will be taken after hospital discharge, including drug name, purpose, dosage, schedule, precautions, drug/drug and food/drug interactions, and potential side effects. Stress that patient will be maintained on long-term antidysrhythmic therapy and that it could be life threatening to stop or skip these medications without the physician's approval because doing so may reduce blood levels effective for suppressing dysrhythmia.
4. Advise patient and significant others about the availability of support groups and counseling; provide appropriate community referrals. Patients who survive sudden cardiac arrest may experience nightmares or other sleep disturbances at home. Explain that anxiety and fear, along with periodic feelings of denial, depression, anger, and confusion, are normal after this experience.
5. Stress the importance of leading a normal, productive life, even though patient may fear breakthrough of life-threatening dysrhyth-

mias. If patient is going on vacation, advise him or her to take along sufficient medication and to investigate health care facilities in the vacation area.

6. Advise patient and significant others to take CPR classes; provide addresses of community programs.
7. Teach the importance of follow-up care; confirm date and time of next appointment. Explain that outpatient Holter monitoring is performed periodically.
8. Explain that individuals with recurrent dysrhythmias should follow a general low-cholesterol diet (see Table 2-3) and reduce intake of products containing caffeine, including coffee, tea, chocolate, and colas.
9. As indicated, teach patient relaxation techniques that reduce stress and enable patient to decrease sympathetic tone (see p. 27).

PATIENT-FAMILY TEACHING AND DISCHARGE PLANNING

See patient's primary diagnosis.

Cardiac Arrest

NURSING DIAGNOSES AND INTERVENTIONS

Decreased cardiac output related to altered mechanical and electrical factors secondary to cardiac arrest

Desired outcome: Within 15 min of arrest, patient has adequate cardiac output, as evidenced by systolic BP $\geq$90 mm Hg, HR 60-100 bpm with regular rhythm, peripheral pulse amplitude $>2+$ on a 0-4+ scale, equal radial/apical pulses, and RR 12-20 breaths/min with normal depth and pattern (eupnea).

1. Ensure adequate oxygenation by maintaining a patent airway; provide O_2 support as prescribed.
2. Maintain closed chest compressions until cardiac rhythm is restored.
3. Maintain or establish an IV line. Typically, 5% dextrose in water (D_5W) is run at a rapid rate unless otherwise prescribed.
4. Assess and document BP at frequent intervals (q5-15min), and immediately report changes in pressure to physician.
5. Administer antidysrhythmic agents (e.g., lidocaine, bretylium, quinidine, and procainamide) and inotropic drugs (e.g., dopamine hydrochloride) as prescribed.
6. Assess and document HR; report irregularities or apical/radial deficit (e.g., apical rate 80 bpm/radial rate 50 bpm).
7. Monitor ventilatory status, and be alert for indicators of hypoxia or inadequate ventilation: changes in breathing rhythm, adventitious breath sounds, breath sounds that are not equal in both lungs. Be alert for ABG results that signal hypoxemia, hypercapnia, or acidosis: low pH (<7.35), low Pao_2 (<80 mm Hg), decreased O_2 saturation ($<90\%$-95%), high $Paco_2$ (>45 mm Hg). Report significant findings.
8. Monitor femoral pulses for peripheral perfusion. Be alert for and report decreasing amplitude of pulse pressures.

Also see psychosocial nursing diagnoses in Appendix One, "Caring for Patients with Cancer and Other Life-Disrupting Illnesses," p. 450.

PATIENT-FAMILY TEACHING AND DISCHARGE PLANNING

See patient's primary diagnosis.

Pulmonary Edema

NURSING DIAGNOSES AND INTERVENTIONS

Impaired gas exchange related to alveolar capillary membrane changes secondary to fluid accumulation in the alveoli

Desired outcome: Within 30 min of treatment/intervention, patient has adequate gas exchange, as evidenced by normal breath sounds and skin color, eupnea, HR ≤ 100 bpm, oxygen saturation $\geq 95\%$, Pao_2 ≥ 80 mm Hg, $Paco_2$ ≤ 45 mm Hg.

1. Auscultate lung fields for breath sounds; be alert for crackles, which signal alveolar fluid congestion.
2. Help patient into high Fowler's position to reduce WOB and enhance gas exchange.
3. Teach patient to take slow, deep breaths to increase oxygenation.
4. Administer O_2 as prescribed. If ABGs are tested, monitor results for hypoxemia (decreased Pao_2) and hypercapnia (increased $Paco_2$). Be alert for O_2 saturation level $<95\%$.
5. Be alert for signs of increasing respiratory distress: increased RR, gasping for air, cyanosis, rapid HR.
6. Administer diuretics as prescribed. Monitor potassium (K^+) levels because of the potential for hypokalemia ($K^+ <3.5$ mEq/L) in patients taking certain diuretics.
7. Administer vasodilators (e.g., nitrates) as prescribed to increase venous capacitance (venous dilatation) and decrease pulmonary congestion.
8. As indicated, have emergency equipment (e.g., airway and manual resuscitator) available and functional.
9. As indicated, prepare to transfer patient to ICU.

Fluid volume excess related to compromised regulatory mechanisms secondary to decreased cardiac output

Desired outcome: Within 2 h of intervention/treatment, patient becomes normovolemic, as evidenced by balanced I&O, normal breath sounds, and urine output ≥ 30 ml/h. Within 1 day of treatment/intervention, edema is $\leq 1+$ on a 0-4+ scale. Within 2-3 days, weight becomes stable.

1. Closely monitor I&O, including insensible losses from diaphoresis and respirations.
2. Record weight daily and report steady gains.
3. Assess for edema (interstitial fluids), especially in dependent areas such as ankles and sacrum.
4. Assess respiratory system for indicators of fluid extravasation: crackles; pink-tinged, frothy sputum.

5. Monitor IV rate of flow to prevent volume overload. Use a commercial infusion controller if possible.
6. Unless contraindicated, provide ice chips or popsicles to help patient control thirst. Record amount on I&O record.
7. Administer diuretics as prescribed, and record patient's response.
8. Administer morphine sulfate if prescribed to induce vasodilatation and reduce venous return to the heart.

Altered cardiopulmonary, peripheral, and cerebral tissue perfusion related to interrupted blood flow secondary to decreased cardiac output

Desired outcome: Within 2 h of intervention/treatment, patient has adequate tissue perfusion, as evidenced by BP within 20 mm Hg of patient's baseline; HR ≤100 bpm with regular rhythm; RR ≤20 breaths/min with normal depth and pattern (eupnea); brisk capillary refill (<2 sec); and orientation to time, place, and person.

1. Monitor BP q15min or more often if unstable. Be alert for decreases of more than 20 mm Hg over patient's baseline or associated changes, such as dizziness and altered mentation.
2. Check pulse rate q15-30min. Monitor for irregularities, increased HR, or skipped beats, which can signal decompensation and decreased function.
3. Monitor for indicators of peripheral vasoconstriction (from SNS compensation): cool extremities, pallor, diaphoresis. Evaluate capillary refill. Optimally, pink color should return within 1-2 sec after applying pressure to nail beds.
4. Monitor for indicators of decreased cerebral perfusion: restlessness, anxiety, confusion, lethargy, stupor, coma. Institute safety precautions accordingly.
5. Administer inotropic drugs (e.g., digitalis) as prescribed.
6. Administer vasodilators as prescribed, and monitor effects closely. Be alert for problems such as hypotension and irregular heartbeats.
7. Implement measures for decreasing venous return and increasing peripheral perfusion, such as placing patient in high Fowler's position.

Fear related to potentially life-threatening situation

Desired outcomes: Within 24 h of this diagnosis, patient communicates fears and concerns and reports increasing physical and psychological comfort.

1. Provide opportunity for patient and significant others to express feelings and fears. Be reassuring and supportive.
2. Help make patient as comfortable as possible with prompt pain relief and positioning, typically high Fowler's position.
3. Keep environment as calm and quiet as possible.
4. Explain all treatments, especially those that may be uncomfortable (e.g., O_2 face mask, rotating tourniquets).
5. Remain with patient if at all possible, providing emotional support for both patient and significant others.
6. Also see this nursing diagnosis in Appendix One, "Caring for Patients with Cancer and Other Life-Disrupting Illness," p. 454.

See "Coronary Artery Disease" for **Knowledge deficit:** Precautions and side effects of nitrates, p. 29.

See "Heart Failure" for **Knowledge deficit:** Precautions and side effects of diuretic therapy, p. 35, **Knowledge deficit:** Precautions and side effects of digitalis therapy, p. 35, and **Knowledge deficit:** Precautions and side effects of vasodilators, p. 36.

See psychosocial nursing diagnoses and interventions in Appendix One, "Caring for Patients with Cancer and Other Life-Disrupting Illnesses," p. 450.

PATIENT-FAMILY TEACHING AND DISCHARGE PLANNING
See patient's primary diagnosis.

SECTION FOUR: SPECIAL CARDIAC PROCEDURES

Pacemakers
NURSING DIAGNOSES AND INTERVENTIONS

Knowledge deficit: Pacemaker insertion procedure, pacemaker function, and precautions to take after hospital discharge
Desired outcomes: Before procedure, patient verbalizes knowledge of insertion procedure and function of pacemaker. Before hospital discharge, patient describes precautions to take at home.
BEFORE PACEMAKER INSERTION
1. Assess patient's knowledge about insertion procedure and function of pacemaker. As appropriate, describe procedure and explain that pacemaker stimulates patient's own heart to beat when the heart becomes lazy or slows down.
2. Begin a teaching program specific to patient's rhythm disorder and type of pacemaker inserted, including normal function of the heart, patient's rhythm disorder that requires a pacemaker, and how patient's pacemaker works.
3. Reinforce physician's explanation about duration of procedure, use of local anesthetic, and postprocedural care.
4. Explain that after the procedure, patient can expect continuous ECG monitoring, stiffness and soreness at the insertion site, and no vigorous activity. Explain that patient should request pain medication as soon as pain is felt.
AFTER PACEMAKER INSERTION
1. Explain activity restrictions as directed by physician (e.g., no heavy lifting [>10 lb]), and give instructions about amount and type of exercise allowed. Resumption of sexual activity probably will not be affected, but this will depend on patient's underlying condition.

2. Teach patient the signs and symptoms that require medical attention: decreasing pulse rate, irregular pulse, dizziness, SOB, ankle
   swelling, passing out, signs of infection. Teach patient the technique
   for measuring radial pulse.
3. Stress the necessity of follow-up care, usually at pacemaker clinic;
   confirm date and time of next appointment. Telephonic monitoring
   of pacemakers frequently is used as a method of assessing patients
   between visits. If this method is to be used, inform patient about
   this type of monitoring.
4. Teach patient the expected life of the pacemaker battery, which is
   approximate and can vary from 5-10 yr, depending on the type of
   battery. It is important to know the manufacturer of the specific
   pacemaker because some start to show signs of battery failure 2 yr
   before absolute failure.

**Altered cardiopulmonary and peripheral tissue perfusion
(or risk for same)** related to interrupted blood flow secondary to
pacemaker malfunction
Desired outcome: On an ongoing basis, patient has adequate perfusion, as evidenced by BP within 20 mm Hg of baseline BP; peripheral pulse amplitude >2+ on a 0-4+ scale; and apical/radial pulses
regular, equal, and at rate $\geq$ that established for pacemaker.

1. Monitor perfusion by assessing BP at frequent intervals.
2. Assess rate and regularity of apical and radial pulses. At minimum,
   it should be the rate established for the pacemaker.
3. Assess for apical/radial deficit, which if present indicates that the
   heart is mechanically contracting but that there is no peripheral perfusion (e.g., the apical pulse rate is 80 bpm with auscultation, but
   the palpable radial pulse is 42 bpm).
4. Be alert for pulse irregularity, which can signal pacemaker malfunction or decreasing patient response.
5. Ensure that patient maintains strict bed rest for prescribed amount
   of time postoperatively to prevent pacemaker dislodgment.
6. Maintain patient's arm in a sling or other immobilizer to prevent
   pacemaker dislodgment caused by arm movement.
7. Alert physician to significant findings.

Pain related to pacemaker insertion
Desired outcomes: Within 1 h of intervention, patient's subjective
perception of pain decreases, as documented by a pain scale. Objective
indicators, such as grimacing, are absent.

1. Assess for pain, using a pain scale of 0 (no pain) to 10 (worst pain),
   and medicate as prescribed. Evaluate relief obtained, using pain scale.
2. Assist patient with positioning for comfort, using pillows for support
   as needed.
3. Adjust sling or shoulder support to avoid incisional pressure and other
   pressure areas.
4. For additional information about pain, see this nursing diagnosis in
   Appendix One, p. 396.

Also see Appendix One, "Caring for Preoperative and Postoperative
Patients," p. 395.

PATIENT-FAMILY TEACHING
AND DISCHARGE PLANNING

Give patient and significant others verbal and written information about the following:

1. Activity restrictions as directed by physician, such as no heavy lifting (>10 lb), and instructions about the amount and type of exercise allowed. Resumption of sexual activity probably will not be affected, but this will depend on patient's underlying condition.
2. Technique for measuring radial pulse.
3. Signs and symptoms that require medical attention: decreasing pulse rate, irregular pulse, dizziness, passing out, signs of infection.
4. Necessity of follow-up care, usually at pacemaker clinic; confirm date and time of next appointment. Telephonic monitoring of pacemakers is used frequently as a method of assessing patients between visits. If this method is to be used, inform patient about this type of monitoring.
5. Medications, including drug name, purpose, dosage, schedule, precautions, drug/drug and food/drug interactions, and potential side effects.
6. Importance of using caution around strong magnetic fields, which can alter the function of the pacemaker (this is not a problem for newer pacemakers). **Note:** Strong magnetic fields such as microwave ovens can convert some pacemakers to a "fixed-rate" mode. Once the patient moves away from the magnetic field, the pacemaker will return to the normal programmed function.
7. Expected life of the pacemaker battery, which is approximate and can vary from 5-10 yr, depending on the type of battery. It is important to know the manufacturer of the specific pacemaker because some start to show signs of battery failure 2 yr before absolute failure.

Cardiac Surgery

NURSING DIAGNOSES AND INTERVENTIONS

Knowledge deficit: Diagnosis, surgical procedure, preoperative routine, and postoperative course
Desired outcome: Before surgery, patient verbalizes knowledge of diagnosis, surgical procedure, and preoperative and postoperative regimens.

1. Assess patient's level of knowledge about diagnosis and surgical procedure, and provide information where necessary. Encourage questions and allow time for verbalization of concerns and fears.
2. If appropriate for patient, provide orientation to ICU and equipment that will be used postoperatively.
3. Provide instructions for deep breathing and coughing in preoperative teaching.
4. Reassure patient that postoperative discomfort will be relieved with medication. **Note:** Pain following a midline sternotomy (the usual incision with cardiac surgery) usually is less than that with conven-

tional thoracotomy because the somatic nerves are not divided by the surgical incision.

5. Advise patient that in the immediate postoperative period, speaking will be impossible because of the presence of an endotracheal tube, which will assist with breathing. Also explain that a chest tube will be present. Teach patient how he or she will move, deep breathe, and cough with a chest tube in place. (See "Pneumothorax/Hemothorax" for care considerations for patients with chest tubes.)

Activity intolerance related to generalized weakness and bed rest secondary to cardiac surgery

Desired outcome: By a minimum of 24 h before hospital discharge, patient rates perceived exertion at ≤3 on a 0-10 scale and exhibits cardiac tolerance to activity after cardiac surgery, as evidenced by HR ≤120 bpm, systolic BP within 20 mm Hg of resting systolic BP, and RR ≤20 breaths/min with normal depth and pattern (eupnea).

1. Ask patient to rate perceived exertion during activity, and monitor for evidence of activity intolerance. For details, see **Risk for activity intolerance** in Appendix One, "Caring for Patients on Prolonged Bed Rest," p. 413. Consult physician about significant findings.

2. Monitor VS at frequent intervals, and be alert for indicators of cardiac failure: hypotension, tachycardia, crackles, tachypnea, decreased amplitude of peripheral pulses. Consult physician about significant findings.

3. Monitor BP and note a decrease of more than 20 mm Hg in resting systolic BP. **Note:** A mean BP of 50 mm Hg is required for adequate brain perfusion.

4. To help minimize myocardial oxygen consumption, make sure patient has frequent rest periods.

5. As prescribed, administer medications that reduce myocardial O_2 consumption, such as beta-blockers or calcium antagonists.

6. Assist patient with ROM and other exercises, depending on tolerance and prescribed activity limitations. Consult physician about patient's readiness to participate in exercises that require increased cardiac tolerance. For a discussion of in-bed exercises that may be used, see **Risk for activity intolerance,** p. 413, and **Risk for disuse syndrome,** p. 416, in Appendix One.

See "Pulmonary Embolus" for **Altered protection** related to risk of prolonged bleeding or hemorrhage secondary to anticoagulant therapy, p. 7.

See "Coronary Artery Disease" for **Altered nutrition:** More than body requirements of calories, sodium, or fats, p. 26, and **Health-seeking behaviors:** Relaxation technique effective for stress reduction, p. 27.

See "Atherosclerotic Arterial Occlusive Disease" for **Altered renal tissue perfusion,** p. 58.

See Appendix One, "Caring for Preoperative and Postoperative Patients," in particular, **Ineffective breathing pattern (or risk for same),** p. 404, and **Risk for infection,** p. 408.

Also see Appendix One, "Caring for Patients on Prolonged Bed Rest," in particular, **Altered peripheral tissue perfusion,** p. 418.

PATIENT-FAMILY TEACHING
AND DISCHARGE PLANNING

Give patient and significant others verbal and written information about the following:

1. Medications, including drug name, purpose, dosage, schedule, precautions, drug/drug and food/drug interactions, and potential side effects.

2. Untoward symptoms requiring medical attention for patients taking warfarin: bleeding from the nose, hemoptysis, hematuria, melena, excessive bruising. In addition, stress the following: take warfarin at the same time every day; notify physician if *any* signs of bleeding occur; keep appointments for prothrombin time (PT) checks; avoid OTC medications unless approved by physician; use a Medic-Alert bracelet or card; avoid constrictive or restrictive clothing; use soft-bristled toothbrushes and electric razors.

3. Maintenance of a diet that is low in sodium (see Table 1-4, p. 18, for a list of high-sodium foods to avoid); fat (Table 2-2), and cholesterol (Table 2-3).

4. Importance of pacing activities at home and allowing for frequent rest periods.

5. Technique for assessing radial pulse, temperature, and weight, if these indicators require monitoring at home, and reporting significant changes to physician.

6. Introduction to local American Heart Association activities.

7. Telephone number of nurse available to discuss concerns and questions or clarify instructions.

8. Importance of follow-up visits with physician; confirm date and time of next appointment.

9. Signs and symptoms that require immediate medical attention: chest pain, dyspnea, SOB, weight gain, decrease in exercise tolerance.

10. Activity restrictions (e.g., no heavy lifting [$\geq$10-20 lb], pushing, or pulling for at least 6 wk); prescribed exercise program; and resumption of sexual activity, work, and driving a car as directed.

11. Care of incision site and importance of assessing for signs of infection: drainage, fever, persistent redness, local warmth and tenderness.

12. Referral to a cardiac rehabilitation program.

13. Discussion of patient's home environment and the potential need for changes or adaptations (e.g., too many steps to climb, ADLs that are too strenuous).

SECTION FIVE: DISORDERS OF THE PERIPHERAL VASCULAR SYSTEM

Atherosclerotic Arterial Occlusive Disease

NURSING DIAGNOSES AND INTERVENTIONS

Impaired extremity tissue integrity related to altered arterial circulation secondary to atherosclerotic process

Desired outcome: Patient's extremity tissue remains intact.

1. Assess legs for ulcerations that can occur with decreased arterial circulation.
2. Teach patient to elevate HOB to increase circulation to lower extremities. Explain that this can be accomplished at home by raising HOB on 6-in blocks.
3. Teach patient that walking and ROM exercises for the hip, knee, and ankle promote collateral circulation.
4. Discuss an exercise program with physician, and describe routine to patient. Often this includes walking to patient's tolerance (without pain).
5. If prescribed, teach patient Buerger-Allen exercises. **Note:** Bed rest without exercise may be prescribed to reduce O_2 demand in acute, severe cases.
   - Teach patient to lie flat in bed with legs elevated above the level of the heart for 2-3 min.
   - Have patient sit on the edge of the bed for 2-3 min with the legs relaxed and dependent.
   - In the same position, have patient flex, extend, invert, and evert the feet, holding each position for 30 sec.
   - Finally, have patient lie flat with legs at heart level for approximately 5 min, keeping legs covered with a warm blanket.
6. Teach patient to assess peripheral pulses, warmth, color, hair distribution, and capillary filling. To check for capillary filling, teach patient to press on a nail bed until blanching occurs and then release pressure. Explain that with normal capillary filling, color (pink) returns in 1-2 sec.
7. As appropriate, teach patient that smoking results in a decrease in blood flow to the extremities and in extremity temperature, particularly in the fingers and toes.
8. Discuss the importance of keeping warm by wearing socks when walking or in bed. Caution patient about using heating pads, which increase metabolism and may promote ischemia if circulation is limited.
9. Caution patient to cover all exposed areas when going outside in cooler weather.
10. Teach patient to maintain moderate room temperature and avoid extremes.

11. Administer antiplatelet agents as prescribed to help prevent platelet adherence.

Chronic pain related to atherosclerotic obstructions

Desired outcomes: By hospital discharge, patient's subjective perception of chronic pain decreases, as documented by a pain scale. Objective indicators, such as grimacing, are absent.

1. Assess for pain using a pain scale of 0 (no pain) to 10 (worst pain). Administer pain medications as prescribed; document effectiveness, using pain scale.
2. Teach patient to rest and stop exercising before claudication (severe, cramping pain) occurs.
3. Because pain may be chronic and continuous, explore alternative methods of pain relief: visualization, guided imagery, biofeedback, meditation, relaxation exercises or tapes. For an example of a relaxation exercise, see "Coronary Heart Disease," **Health-seeking behaviors,** p. 27.
4. Institute measures to increase circulation to ischemic extremities, such as Buerger-Allen exercises and walking.
5. Administer calcium channel blockers (e.g., diltiazem hydrochloride) as prescribed to reduce vasospasm.
6. Advise patient about the possibility of "rest" pain, which occurs at night when recumbent and decreases when the legs are in a dependent position.

Knowledge deficit: Potential for infection and impaired tissue integrity due to decreased arterial circulation

Desired outcome: By hospital discharge, patient verbalizes knowledge of the potential for infection and impaired tissue integrity, as well as measures to prevent these problems.

1. Teach patient how to assess for signs of infection or problems with skin integrity and to report significant findings to physician.
2. Caution patient about increased potential for easily traumatizing the skin (e.g., from bumping the lower extremities).
3. Stress the importance of wearing shoes or slippers that fit properly.
4. Instruct patient to cut toenails straight across to prevent ingrown toenails.
5. Advise patient to cover corns or calluses with pads to prevent further injury.
6. Encourage patient to keep the feet clean and dry, using mild soap and warm water for cleansing and applying a mild lotion to prevent dryness.
7. Advise patient not to scratch or rub the skin on the feet, because this can result in abrasions that easily can become infected.
8. Suggest that patient keep the feet warm with loose-fitting socks and warm soaks. Caution patient to check temperature of warm soaks and bathwater carefully to protect skin from burns.
9. Discuss potential surgical interventions: endarterectomy, bypass vascular grafting, angioplasty.

Altered peripheral tissue perfusion (or risk for same) related to interrupted arterial flow with postsurgical graft occlusion

Desired outcome: Patient has adequate peripheral perfusion, as evidenced by peripheral pulse amplitude >2+ on a 0-4+ scale, BP within 20 mm Hg of baseline BP, and absence of the six P's in the involved extremities.

1. Assess peripheral pulses and involved extremity for the six P's: *p*ain, *p*allor, *p*ulselessness, *p*aresthesia, *p*olar (coolness), and *p*aralysis. Report significant findings.
2. Monitor BP, another indicator of peripheral perfusion pressure. Report to physician any significant increase or decrease (>15-20 mm Hg, or as directed).
3. If necessary, use Doppler ultrasonic probe to check pulses, holding probe to the skin at a 45-degree angle to blood vessel. In the presence of blood flow, wavelike "whooshing" sounds will be heard. Record presence or absence of pulsations, as well as rate, character, frequency, and intensity of sounds.
4. To prevent pressure on tissue, use foam protectors to keep sheets and blankets off legs and feet.
5. For the first 48-72 h after surgery (or as directed), prevent acute joint flexion in the presence of a graft, which can occlude blood flow.

Altered renal tissue perfusion related to interrupted blood flow during surgery and potential embolization

Desired outcome: Within 1 h after surgery, patient has adequate renal perfusion, as evidenced by urinary output ≥30 ml/h.

N O T E : During many vascular surgical procedures, the aorta is clamped temporarily to facilitate endarterectomy and grafting. Although all body systems are affected to a degree, the renal system is especially sensitive to the lack of blood flow.

1. Monitor I&O. Report output <30 ml/h.
2. Monitor results of renal function tests. Be alert for increases in serum creatinine (>1.5 mg/dl) and BUN (>20 mg/dl), which occur with decreasing renal function.
3. Monitor for signs of fluid retention (e.g., distended neck veins, crackles [rales], and peripheral edema).
4. In the absence of acute cardiac or renal failure, encourage adequate fluid intake (2-3 L/day) to help maintain adequate renal blood flow and promote fluid balance.

As appropriate, also see Appendix One, "Caring for Preoperative and Postoperative Patients," p. 395.

PATIENT-FAMILY TEACHING
AND DISCHARGE PLANNING

Give patient and significant others verbal and written information about the following:

1. "Stop smoking" programs, if appropriate.

2. Importance of avoiding factors and activities that cause vasoconstriction (e.g., tight clothing and crossing the legs at the knee).
3. Exercise program as prescribed by physician; importance of rest periods if claudication occurs.
4. Skin and foot care.
5. Measures that optimize arterial blood flow: keeping warm and raising HOB on blocks to promote circulation to lower extremities.
6. Medications, including drug name, purpose, dosage, schedule, precautions, drug/drug and food/drug interactions, and potential side effects.

Aneurysms: Abdominal, Thoracic, and Femoral

NURSING DIAGNOSES AND INTERVENTIONS

Risk for fluid volume deficit related to bleeding/hemorrhage after surgical repair/graft
Desired outcome: Patient is normovolemic, as evidenced by systolic BP ≥90 mm Hg (or within 20 mm Hg of patient's baseline) and <180 mm Hg, HR ≤100 bpm, peripheral pulse amplitude >2+ on a 0-4+ scale, balanced I&O, and urine output ≥30 ml/h.

1. After patient has been transferred from the ICU, monitor BP and peripheral pulses q30min during the first hour; then q2h or as necessary.
2. Check operative site for frank bleeding.
3. Assess apical and peripheral pulses, and report tachycardias or a decreased amplitude of peripheral pulses, which can occur with bleeding.
4. Monitor abdomen for increasing girth.
5. Be alert for patient complaints of low back pain, which, in addition to signs of hypovolemic shock, may signal retroperitoneal hemorrhage.
6. Monitor urine output qh and report volume <30 ml/h.
7. Instruct patient to alert staff members promptly to signs and symptoms such as dizziness, lightheadedness, or palpitations (tachycardia), which may occur with hemorrhage due to SNS compensation.

Altered peripheral tissue perfusion (or risk for same) related to interrupted arterial flow secondary to postoperative embolization
Desired outcome: Patient has adequate peripheral perfusion, as evidenced by peripheral pulse amplitude >2+ on a 0-4+ scale, brisk capillary refill (<2 sec), and baseline extremity sensation, motor function, color, and temperature.

1. Assess peripheral pulses at least qh, and report decreases in amplitude or absence of a pulse.
2. Report to physician any changes in color, capillary refill, temperature, sensation, and motor function of extremities.
3. Maintain patient on bed rest until otherwise directed.
4. Keep patient flat to maintain graft patency and ensure healing with reduced risk of embolization.
5. Instruct patient to report impaired sensation promptly to staff members.

Also see Appendix One, "Caring for Preoperative and Postoperative Patients," p. 395.

PATIENT-FAMILY TEACHING
AND DISCHARGE PLANNING

Give patient and significant others verbal and written information about the following:

1. Importance of regular medical follow-up to ensure graft patency and prompt identification of development of a new aneurysm.
2. Prevention of recurrence of aneurysm by avoiding factors that accelerate atherosclerosis: cigarette smoking, obesity, hypertension.
3. Necessity of a regularly scheduled exercise program that alternates exercise with rest.
4. Indicators of wound infection and thrombus or embolus formation, and the need to report them promptly to physician should they occur.
5. Medications, including drug name, purpose, dosage, schedule, precautions, drug/drug and food/drug interactions, and potential side effects.
6. Telephone number of nurse available to discuss concerns and questions or clarify instructions.
7. Importance of follow-up visits with physician; confirm date and time of next appointment.
8. Potential for aneurysm rupture if surgery is not immediately planned.
   - Teach patient and significant others the symptoms of rupture: sudden onset of severe pain, often described as tearing or ripping; pallor; diaphoresis; sudden loss of consciousness.
   - Emphasize the importance of seeking immediate medical attention should any signs and symptoms of rupture occur. Provide numbers of emergency services in the area.
9. Potential need for ultrasound for other family members to rule out aneurysm.

Arterial Embolism

NURSING DIAGNOSES AND INTERVENTIONS

Altered peripheral tissue perfusion related to interrupted arterial flow secondary to embolization (preoperative period)

Desired outcome: Optimally, patient's peripheral perfusion is adequate, as evidenced by peripheral pulse amplitude >2+ on a 0-4+ scale and normal extremity color, temperature, sensation, and motor function.

1. Maintain patient on bed rest to prevent further embolization.
2. Monitor peripheral circulation. Keep extremities warm (room temperature). Advise patient to avoid chilling by wearing socks or slippers.
3. Protect extremities from trauma. Provide foam protectors to keep sheets and blankets off tissue that has reduced circulation.

4. If prescribed, keep lower extremities slightly dependent (but not >45 degrees) to promote circulation.
5. Teach patient and significant others signs and symptoms of embolization, which require immediate medical attention: sudden onset of severe pain and a gradual decrease in sensory and motor functioning; tingling; numbness; coolness; cyanosis.

See "Pulmonary Embolus" for **Altered protection** related to risk of prolonged bleeding or hemorrhage secondary to anticoagulant therapy, p. 7.

Also see Appendix One, "Caring for Preoperative and Postoperative Patients," p. 395, as appropriate.

PATIENT-FAMILY TEACHING
AND DISCHARGE PLANNING

Give patient and significant others verbal and written information about the following:
1. Prescribed exercise plan to prevent stasis of the blood.
2. Signs and symptoms that require immediate medical attention: extremity pain, coolness, pallor, cyanosis.
3. Indicators of wound infection, if surgery was performed.
4. With oral anticoagulant therapy: need for regular medical checkups and immediate reporting of epistaxis, ecchymosis, hemoptysis, melena, or hematuria; administration at the same time every day; not changing regular dietary habits (e.g., becoming a vegetarian without first consulting physician or nurse because many green, leafy vegetables are high in vitamin K, which reverses the effect of warfarin; vegetarian diets may necessitate an increase in warfarin dosage to achieve therapeutic anticoagulation); importance of consulting with physician before taking any OTC medications, especially aspirin products, which affect platelet aggregation and potentiate the anticoagulant effect of warfarin.
5. Other medications, including drug name, purpose, dosage, schedule, precautions, drug/drug and food/drug interactions, and potential side effects.
6. Risk-factor modification: quitting smoking, controlling hypertension, modifying diet to reduce potential for atherosclerosis and acute arterial occlusion.

Venous Thrombosis/Thrombophlebitis

NURSING DIAGNOSES AND INTERVENTIONS

Altered peripheral and cardiopulmonary tissue perfusion (or risk for same) related to interrupted blood flow secondary to embolization from thrombus formation
Desired outcome: Patient has adequate peripheral and cardiopulmonary perfusion, as evidenced by normal extremity color, temperature, and sensation; RR 12-20 breaths/min with normal depth and pattern (eupnea); HR ≤100 bpm; BP within 20 mm Hg of baseline BP; and normal breath sounds.

1. Be alert for and promptly report early indicators of peripheral thrombus formation: pain, edema, erythema, impaired sensation. If indicators appear, maintain patient on bed rest and notify physician promptly.
2. Monitor for and immediately report signs of pulmonary embolus (PE): sudden onset of chest pain, dyspnea, tachypnea, tachycardia, hypotension, hemoptysis, shallow respirations, crackles, decreased breath sounds, diaphoresis. Should they occur, prompt medical attention is crucial.
3. Administer anticoagulants as prescribed. Double-check drip rates and doses with a colleague.
4. Minimize risk of PE by keeping patient on bed rest, providing ROM exercises, and applying support hose as prescribed.

Pain related to inflammatory process caused by thrombus formation

Desired outcomes: Within 1 h of intervention, patient's subjective perception of pain decreases, as documented by a pain scale. Objective indicators, such as grimacing, are absent.

1. Monitor patient for pain. Document degree of pain, using a pain scale from 0 (no pain) to 10 (worst pain). Administer analgesics as prescribed; document relief obtained, using pain scale.
2. Ensure that patient maintains bed rest during acute phase to minimize painful engorgement and the potential for embolization.
3. If prescribed, apply warm, moist packs. Be sure that packs are warm (but not extremely so) and are not allowed to cool. If appropriate, use a Kock-Mason dressing (warm towel covered by plastic wrap and a K-pad to provide continuous moist heat).
4. To promote venous drainage and reduce engorgement, keep legs elevated above heart level (but not >45 degrees).

Altered peripheral tissue perfusion (or risk for same) related to interrupted venous flow secondary to venous engorgement or edema

Desired outcome: Patient has adequate peripheral perfusion, as evidenced by absence of discomfort, and normal extremity temperature, color, sensation, and motor function.

1. Assess for signs of inadequate peripheral perfusion: pain; changes in skin temperature or color; changes in motor or sensory function. Be alert for venous engorgement (prominence) in lower extremities.
2. Elevate patient's legs above heart level (but not >45 degrees) to promote venous drainage.
3. As prescribed for patients without evidence of thrombus formation, apply antiembolic hose, which compress superficial veins to increase blood flow to deeper veins. Remove stockings for approximately 15 min q8h. Inspect skin for evidence of irritation.
4. Encourage patient to perform ankle circling and active or assisted ROM exercises of the lower extremities to prevent venous stasis. Perform passive ROM if patient cannot.

C A U T I O N :   If any signs of acute thrombus formation are present, such as calf hardness or tenderness, exercises are contraindicated because of the risk of embolization. Notify physician.

5. Encourage deep breathing, which creates increased negative pressure in the lungs and thorax to assist in emptying of large veins.
6. Arterial circulation usually will not be impaired except with arterial disease or severe edema compressing arterial flow. However, assess pulses regularly to confirm good arterial flow.

Impaired tissue integrity related to altered circulation secondary to venous engorgement
Desired outcome: Patient's tissue remains intact.

1. Put on elastic stockings when veins are most likely to be empty (e.g., after patient has been recumbent or legs have been elevated for 20 min). This will help minimize distention.
2. Remove stockings at prescribed intervals to minimize swelling proximal to hose. Assess skin while hose are off, and be alert for signs of stasis dermatitis (i.e., skin that is thin, shiny, and bluish in color) and for ulcerations. Be sure patient's skin is cleansed and dried thoroughly before putting stockings back on.
3. Ensure that tops of stockings do not roll, because this would cause a tourniquet effect and further compromise circulation. Also be sure that there are no creases or wrinkles in the hose, which would cause pressure areas.
4. Protect extremities from trauma. If indicated, use foam protectors to keep bedding off compromised tissues.
5. Teach patient not to cross legs, which worsens venous stasis.

Knowledge deficit: Disease process with venous thrombosis/thrombophlebitis and treatment/management measures after hospital discharge
Desired outcome: Before hospital discharge, patient verbalizes knowledge of the disease process and treatment/management measures that are to occur after hospital discharge.

1. Discuss the process of venous thrombosis/thrombophlebitis and ways to prevent thrombosis and discomfort: avoiding restrictive clothing, avoiding prolonged periods of standing, elevating legs above heart level when sitting.
2. Teach patient the signs of venous stasis ulcers, such as redness and skin breakdown. Stress the importance of avoiding trauma to extremities and keeping the skin clean and dry.
3. Discuss prescribed exercise program. Walking usually is considered the best exercise.
4. Teach patient how to wear antiembolic hose if prescribed. Hose must fit properly without wrinkling and should be snug over feet and progressively less snug as they reach the knee or thigh.
5. Describe indicators that require medical attention: persistent redness, swelling, tenderness, weak or absent pulses, ulcerations on extremities.

See "Pulmonary Embolus" for **Altered protection** related to prolonged bleeding or hemorrhage secondary to anticoagulant therapy, p. 7.

PATIENT-FAMILY TEACHING
AND DISCHARGE PLANNING

See **Knowledge deficit,** p. 63, for topics to discuss (both verbally and through written information) with patient and significant others.

IN ADDITION

If patient is discharged from the hospital on warfarin therapy, provide information about the following:

- As directed, see physician for scheduled prothrombin time (PT) checks.
- Take warfarin at the same time each day; do not skip days unless directed to do so by physician.
- Wear a Medic-Alert bracelet.
- Avoid alcohol consumption and changes in diet (e.g., changing to a vegetarian diet), both of which can alter the body's response to warfarin.
- When making appointments with other physicians and dentists, inform them of warfarin treatment.
- Be alert for indicators that require immediate medical attention: hematuria, melena, epistaxis, ecchymosis, hemoptysis, dizziness, weakness.
- Avoid taking OTC medications (e.g., aspirin, which potentiates the anticoagulant effect of warfarin) without consulting physician or nurse.

Renal-Urinary Disorders

3

SECTION ONE: RENAL DISORDERS

Acute Pyelonephritis

NURSING DIAGNOSES AND INTERVENTIONS

Pain related to dysuria secondary to infection
Desired outcomes: Within 1 h of intervention, patient's subjective perception of discomfort decreases, as documented by a pain scale. Objective indicators, such as grimacing, are absent or diminished.
1. Monitor patient for costovertebral angle (CVA) pain and tenderness, abdominal pain, and dysuria. Devise a pain scale with patient, rating pain from 0 (absent) to 10 (worst pain). As appropriate, administer prescribed analgesics and document their effectiveness, using pain scale.
2. If not contraindicated, increase patient's fluid intake to help relieve dysuria.
3. Consult physician about unrelieved or increasing flank pain.
4. As appropriate, assist patient with repositioning if it helps relieve discomfort.
5. Use nonpharmacologic interventions when possible (e.g., relaxation techniques, guided imagery, distraction).

Risk for infection (or its recurrence) related to chronic disease process
Desired outcomes: Patient is free of infection, as evidenced by normothermia; urine that is clear and of normal odor; HR ≤100 bpm; BP ≥90/60 mm Hg (or within patient's normal range); absence of flank, CVA, and labial pain; and absence of dysuria, urgency, and frequency. Within the 24 h before hospital discharge, patient verbalizes knowledge about the signs and symptoms of infection and the importance of reporting them promptly if they occur.
1. Monitor patient's temperature at least q4h. Report temperature >38° C (100° F) to physician. Monitor for flank, CVA, and labial pain; foul-smelling or cloudy urine; malaise; headache; and frequency and urgency of urination. Teach patient about these indicators and stress the importance of reporting them promptly to physician or staff if they occur.

2. Monitor BP and pulse at least q4h. Hypotension and tachycardia can indicate sepsis and bacteremic shock.
3. Administer prescribed antibiotics as scheduled. Draw prescribed antibiotic serum levels at correct times to ensure reliable results. **Note:** Most antibiotics are measured at peak level (30-60 min after infusion) and trough level (30-60 min before the next dose).
4. Use urinary catheters only when mandatory. Use meticulous sterile technique when inserting, irrigating, or obtaining specimens. Provide perineal care daily. For indwelling catheters, maintain unobstructed flow, and always keep urinary collection container below level of patient's bladder to prevent reflux of urine. Tape catheter to the thigh or abdomen to reduce meatal irritation. **Note:** Intermittent catheterization carries less of a risk of UTI than indwelling catheterization.
5. Offer cranberry, plum, or prune juices, which leave an acid ash in the urine and inhibit bacteriuria.
6. Treat fever with prescribed antipyretics and tepid baths as needed.
7. Teach women patients the importance of wiping the perianal area from front to back, wearing undergarments with a cotton crotch, and voiding before and immediately after sexual intercourse to minimize the risk of introducing bacteria into the urinary tract.
8. Stress the importance of emptying the bladder at least q3-4h and once during the night to help prevent UTI caused by residual urine.

Altered nutrition: Less than body requirements, related to nausea and anorexia

Desired outcome: Within 24 h of admission, patient maintains an adequate diet.

1. Provide nauseated or anorectic patient with frequent small meals and carbonated beverages.
2. Treat nausea and vomiting with prescribed medications.
3. Record accurate calorie intake, and weigh patient daily.
4. Consult physician about inadequate nutritional intake.
5. For additional information, see "Providing Nutritional Support," p. 378.

Fluid volume deficit related to decreased intake secondary to anorexia or active loss secondary to vomiting and diaphoresis

Desired outcomes: After treatment, patient becomes normovolemic, as evidenced by balanced I&O, stable weight, urinary output ≥30-60 ml/h, and BP and HR within patient's normal range. Within 24 h of admission, patient verbalizes knowledge of the importance of a fluid intake of at least 2-3 L/day.

1. Maintain adequate fluid intake to prevent fluid volume deficit. An intake of at least 2-3 L/day usually is indicated; however, the appropriate amount depends on patient's output, which includes gastric, fecal, urinary, sensible, and insensible losses. Obtain guidelines for desired amount of fluid intake/restriction from physician. Teach nonrestricted patients the importance of maintaining a fluid intake of at least 2-3 L/day.
2. Monitor I&O and daily weight as indicators of hydration status.
3. Report indicators of volume deficit: poor skin turgor, thirst, dry mucous membranes, tachycardia, or orthostatic hypotension.

PATIENT-FAMILY TEACHING
AND DISCHARGE PLANNING

Give patient and significant others verbal and written information about the following:

1. Medications, including drug name, purpose, dosage, schedule, precautions, drug/drug and food/drug interactions, and potential side effects.
2. Importance of taking medications for prescribed length of time, even if feeling "well."
3. Necessity of reporting the following indicators of UTI to physician: urgency, frequency, dysuria, flank pain, cloudy or foul-smelling urine, fever.
4. Importance of perineal hygiene for women patients and of wiping from front to back, wearing undergarments with a cotton crotch, and voiding before and after intercourse.
5. Importance of emptying the bladder at least q3-4h and once during the night to help prevent UTI caused by residual urine.
6. Necessity of maintaining a fluid intake of at least 2-3 L/day and of drinking fruit juices (cranberry, plum, prune) that leave an acid ash in the urine.
7. Importance of continued medical follow-up because of the high incidence of recurrence.

Renal Calculi

NURSING DIAGNOSES AND INTERVENTIONS
FOR THE SURGICAL PATIENT

Risk for fluid volume deficit related to postoperative bleeding after pyelolithotomy or nephrolithotomy

Desired outcome: Patient remains normovolemic, as evidenced by balanced I&O, stable weight, good skin turgor, and BP and HR within patient's normal range.

1. Monitor I&O, daily weight, VS, and skin turgor as indicators of volume status. **Note:** Skin turgor is not a reliable indicator of volume deficit in older adults because of the decreased elasticity of their skin.
2. Observe for signs of hemorrhage. Urine usually is dark red or pink for approximately 48 h postoperatively in a patient who has had a pyelolithotomy or nephrolithotomy. Urine should not be bright red or contain clots.
3. For additional information, see this nursing diagnosis in Appendix One, "Caring for Preoperative and Postoperative Patients," p. 405.

Risk for impaired skin integrity related to wound drainage

Desired outcome: Patient's skin remains clear and intact.

1. After a pyelolithotomy, urine can drain from the incision for several days. Apply an ostomy pouch with a skin barrier to collect drainage and protect skin.
2. Closely monitor skin integrity, especially in older adults, who are at increased risk for skin breakdown.

3. Ensure that wound drainage tube remains in proper position; notify physician immediately if it dislodges because it can be difficult to reinsert after 30 min.

Knowledge deficit: Potential for recurrence of calculi and interventions that can be taken to prevent it

Desired outcome: Within the 24 h before hospital discharge, patient verbalizes knowledge about the potential for recurrence of calculi and steps that can be taken to prevent it.

1. When appropriate, teach patient a diet that prevents recurrence of stones. Provide lists of foods that should be limited or avoided, including those that are high in calcium (e.g., dairy products), purine (e.g., meats, fish, poultry), and oxalate (e.g., beets, figs, nuts, spinach, black tea, chocolate, instant and decaffeinated coffee, carbonated beverages), depending on the type of stone and its cause.
2. Encourage a daily fluid intake of at least 3 L/day in nonrestricted patients. A high fluid intake is especially important in preventing recurrent stones in patients with cystinuria.
3. Teach patient about the need for continued use of medications and medical follow-up because of the high rate of recurrence.
4. Teach patient about the importance of maintaining the prescribed urinary pH to prohibit stone precipitation and the necessity of urine pH testing. Demonstrate urine pH testing as appropriate.
5. Caution patient about the importance of seeking prompt medical treatment for signs and symptoms of UTI (e.g., fever, flank or labial pain, cloudy or foul-smelling urine), obstruction (e.g., anuria, oliguria, and pain that is dull and aching or sharp and sudden), and recurrence of stones (e.g., renal colic, hematuria, nausea, vomiting).

See "Ureteral Calculi," p. 87, for more information about stone formation. Also see nursing diagnoses and interventions in Appendix One, "Caring for Preoperative and Postoperative Patients," p. 395.

PATIENT-FAMILY TEACHING AND DISCHARGE PLANNING

Give patient and significant others verbal and written information about the following:

1. Medications, including drug name, purpose, dosage, schedule, precautions, drug/drug and food/drug interactions, and potential side effects.
2. When appropriate, a diet that prevents recurrence of stones. Provide lists of foods that should be limited or avoided, including those that are high in calcium (e.g., dairy products), purine (e.g., meats, fish, poultry), and oxalate (e.g., beets, figs, nuts, spinach, black tea, chocolate, instant and decaffeinated coffee, and carbonated beverages). Encourage a daily fluid intake of at least 3 L/day in nonrestricted patients. A high fluid intake is especially important in preventing recurrent stones in patients with cystinuria.
3. Need for continued use of medications and medical follow-up because of the high rate of recurrence.

4. Requirements for maintaining alterations in urinary pH to prohibit stone precipitation and the necessity of urine pH testing.
5. Importance of seeking prompt medical treatment for signs and symptoms of UTI (e.g., fever, flank or labial pain, cloudy or foul-smelling urine) or obstruction (e.g., anuria, oliguria, and pain that is dull and aching or sharp and sudden).
6. Care of drains or catheters if patient is discharged with them.
7. Care of the surgical incision and indicators of wound infection, which require medical attention: persistent erythema, swelling, pain, local warmth, and purulent drainage.
8. Postoperative activity precautions: avoiding heavy lifting (>10 lb) for the first 6 wk, avoiding fatigue, getting maximum amounts of rest, and gradually increasing activities to tolerance.

Hydronephrosis

NURSING DIAGNOSES AND INTERVENTIONS

Risk for infection related to invasive procedure (insertion/presence of nephrostomy tube)
Desired outcome: Patient is free of infection, as evidenced by normothermia, BP and HR within patient's normal range, urine that is clear and normal in odor and color, absence of dysuria.
1. Maintain sterile technique when performing dressing changes and nephrostomy tube care.
2. Observe for and report indicators of infection (e.g., fever, pain, purulent drainage, tachycardia). Document changes in color, odor, or clarity of urine. Infection is common with hydronephrosis.
3. Do not change, clamp, or irrigate nephrostomy tube unless specifically prescribed by physician.

C A U T I O N :   Because the renal pelvis is tiny, never inject >5 ml at one time into the tube unless a larger amount has been specifically prescribed by the physician.

---

4. Keep urine collection container and tubing in a dependent position. Do not allow kinks to form in the tubing.

Risk for injury related to insertion/presence of nephrostomy tube
Desired outcome: Patient remains free of signs of nephrostomy tube complications, as evidenced by urine that is clear and of normal color after the first 24-48 h, a urine output of 30-60 ml/h, and absence of discomfort/pain.
1. Report gross hematuria (urine that is bright red, possibly with clots). Transient hematuria can be expected for 24-48 h after tube insertion.
2. Consult physician about leakage around the catheter, which can occur with blockage, as well as about a sudden decrease in urine output, which can signal a dislodged catheter.
3. Report a sudden onset of or increase in pain, which can indicate perforation of a body organ by the catheter.

4. Keep the tube securely taped to the patient's flank with elastic tape. If the tube becomes accidentally dislodged, cover the site with a sterile dressing; notify physician immediately.

N O T E :   Before removing the nephrostomy tube, the physician may request that it be clamped for several hours at a time to evaluate the patient's tolerance. While the tube is clamped, monitor the patient for indications of ureteral obstruction: flank pain, diminished urinary output, fever.

Fluid volume deficit related to active loss secondary to postobstructive diuresis
Desired outcome: With intervention/treatment, patient becomes normovolemic, as evidenced by stable weight, good skin turgor, BP $\geq$90/60 mm Hg, HR $\leq$100 bpm, and CVP $\geq$5 cm H_2O (or VS within patient's normal range).
1. Monitor I&O hourly. Initially, output should exceed intake.
2. Monitor weight daily. Alert physician to steady weight loss.
3. Observe for and report indicators of volume depletion, including postural hypotension, tachycardia, poor skin turgor, elevated Hct, and decreased CVP. Monitor VS q30min for the first few hours after release of obstruction.
4. As prescribed, encourage fluids in nonrestricted patients who are hypovolemic.

PATIENT-FAMILY TEACHING
AND DISCHARGE PLANNING

Give patient and significant others verbal and written information about the following:
1. Medications, including drug name, purpose, dosage, schedule, precautions, drug/drug and food/drug interactions, and potential side effects.
2. Care of the nephrostomy catheter, if patient is discharged with one, and the procedure to follow should the catheter become dislodged.
3. Frequency of and procedure for dressing changes. Patient or significant others should demonstrate safe dressing-change technique before hospital discharge.
4. Need for continued medical follow-up; confirm date and time of patient's next appointment with physician, if known.
5. Signs and symptoms that require medical attention: fever, cloudy or foul-smelling urine, flank or labial pain, increased catheter drainage, and drainage around the catheter site.

Renal Artery Stenosis

NURSING DIAGNOSES AND INTERVENTIONS

Knowledge deficit: Rationale for frequent assessments after aortorenal bypass graft, angioplasty, or endarterectomy, and the technique for measuring BP

Desired outcome: Before procedure, patient verbalizes knowledge of renal procedure he or she will undergo and the rationale for frequent VS checks; patient demonstrates BP measurement technique before hospital discharge.

1. Monitor BP frequently during the first 48 h after aortorenal bypass graft procedure. Explain to patient and significant others that hypertension during this period usually is temporary but may require treatment. When angioplasty is successful, hypertension should decrease within 4-6 h postprocedure.
2. Explain the rationale for measuring VS q15min immediately after angioplasty. Monitor integrity of pulses distal to angioplasty site.
3. Alert patient and significant others to potential for bleeding and hematoma formation at angioplasty site, as well as to symptoms of hidden bleeding, including hypotension and tachycardia. Explain that if a hematoma is noted, it will be circled with ink and the time will be noted so that further bleeding can be detected.
4. Explain the rationale for measuring BP under the same conditions each day: sitting, standing, lying down. Teach patient and significant others the technique for measuring BP before hospital discharge.
5. Explain that BP may remain elevated after the renal procedure and that antihypertensive medication still may be required. Review the purpose, action, dosage, and potential side effects of all medications with patient and significant others before hospital discharge. See Table 3-1.
6. Stress the need for continued medical evaluation of BP and renal function.

See nursing diagnoses and interventions in Appendix One, "Caring for Preoperative and Postoperative Patients," p. 395.

PATIENT-FAMILY TEACHING AND DISCHARGE PLANNING

Give patient and significant others verbal and written information about the following:

1. Medications, including drug name, purpose, dosage, schedule, precautions, drug/drug and food/drug interactions, and potential side effects.
2. Diet: low in sodium (see Table 1-4, p. 18, for a list of high-sodium foods that should be avoided); include a list of foods high in potassium (see Table 3-2) if patient is taking diuretics that cause hypokalemia. Provide sample menus, and have patient demonstrate understanding of diet by planning meals for 3 days.
3. Technique for measuring BP. Patient or significant others should demonstrate proficiency before discharge.
4. Care of incision or angioplasty site. Teach patient the indicators of wound infection (e.g., erythema, purulent discharge, local warmth, fever) and the importance of reporting them promptly to the physician.

Table 3-1 Drug usage in renal failure

Drugs handled primarily by the kidneys have an increased effect in
patients with renal failure. Usually either the dosage or scheduling
of these drugs must be modified.
Drugs that require modification of dosage or scheduling:

Antibiotics	**Antihypertensives**	**H$_2$-Receptor Blockers**
carbenicillin*	atenolol*	cimetidine
cefazolin*	enalapril*	famotidine
gentamicin*		ranitidine
kanamycin*	**Hypoglycemic Agent**	
tobramycin*	insulin	
vancomycin		
Antidysrhythmics	**Sedative**	
digoxin	phenobarbital*	
procainamide*		

Drugs that usually do not require modification of dosage or scheduling:

Antibiotics	**Antihypertensives**	**Hypoglycemic Agent**
chloramphenicol*	clonidine HCl	glipizide
clindamycin	hydralazine	
dicloxacillin	methyldopa*	**Narcotics**
erythromycin	minoxidil	codeine
nafcillin sodium	prazosin HCl	morphine
Anticoagulant	**Antiinflammatory Agent**	**Sedatives**
heparin	indomethacin	chlordiazepoxide HCl
Antidysrhythmics	**Diuretics**	diazepam
propranolol	furosemide	
quinidine gluconate*	metolazone	

*Dialyzable drug, which may require increased dosage after dialysis.

Table 3-2 Foods high in potassium

Apricots	Nuts
Artichokes	Oranges, orange juice
Avocados	Peanuts
Bananas	Potatoes
Cantaloupe	Prune juice
Carrots	Pumpkin
Cauliflower	Spinach
Chocolate	Sweet potatoes
Dried beans, peas	Swiss chard
Dried fruit	Tomatoes, tomato juice, tomato sauce
Mushrooms	Watermelon

5. Need for continued medical follow-up to evaluate effectiveness of treatment.
6. Importance of avoiding other risk factors for hypertension: obesity, smoking, stress, and poorly controlled diabetes mellitus.

SECTION TWO: RENAL FAILURE

Acute Renal Failure

NURSING DIAGNOSES AND INTERVENTIONS

Fluid volume excess related to compromised regulatory mechanisms secondary to renal dysfunction: *oliguric phase*
Desired outcome: Patient adheres to prescribed fluid restrictions and becomes normovolemic, as evidenced by decreasing or stable weight, normal breath sounds, edema $\leq 1+$ on a 0-4+ scale, CVP ≤ 12 cm H_2O, and BP and HR within patient's normal range.

1. Closely monitor and document I&O.
2. Monitor weight daily. Patient should lose 0.5 kg/day if not eating; a sudden weight gain suggests excessive fluid volume.
3. Observe for indicators of fluid volume excess, including edema, hypertension, crackles, tachycardia, distended neck veins, SOB, and increased CVP.
4. Carefully adhere to prescribed fluid restriction. Provide oral hygiene at frequent intervals, and offer fluids in the form of ice chips or popsicles to minimize thirst. Hard candies also may be given to reduce thirst. Spread allotted fluids evenly over a 24-h period, and record the amount given. Instruct patient and significant others about the need for fluid restriction. **Note:** Patients nourished by means of TPN are at increased risk for fluid overload because of the necessary fluid volume involved.

Risk for fluid volume deficit related to active loss secondary to excessive urinary output: *diuretic phase*
Desired outcome: Patient remains normovolemic, as evidenced by stable weight, balanced I&O, good skin turgor, CVP ≥ 5 cm H_2O, and BP and HR within patient's normal range.

1. Closely monitor and document I&O.
2. Monitor weight daily. A weight loss ≥ 0.5 kg/day may reflect excessive volume loss.
3. Observe for indicators of volume depletion, including poor skin turgor, hypotension, tachycardia, and decreased CVP.
4. As prescribed, encourage fluids in a dehydrated patient.
5. Report significant findings to physician.

Altered nutrition: Less than body requirements, related to nausea, vomiting, anorexia, and dietary restrictions
Desired outcome: Within 2 days of admission, patient has stable weight and demonstrates normal intake of food within restrictions, as indicated.

1. Nausea, vomiting, and anorexia may signal increased uremia. Alert physician to symptoms, and monitor BUN levels. BUN levels >80-100 mg/dl usually require dialytic therapy.
2. Provide frequent small meals.
3. Administer prescribed antiemetics as necessary.
4. Coordinate meal planning and dietary teaching with patient, significant others, and renal dietitian. Dietary restriction may include reduced intakes of protein, sodium, potassium, and fluid.

Activity intolerance related to generalized weakness secondary to uremia and anemia

Desired outcome: After intervention/treatment, patient rates perceived exertion at ≤3 on a 0-10 scale and exhibits improving endurance during activity, as evidenced by HR ≤20 bpm over resting HR, systolic BP ≤20 mm Hg over or under resting systolic BP, and RR ≤20 breaths/min with normal depth and pattern (eupnea).

1. Monitor patient during activity for signs of activity intolerance, and ask patient to rate perceived exertion. For details, see **Risk for activity intolerance,** p. 413, in Appendix One, "Caring for Patients on Prolonged Bed Rest."
2. Anemia is common in renal failure. Administer epoetin alfa (Epogen) as prescribed. Monitor BP, and consult physician about increases because hypertension is a common complication of erythropoietin therapy.
3. Patients usually are not transfused unless the Hct drops below 20%-25% or the anemia is poorly tolerated. Consult physician if increased weakness, fatigue, dyspnea, or chest pain or a further decrease in Hct occurs.

C A U T I O N :   Muscle weakness can be an indicator of dangerous hyperkalemia and should be reported immediately.

4. Assist with ADLs as necessary; encourage independence to patient's tolerance.
5. Establish a progressive activity regimen within patient's activity limitations that will help him or her return to normal activities without complications. For more information, see Appendix One, "Caring for Patients on Prolonged Bed Rest," **Risk for activity intolerance,** p. 413, and **Risk for disuse syndrome,** p. 416.

Altered protection related to neurosensory, musculoskeletal, and cardiac changes secondary to uremia, electrolyte imbalance, and metabolic acidosis

Desired outcomes: After treatment, patient verbalizes orientation to time, place, and person and is free of injury caused by neurosensory, musculoskeletal, or cardiac disturbances. Within the 24 h before hospital discharge, patient verbalizes the signs and symptoms of electrolyte imbalance and metabolic acidosis and the importance of reporting them promptly should they occur.

1. Assess for and alert patient to indicators of the following:
   - *Hypokalemia* (may occur during the diuretic phase): Muscle weakness, lethargy, dysrhythmias, and nausea and vomiting (secondary to ileus).

- *Hyperkalemia:* Muscle cramps, dysrhythmias, muscle weakness, peaked T waves on ECG.

NOTE: A normal serum potassium (K^+) is necessary for normal cardiac functioning. Hyperkalemia is a common and potentially fatal complication of acute renal failure (ARF) during the oliguric phase.

- *Hypocalcemia:* Neuromuscular irritability, paresthesia.
- *Hyperphosphatemia:* Soft tissue calcifications.
- *Uremia:* Anorexia, nausea, metallic taste in the mouth, irritability, confusion, lethargy, restlessness, itching.
- *Metabolic acidosis:* Rapid, deep respirations; confusion.

2. Do not give patient foods high in potassium (see Table 3-2). Salt substitutes also contain potassium and should not be used.
3. Minimize tissue catabolism by controlling fevers, maintaining adequate nutritional intake (especially calories), and preventing infections. If caloric intake is inadequate, body protein will be used for energy. A high-carbohydrate diet helps minimize tissue catabolism and production of nitrogenous wastes.
4. Prepare patient for the possibility of altered taste and smell.
5. Patients with renal failure are at risk for increased magnesium levels because of decreased urinary excretion of dietary magnesium, and thus magnesium-containing medications should be avoided (e.g., patients using magnesium-containing antacids such as Maalox typically are switched to aluminum hydroxide preparations, such as AlternaGel or Amphojel, or calcium carbonate antacids such as Tums).
6. Administer antacids as prescribed to control hyperphosphatemia. Experiment with different brands or try capsules for patients who refuse certain liquid antacids. However, phosphate binders vary in their aluminum or calcium content, and one may not be exchanged for another without first ensuring that the patient is receiving the same amount of elemental aluminum or calcium.
7. Reassure patient and significant others that irritability, restlessness, and altered thinking are temporary. Facilitate orientation through calendars, radios, familiar objects, and frequent reorientation.
8. Ensure safety measures (e.g., padded side rails, airway) for patients who are confused or severely hypocalcemic. For patients who exhibit signs of hyperkalemia, have emergency supplies available (e.g., manual resuscitator bag, crash cart, emergency drug tray).

Risk for infection related to uremia

Desired outcome: Patient is free of infection, as evidenced by normothermia, WBC count $\leq 11,000/\mu l$, urine that is clear and of normal odor, normal breath sounds, and absence of erythema, swelling, and drainage at the catheter sites.

NOTE: One of the primary causes of death in ARF is sepsis.

1. Monitor temperature and secretions for indicators of infection. Even minor increases in temperature can be significant, because uremia masks the febrile response and inhibits the body's ability to fight infection.

2. Use meticulous aseptic technique when changing dressings or manipulating venous catheters, IV lines, or indwelling catheters.
3. Avoid use of indwelling urinary catheters, because they are a common source of infection. When catheterization is indicated, use intermittent catheterization instead.
4. Provide oral hygiene and skin care at frequent intervals. Use emollients and gentle soap to avoid drying and cracking of skin, which can lead to breakdown and infection. Take care to rinse off all soap when bathing patient, because soap residue may further irritate skin.

Constipation related to restriction of fresh fruit and fluids; to prolonged bed rest; and to side effects of medications (e.g., phosphate-binding antacids)

Desired outcomes: Within 1-3 days of intervention, patient states that bowel movements are within normal pattern. Before hospital discharge, patient verbalizes foods and activities that promote bowel movements.

1. Monitor and record the quality and number of bowel movements.
2. Provide prescribed stool softeners and bulk-building supplements (e.g., Metamucil) as necessary.
3. Suggest alternate dietary sources of fiber, such as unsalted popcorn or unprocessed bran.
4. Encourage exercise and activity as appropriate.
5. Provide Fleet, oil retention, or tap water enemas as prescribed *only* if the previous measures fail. Avoid use of large-volume water enemas, because excess fluid can be absorbed from the GI tract.

PATIENT-FAMILY TEACHING
AND DISCHARGE PLANNING

Give patient and significant others verbal and written information about the following:

1. Medications, including drug name, purpose, dosage, schedule, precautions, drug/drug and food/drug interactions, and potential side effects.
2. Diet: Include fact sheet that lists foods to restrict.
3. Care and observation of dialysis access if patient is being discharged with one.
4. Importance of continued medical follow-up of renal function.
5. Signs and symptoms of potential complications. These should include indicators of infection (see **Risk for infection,** p. 75), electrolyte imbalance (see **Altered protection,** p. 74), **Fluid volume excess** (see p. 73), and bleeding (especially from the GI tract for patients who are uremic).

IN ADDITION
6. If patient requires dialysis after discharge, coordinate discharge planning with dialysis unit staff. Arrange visit to dialysis unit if possible.

Chronic Renal Failure
NURSING DIAGNOSES AND INTERVENTIONS

Activity intolerance related to generalized weakness secondary to anemia and uremia
Desired outcome: After treatment, patient rates perceived exertion at ≤3 on a 0-10 scale and exhibits improving endurance to activity, as evidenced by HR ≤20 bpm over resting HR, systolic BP ≤20 mm Hg over or under resting systolic pressure, and RR ≤20 breaths/min with normal depth and pattern (eupnea).

N O T E :   Anemia is better tolerated in uremic than in nonuremic patients.

1. Anemia usually is proportional to the degree of azotemia. Hct can be as low as ≤20% but usually stabilizes at about 20%-25% without treatment. Typically these patients are not transfused unless the Hct drops <20% or the anemia is poorly tolerated. Monitor patient during activity, and ask him or her to rate perceived exertion (for details, see **Risk for activity intolerance,** p. 413, in Appendix One, "Caring for Patients on Prolonged Bed Rest"). Consult physician if increased weakness, fatigue, dyspnea, chest pain, or further decreases in Hct occur. In addition:
   - Provide and encourage optimal nutrition.
   - Administer epoetin alfa (Epogen) if prescribed. Monitor BP and alert physician to elevations, because hypertension can be a complication of erythropoietin therapy.
   - Administer anabolic steroids (e.g., nandrolone) if prescribed. Prepare women patients for side effects, including increasing facial hair, deepening voice, and menstrual irregularities.
   - Coordinate laboratory studies to minimize blood drawing.
   - Observe for and report evidence of occult blood and blood loss.
   - Report symptomatic anemia: weakness, SOB, chest pain.
   - Do not administer ferrous sulfate at the same time as antacids. The two medications should be given at least 1 h apart to maximize absorption of the ferrous sulfate.
   - Administer parenteral iron if prescribed. Anaphylaxis is a possible complication.
2. Help patient to identify activities that increase fatigue and to adjust those activities accordingly.
3. Assist patient with ADLs while encouraging maximum independence to patient's tolerance.
4. Establish with patient realistic, progressive exercises and activity goals designed to increase endurance. Ensure that they are within patient's prescribed limitations. Examples are found in **Risk for activity intolerance,** p. 413, and **Risk for disuse syndrome,** p. 416, in Appendix One, "Caring for Patients on Prolonged Bed Rest."

Impaired skin integrity related to pruritus and dry skin secondary to uremia and edema

Desired outcome: Patient's skin remains intact and free of erythema and abrasions.

1. Pruritus is common in uremic patients, causing frequent and intense scratching. Pruritus often eases with a reduction in BUN and improved phosphorus control. Encourage use of phosphate binders and reduction of dietary phosphorus if elevated phosphorus level is a problem. Foods high in phosphorus include meats (especially organ meats—brain, kidney, liver), fish, poultry, milk and milk products (e.g., cheese, ice cream, cottage cheese), whole grains (e.g., oatmeal, bran, barley), seeds (e.g., pumpkin, sesame, sunflower), nuts (e.g., Brazil nuts, peanuts), eggs and egg products (e.g., eggnog, soufflés), and dried peas and beans. Give phosphate binders with meals for maximum effects. If necessary, administer antihistamines as prescribed. Keep patient's fingernails short.
2. Because uremia retards wound healing, instruct patient to monitor scratches for evidence of infection and seek early medical attention should signs and symptoms of infection appear.
3. Uremic skin often is dry and scaly because of reduced oil gland activity. Encourage use of skin emollients. Patient should avoid hard soaps and excessive bathing. Advise patient to bathe every other day and to use bath oils as needed if dry skin is a problem.
4. Clotting abnormalities and capillary fragility place the uremic patient at increased risk for bruising. Advise patient and significant others that this can occur.
5. Provide scheduled skin care and position changes for individuals with edema.

Knowledge deficit: Need for frequent BP checks and adherence to antihypertensive therapy and potential for change in insulin requirements for individuals who are diabetic

Desired outcomes: Within the 24 h before hospital discharge, patient verbalizes knowledge about the importance of frequent BP checks and adherence to antihypertensive therapy. Patient with diabetes mellitus (DM) verbalizes knowledge about potential for change in insulin requirements.

N O T E :   Patients with chronic renal failure (CRF) may develop hypertension because of fluid overload, excess renin secretion, or arteriosclerotic disease.

---

1. Teach patient about the importance of getting BP checked at frequent intervals and of adhering to prescribed antihypertensive therapy. Control of hypertension may slow progression of chronic renal insufficiency.
2. Teach patients with DM that insulin requirements often decrease as renal function decreases. Instruct these patients to be alert for indicators of hypoglycemia, including confusion, blurred vision, diaphoresis, and tachycardia.

Altered protection related to neurosensory, musculoskeletal, and cardiac changes secondary to electrolyte and acid-base imbalances

Desired outcomes: After treatment, patient verbalizes orientation to time, place, and person and remains free of injury caused by neurosensory, musculoskeletal, and cardiac disturbances. Within the 24 h before hospital discharge, patient verbalizes the importance of avoiding foods and products high in potassium in particular and, if indicated, those high in sodium, phosphorus, and protein.

N O T E : Potassium is limited because of the kidneys' inability to excrete excessive K^+ (for a list of foods high in potassium, see Table 3-2, p. 72). Depending on existing renal function, sodium is limited to prevent thirst and fluid retention (for a list of foods high in sodium, see Table 1-4, p. 18). Dietary restriction of protein and phosphorus early in the course of the disease may slow the progression of chronic renal insufficiency (for foods high in phosphorus, see **Impaired skin integrity**, above). Protein intake often is limited to that of high biologic value. Carbohydrates are increased for patients on protein restriction to ensure adequate caloric intake and to prevent catabolism.

---

1. Hyperkalemia is a common complication of end-stage renal disease (ESRD). Avoid salt substitutes (potassium chloride [KCl]), "light" salt (which contains KCl), and medications containing potassium, such as potassium penicillin G. Teach patient and significant others to read the labels on all OTC drugs.
2. If patient requires multiple blood transfusions, observe for indicators of hyperkalemia because old banked blood may contain as much as 30 mEq/L of potassium. Use fresh-packed cells when possible.
3. Compliance with the prescribed dietary restrictions on potassium, sodium, protein, and phosphorus should ease symptoms and limit complications. To promote dietary compliance, encourage use of spices such as garlic, onions, and oregano to enhance the flavor of foods the patient is allowed. Provide fact sheets listing foods to be restricted or limited. Inform patient that diet and fluid restrictions may be altered as renal function decreases. Provide sample menus, and have patient demonstrate understanding by planning 3-day menus that incorporate dietary restrictions.
4. For other interventions, see this nursing diagnosis in "Acute Renal Failure," p. 74.

See "Acute Renal Failure" for **Fluid volume excess** (oliguric phase), p. 73, **Altered nutrition,** p. 73, **Risk for infection,** p. 75, and **Constipation,** p. 76. See psychosocial nursing diagnoses and interventions in Appendix One, "Caring for Patients with Cancer and Other Life-Disrupting Illnesses," p. 450.

PATIENT-FAMILY TEACHING
AND DISCHARGE PLANNING

Give patient and significant others verbal and written information about the following:
1. Medications, including drug name, purpose, dosage, schedule, precautions, drug/drug and food/drug interactions, and potential side effects.
2. Diet, including fact sheet listing foods to be restricted or limited. Inform patient that diet and fluid restrictions may be altered as renal function decreases. Provide sample menus and have the patient

demonstrate understanding by planning 3-day menus that incorporate dietary restrictions.

3. Care and observation of dialysis access if patient has one.

4. Signs and symptoms that require medical attention: irregular pulse, fever, unusual SOB or edema, sudden change in urine output, and unusual muscle weakness.

5. Need for continued medical follow-up; confirm date and time of patient's next appointment with physician.

6. Importance of preventing infections and of seeking treatment promptly should one develop. Teach patient the indicators of frequently encountered infections, including upper respiratory infection (URI), urinary tract infection (UTI), impetigo, and otitis media. For details, see **Risk for infection,** p. 86, under "Care of the Renal Transplant Recipient"; also see Table 2-5, p. 39.

IN ADDITION

7. For patients with or approaching ESRD, provide information about the various treatment options and support groups. The local chapter of the National Kidney Foundation can be helpful in identifying support groups and organizations in the area. Patient and significant others should meet with the renal dietitian and social worker before discharge.

8. Coordinate discharge planning and teaching with the dialysis unit or facility. If possible, have patient visit dialysis unit before discharge.

9. For an individual with ESRD, the importance of coordinating all medical care through the nephrologist and of alerting all medical and dental personnel to ESRD status, owing to increased risk of infection and need to adjust medication dosages. In addition, dentists may want to premedicate ESRD patients with antibiotics before dental work and avoid scheduling dental work on the day of dialysis, owing to heparinization used in dialytic therapy.

Care of the Patient Undergoing Peritoneal Dialysis

Peritoneal dialysis uses the peritoneum as the dialysis membrane. Dialysate is instilled into the peritoneal cavity *via* a special catheter, and movement of solutes and fluid occurs between the patient's capillary blood and the dialysate. At set intervals the peritoneal cavity is drained and new dialysate is instilled.

COMPONENTS OF PERITONEAL DIALYSIS

Catheter: Silastic tube that is either implanted as a surgical procedure for chronic patients or inserted at the bedside for acute dialysis.

Dialysate: Sterile electrolyte solution similiar in composition to normal plasma. The electrolyte composition of the dialysate can be adjusted according to individual need. The most commonly adjusted electrolyte is K^+. Glucose is added to the dialysate in varying concentrations to remove excess body fluid *via* osmosis. **Note:** Some glucose crosses the peritoneal membrane and enters the patient's blood. Patients with diabetes mellitus may require additional insulin. Observe for and report indicators of hyperglycemia (e.g., complaints of thirst or changes in sensorium).

NURSING DIAGNOSES AND INTERVENTIONS

Risk for infection related to invasive procedure (direct access of catheter to peritoneum)

Desired outcomes: Patient is free of infection, as evidenced by normothermia and absence of abdominal pain, cloudy outflow, nausea, and malaise, as well as erythema, drainage, and tenderness at the exit site. Before hospital discharge, patient verbalizes signs and symptoms of infection and demonstrates sterile technique for bag, tubing, and dressing changes.

1. The most common complication of peritoneal dialysis is peritonitis. Monitor for and report indications of peritonitis, including fever, abdominal pain, cloudy outflow, nausea, and malaise.

C A U T I O N : To minimize the risk of peritonitis, it is essential that sterile technique be used when connecting and disconnecting the catheter from the dialysis system.

2. The dialysate must remain sterile, because it is instilled directly into the body. Maintain sterile technique when adding medications to the dialysate.
3. Follow agency policy for dressing the catheter exit site.
4. Observe for and report redness, drainage, or tenderness at exit site. Culture any exudate, and report the results to the physician.
5. Consult physician if dialysate leaks around the catheter exit site. This can indicate an obstruction or the need for another purse-string suture around the catheter site. Continued leakage at the site can lead to peritonitis.
6. Instruct the patient in the preceding interventions and observations if peritoneal dialysis will be performed after discharge.

Risk for fluid volume deficit related to hypertonicity of the dialysate; *or*

Fluid volume excess related to inadequate exchange

Desired outcomes: Postdialysis, patient is normovolemic, as evidenced by balanced I&O, stable weight, good skin turgor, CVP 5-12 cm H_2O, RR 12-20 breaths/min with normal depth and pattern (eupnea), and BP and HR within patient's normal range. Dialysate outflow equals or exceeds inflow.

1. Fluid retention can occur because of catheter complications that prevent adequate outflow or because of a severely scarred peritoneum that prevents adequate exchange. Observe for and report indicators of fluid overload, such as hypertension, tachycardia, distended neck veins, or increased CVP. Also be alert for incomplete dialysate returns. Accurate measurement and recording of outflow are critical.
2. Outflow problems can occur because of the following:
   - *Full colon:* Use stool softeners, high-fiber diet, or enemas if necessary.

- *Catheter occlusion by fibrin* (usually occurs soon after insertion): Obtain prescription to irrigate with heparinized saline.
- *Catheter obstruction by omentum:* Turn patient from side to side, elevate HOB, or apply firm pressure to the abdomen. **Note:** Consult physician about unresolved outflow problems.

3. Monitor I&O and weight daily. A steady weight gain indicates fluid retention.
4. Respiratory distress can occur because of compression of the diaphragm by the dialysate. If this occurs, elevate HOB, drain dialysate, and consult physician.
5. Bloody outflow may appear with initial exchanges. Report gross bloody outflow.
6. Coordinate laboratory studies to limit blood drawing because patients with renal failure are anemic owing to altered RBC production and longevity.
7. Volume depletion can occur with excessive use of hypertonic dialysate. Observe for and report indicators of volume depletion, including poor skin turgor, hypotension, tachycardia, and decreased CVP.

Altered nutrition: Less than body requirements, related to protein loss in the dialysate

Desired outcomes: At least 24 h before hospital discharge, patient exhibits adequate nutrition, as evidenced by stable weight and serum albumin 3.5-5.5 g/dl. Patient's protein intake is 1.2-1.5 g/kg body weight/day.

1. Protein crosses the peritoneum, and a significant amount is lost in dialysate. Increased intake of protein is necessary to prevent excessive tissue catabolism. Protein loss increases with peritonitis. Ensure adequate dietary intake of protein: 1.2-1.5 g/kg body weight/day.
2. Peritoneal dialysis patients typically have fewer dietary restrictions than those on hemodialysis. Ensure that dietary evaluation and teaching are performed when patient changes from one type of dialysis to the other.
3. Provide a list of restricted and encouraged foods, with menus that illustrate their integration into the daily diet. Ensure patient's understanding by having him or her plan a 3-day menu that incorporates the appropriate foods and restrictions.

Altered protection related to neurosensory, musculoskeletal, or cardiac changes secondary to uremia and serum electrolyte imbalance

Desired outcome: Patient verbalizes orientation to time, place, and person and remains free of injury caused by neurosensory, musculoskeletal, or cardiac changes.

1. Instruct patient and staff to observe for and report indications of the following:
    - *Increased uremia:* Confusion, lethargy, and restlessness. Monitor BUN and serum creatinine values; increases can signal a need for increased dialysis. BUN should be <80-100 mg/dl. Serum creatinine values will vary, depending on individual's muscle mass.
    - *Hyperkalemia:* Muscle cramps, muscle weakness. Monitor serum potassium (K^+) values (normal range is 3.5-5 mEq/L).

■ *Hypokalemia* (secondary to dialysis): Abdominal pain, lethargy, and dysrhythmias. Monitor serum K^+ values (normal range is 3.5-5 mEq/L).

N O T E : Alert physician to the development of an irregular pulse because it could indicate dangerous hypokalemia. This is especially important for patients taking digitalis, because hypokalemia potentiates digitalis toxicity.

---

2. Promptly report abnormal laboratory values to physician. The dialysate or length of dialysis time may require adjustment to compensate for abnormal values.
3. For other interventions, see this nursing diagnosis, p. 74. As appropriate, also see nursing diagnoses and interventions in "Care of the Patient Undergoing Hemodialysis," below.

Care of the Patient Undergoing Hemodialysis

During hemodialysis, blood is removed *via* a special vascular access, heparinized, pumped through an artificial kidney (dialyzer), and returned to the patient's circulation. Either hemodialysis is a temporary, acute procedure performed as needed, or it is performed chronically 2-4 ×/wk, with each treatment lasting 2-5 h.

COMPONENTS OF HEMODIALYSIS

Artificial kidney (dialyzer): A unit composed of a blood compartment and a dialysate compartment, which are separated by a semipermeable membrane that allows the diffusion of solutes and the filtration of water. Protein and bacteria do not cross the artificial membrane.

Dialysate: An electrolyte solution similar in composition to normal plasma. Each component of the dialysate can be varied according to the patient's needs. The most commonly altered component is potassium. Glucose may be added to prevent sudden drops in serum osmolality and serum glucose during dialysis.

Vascular access: The route required to obtain a blood flow rate of 200-500 ml/min, the rate needed for effective dialysis.

NURSING DIAGNOSES AND INTERVENTIONS

Risk for fluid volume deficit related to excessive fluid removal or bleeding resulting from dialysis; *or*
Fluid volume excess related to compromised regulatory mechanism resulting in fluid retention secondary to renal failure
Desired outcomes: Postdialysis, patient is normovolemic, as evidenced by balanced I&O, stable weight, RR 12-20 breaths/min with normal depth and pattern (eupnea), CVP 5-12 cm H_2O, HR and BP within patient's normal range, and absence of abnormal breath sounds and abnormal bleeding. After instruction, patient knows signs and symptoms of fluid volume excess and deficit.
1. Monitor I&O and daily weight as indicators of fluid status. A steady weight gain indicates retained fluid. Patient's weight is an important

guideline for determining the quantity of fluid that needs to be removed during dialysis. Weigh patient at the same time each day, using the same scale and having patient wear the same amount of clothing (or with same items on bed if using a bed scale).

2. Instruct patient and staff to observe for and report indications of fluid volume excess: edema, hypertension, crackles, tachycardia, distended neck veins, SOB, and increased CVP.

3. After dialysis, observe for and report indicators of fluid volume deficit, including hypotension, decreased CVP, and tachycardia. Describe the signs and symptoms to the patient and explain the importance of reporting them promptly should they occur. Be aware that because of autonomic neuropathy, a patient with uremia may not develop a compensatory tachycardia when hypovolemic. **Note:** Antihypertensive medications usually are held before and during dialysis to help prevent hypotension during dialysis. Clarify medication prescriptions with physician.

4. Monitor for postdialysis bleeding (gums, needle sites, incisions), which can occur because of use of heparin during dialysis. Alert patient to potential for bleeding from these areas.

5. To prevent hematoma formation, do not give IM injection for at least 1 h after dialysis.

6. GI bleeding is common in patients with renal failure, especially after heparinization. Test all stools for blood and report significant finding.

Risk for fluid volume deficit related to bleeding/hemorrhage that can occur with vascular access puncture or disconnection

Altered peripheral tissue perfusion (or risk for same) related to interrupted blood flow that can occur with clotting in the vascular access; *and*

Risk for infection related to invasive procedure (creation of the vascular access for hemodialysis)

Desired outcomes: Patient's vascular access remains intact and connected, and patient is normovolemic (see description in preceding nursing diagnosis). Patient has adequate tissue perfusion, as evidenced by normal skin temperature and color and brisk capillary refill (<2 sec) distal to the vascular access. Patient's access is patent, as evidenced by bright red blood within shunt tubing or by thrill with palpation and bruit with auscultation of fistula or graft. Patient is free of infection, as evidenced by normothermia and absence of erythema, local warmth, exudate, swelling, and tenderness at exit site.

1. After surgical creation of the vascular access, assess for patency, auscultate for bruit, and palpate for thrill. Report severe or unrelieved pain, and observe for and report numbness, tingling, and swelling of the extremity distal to the access, any of which can signal impaired tissue perfusion. Expect postoperative swelling along fistula, and elevate extremity accordingly.

2. Consult physician if extremity distal to vascular access becomes cool, has decreased capillary refill, or is discolored, because these problems can occur with vascular insufficiency.

3. Follow the three principles of nursing care common to all types of vascular access: prevent bleeding, prevent clotting, and prevent infection. Explain monitoring and care procedures to patient. Remember that the vascular access is the patient's lifeline; monitor it closely and handle it with care. Vascular accesses include the following:

- **Subclavian or femoral lines:** External, temporary catheters inserted into a large vein.
  - *Prevent bleeding:* Anchor catheter securely because it might not be sutured in. Tape all connections. Keep clamps at bedside in case line becomes disconnected. If line is removed or accidentally pulled out, apply firm pressure to site for at least 10 min.

C A U T I O N :   An air embolus can occur if a subclavian line accidentally becomes disconnected. If this occurs, immediately clamp the line. Turn the patient onto a left side-lying position to help prevent air from blocking the pulmonary artery, and lower HOB into Trendelenburg's position to increase intrathoracic pressure. This will reduce the flow of inspiratory air into the vein. Administer 100% oxygen by mask, and obtain VS. Notify physician *stat!*

- *Prevent clotting:* Keep line patent by priming with heparin or by constant infusion with a heparinized solution. Follow protocol, or obtain specific prescription from physician. Attach a label to all lines that are primed with heparin to alert other personnel.
  - *Prevent infection:* Perform aseptic dressing changes according to agency protocol. Observe for and report indications of infection, including erythema, local warmth, exudate, swelling, and tenderness at exit site. Report and culture any drainage.
- **Fistula or graft:** Internal, permanent connection between an artery and a vein, or the insertion of an internal graft that is joined to an artery and vein. Grafts can be straight or U-shaped. They are located in the arm or thigh.
  - *Prevent bleeding:* Inspect needle puncture sites for postdialysis bleeding. If bleeding occurs, apply just enough pressure over site to stop it. Release pressure and check for bleeding q5-10min.
  - *Prevent clotting:* Do not take BP, start IV, or draw blood in arm with graft or fistula. Have patient avoid tight clothing, jewelry, name bands, or restraint on affected extremity. Palpate for thrill and auscultate for bruit at least every shift and after hypotensive episodes. Consult physician *stat* if bruit or thrill is absent.
  - *Prevent infection:* Observe for and report indications of infection: erythema, local warmth, swelling, exudate, unusual tenderness at fistula site. Culture and report any drainage.

SECTION THREE: CARE OF THE RENAL TRANSPLANT RECIPIENT

NURSING DIAGNOSES AND INTERVENTIONS

Risk for infection related to invasive procedures, exposure to infected individuals, and immunosuppression

Desired outcomes: Patient is free of infection, as evidenced by normothermia, HR ≤100 bpm (or within patient's normal range), and absence of erythema or purulent drainage at wounds or catheter exit sites. Patient verbalizes indicators of infection and the importance of reporting them promptly to physician or staff.

1. Observe for indicators of infection, such as fever and unexplained tachycardia. Instruct patient to be alert for signs and symptoms of commonly encountered infections, and stress the importance of reporting them promptly. These include UTI—cloudy and malodorous urine; urinary burning, frequency, and urgency; URI—malodorous, purulent, colored, and copious secretions; productive cough; otitis media—malaise, earache; impetigo—inflamed or draining areas on the skin.
2. Teach patient to avoid exposure to individuals known to have infections.
3. Use aseptic technique with all invasive procedures and dressing changes.

Knowledge deficit: Signs and symptoms of rejection, side effects of immunosuppressive agents, transplantation complications, and importance of protecting existing hemodialysis vascular access

Desired outcome: Within the 24 h before hospital discharge, patient verbalizes knowledge of signs and symptoms of rejection, side effects of immunosuppressive therapy, complications of transplantation, and the importance of protecting the hemodialysis vascular access.

1. Explain the importance of renal function monitoring: I&O, daily weight, and BUN and serum creatinine values. As renal function decreases, BUN and creatinine values will increase.
2. Alert patient to the following signs and symptoms of rejection: oliguria, tenderness over the kidney (located in the iliac fossa), sudden weight gain, fever, malaise, hypertension, and increased BUN (>20 mg/dl) and serum creatinine (>1.5 mg/dl). Provide patient with a notebook in which to record daily VS and weight measurements. Remind patient to bring the notebook to all outpatient visits and to report abnormal values promptly should they occur.
3. Explain that significant decreases in WBC and platelet counts can be a side effect of immunosuppressive agents, and therefore serial monitoring is essential.
4. Explain that GI bleeding is a potential side effect of immunosuppressive agents. Alert patient to the signs and symptoms of GI bleeding (e.g., tarry stools, "coffee-ground" emesis, increasing fatigue and weakness) and to the importance of reporting them promptly should they occur.

5. In a patient who has undergone renal transplantation, hypertension may develop for a variety of reasons, including cyclosporine or steroid use, rejection, or renal artery stenosis. Teach patient and/or significant others how to measure BP, and provide guidelines for values that require notification of physician or staff member.
6. If patient has a patent fistula or graft (hemodialysis vascular access), explain that it must be handled with care, because the patient will need it if a return to dialysis is indicated. Explain that taking BP, drawing blood, and starting IVs are contraindicated in the fistula arm, and patient should warn others about these contraindications.
7. Stress the need for continued medical evaluation of the transplant.

SECTION FOUR: URINARY TRACT DISORDERS

Ureteral Calculi

NURSING DIAGNOSES AND INTERVENTIONS

Pain related to presence of calculus or surgical procedure to remove it
Desired outcomes: Within 1 h of intervention, patient's subjective perception of pain decreases, as documented by a pain scale. Objective indicators, such as grimacing, are absent or diminished.
1. Assess and document quality, location, intensity, and duration of pain. Devise a pain scale with patient that ranges from 0 (no pain) to 10 (worst pain). Notify physician of sudden and/or severe pain.
2. Notify physician of a sudden cessation of pain, which can signal passage of the stone. (Strain all urine for solid matter, and send it to the laboratory for analysis.)
3. Medicate patient with prescribed analgesics, narcotics, and antispasmodics; evaluate and document response based on the pain scale.
4. Provide warm blankets, heating pad to affected area, or warm baths to increase regional circulation and relax tense muscles.
5. Provide back rubs. These are especially helpful for postoperative patients who were in the lithotomy position during surgery.

Altered urinary elimination (dysuria, urgency, or frequency) related to obstruction caused by ureteral calculus
Desired outcomes: Within 2 days, patient reports return of normal voiding pattern. Patient demonstrates ability to record I&O and strain urine for stones.
1. Determine and document patient's normal voiding pattern.
2. Monitor quality and color of urine. Optimally it is straw colored and clear and has a characteristic urine odor. Dark urine often indicates dehydration, and blood-tinged urine can result from the rupture of ureteral capillaries as the calculus passes through the ureter.

3. In patients for whom fluids are not restricted, encourage a fluid intake of at least 2 L/day to help flush calculus through the ureter into the bladder and out through the system.
4. Record accurate I&O; teach patient how to record I&O.
5. Strain urine for evidence of solid matter; teach patient the procedure.
6. Send any solid matter to the laboratory for analysis.

Altered urinary elimination related to obstruction or positional problems of the ureteral catheter

Desired outcome: After intervention, patient has output from the ureteral catheter and is free of spasms or flank pain, which could signal obstruction or dislodgment.

1. Occasionally patients return from surgery with a ureteral catheter. If patient has more than one catheter, label one *right* and the other *left;* keep all drainage records separate.
2. Monitor output from ureteral catheter. Amount will vary with each patient and depend on catheter dimension. If drainage is scanty or absent, milk catheter and tubing gently to try to dislodge obstruction. If this fails, consult physician.

C A U T I O N :   Never irrigate the catheter without specific instructions from the physician to do so. If irrigation is prescribed, use gentle pressure and aseptic technique. Always aspirate with a sterile syringe before instillation to prevent ureteral damage from overdistention. Use another sterile syringe to inject amounts no greater than 3 ml per instillation.

---

3. Typically patient requires bed rest if ureteral catheter is indwelling. Explain to patient that semi-Fowler's and side-lying positions are acceptable. Fowler's position should be avoided because sutures are seldom used and gravity can cause the catheter to move into the bladder.
4. Ureteral catheters often are attached to the urethral catheter after placement in the ureters. Carefully monitor the urethral catheter for movement and ensure that it is securely attached to the patient. **Note:** After ureteral catheters have been removed (usually simultaneously with the urethral catheter), monitor for indicators of ureteral obstruction, including flank pain, nausea, and vomiting.

Risk for impaired skin integrity related to wound drainage

Desired outcome: Skin surrounding wound site remains intact.

1. Monitor incisional dressings frequently during the first 24 h and change or reinforce as needed. Excoriation can result from prolonged contact of urine with skin.
2. Note and document odor, consistency, and color of drainage. Immediately after surgery, drainage may be red.
3. To facilitate frequent dressing changes, use Montgomery straps rather than tape to secure dressing.
4. If drainage is copious after drain removal, apply wound drainage or ostomy pouch with a skin barrier over incision. Use a pouch with an antireflux valve to prevent contamination from reflux.

Health-seeking behaviors: Dietary regimen and its relationship to stone formation

Desired outcome: Within the 24 h before hospital discharge, patient verbalizes knowledge about foods and liquids to limit to prevent stone formation and demonstrates this knowledge by planning a 3-day menu that excludes or limits these foods.

1. Assess patient's knowledge about diet and its relationship to stone formation.
2. Advise patient to maintain a urine output of >2 L/day. Increasing urine output reduces saturation of stone-forming solutes.
3. Teach patient to maintain adequate hydration of 2-3 L/day. Good hydration after meals and exercise is important, because solute load is highest at these times. **Caution:** Persons with cardiac or renal disease require special fluid intake instructions from their physician.
4. Teach patient the technique for measuring urine specific gravity *via* a hydrometer. Explain that to minimize stone formation, specific gravity should remain <1.010.
5. As appropriate, provide the following information:
   - *For uric acid stones:* Limit intake of foods high in purines, such as lean meat, legumes, and whole grains. Limit protein intake to 90 g/day.
   - *For calcium stones:* Limit intake of foods high in calcium, such as milk, cheese, green leafy vegetables, and yogurt. Limit sodium intake (see Table 1-4 for a list of foods high in sodium). Explain to patient that a low-sodium diet helps reduce intestinal absorption of calcium. Limit intake of refined carbohydrates and animal proteins, which cause hypercalciuria. Encourage patient to eat foods high in natural fiber (e.g., bran, prunes, apples). Foods high in natural fiber provide phytic acid, which binds dietary calcium. Explain that sodium cellulose phosphate, 5 g tid, may be given to bind with intestinal calcium and increase excretion of calcium.
   - *For oxalate stones:* Limit intake of foods high in oxalate, such as chocolate, caffeine-containing drinks (including instant and decaffeinated coffees), beets, spinach, and peanuts. Large doses of pyridoxine may help with certain types of oxalate stones, and cholestyramine, 4 g qid, may be prescribed to bind with oxalate enterally. Explain that vitamin C supplements should be avoided because as much as half is converted to oxalic acid.

Also see nursing diagnoses and interventions in Appendix One, "Caring for Preoperative and Postoperative Patients," p. 395.

PATIENT-FAMILY TEACHING AND DISCHARGE PLANNING

Give patient and significant others verbal and written information about the following:

1. Medications, including drug name, purpose, dosage, schedule, precautions, drug/drug and food/drug interactions, and potential side effects.
2. Indicators of UTI or recurrent calculi, which require medical attention: chills, fever, hematuria, flank pain, cloudy and foul-smelling urine, frequency, and urgency.
3. Care of incision, including cleansing and dressing. Teach patient

signs and symptoms of local infection: redness, swelling, local warmth, tenderness, purulent drainage.
4. Care of drains or catheters if patient is discharged with them.
5. Importance of daily fluid intake of at least 3 L/day in nonrestricted patients.
6. Dietary changes as specified by physician.
7. Activity restrictions as directed for patient who has had surgery: avoid lifting heavy objects (>10 lb) for the first 6 wk, be alert for fatigue, get maximum rest, increase activities gradually to tolerance.
8. Use of nitrazine paper to assess pH of urine. Desired pH will be determined by type of stone formation to which patient is prone. Instructions for use are on nitrazine container.
9. Importance of walking or other exercise to reduce risk of stone formation.

Urinary Tract Obstruction

NURSING DIAGNOSES AND INTERVENTIONS

Risk for fluid volume deficit related to postobstructive diuresis
Desired outcomes: Patient is normovolemic, as evidenced by HR ≤100 bpm (or within patient's normal range), BP ≥90/60 mm Hg (or within patient's normal range), RR ≤20 breaths/min, and orientation to time, place, and person (within patient's normal range). Within 2 days after bladder decompression, output approximates input, patient's urinary output is normal for patient (or ≥30-60 ml/h), and weight becomes stable.
1. Using sterile technique, insert urinary catheter to drain patient's bladder. Monitor patient carefully during catheterization; clamp catheter if patient complains of abdominal pain or has a symptomatic drop in systolic BP of ≥20 mm Hg. Current research suggests that rapid bladder decompression of >750-1,000 ml does not result in shock syndrome, as previously believed.
2. Monitor I&O hourly for 4 h and then q2h for 4 h after bladder decompression. Consult physician if output exceeds 200 ml/h or 2 L over an 8-h period; this can signal postobstructive diuresis, which can lead to major electrolyte imbalance. If this occurs, anticipate initiation of IV infusion.
3. Monitor VS for signs of shock: decreasing BP, changes in LOC or mentation, tachycardia, tachypnea, thready pulse.
4. Anticipate need for urine specimens for analysis of electrolytes and osmolality and blood specimens for analysis of electrolytes.
5. Observe for and report indicators of the following:
   ▪ *Hypokalemia:* Abdominal cramps, lethargy, dysrhythmias.
   ▪ *Hyperkalemia:* Diarrhea, colic, irritability, nausea, muscle cramps, weakness, irregular apical or radial pulses.
   ▪ *Hypocalcemia:* Muscle weakness and cramps, complaints of tingling in fingers, positive Trousseau's and Chvostek's signs.
   ▪ *Hyperphosphatemia:* Excessive itching.
6. Monitor mentation, noting signs of disorientation, which can occur with electrolyte disturbance.

7. Weigh patient daily using the same scale and at the same time of day (e.g., before breakfast). Weight fluctuations of 0.9-1.8 kg (2-4 lb) per day are normal in a patient undergoing diuresis.

Pain related to bladder spasms

Desired outcomes: Within 1 h of intervention, patient's subjective perception of discomfort decreases, as documented by a pain scale. Objective indicators, such as grimacing, are absent or diminished.

1. Assess for and document complaints of pain in suprapubic or urethral area. Devise a pain scale with patient, rating pain from 0 (no pain) to 10 (worst pain). Reassure patient that spasms are normal with obstruction.
2. Medicate with antispasmodics or analgesics as prescribed. Document pain relief obtained, using pain scale.
3. Teach patient the procedure for slow diaphragmatic breathing.
4. If patient is losing urine around catheter and has a distended bladder (with or without bladder spasms), check catheter and drainage tubing for evidence of obstruction. Inspect for kinks and obstructions in drainage tubing, compress and roll catheter gently between fingers to assess for gritty matter within catheter, milk drainage tubing to release obstructions, or instruct patient to turn from side to side. Obtain prescription for catheter irrigation if these measures fail to relieve obstruction.
5. In nonrestricted patients, encourage intake of fluids of at least 2-3 L/day to help reduce frequency of spasms.
6. Instruct patient in the use of nonpharmacologic methods of pain relief, such as guided imagery, relaxation techniques, and distraction. See relaxation technique described under "Coronary Artery Disease," **Health-seeking behaviors,** p. 27.

See "Hydronephrosis" for **Risk for injury** related to insertion/presence of nephrostomy tube, p. 69.

See "Ureteral Calculi" for **Risk for impaired skin integrity** related to wound drainage, p. 88.

See nursing diagnoses and interventions in Appendix One, "Caring for Preoperative and Postoperative Patients," p. 395.

PATIENT-FAMILY TEACHING
AND DISCHARGE PLANNING

Give patient and significant others verbal and written information about the following:

1. Medications, including drug name, purpose, dosage, schedule, precautions, drug/drug and food/drug interactions, and potential side effects.
2. Indicators that signal recurrent obstruction and require prompt medical attention: pain, fever, decreased urinary output.
3. Necessity of limiting activities during postoperative period.
4. Care of drains or catheters if patient is discharged with them; care of surgical incision if present.
5. Indicators of (1) *wound infection:* persistent redness, local warmth

and tenderness, drainage, swelling; and (2) *UTI:* dysuria, flank or suprapubic pain, cloudy or foul-smelling urine, chills, fever.

Cancer of the Bladder

NURSING DIAGNOSES AND INTERVENTIONS

Risk for fluid volume deficit related to postsurgical hemorrhage after transurethral resection of bladder and tumor (TURBT) or segmental resection; *or*

Fluid volume excess (or risk for same) related to excessive fluid intake secondary to irrigation

Desired outcome: Patient is normovolemic, as evidenced by BP ≥90/60 mm Hg (or within patient's normal range), HR ≤100 bpm (or within patient's normal range), and orientation to time, place, and person (within patient's normal range).

1. Monitor and record VS and I&O; record color and consistency of catheter drainage at least q8h. Drainage may be dark red after surgery, but it should lighten to pink or blood tinged within 24 h. **Note:** Patients who have undergone TURBT may have clots passing through the drainage tubing. Continuous bladder irrigation (CBI) often is used to flush bloody drainage from the bladder to prevent clot formation, which can occlude the urethral catheter. For more information about patient care after a transurethral resection, see "Benign Prostatic Hypertrophy," p. 358.

2. Be alert for hypotension and rapid HR, and watch for bright red, thick drainage or drainage that does not lighten after irrigation, any of which can signal arterial bleeding within the operative area and require immediate surgical intervention.

3. Monitor TURBT patient's postoperative mental status, being alert for changes in mentation, such as confusion, which can denote a change in electrolyte balance and require medical intervention. Water intoxication and hyponatremia (as evidenced by headache, lassitude, apathy, confusion, weakness, hypertension, muscle spasms, convulsions, and coma) can occur because of the high volumes of irrigation fluid used with a transurethral resection.

Risk for infection related to invasive procedure (presence of suprapubic catheter), increased environmental exposure (opening of a closed drainage system), or use of intravesical chemotherapy

Desired outcome: Patient is free of infection, as evidenced by WBC ≤11,000/µl, normothermia, and orientation to time, place, and person (within patient's normal range).

1. Using aseptic technique, cleanse area surrounding suprapubic catheter with an antimicrobial solution, such as povidone-iodine. Apply one or more sterile 4×4 gauze pads over catheter exit site and tape securely. Change dressing as soon as it becomes wet, and use a pectin wafer skin barrier to protect insertion site if indicated. **Note:** If a trocar system is used, clean around plastic cover and keep area dry. Tape plastic edges securely to skin to prevent accidental removal.

2. Wash hands *before* and *after* manipulating catheter, and use aseptic

technique when opening closed drainage system, changing dressings, and irrigating catheter.

3. Irrigate catheter *only* if an obstruction is present and by physician's prescription.
4. Protect catheter by keeping it securely taped to patient's lateral abdomen.
5. If catheter is accidentally pulled out of insertion site, immediately cover site with a sterile 4×4 gauze pad and consult physician.
6. To keep urine dilute to help prevent UTI, encourage a fluid intake of at least 2-3 L/day in nonrestricted patients.
7. Keep drainage collection container below level of patient's bladder to prevent infection from reflux of urine.

Altered urinary elimination related to obstruction of suprapubic catheter or anuria/dysuria secondary to removal of catheter
Desired outcome: By postoperative day 3, patient's urinary output is appropriate for amount of intake.

1. Keep drainage records from suprapubic catheter separate from those of other catheters and drains.
2. Prevent external obstruction of catheter, assessing frequently for patency. Irrigate *only* if internally obstructed and with physician's order.
3. Before removal of suprapubic catheter, physician may request a 3- to 4-h clamping routine to assess patient's ability to void normally. After patient has voided, unclamp catheter and measure residual urine that flows into drainage collection container. Once residual urine is <100 ml after each of two successive voidings, consult physician. Usually the catheter can be removed at that time.
4. After removal of catheter, evaluate patient's ability to void by recording time and amount during the first 24 h. Patients with segmental resections will void frequently and in small amounts at first because the bladder capacity is approximately 60 ml. Explain to patient that the bladder will expand to 200-400 ml within a few months.
5. If patient cannot void 8-12 h after catheter removal and experiences abdominal pain or has a distended bladder, consult physician for intervention.
6. If patient experiences burning with urination, encourage an increased intake of fluids and apply heat over the bladder area, using a warm blanket, heating pad, or sitz bath, any of which will increase circulation to the area and relax the muscles.
7. Obtain specimen for urine culture as prescribed if patient complains of burning, urgency, or frequency. The culture will differentiate between sterile pyuria and bacterial cystitis.

See "Urinary Tract Obstruction" for **Pain** related to bladder spasms, p. 91.

See Appendix One, "Caring for Preoperative and Postoperative Patients," p. 395, and "Caring for Patients with Cancer and Other Life-Disrupting Illnesses," p. 423, particularly **Altered urinary elimination** related to hemorrhagic cystitis secondary to cyclophosphamide treatment; oliguria or renal toxicity secondary to cisplatinum or high-dose methotrexate administration; or dysuria secondary to cystitis, p. 449).

Renal-Urinary

PATIENT-FAMILY TEACHING AND DISCHARGE PLANNING

Give patient and significant others verbal and written information about the following:
1. Medications, including drug name, purpose, dosage, schedule, precautions, drug/drug and food/drug interactions, and potential side effects.
2. Indicators of complications from photodynamic therapy, such as redness or swelling over areas exposed to sun, the importance of reporting them to health care provider, and the necessity of avoiding sun exposure for 4-6 wk after the last treatment.
3. Expectations of severe urinary frequency and urgency, blood-tinged urine, and dysuria during the first week after cauterization.

SECTION FIVE: URINARY DISORDERS SECONDARY TO OTHER DISEASE PROCESSES

Urinary Incontinence

NURSING DIAGNOSES AND INTERVENTIONS

N O T E :   Patients with urinary incontinence may have overlapping conditions. For example, they may have functional incontinence, which is aggravated by UTI superimposed on urge incontinence.

Stress incontinence related to degenerative changes or weakness in pelvic muscles and structural supports secondary to menopause, childbirth, obesity, or surgical procedure interfering with normal vesicourethral structure

Desired outcome: After implementation of bladder training program, patient becomes continent.

BLADDER TRAINING PROGRAM
1. Assess and document patient's voiding pattern: time, amount voided, amount of fluid intake, timing of fluid intake followed by voiding, and related information, such as the degree of wetness experienced (e.g., number of incontinence pads used in a day, degree of underwear dampness) and the exertion factor causing the wetness (e.g., laughing, sneezing, bending, lifting). Teach patient to keep a voiding diary that incorporates this information.
2. Determine the amount of time between voidings to estimate how long patient can hold urine. Establish a voiding schedule that does not exceed this interval.

3. Assist patient with scheduling times for emptying the bladder, such as (initially) q1-2h when awake and q4h at night. If successful, attempt to lengthen intervals between voiding. Provide patient and significant others with a written copy of the schedule. **Note:** Patients need to empty their bladders at least q4h during the day to reduce the risk of UTI caused by urinary stasis.

4. Estimate and document urinary output when patient is incontinent in clothes or bed linens. For example, a wet spot approximately 2 in in diameter is equal to approximately 5 ml of urine.

5. Teach patient techniques that strengthen sphincter and structural supports of the bladder, such as Kegel exercises (see **Knowledge deficit,** p. 97).

6. In nonrestricted patients, encourage a fluid intake of at least 2-3 L/day. Be aware that patients with urinary incontinence often reduce their fluid intake to avoid incontinence, at the risk of dehydration and UTI.

7. Teach patient about dietary irritants (e.g., caffeine, alcoholic beverages) that may increase stress incontinence.

Urge incontinence related to bladder irritation or reduced bladder capacity secondary to radiation treatment for bladder cancer, UTI, increased urine concentration, use of caffeine or alcohol, or enlarged prostate

Desired outcome: After implementation of toileting program, patient becomes continent.

1. Assess and document patient's usual pattern of voiding, including frequency and timing of incontinent episodes.

2. Adhere to toileting program (see interventions with **Stress incontinence,** above).

3. Teach nonrestricted patient to increase fluid intake to ≥3 L/day but to avoid caffeinated drinks or alcohol, which are natural diuretics and bladder irritants.

4. Explain the types of fluids patient should drink that are not irritating to the bladder (e.g., water, fruit juices, herbal drinks, and decaffeinated sodas, teas, and coffees).

5. Encourage patient to consume cranberry juice, prunes, and plums, which leave an acid ash in the urine, to minimize the occurrence of UTI.

6. Teach patient to keep a voiding record for at-home use, documenting accurate information about frequency and timing of incontinent episodes.

7. Encourage patient to reduce fluid intake a few hours before bedtime and to void before sleep.

8. Keep a urinal or bedpan at bedside and instruct patient in its use.

9. Teach patient deep, slow breathing technique, which can be used when urge to void occurs prematurely.

10. If patient is ambulatory but has a cognitive impairment, label bathroom door with signs that denote *toilet* to patient (e.g., picture of a commode). Adhere closely to toileting program, reminding patient to void at scheduled intervals.

11. Administer prescribed anticholinergics or smooth muscle relaxants, which inhibit detrusor contractions or reduce detrusor instability.

Functional incontinence related to sensory, cognitive, or mobility deficits or environmental changes

Desired outcome: After implementation of habit training program, patient becomes continent.

1. Assess and document patient's pattern of voiding: time, amount voided, amount of fluid intake, timing of fluid intake followed by voiding, and other related factors.
2. Determine environmental obstacles that would prevent patient from toileting appropriately and intervene accordingly. For example, remove obstacles between bed and bathroom, leave light on in bathroom, and attach call light to bed sheet.
3. Assess patient's bowel status for the potential for constipation, which causes straining and weakens sphincter tone.
4. Monitor patient for increased need to void after taking medications such as diuretics, which increase urine production or the sensation of urgency.

Habit Training

5. Based on assessed pattern of incontinence, establish a planned schedule for voiding.
6. Offer bedpan, urinal, or assistance to bathroom at least q2h.
7. Maintain planned schedule for voiding, and note time of any incontinent episode that occurs between scheduled voidings. If patient's incontinence pattern consistently does not match voiding schedule, change voiding schedule

In Addition

8. Administer diuretics in the morning or early afternoon to reduce the risk of nighttime incontinence.
9. If patient has an intravenous infusion, consult physician about advisability of reducing infusion rate at night.
10. For bedridden patients, keep call light within patient's reach and answer call quickly.
11. For confused patients, keep a clock and calendar in room and remind patient of time and date as appropriate. Toilet patient as described above. If patient is acutely confused, calmly let patient know that you do not see or hear what he or she does, but do not argue (e.g., if patient cries, "Help, I'm in jail," you might say, "It must feel like jail being tied to all these tubes"). This approach, rather than constantly trying to reorient the patient, will minimize his or her agitation until the underlying cause of the disorientation has been resolved. When patient is calm, you can reorient him or her to environment, but if patient becomes agitated, stop attempt to reorient.
12. If patient has permanent or severe cognitive impairment, reorient to his or her baseline and toilet patient as described previously.
13. Monitor patient's bowel function and status, inasmuch as constipa-

tion or impaction can cause symptoms of incontinence (e.g., dribbling).

Risk for impaired skin integrity related to incontinence of urine
Desired outcome: Patient's perineal skin remains intact.
1. Assess patient for wetness of perineal area at frequent intervals. Inform patient that prolonged exposure to urine can cause maceration, and instruct him or her to alert staff as soon as wetness occurs.
2. Keep bed linen dry. As necessary, use and change absorbent materials (e.g., protective underwear or underpads).
3. Keep perineum clean with mild soap and water; dry well.
4. Expose perineum to air whenever possible by using a sheet draped over a bed cradle; ensure patient's privacy.
5. Use sealants and moisture-barrier ointments to protect patient's skin.
6. Make sure plastic pads or sheet protectors do not contact patient's skin directly, because maceration can result from the increased perspiration they cause. Cover these pads with pillow cases or place them under sheets.
7. Educate patient in the use of containment devices (e.g., briefs with pads, adult absorptive briefs, and external catheters).
8. Initiate habit or bladder training to reduce episodes of incontinence.

Body image disturbance related to odor, discomfort, and embarrassment secondary to incontinence
Desired outcomes: After interventions, patient verbalizes feelings and frustrations without self-deprecating statements. Within the 24 h before hospital discharge, patient verbalizes knowledge about actions that will control either incontinence or odor and discomfort.
1. Encourage patient to discuss feelings and frustrations.
2. Offer reassurance and encouragement and provide information about treatment, especially about activities within patient's control.
3. Be realistic with patient; if incontinence cannot be controlled, reassure patient that odor and discomfort *can* be controlled.
4. Explore with patient methods for relieving discomfort and controlling odor: maintaining good hygiene, changing undergarments often, and using and frequently changing incontinence pads.
5. Although fluid intake of at least 2-3 L/day is essential for minimizing the risk of UTI, suggest that patient limit fluids when away from home and increase them on return. A reduction also should be incorporated into evening hours to prevent nighttime incontinence.
6. Refer patient to support groups, such as HIP (Help for Incontinent People): Box 544, Union, SC 29379, (803)-579-7900; and the Simon Foundation: Box 835, Wilmette, IL 60091, (800)-23-SIMON.
7. For additional information, see this nursing diagnosis in Appendix One, "Caring for Patients with Cancer and Other Life-Disrupting Illnesses," p. 459.

Knowledge deficit: Pelvic muscle (Kegel) exercise program to strengthen perineal muscles (effective for individuals with mild to moderate stress incontinence or for those with functional incontinence who can participate)
Desired outcome: Within the 24 h before hospital discharge, pa-

tient verbalizes and demonstrates knowledge about pelvic muscle (Kegel) exercise program.
1. Explain that Kegel exercises strengthen pelvic area muscles, which will help regain bladder control.
2. Help patient identify correct muscle group:
   ■ To strengthen proximal muscle, instruct patient to attempt to shut off urinary flow after beginning urination, hold for a few seconds, and then start stream again. Explain to patient that if this can be accomplished, the correct muscle is being exercised.
   ■ To strengthen distal muscle, teach patient to contract muscle around the anus, as though to stop a bowel movement.

N O T E :   A common error when attempting to identify the correct muscle group is contraction of the buttocks, quadriceps, and abdominal muscles.

3. Teach patient to repeat these exercises 10-20 times, 4 ×/day. Advise patient that these exercises may need to be done for 2-9 mo before any benefit is obtained.

Knowledge deficit: Use of external (condom) catheter
Desired outcomes: Within the 24 h before hospital discharge, patient or significant other successfully returns demonstration of condom catheter application and verbalizes knowledge about rationale for its use.

N O T E :   Both internal and external catheters should be used only if other methods of achieving urinary continence have failed, because both lead to increased incidence of UTI.

1. Instruct men patients or significant others in procedure for applying condom catheter.
2. Teach the importance of keeping pubic hair trimmed or moved away from penis to avoid contact with adhesive used with catheter.
3. Instruct patient to cleanse and dry penis thoroughly before and after every condom application. In uncircumcised patients, the foreskin should be retracted to cleanse area under prepuce and then returned to its original position.
4. Teach patient or significant other to monitor skin under external device daily for redness, rashes, or open areas.
5. For ambulatory patients, demonstrate connecting condom catheter to a leg drainage bag; for patients on bed rest, demonstrate connecting catheter to a bedside urinary collection container, such as that used with an indwelling catheter.
6. Advise patient to remove and replace catheter as directed. Most manufacturers recommend that external catheters be changed and replaced daily.
7. If appropriate for patient, suggest that condom catheter be used only during the night.

See "Neurogenic Bladder" for **Reflex incontinence,** p. 101.
   For surgical patients, see nursing diagnoses and interventions in Appendix One, "Caring for Preoperative and Postoperative Patients,"

p. 395, particularly **Risk for infection** as it relates to presence of indwelling urinary catheter, p. 408.

PATIENT-FAMILY TEACHING
AND DISCHARGE PLANNING

Give patient and significant others verbal and written information about the following:

1. Medications, including drug name, purpose, dosage, schedule, precautions, drug/drug and food/drug interactions, and potential side effects.
2. Diet: importance of increasing dietary fiber to help prevent constipation and keep stools soft.
3. Indicators of UTI, which require medical attention: fever, chills, cloudy or foul-smelling urine, frequency, urgency, burning with urination, hematuria, increasing or recurring incontinence.
4. Care of catheters and drains if patient is discharged with them.
5. Importance of maintaining fluid intake of at least 3 L/day and avoiding caffeine and alcohol, which act as bladder irritants and increase the risk of urgency.
6. Maintaining schedule for bladder training program.
7. Use of perineal muscles to improve bladder tone.
8. Care of perineal skin.
9. Support groups (see **Body image disturbance,** p. 97).

SURGICAL PATIENTS

10. Care of incision, including cleansing and dressing; and indicators of infection: purulent drainage, persistent redness, swelling, warmth along incision line.
11. Activity restrictions: no heavy lifting ($>$10 lb) and resting when fatigued. Explain that prolonged periods of sitting can cause relaxation of musculature of bladder and sphincter, leading to incontinence. Encourage mild activity, such as walking, to improve muscle tone.

Urinary Retention

NURSING DIAGNOSES AND INTERVENTIONS

Urinary retention related to weak detrusor muscle, blockage, inhibition of reflex arc, or strong sphincter

Desired outcome: Within 2 days, patient reports a normal voiding pattern or, if appropriate, demonstrates self-catheterization before hospital discharge.

1. Assess bladder for distention by inspection, percussion, and palpation; measure and document I&O.
2. If appropriate, try noninvasive measures for release of urine: position patient in a normal position for voiding; have patient listen to the sound of running water or place hands in a basin of warm water. If these measures are ineffective, try pouring warm water over perineum. Unless contraindicated, Credé's method (pressure applied

from the umbilicus to the pubis) may be used to stimulate a weak micturitional reflex.

3. Maintain privacy for patient who is trying to use the commode, bedpan, or urinal. Remember that cold bedpans can cause muscle tension, so use a plastic bedpan or warm a metal bedpan before giving it to the patient. Encourage relaxation technique, such as deep breathing or visualization, to relax the body.

4. Provide an adequate amount of time for patient's urge to void to occur. Do not rush patient.

5. Consult physician if patient cannot void, has a distended bladder, or has suprapubic or urethral pain.

6. Monitor patient's bowel function and status, inasmuch as constipation or impaction can cause urinary retention.

7. If catheterization is prescribed, monitor patient's BP and HR during the procedure. If the patient complains of abdominal pain or has a symptomatic drop of >20 mm Hg systolic BP, clamp catheter until patient's BP returns to within normal limits. For additional information see **Risk for fluid volume deficit** related to postobstructive diuresis in "Urinary Tract Obstruction," p. 90.

8. Catheterization may be difficult beyond the prostatic gland in men with benign prostatic hypertrophy (BPH) or in those over age 65, a large percentage of whom have undiagnosed BPH. For these patients, use a coudé (bent tip) catheter instead of a straight catheter. The tip on this catheter is stiff and does not bend against an obstacle. Lubricate the catheter tip generously with a minimum of 5 ml of lubricating jelly before insertion.

9. Teach patient the technique for intermittent self-catheterization, if appropriate. Catheterization should be accomplished on a set q4h schedule to prevent bladder distention, which can injure the bladder mucosa and increase the risk of infection. Teach patient clean technique for use at home.

See "Urinary Tract Obstruction" for **Risk for fluid volume deficit** related to postobstructive diuresis, p. 90, and **Pain** related to bladder spasms, p. 91.

Also see "Neurogenic Bladder" for **Dysreflexia** related to distended bladder, p. 102.

PATIENT-FAMILY TEACHING
AND DISCHARGE PLANNING

Give patient and significant others verbal and written information about the following:

1. Medications, including drug name, purpose, dosage, schedule, precautions, drug/drug and food/drug interactions, and potential side effects.

2. Indicators of UTI and recurrent retention, which require medical attention: suprapubic or urethral pain, fever, recurring or increasing difficulty with voiding.

3. Self-catheterization technique, if appropriate.

Neurogenic Bladder

NURSING DIAGNOSES AND INTERVENTIONS

Reflex incontinence related to neurologic impairment secondary to injury or disease that affects transmission of signals from reflex arc to cerebral cortex

Desired outcomes: Patient or significant other participates in a habit training program. Patient has fewer or no incontinent episodes.

Habit Training Program

1. Assess patient's voiding pattern: time, amount voided, amount of fluid intake, timing of fluid intake followed by voiding, and other related factors.

2. Determine amount of time between voidings to estimate amount of time patient can hold urine. Establish a voiding schedule that does not exceed this period.

3. Regulate fluids to achieve adequate hydration and a desirable voiding pattern. For example, teach patient to drink measured amounts of fluids (e.g., 8 oz q2h) and attempt to void 30 min later, based on voiding schedule.

4. Help patient schedule times for emptying bladder, such as q1-2h when awake and q4h at night. If successful, attempt to lengthen intervals between voidings. Provide patient and significant others with a written copy of the schedule.

In Addition

5. Monitor for bladder retention by assessing I&O, inspecting suprapubic area, and percussing and palpating bladder. Be alert for swelling proximal to the symphysis pubis, a "kettle drum" sound with percussion, and dribbling of urine.

6. As appropriate, teach patient techniques that stimulate voiding reflex. Examples include tapping the suprapubic area with the fingers, pulling the pubic hair, or digitally stretching the anal sphincter. This last method is effective because the rectal nerves follow basically the same path as the urethral nerves; however, the maneuver is contraindicated in patients with a spinal cord injury (SCI) at or above T6, because it can cause autonomic dysreflexia (see next nursing diagnosis). The Valsalva maneuver also can be used to stimulate voiding: Patient bears down as though having a bowel movement to increase intrathoracic and intraabdominal pressure.

7. If an artificial inflatable sphincter is used, instruct patient to deflate the valve q4h, which allows the bladder to empty. Remind patient to wear a Medic-Alert tag or bracelet to alert emergency personnel to presence and use of the device.

8. If a condom catheter is used, see **Knowledge deficit:** Use of external (condom) catheter in "Urinary Incontinence," p. 98, for appropriate nursing interventions.

9. For men with extensive sphincter damage, a penile clamp might be prescribed. Before and after use, instruct patient (or significant other) to cleanse the penis with soap and water, dry it thoroughly, and sprinkle powder along the shaft. Explain that the clamp is placed horizontally behind the glans after voiding and removed q3h. Stress the importance of inspecting the skin for redness along the area in which the clamp presses. If breakdown occurs (i.e., redness does not disappear after massage), the clamp must be discontinued. If swelling appears along the glans, advise patient to set the clamp at a looser setting. **Caution:** Minimize the potential for injury by alternating the penile clamp with a condom catheter.

10. If intermittent catheterization is prescribed, teach the procedure to patient or significant other. Emphasize the need to follow a routine (e.g., q4h) to minimize potential for UTI caused by stasis and bladder distention.

11. If Credé's method is prescribed, patients with arm and hand strength should be taught the procedure as an alternative to self-catheterization: Place ulnar surface of hand horizontally along umbilicus; while bearing down with abdominal muscles, press hand downward and toward bladder in a kneading motion until urination is initiated; continue q30sec until urination ceases.

12. In nonrestricted individuals, encourage a fluid intake of at least 3 L/day, which dilutes the urine and increases output, thereby minimizing the risk of infection and calculi.

13. To help prevent urinary stasis, which can lead to UTI, and to increase cardiac output, which nourishes kidneys, encourage as much mobility as patient can tolerate.

14. If diuretics are prescribed, administer them in the morning or early afternoon to reduce the risk of nighttime incontinence.

15. If patient has an IV infusion, consult physician about advisability of reducing infusion rate at night to minimize risk of nighttime incontinence.

16. If patient has a permanent cognitive impairment, use visual clues, such as a sign on the bathroom door that says *toilet* or a picture of a toilet.

Dysreflexia (or risk for same) related to distended bladder

Desired outcomes: Patient is free of indicators of autonomic dysreflexia (AD), as evidenced by HR $\geq$60 bpm, BP within patient's normal limits, skin dry and of normal color above level of SCI (if appropriate), normal vision, and absence of headache, nausea, piloerection (goose bumps) below level of injury (if appropriate), and nasal congestion. Patient and/or significant others verbalize understanding of indicators, prevention, and treatment of AD.

N O T E : Autonomic dysreflexia is a life-threatening condition that can occur in patients with neurogenic bladder, especially those with SCI at or above T8.

1. Be alert for indicators of AD: headache, bradycardia, excessively high BP, blurred vision, flushing and sweating above level of injury, piloerection and pallor below level of injury, and nausea.
2. If signs of AD occur, raise HOB immediately to help lower BP, and assess for bladder distention. Have patient empty bladder in accustomed manner, or check for patency of the indwelling catheter. **Caution:** Irrigation of the urinary catheter can increase bladder pressure and intensify AD. If catheter is obstructed, either recatheterize patient, using liberal amounts of anesthetic jelly, or irrigate catheter gently, using ≤30 ml of normal saline. Follow agency policy.
3. Monitor patient's BP for trends. Be aware that continuing increases in BP can be life threatening, leading to CVA, status epilepticus, and death.
4. Administer appropriate medications as prescribed, such as phenoxybenzamine hydrochloride, a long-acting vasodilator that increases blood flow to the skin, mucosa, and abdominal viscera and lowers both supine and standing BP. Consult physician if symptoms do not disappear after bladder is emptied, if bladder is full and cannot be emptied, or if medication does not relieve symptoms.
5. Encourage a fluid intake of at least 3 L/day, which dilutes urine and increases output, thereby minimizing the risk of infection, calculi, and ultimately AD.
6. To help prevent urinary stasis, which can lead to UTI and consequently to AD, encourage as much mobility as patient can tolerate.
7. Teach patient and significant others the indicators, prevention, and treatment of AD and the importance of seeking help immediately if indicators are noted.
8. For additional information about AD, see **Dysreflexia (or risk for same)** in "Spinal Cord Injury," p. 142.

Total incontinence related to neuropathy preventing transmission of reflex indicating bladder fullness or related to lower motor neuron disturbance secondary to SCI below S3-S4

Desired outcomes: Patient or significant other follows habit training program; incontinent episodes decrease to less than 3/wk.

Habit Training Program

1. Assess and document patient's voiding pattern: time, amount voided, amount of fluid intake, timing of fluid intake followed by voiding, and other related factors.
2. Determine amount of time between voidings to estimate how long patient can hold urine. Establish a voiding schedule that does not exceed this interval.
3. Help patient schedule times for emptying the bladder, such as q1-2h when awake and q4h at night. If successful, attempt to lengthen intervals between voiding. Provide patient and significant other with a written copy of the schedule.
4. If patient takes fluids orally, provide necessary amounts for optimal hydration (3 L/day) during the day and reduce amount given during the evening and nighttime hours.

5. Provide information about incontinence aids (e.g., incontinence pads and clothing that is easy to remove).
6. For men patients, demonstrate use of external (condom) catheters for nighttime use (see p. 98).

In Addition

7. Administer diuretics in the morning or early afternoon to reduce the risk of nighttime incontinence.
8. If patient has an IV infusion, consult physician about advisability of reducing infusion rate at night.

Knowledge deficit: Function and care of long-term indwelling catheters after continent vesicostomy (continent urinary reservoir)

Desired outcomes: Before continent vesicostomy, patient verbalizes rationale for use of a suprapubic catheter and vesicostomy tube, including approximate amount of time they will be indwelling. Within the 24 h before hospital discharge, patient or significant other demonstrates proficiency with intermittent catheterization, tube irrigation, and dressing changes.

1. Preoperatively, explain that patient will return from surgery with a suprapubic catheter and vesicostomy tube in place.
2. Explain that patient will be discharged with catheter and readmitted for catheter removal in approximately 6 wk. After removal of indwelling catheter, intermittent catheterization will be performed hourly, progressing to 2-4 h and ultimately to 4-6 h. Continuous drainage will be used overnight. After removal of indwelling catheter, make sure patient or significant other demonstrates proficiency with the following:
   - Washing hands with soap and water before catheterization.
   - Selecting a clean catheter and placing it on a clean paper towel.
   - Cleaning the stoma site with povidone-iodine solution and removing mucus that has drained from the stoma.
   - Inserting the catheter carefully into the stoma and draining the bladder of urine. Lubricants usually are not necessary. If lubrication is needed, however, teach patient to use one that is water soluble, *never* products made from petroleum jelly, which can damage the catheter.
   - If mucus clogs the catheter, removing the catheter from the stoma, rinsing it with hot water, and reinserting the catheter to continue the drainage.
3. Encourage patient to participate in care, including tube irrigation, which removes mucus from the pouch, and dressing changes. Demonstrate procedure for irrigation once it has been prescribed. Typically, sterile normal saline (30-50 ml) is used for irrigation. Instruct patient to wash hands before handling catheters to help prevent contamination and to cleanse around catheter site daily with an antimicrobial solution (e.g., povidone-iodine).

As appropriate, see "Urinary Incontinence" for **Risk for impaired skin integrity,** p. 97, and **Body image disturbance,** p. 97.

PATIENT-FAMILY TEACHING
AND DISCHARGE PLANNING

Give patient and significant others verbal and written information about the following:
1. For patients with artificial sphincters, the indicators of UTI and erosion: pain, fever, swelling, urinary retention, or incontinence.
2. For more information, see this discussion in "Urinary Incontinence," p. 99.

SECTION SIX: URINARY DIVERSIONS

NURSING DIAGNOSES AND INTERVENTIONS

Anxiety related to threat to self-concept, interaction patterns, or health status secondary to urinary diversion surgery
Desired outcome: Before surgery, patient communicates fears and concerns, relates attainment of increased psychologic and physical comfort, and exhibits effective coping mechanisms.
1. Assess patient's perceptions of his or her impending surgery and the resulting changes in body function. Provide opportunities for patient to express fears and concerns (e.g., "You seem very concerned about next week's surgery"). Listen actively to patient. Recognize that anger, denial, withdrawal, and demanding behavior may be coping responses.
2. Acknowledge patient's fears and concerns.
3. Provide brief, basic information regarding physiology of the procedure and the equipment that will be used after surgery, including tubes and drains.
4. Show patient pouches that will be used after surgery. Assure patient that the pouch usually cannot be seen through clothing and that it is odor resistant.
5. For patient about to undergo a continent urostomy, explain that a pouching system may be needed for a short time after surgery. Reassure patient that teaching about accessing the continent urostomy will be done before hospital discharge.
6. Discuss ADLs with patient. Inform patient that showers, baths, and swimming can continue and that diet is not affected after the early postoperative period.
7. As appropriate, ask patient what information has been relayed by the surgeon about the sexual implications of the surgery. This will help establish an open relationship between the patient and primary nurse and inform the nurse if the patient has understood the information given by the surgeon. Some men undergoing radical cystectomy with urinary diversion may become impotent, but recent surgical advances have enabled preservation of potency for others. The pelvic plexus, which innervates the corpora cavernosa, will be dam-

Renal-Urinary

aged permanently. Autonomic nerve damage results in loss of erection and ejaculation; however, because sensation and orgasm are mediated by the pudendal nerve (sensorimotor), they are not affected.

8. Arrange for a visit by the enterostomal therapy (ET) nurse during the preoperative period. Collaborate with the surgeon, ET nurse, and patient to identify and mark the most appropriate site for the stoma. Showing the patient the actual spot for placement may help alleviate anxiety by reinforcing that the impact on life-style and body image will be minimal.

Altered protection related to neurosensory, musculoskeletal, and cardiac changes secondary to hyperchloremic metabolic acidosis with hypokalemia (can occur secondary to reabsorption of Na^+ and Cl^- from the urine in the ileal segment, which results in compensatory loss of K^+ and HCO_3^-)

Desired outcome: Patient verbalizes orientation to time, place, and person (within patient's normal range) and remains free of injury caused by neurosensory, musculoskeletal, and cardiac changes.

1. For patients with ileal conduits, assess for indicators of hypokalemia and metabolic acidosis, including nausea and changes in LOC (from sleepy to combative), muscle tone (convulsions to flaccidity), and irregular HR.

2. If patient is confused or exhibits signs of motor dysfunction, keep bed in lowest position and raise side rails. Consult physician about significant findings.

3. Encourage oral intake as directed, and assess for need for IV management. Physician may prescribe IV fluids with potassium supplements.

4. If patient is hypokalemic and allowed to eat, encourage foods high in potassium (e.g., bananas, cantaloupes, and apricots). See Table 3-2 for other high-potassium foods.

5. Encourage patient to ambulate by second or third day after surgery. Mobility helps prevent urinary stasis, which increases the risk of electrolyte problems.

Risk for impaired skin integrity related to presence of urine or sensitivity to appliance material

Desired outcome: Patient's peristomal skin remains nonerythematous and intact.

1. For patient with significant allergy history, patch test skin for a 24-h period at least 24 h before ostomy surgery, to assess for allergies to different tapes that might be used on postoperative appliance. If erythema, swelling, itching, weeping, or other indicators of tape allergy occur, document type of tape that caused the reaction and note on the cover of the chart "Allergic to _____ tape."

2. Inspect integrity of peristomal skin with each pouch change, and question patient about itching or burning, which can signal leakage. Change pouch routinely (per agency or surgeon's preference) or immediately if leakage is suspected.

3. Assess for inflamed hair follicles (folliculitis) or a reaction to the

tape. Report rash to physician, since this often occurs with a yeast infection and requires topical medication.

4. Assess stoma, pouch, or skin for crystalline deposits, which are signals of alkaline urine.
   - Teach patient to monitor urine pH every week and to maintain pH <6.
   - Teach patient to decrease urine pH by drinking acetic fluids (e.g., cranberry or orange juice) or by taking ascorbic acid in a dosage consistent with patient's size.
   - Teach patient signs of ascorbic acid toxicity: nausea, vomiting, heartburn, diarrhea, flushing, and insomnia.

5. When changing pouch, measure stoma with a measuring guide and ensure that opening of the skin barrier is cut to the exact size of the stoma to protect the peristomal skin. Protect skin from maceration caused by pooling of urine on skin:
   - *For patient using a two-piece system or pouch with a barrier:* Size barrier to fit snugly around stoma. If using a barrier and attaching an adhesive pouch, size barrier to fit snugly around stoma, and size pouch to clear stoma by at least ⅛ in.
   - *For patient using a one-piece "adhesive-only" pouch:* If pouch has an antireflux valve, size pouch to clear stoma and any peristomal creases so that pouch adheres to a flat, dry surface. An antireflux valve prevents pooling of urine on skin. If pouch does not have an antireflux valve, size pouch so that it clears stoma by ⅛ in, to prevent stomal trauma while minimizing the amount of exposed skin. Use a copolymer film sealant wipe on peristomal skin before applying adhesive-only pouch; this provides a moisture barrier and reduces epidermal trauma when pouch is removed.

6. Wash peristomal skin with water or a special cleansing solution marketed by ostomy supply companies. Dry skin thoroughly before applying skin barrier and pouch.

7. When changing pouch, instruct patient to hold a gauze pad on (but not in) the stoma to absorb urine and keep skin dry.

8. After applying pouch, connect it to bedside drainage system if patient is on bed rest. When patient is no longer on bed rest, empty pouch when it is one third to one half full by opening the spigot at the bottom of the pouch and draining the urine into the patient's measuring container. Do not allow pouch to become too full, because this could break the appliance's seal with the patient's skin. Instruct patient accordingly.

9. Change incisional dressing as often as it becomes wet, using sterile technique.

10. Teach patient to treat peristomal skin irritation in the following ways after hospital discharge:
    - Dry skin with a hair dryer on a cool setting.
    - Dust peristomal skin with absorptive powder (e.g., Karaya or Stomahesive).
    - If desired, blot skin with water or a sealant wipe to "seal in" powder.
    - Use porous tape to prevent moisture trapping.

- Consult physician or ET nurse about any severe or nonresponsive skin problems.

Impaired stomal tissue integrity (or risk for same) related to altered circulation

Desired outcomes: Patient's stoma is pink or bright red and shiny. Stoma of a cutaneous urostomy is raised, moist, and red.

1. Inspect stoma at least q8h and as indicated. The stoma of an ileal conduit will be edematous and should be pink or red with a shiny appearance. A stoma that is dusky or cyanotic indicates insufficient blood supply and impending necrosis and must be reported to the physician immediately.

2. Also assess degree of swelling, and inform patient that stoma will shrink considerably over the first 6-8 wk and less significantly over the next year. For patients with ileal conduit, evaluate stomal height and plan care accordingly (see **Risk for impaired skin integrity,** p. 106). The stoma formed by a cutaneous ureterostomy usually is raised during the first few weeks after surgery, red, and moist.

Altered urinary elimination related to postoperative use of ureteral stents, catheters, or drains and to urinary diversion surgery

Desired outcome: Patient's urinary output is ≥ 30 ml/h, and urine is clear and straw colored and has normal odor.

1. Monitor color, clarity, and volume of urine output *via* stoma, stents, and/or catheter.
   - *Ureterostomy:* Urine drainage *via* stoma and/or ureteral stents.
   - *Intestinal conduit:* Urine drainage *via* stoma. Patient also may have ureteral stents and/or conduit catheter/stent in early postoperative period to stabilize ureterointestinal anastomoses and maintain drainage from conduit during early postoperative edema.
   - *Continent urinary diversions or reservoirs:* The Kock urostomy usually has a reservoir catheter and also may have ureteral stents. The Indiana (ileocecal) reservoir usually has ureteral stents exiting from the stoma through which most of the urine drains, and it may have a reservoir catheter exiting from a stab wound, which serves as an overflow catheter. The continent urinary diversion with urethral anastomosis has a urethral catheter in place that drains urine, which initially is light red to pink and has mucus but should clear in 24-48 h. This catheter remains in place for 21 days to ensure adequate healing of the anastomosis.

2. Monitor for evidence of anastomotic breakdown/intraabdominal urine leakage, which may occur in an individual with intestinal conduit or continent diversion: decreasing urinary output from stoma or stents, flank pain, increasing abdominal girth, and increasing drainage from Penrose drains.

3. Monitor functioning of ureteral stents, which protrude from the stoma under the pouch. These stents maintain patency of ureters and assist healing of the anastomosis. Right stents usually are cut at a 90-degree angle, whereas left stents are cut at a 45-degree angle. Each usually produces approximately the same amount of urine, although the amount produced by each is not important as long as

each drains adequately and total drainage from all sources is ≥30 ml/h. Urine should be pink for the first 24-48 h and become straw colored by postoperative day 3. Absent or declining amounts of urine may indicate a blocked stent or ureteral problems. **Note:** Stents may become blocked with mucus. As long as urine is draining adequately around the stent and the volume of output is adequate, this is not a problem.

4. Monitor functioning of stoma catheters. In continent urinary diversions, a catheter is placed in the reservoir to prevent distention and promote healing of suture lines. This new reservoir exudes large amounts of mucus, requiring irrigation of the catheter with 30-50 ml of normal saline; this is instilled gently and allowed to empty *via* gravity. Expect output to include pink or light red urine with mucus and small red clots for the first 24 h. Urine should become amber colored with occasional clots in 3 postoperative days. Mucus production will continue but should decrease in volume.

5. Monitor functioning of drains. Any urinary diversion may have Penrose drains in place to maintain integrity of ureterointestinal anastomosis. Excessive lymph fluid and urine can be removed *via* these drains without putting pressure on the suture lines. Drainage from the Penrose drain may be light red to pink for the first 24 h and then lighten to amber and diminish in amount. In a continent urinary diversion, an increase in drainage after amounts have been low might signal reservoir leakage. Consult physician if this occurs.

6. Monitor I&O, and record total amount of urine output from urinary diversion for the first 24 h postoperatively. Differentiate and record separately amounts from all drains, stents, and catheters. Consult physician about an output <60 ml during a 2-h period, because in the presence of adequate intake, this can indicate a ureteral obstruction, a leak in the urinary diversion, or impending renal failure. Assess for other indicators of ureteral obstruction: flank pain, nausea, vomiting, anuria.

7. Monitor drainage from Foley catheter or urethral drain, if present. Patients who have had a cystectomy may have a urethral drain, whereas those with a cystectomy will have a Foley catheter in place. Note color, consistency, and volume of drainage, which may be red or pink with mucus. Report sudden increase (which would occur with hemorrhage) or decrease (which can signal blockage that can lead to infection). Report significant findings to physician.

8. Advise patient that after removal of urethral catheter or drain, mucus drainage will continue from the urethral meatus for several months.

9. To keep the urinary tract well irrigated, encourage a fluid intake of at least 2-3 L/day in nonrestricted patient.

Risk for infection related to invasive surgical procedure and risk of ascending bacteriuria with urinary diversion

Desired outcome: Patient is free of infection, as evidenced by normothermia, WBC count ≤11,000/µl, and absence of purulent drainage, erythema, puffiness, warmth, and tenderness along incision.

1. Monitor patient's temperature q4h during the first 24-48 h after surgery. Consult physician about fever spikes.
2. Inspect dressing frequently after surgery. Infection is most likely to become evident after the first 72 h. Assess for purulent drainage on dressing, and consult physician accordingly. Change dressing when it becomes wet, using sterile technique. Use extra care to prevent disruption of drains.
3. Note condition of incision. Be alert for indicators of infection, including erythema, tenderness, local warmth, puffiness, and purulent drainage.
4. Monitor and record character of urine at least q8h. Mucus particles are normal in urine of patients with ileal conduits and continent urinary diversions because of the nature of the bowel segment used. However, cloudy urine is abnormal and can signal an infection. Urine should be yellow or pink tinged during the first 24-48 h after surgery. Assess for other indicators of UTI, including flank pain, chills, and fever.
5. Note position of stoma relative to incision. If they are close together, apply pouch first to avoid overlapping pouch onto suture line, which can increase the risk of infection. If necessary, cut pouch down on one side, or place it at an angle to avoid contact with drainage, which may loosen adhesive. To help prevent contamination and cross-contamination, wash your hands before and after caring for patient.
6. Patients with cystectomies without anastomosis to the urethra may have an indwelling urethral catheter to drain serosanguineous fluid from the peritoneal cavity. **Caution:** Do not irrigate this catheter, because irrigation can result in peritonitis.
7. Encourage a fluid intake of at least 2-3 L/day, because this helps flush urine through the urinary tract, preventing stasis.

Risk for fluid volume deficit related to postsurgical bleeding/hemorrhage

Desired outcomes: Patient is normovolemic, as evidenced by balanced I&O; urinary output ≥30 ml/h; and BP, HR, and RR within patient's baseline range. Urine becomes amber to straw colored after 2-3 postoperative days.

1. Monitor I&O, and note amount and character of urine output at least q4h. Initially urinary output will be blood tinged, but it should become clear within 2-3 days. Amount of urinary output should be normal (≥30 ml/h for 2 consecutive hours).
2. Be alert for gross hematuria, along with decreasing BP, tachycardia, and tachypnea, which can signal hemorrhage.
3. Report significant findings to physician.

Knowledge deficit: Self-care regarding urinary diversion

Desired outcome: Patient or significant other demonstrates proper care of stoma and urinary diversion before hospital discharge.

1. Assess patient's or significant other's readiness to participate in care.
2. Involve ET nurse in patient teaching if available.
3. Help patient organize equipment and materials needed for accomplishing home care. Usually patient is discharged with disposable

pouching systems. Most of these patients remain in disposable systems for the long term; those who will use reusable systems usually are not fitted for 6-8 wk after surgery.

4. Teach patient how to remove and reapply pouch, how to empty it, and how to use gravity drainage system at night, including procedures for rinsing and cleansing drainage system.

5. Teach patient the signs and symptoms of UTI, peristomal skin breakdown, and appropriate therapeutic responses, including maintenance of an acidic urine (if not contraindicated), the importance of adequate fluid intake, and techniques for checking urine pH, which should be assessed weekly. Explain that urine pH should remain ≤6. Individuals with urinary diversions have a higher incidence of UTIs than the general public, so it is important to keep their urinary pH acidic. If it is >6, advise patient to increase fluid intake and, with physician's approval, to increase vitamin C intake to 500-1,000 mg/day, which will increase urine acidity.

6. Teach patient with continent diversion the technique for irrigating the reservoir catheter.

7. Teach patient with continent urinary diversion with urethral anastomosis the signals of urge to void: (1) feeling of vague abdominal discomfort and (2) feeling of abdominal pressure or cramping.

8. Instruct patient with continent urinary diversion with urethral anastomosis about the procedure to void: relax perineal muscles and use Valsalva maneuver.

9. Emphasize the importance of follow-up visits, particularly for patients with continent urinary diversions, who will be taught how to catheterize the reservoir and use a small dressing over the stoma rather than an appliance.

10. Provide patient with a list of ostomy groups and ET nurses in the area for referral and assistance.

11. Provide patient with enough equipment and materials for the first week after hospital discharge. Remind patient that proper cleansing of ostomy appliances reduces the risk of bacterial growth and UTI.

See "Fecal Diversions" for **Body image disturbance,** p. 263.

See nursing diagnoses and interventions in Appendix One, "Caring for Preoperative and Postoperative Patients," p. 395, and "Caring for Patients with Cancer and Other Life-Disrupting Illnesses," p. 423.

PATIENT-FAMILY TEACHING AND DISCHARGE PLANNING

Give patient and significant others verbal and written information about the following:

1. Medications, including drug name, purpose, dosage, schedule, precautions, drug/drug and food/drug interactions, and potential side effects.

2. Indicators that require medical intervention: fever, chills, nausea, vomiting, abdominal pain and distention, cloudy urine, incisional pain or redness, peristomal skin irritation, or abnormal changes in

stoma shape or color from the normal bright, shiny red.

3. Community resources, including local United Ostomy Association, the American Cancer Society, and an ET nurse in the area, if appropriate.

4. Maintaining fluid intake at least 2-3 L/day to ensure adequate kidney function.

5. Monitoring of urine pH, which should be checked weekly. Urine pH should remain at 6 or less. Individuals with urinary diversions have a higher incidence of UTIs than the general public, so it is important to keep their urinary pH acidic. If it is above 6, advise patient to increase fluid intake and, with physician's approval, to increase vitamin C intake to 500-1,000 mg/day, which will increase urine acidity.

6. Care of stoma and application of urostomy appliances. Patient should be proficient in application technique before hospital discharge.

7. Care of urostomy appliances. Remind patient that proper cleansing reduces the risk of bacterial growth, which would contaminate the urine and increase the risk of UTI.

8. Importance of follow-up care with physician and ET nurse. Confirm date and time of next appointment.

Neurologic Disorders

4

SECTION ONE: INFLAMMATORY DISORDERS OF THE NERVOUS SYSTEM

Multiple Sclerosis

NURSING DIAGNOSES AND INTERVENTIONS

Knowledge deficit: Factors that aggravate and exacerbate symptoms of multiple sclerosis (MS)

Desired outcome: By day 3 (or before hospital discharge), patient and significant others verbalize knowledge about factors that exacerbate, prevent, or ameliorate symptoms of MS.

1. Inform patient and significant others that heat, both external (hot weather, bath) and internal (fever), tends to aggravate weakness and other symptoms of MS.

2. Teach preventive measures (e.g., avoiding hot baths, using acetaminophen or aspirin to reduce fever).

3. Because infection often precedes exacerbations, caution patient to avoid exposure to persons known to have infections of any kind.

4. Teach the indicators of common infections (see "Care of the Renal Transplant Recipient," p. 86, and Table 2-5, p. 39) as well as the importance of seeking prompt medical treatment should these signs appear. For example, the MS patient is susceptible to UTI because of urinary retention. As a result of the disease process, the patient may not feel any pain with urination. Teach patient to monitor for increased frequency, urgency, or incontinence and to check the urine for changes in odor, cloudiness, or blood. Instruct patient to check body temperature periodically for fever. Signals that a UTI has reached the kidneys include chills and flank pain.

5. Teach patient that stress and fatigue are related to exacerbations. Encourage patient to get sufficient rest, stop activity short of fatigue, schedule activity and rest periods, and reduce factors that cause stress. To reduce fatigue, encourage patient to conserve en-

ergy in ADLs by sitting while getting dressed, rather than standing; by sliding heavy items along work surfaces, rather than lifting them; by using a wheeled cart to transport items; and by having work surfaces at the proper height. The drug amantadine (see "Parkinsonism," p. 128) also may help manage fatigue. (Also see "Coronary Artery Disease" for **Health-seeking behaviors:** Relaxation technique effective for stress reduction, p. 27.)

6. As appropriate, explain to patient that exacerbations may increase postpartum. Provide information about birth control measures to women patients who desire counseling.

7. As appropriate, reassure patient and significant others that most people with MS do not become severely disabled. Encourage continued activity and normal life-style even when limitations are necessary.

Knowledge deficit: Precautions and potential side effects of prescribed medications

Desired outcome: By day 3 (or before hospital discharge), patient verbalizes accurate information about prescribed medications.

1. Provide patient with verbal instructions and written handouts that describe the name, purpose, dosage, drug/drug and food/drug interactions, and schedule of the prescribed medications.

2. For patients taking ACTH, prednisone, or dexamethasone, provide additional instructions for the following:
   - Common side effects: sodium and fluid retention, hypertension, gastric ulcers, stomach upset, weakness, hypokalemia, mood changes, impaired wound healing, and masking of infections.
   - Importance of monitoring weight and BP for evidence of fluid retention; taking the medication with food, milk, or buffering agents to help prevent gastric irritation; avoiding aspirin, indomethacin, caffeine, or other gas GI irritants while taking the medication; and tapering rather than abruptly stopping the drug when it is to be discontinued. Advise patient to report symptoms of potassium deficiency (e.g., anorexia, nausea, muscle weakness) and to eat foods high in potassium (see Table 3-2, p. 72). Encourage patient also to keep his or her diet low in sodium (see Table 1-4, p. 18, for a list of high-sodium foods that should be avoided) to minimize the potential for fluid retention. Monitor for and report black, tarry stools, which may signal occult blood. Follow-up with physician is important while patient is taking these drugs.

3. If patient is taking baclofen or dantrolene, provide instructions for the following:
   - Common side effects: drowsiness, dizziness, fatigue, nausea. In addition, dantrolene can cause diarrhea, muscle weakness, hepatitis, and photosensitivity.
   - Importance of taking the medication with food, milk, or a buffering agent to reduce gastric upset or nausea. Explain that although drowsiness is usually transient, patient should avoid activities that require alertness until the drug's effect on the central nervous system (CNS) is known. The patient also should avoid alcohol intake because of its additive CNS depression effects. Ba-

clofen can lower a person's seizure threshold and should be used cautiously in susceptible patients. Baclofen also may raise blood glucose levels, and individuals with diabetes mellitus may need an insulin dose adjustment. Monitor patients during transfers/ambulation initially, because some weak patients cannot tolerate the loss in spasticity that may be permitting them to bear weight. Patients taking dantrolene should monitor for and report fever, jaundice, dark urine, clay-colored stools, and itching (all of which signal hepatitis) or severe diarrhea; avoid exposure to the sun; and use sunscreens if exposure is unavoidable.

4. If bethanechol chloride has been prescribed, provide instructions for the following:
   - Common side effects: hypotension, diarrhea, abdominal cramps, urinary urgency, bronchoconstriction.
   - Importance of taking the drug on an empty stomach to avoid nausea and vomiting; notifying physician if lightheadedness occurs, because this can signal hypotension; and seeking medical attention if an asthmatic attack occurs. Caution patient to make position changes slowly and in stages to prevent fainting caused by orthostatic hypotension.

5. If patient is taking propantheline bromide, provide instructions for the following:
   - Common side effects: dryness of the mouth, blurred vision, constipation, palpitations, tachycardia, decreased sweating, and urinary retention or overflow incontinence.
   - Measures that relieve constipation; measures for remaining cool in hot or humid weather because heat stroke is more likely to develop with this medication; importance of notifying physician immediately if urinary retention or overflow incontinence occurs. In addition, if patient can chew and swallow effectively, explain that sugarless gum, hard candy, or artificial saliva products may reduce mouth dryness. Encourage slow position changes and monitoring for dizziness because postural hypotension may occur when the drug is first started.

Chronic pain and spasms related to motor and sensory nerve tract damage

Desired outcomes: Within 1-2 h of intervention, patient's subjective evaluation of pain and spasms improves, as documented by a pain scale. Objective indicators, such as grimacing, are absent or reduced.

1. Because heat tends to aggravate MS symptoms, maintain a comfortable room temperature. Advise patient to keep environment cool in warm weather and to avoid hot baths.

2. To reduce muscle tightness and spasms, provide passive, assisted, or active ROM exercises q2h and periodic stretching exercises. Teach these exercises to patient and significant others and encourage their performance several times daily. Explain that sleeping in a prone position may help reduce flexor spasms of the hips and knees.

3. Administer antispasmodics as prescribed.

4. For other interventions, see **Pain,** p. 201, in "General Care of Patients with Neurologic Disorders."

For patients undergoing plasmapheresis, see "Guillain-Barré Syndrome" for **Knowledge deficit:** Therapeutic plasma exchange procedure, p. 119.

See "Spinal Cord Injury" for **Constipation,** p. 143; **Risk for disuse syndrome,** p. 145; **Urinary retention** *or* **Reflex incontinence,** p. 148; and **Sexual dysfunction,** p. 152.

See "General Care of Patients with Neurologic Disorders" for **Risk for trauma,** p. 187; **Risk for injury,** p. 189; **Impaired corneal tissue integrity,** p. 189; **Altered nutrition:** Less than body requirements, p. 190; **Risk for fluid volume deficit,** p. 191; **Risk for aspiration,** p. 192; **Self-care deficit** related to spasticity, tremors, weakness, paresis, paralysis, or decreasing LOC secondary to sensorimotor deficits, p. 193; **Self-care deficit** (oral hygiene), p. 195; **Impaired verbal communication,** p. 195; **Constipation,** p. 196; **Sensory/perceptual alterations** (visual), p. 200; **Impaired swallowing,** p. 201; and **Knowledge deficit:** Neurologic diagnostic tests (for discussion of EEG, MRI study, CT scan, evoked potential studies, PET, and LP), p. 205.

For patients with impaired nutrition, see "Providing Nutritional Support," p. 378.

For patients who are immobile, see related nursing diagnoses in "Pressure Ulcers," p. 390, and in Appendix One, "Caring for Patients on Prolonged Bed Rest," p. 413.

For patients undergoing immunosuppressive drug or radiation therapy, see Appendix One, "Caring for Patients with Cancer and Other Life-Disrupting Illnesses," p. 423, and related psychosocial nursing diagnoses (p. 450) as appropriate.

PATIENT-FAMILY TEACHING
AND DISCHARGE PLANNING

The patient with MS may have a wide variety of symptoms that cause disability, ranging from mild to severe. Give patient and significant others verbal and written information about the following, as appropriate:

1. Remission/exacerbation aspects of the disease process. Explain the effects of demyelinization on sensory and motor function and factors that aggravate symptoms.
2. Referrals to community resources, such as local and national MS society chapters, public health nurse, Visiting Nurse Association, community support groups, social workers, psychological therapists, vocational rehabilitation agencies, home health agencies, extended and skilled care facilities, and financial counseling. The National Multiple Sclerosis Society can be reached at 733 Third Avenue, New York, NY 10017; phone: (800)-344-4867.
3. Safety measures relative to diminished sensation, visual disturbances, and motor deficits.
4. Medications, including drug name, purpose, dosage, schedule, precautions, drug/drug and food/drug interactions, and potential side effects.

5. Exercises that promote muscle strength and mobility; measures for preventing contractures and skin breakdown; transfer techniques and proper body mechanics; use of assistive devices and other measures to minimize neurologic deficits.

6. Measures for relieving pain, muscle spasms, or other discomfort.

7. Indications of constipation, urinary retention, or UTI; implementation of bowel and bladder training programs; self-catheterization technique or care of indwelling urinary catheters.

8. Indications of upper respiratory infection; implementation of measures that help prevent regurgitation, aspiration, and respiratory infection.

9. Dietary adjustments that may be appropriate for neurologic deficit (e.g., soft, semisolid foods for patients with chewing difficulties, or a high-fiber diet for patients experiencing constipation).

10. Importance of follow-up care, including visits to physician, PT, and OT, as well as speech, sexual, or psychologic counseling.

Guillain-Barré Syndrome

NURSING DIAGNOSES AND INTERVENTIONS

Ineffective breathing pattern related to neuromuscular weakness or paralysis of facial, throat, and respiratory muscles (severity of symptoms peaks around wk 1-3)

Desired outcome: Deterioration in patient's breathing pattern (e.g., Pao_2 <80 mm Hg, vital capacity <1 L [or <12-15 ml/kg], and tidal volume <75% of predicted value) is detected and reported promptly, resulting in immediate treatment.

1. Test for ascending loss of sensation by touching patient lightly with a pin or fingers at frequent intervals (hourly or more frequently initially). Assess from the level of the iliac crest upward toward the shoulders. Measure the highest level at which decreased sensation occurs. Decreased sensation frequently precedes motor weakness, so if it ascends to the level of the T8 dermatome, anticipate that intercostal muscles (used with respirations) soon will be impaired. Also monitor for upper arm and shoulder weakness, which precedes respiratory failure, by checking patient for arm drift and the ability to shrug the shoulders. To detect arm drift: Have patient hold both arms out in front of the body, level with the shoulders and with palms up. Instruct patient to close his or her eyes while holding this position. Weakness is present if one arm pronates or drifts down or out from its original position. Alert physician to significant findings.

2. Assist patient with oral intake to detect changes or difficulties that may indicate ascending paralysis. Assess patient q8h and before oral intake for cough reflexes, gag reflexes, and difficulty swallowing.

3. Observe patient for changes in LOC and orientation, which may signal reduced oxygenation to the brain. Monitor patient's respiratory rate, rhythm, and depth. Watch for use of accessory muscles, nasal flaring, dyspnea, shallow respirations, apnea, and loss of abdominal breathing. Auscultate for diminished breath sounds. Monitor patient for breathlessness while speaking. To ob-

Neurologic

serve for breathlessness, ask patient to take a deep breath and slowly count as high as possible. A reduced ability to count to a higher number before breathlessness occurs may signal grossly reduced ventilatory function. Alert physician to significant findings.

4. Monitor effectiveness of breathing by checking serial vital capacity results on pulmonary function tests. If vital capacity is <1 L or is rapidly trending downward, or if patient exhibits signs of hypoxia (e.g., tachycardia, increasing restlessness, mental dullness, or cyanosis), report findings immediately to physician.

5. Monitor ABGs and pulse oximetry to detect hypoxia or hypercapnia.

6. Raise HOB to promote optimal chest excursion.

7. Patient may require tracheostomy, endotracheal intubation, or mechanical ventilation to support respiratory function. Prepare patient emotionally for such procedures or for eventual transfer to ICU or transition care unit for closer monitoring.

8. For other interventions, see **Risk for aspiration** in "General Care of Patients with Neurologic Disorders," p. 192.

Risk for disuse syndrome related to paralysis/immobilization secondary to neuromuscular impairment and prolonged bed rest

Desired outcome: Patient exhibits complete (or baseline) ROM in all joints without subjective or objective indicators of pain.

1. Assess functional ability on a regular basis and at least daily; compare to baseline. Consult physician about significant findings.

2. Perform passive ROM and avoid active exercise during acute phase of Guillain-Barré syndrome (G-BS). Vigorous exercise may exacerbate symptoms and prolong recovery by increasing the time needed for remyelinization.

3. Coordinate care to ensure a balance between activity and rest.

4. Elevate extremities above heart level, if possible, to prevent or reduce edema.

5. For other interventions, see this nursing diagnosis in Appendix One, "Caring for Patients on Prolonged Bed Rest," p. 416.

Pain related to muscle tenderness; hypersensitivity to touch; or discomfort in shoulders, thighs, and back

Desired outcomes: Within 1-2 h of intervention, patient's subjective perception of discomfort decreases, as documented by a pain scale. Objective indicators, such as grimacing, are absent or diminished.

1. For patients with muscle tenderness, consider use of massage, moist heat packs, cold application, or warm baths, which may be very soothing for muscles.

2. For patients with hypersensitivity, assess amount of touch that can be tolerated and incorporate this information into patient's plan of care.

3. Reposition patient often to reduce muscle tension and fatigue. Some individuals find that a supine "frog leg" position is particularly comfortable.

4. Provide passive ROM to reduce joint stiffness.

5. For other interventions, see this nursing diagnosis in "General Care of Patients with Neurologic Disorders," p. 201.

Altered cardiopulmonary and cerebral tissue perfusion (or risk for same) related to interrupted sympathetic outflow with concomitant BP fluctuations secondary to autonomic dysfunction

Desired outcomes: When underlying autonomic dysfunction ceases (usually in about 2 wk), patient has optimal cardiopulmonary and cerebral tissue perfusion, as evidenced by systolic BP $\geq$90 mm Hg and $\leq$160 mm Hg, and orientation to time, place, and person. BP fluctuations, if they occur, are detected and reported promptly.

1. Monitor BP, noting wide fluctuations; report significant findings to physician. Changes in BP that result in severe hypotension or hypertension may occur because of unopposed sympathetic outflow or loss of outflow to the peripheral nervous system, causing changes in vascular tone. Short-acting hypertensive agents may be required for persistent hypertension.
2. Monitor carefully for changes during activities such as coughing, suctioning, position changes, or straining at stool.
3. For patients with hypotension or postural hypotension, see this nursing diagnosis in "Spinal Cord Injury," p. 150.

Altered nutrition: Less than body requirements, related to adynamic ileus

Desired outcome: Patient has adequate nutrition as evidenced by maintenance of baseline body weight.

1. Auscultate abdominal sounds, noting presence, absence, or changes that may signal onset of ileus. Be alert for abdominal distention or tenderness, nausea and vomiting, and absence of stool output. Consult physician about significant findings.
2. Patients with adynamic ileus generally require gastric suctioning to decompress the stomach. Because these patients cannot take foods orally, parenteral nutrition may be required (see "Providing Nutritional Support," p. 378).
3. For general interventions, see **Altered nutrition,** p. 190, in "General Care of Patients with Neurologic Disorders."

Fear related to threat to biologic integrity

Desired outcome: Within 24 h of this diagnosis, patient verbalizes known sources of fear and attainment of increased psychologic and physical comfort.

1. For a patient in whom the neurologic deficit is still progressing, arrange for a transfer to a room close to the nurses' station to help alleviate the fear of being suddenly incapacitated and helpless.
2. Be sure patient's call light is within easy reach. Frequently assess patient's ability to use it.
3. Provide continuity of patient care through assignment of staff and use of care plan.
4. Perform assessments at frequent intervals, letting patient know you are there. Provide care in a calm, reassuring manner.
5. For other interventions, see **Fear** in Appendix One, "Caring for Patients with Cancer and Other Life-Disrupting Illnesses," p. 454.

Knowledge deficit: Therapeutic plasma exchange procedure

Desired outcome: Before scheduled date of each procedure, patient verbalizes accurate information about plasma exchange procedure.

Neurologic

1. Before plasma exchange procedure, patient's physician will explain the reason for the procedure, its risks, and anticipated benefits or outcome. Determine patient's level of understanding of physician's explanation and clarify or reinforce information accordingly.

2. Determine patient's past experience with plasmapheresis, the positive or negative effects, and the nature of any fears or concerns. Document and communicate this information to others involved in patient's care.

3. Explain in words patient can understand that the goal of plasma exchange is to remove autoimmune factors from the blood to reduce or eliminate patient's symptoms. The antibodies to the patient's peripheral and cranial nerve tissue are reduced by the removal of the plasma portion of the blood, which contains the circulating antibodies. The procedure is similar to hemodialysis. Blood is removed from the patient and separated into its components. Patient's plasma is discarded, and the other blood components (e.g., RBCs, WBCs, platelets) are saved and returned to the patient with donor plasma or replacement fluid. If started within 1-2 wk of the onset of G-BS symptoms, the exchange process seems to reduce the duration and severity of the disease. Multiple exchanges over a period of weeks can be expected.

4. Patient is at risk for the following complications during this procedure: fluid volume deficit, hypotension, hypokalemia, hypocalcemia, cardiac dysrhythmias, clotting disorders, anemia, phlebitis, infection, hypothermia, and air embolism. Explain these complications accordingly.

5. This procedure requires good blood flow. Inform patient that the antecubital vein most often is used as the access site, but if patient has poor peripheral veins, the physician may need to insert a central intravenous line or a femoral catheter. If the antecubital site is used, post a sign alerting others not to use this site for routine laboratory sticks.

6. Explain that patient can expect the procedure to take 2-4 h, although it may take considerably longer, depending on the condition of patient's veins, blood flow, and Hct level.

7. Explain that patient can expect preprocedural and postprocedural blood work for clotting factors and electrolyte levels. Patient may be placed on cardiac monitoring to assess for electrolyte imbalance, particularly if he or she is taking prednisone or digitalis. Weight and VS will be checked before and after the procedure, with frequent VS checks during the process. Calcium gluconate or potassium chloride may be administered to correct electrolyte imbalances.

8. Instruct patient to report chills, fever, hives, sweating, or lightheadedness, which may signal reaction to donor plasma.

9. Teach patient to report thirst, faintness, or dizziness, which can occur with hypotension or hypovolemia. Patient should take oral fluids during procedure, if possible.

10. Instruct patient to report numbness or tingling around lips or in the hands, arms, and legs; muscle twitching; cramping; or tetany,

which can occur with hypocalcemia. Fatigue, nausea, weakness, or cramping may signal hypokalemia.

11. Inform patient that medications may be held until after procedure to prevent their removal from the blood.

12. If patient does not have a urinary catheter, remind him or her to void before and during the procedure, if necessary, to avoid any mild hypotension caused by a full bladder. I&O will be monitored closely, because decreased urine output may signal hypovolemia.

13. Explain that patient's temperature will be checked during the procedure, and warm blankets will be provided to prevent hypothermia.

14. Explain that patient probably will feel fatigued 1-2 days after procedure because of decreased plasma protein levels. Encourage extra rest and a high-protein diet during this time.

15. Teach patient to monitor IV access site for signs of infection (e.g., warmth, redness, swelling, or drainage) and to report significant findings.

16. Teach patient to monitor for signs of bruising or bleeding. The anticoagulant citrate dextrose, used in the extracorporeal machine circuitry to prevent clotting, may cause excessive bleeding at the access site. A pressure dressing may be kept in place over the access site for 2-4 h after the procedure. Caution patient to avoid cutting himself or herself or bumping into objects and to sustain pressure over cuts. Inform patient that black, tarry stools usually signal the presence of blood and should be reported.

For patients with urinary incontinence or retention, neurogenic bladder, or urinary tract infection (UTI), see related discussions in Chapter 3, "Renal-Urinary Disorders."

For patients with autonomic dysfunction, see "Spinal Cord Injury" for **Altered peripheral and cardiopulmonary tissue perfusion,** p. 151. See "General Care of Patients with Neurologic Disorders" for **Risk for trauma,** p. 187; **Risk for injury,** p. 189; **Impaired corneal tissue integrity,** p. 189; **Risk for fluid volume deficit,** p. 191; **Self-care deficit** related to spasticity, tremors, weakness, paresis, paralysis, or decreasing LOC secondary to sensorimotor deficits, p. 193; **Self-care deficit** (oral hygiene), p. 195; **Impaired verbal communication,** p. 195; **Constipation,** p. 196; **Sensory/perceptual alterations** (visual), p. 200; **Impaired swallowing,** p. 201; **Altered body temperature,** p. 204; and **Knowledge deficit:** Neurologic diagnostic tests, p. 205.

For patients who are immobile, see related nursing diagnoses in "Pressure Ulcers," p. 390, and in Appendix One, "Caring for Patients on Prolonged Bed Rest," p. 413.

For patients undergoing immunosuppressive drug therapy, see Appendix One, "Caring for Patients with Cancer and Other Life-Disrupting Illnesses," p. 423, and related psychosocial nursing diagnoses (p. 450) as appropriate.

PATIENT-FAMILY TEACHING
AND DISCHARGE PLANNING

Most patients with G-BS eventually recover fully, but because the recovery can be prolonged, the patient often goes home with some degree of neurologic deficit. Discharge planning and teaching will vary according to the degree of disability. Give patient and significant others verbal and written information about the following, as appropriate:

1. The disease process, expected improvement, and importance of continuing in the rehabilitation or PT program to promote as full a recovery as possible.
2. Referrals to community resources, such as public health nurse, Visiting Nurse Association, community support groups, social workers, psychologic therapy, home health agencies, and extended and skilled care facilities. The Guillain-Barré Syndrome Foundation International can be contacted at Box 262, Wynnewood, PA 19096, (215)-667-0131.
3. Safety measures relative to the sensorimotor deficit.
4. Exercises that promote muscle strength and mobility; measures for preventing contractures and skin breakdown; transfer techniques and proper body mechanics; and use of assistive devices.
5. Indications of constipation, urinary retention, or UTI; implementation of bowel and bladder training programs; and, if appropriate, care of indwelling catheters or self-catheterization technique.
6. Indications of URI; measures for preventing regurgitation, aspiration, and respiratory infection.
7. Medications, including drug name, purpose, dosage, schedule, precautions, drug/drug and food/drug interactions, and potential side effects.
8. Importance of follow-up care, including visits to physician, PT, and OT.

Bacterial Meningitis

NURSING DIAGNOSES AND INTERVENTIONS

Knowledge deficit: Side effects and precautions for prescribed antibiotics

Desired outcome: Before beginning medication regimen, patient and significant others verbalize knowledge about potential side effects and precautions for prescribed antibiotics.

1. For significant others and contacts placed on prophylactic rifampin, explain the prescribed dosage and schedule. Rifampin should be taken 1 h before meals for maximum absorption. Emphasize the importance of taking this drug as a preventive measure against meningitis, and describe potential side effects (e.g., nausea, vomiting, diarrhea, orange urine, headache, dizziness). Caution against wearing contact lenses, because the drug will permanently color them orange. In addition, rifampin reduces the effectiveness of oral contraceptives and is contraindicated during pregnancy.
2. Instruct significant others and patient's other contacts who are taking rifampin to report the onset of jaundice (yellow skin or sclera), allergic reactions, and persistence of GI side effects.
3. For other interventions, see **Knowledge deficit:** Side effects of prolonged use of potent antibiotics, p. 317, in "Osteomyelitis."

Knowledge deficit: Rationale and procedure for proper infection management techniques

Desired outcome: Before visitation, patient and significant others verbalize knowledge about rationale for infection management and comply with prescribed restrictions and precautions.

N O T E : Patients with meningitis caused by *Neisseria meningitidis, Haemophilus influenzae,* or an unidentified organism are placed in private rooms and require special isolation precautions for 24 h after appropriate antibiotic therapy is begun. Masks should be worn and other infection management procedures observed.

---

1. For patients with meningitis caused by *H. influenzae* or *N. meningitidis,* explain the method of disease transmission *via* airborne droplets and oral secretions and the rationale for private room and special precautions.
2. Provide instructions for covering the mouth before coughing or sneezing and for properly disposing of tissue.
3. Instruct patients with specific respiratory precautions to stay in their rooms. If they must leave the room for a procedure or test, explain that a mask must be worn to protect others from contact with airborne droplets.
4. For individuals in contact with the patient, explain the importance of wearing a surgical mask and using good handwashing technique. Gloves should be worn when handling any body fluid, especially oral secretions. For more information, see Appendix Two, "Infection Prevention and Control," p. 479.
5. Reassure patient that special respiratory precautions are temporary and will be discontinued after patient has been taking the appropriate antibiotic for 24-48 h.

Pain related to headache, photophobia, and neck stiffness secondary to meningitis

Desired outcomes: Within 1-2 h of intervention, patient's subjective perception of discomfort decreases, as documented by a pain scale. Objective indicators, such as grimacing, are absent or diminished.

1. Provide a quiet environment and darken room. Restrict visitors as necessary to reduce noise. Sunglasses may promote relief from photophobia.
2. Promote bed rest and assist with ADLs as needed to reduce movement that may cause pain.
3. Apply an ice bag to the head or cool cloth to the eyes to help diminish headache.
4. Support patient in a comfortable position. Many patients with meningitis are comfortable in a position with the head in extension and the body slightly curled. HOB elevated to 30 degrees also may help. Keep neck in alignment during position changes.
5. Provide gentle, passive ROM and massage to neck and shoulder joints and muscles to help relieve stiffness. If patient is afebrile, apply moist heat to neck and back to promote muscle relaxation and reduce pain.

6. Patients tend to be hyperirritable, with hyperalgesia. Sounds are loud. Keep communication simple and direct, using a soft, calm tone of voice. Touching startles the patient. Avoid needless stimulation; consolidate activities. Loosen constricting bed clothing. Avoid restraining patient. Reduce stimulation to minimal amount needed to accomplish required activity.
7. For other interventions, see this nursing diagnosis in "General Care of Patients with Neurologic Disorders," p. 201.

Risk for trauma related to oral, musculoskeletal, and airway vulnerability secondary to seizure activity

Desired outcomes: Patient shows no signs of oral or musculoskeletal injury or airway compromise after seizure. Significant others verbalize knowledge of actions necessary during seizure activity.
1. Monitor for twitching of hands, feet, or mouth. Twitching signals generalized CNS irritability and may herald the onset of seizures. This sign requires further evaluation and possible intervention to prevent complications.
2. For other interventions, see this nursing diagnosis in "Seizure Disorders," p. 179.

See "Head Injury" for **Risk for disuse syndrome**, p. 156, and **Fluid volume excess**, p. 158. See "Seizure Disorders" for **Impaired tissue integrity**, p. 181.

See "General Care of Patients with Neurologic Disorders" for **Risk for trauma**, p. 187; **Risk for injury**, p. 189; **Impaired corneal tissue integrity**, p. 189; **Altered nutrition:** Less than body requirements, p. 190; **Risk for fluid volume deficit**, p. 191; **Risk for aspiration**, p. 192; **Self-care deficit** related to spasticity, tremors, weakness, paresis, paralysis, or decreasing LOC secondary to sensorimotor deficits, p. 193; **Self-care deficit** (oral hygiene), p. 195; **Constipation**, p. 196; **Decreased adaptive capacity:** Intracranial, p. 197; **Impaired swallowing**, p. 201; **Altered body temperature**, p. 204; and **Knowledge deficit:** Neurologic diagnostic tests, p. 205.

For patients who need nutritional support, see nursing diagnoses in "Providing Nutritional Support," p. 378.

For patients who are immobile, see related nursing diagnoses in "Pressure Ulcers," p. 390, and in Appendix One, "Caring for Patients on Prolonged Bed Rest," p. 413. Also see Appendix One, "Caring for Patients with Cancer and Other Life-Disrupting Illnesses," p. 450, for appropriate patient and family psychosocial nursing diagnoses and interventions.

PATIENT-FAMILY TEACHING
AND DISCHARGE PLANNING

The extent of teaching and discharge planning will depend on whether the patient has any residual damage. As appropriate, give patient and significant others verbal and written information about the following:
1. Referrals to community resources, such as public health nurse, Visiting Nurse Association, community support groups, social workers,

psychologic therapy, vocational rehabilitation agency, home health agencies, and extended and skilled care facilities.

2. Importance of reporting promptly the following indicators of meningitis: severe headache, fever, photophobia, neck stiffness.

3. Drug name, purpose, dosage, schedule, precautions, drug/drug and food/drug interactions, potential side effects for patient's medications and for antibiotics taken prophylactically by family and significant others.

IN ADDITION

4. For patients with residual neurologic deficits, teach the following as appropriate: exercises that promote muscle strength and mobility; measures for preventing contractures and skin breakdown; transfer techniques and proper body mechanics; safety measures if patient has decreased pain and sensation or visual disturbances; use of assistive devices; indications of constipation, urinary retention, or UTI; bowel and bladder training programs; self-catheterization technique or care of indwelling catheters; and seizure precautions if indicated.

SECTION TWO: DEGENERATIVE DISORDERS OF THE NERVOUS SYSTEM

Parkinsonism

NURSING DIAGNOSES AND INTERVENTIONS

Risk for trauma related to unsteady gait secondary to bradykinesis, tremors, and rigidity

Desired outcome: After instruction, patient demonstrates effective ambulatory techniques and measures to prevent falls and remains free of trauma

1. During ambulation, encourage patient to swing arms to assist gait, and to raise feet and elevate toes with each step to help prevent falls. Instruct these patients to step over an imaginary object or line, which will help them raise their feet higher and increase their stride.

2. Have patient practice movements that are especially difficult (e.g., turning). Teach patient to walk in a wide arc, rather than pivoting, when turning and to avoid crossing one leg over the other.

3. Teach patient head and neck exercises to help improve posture. Remind patient repeatedly to maintain an upright posture, especially when walking.

4. Advise patient to stop occasionally to slow down walking speed. Teach patients to concentrate on listening to their feet as they touch the floor and to count the cadence to prevent too fast a gait.

Encourage patient to lift toes and to walk with the heel touching the floor first.

5. Remind patient to maintain a wide-based gait.
6. Provide a clear pathway while patient is walking. Teach patient to avoid crowds, scatter rugs, uneven surfaces, fast turns, narrow doorways, and obstructions.
7. Encourage patient to perform ROM and stretching exercises daily and to exercise for flexibility, strength, gait, and balance. Emphasize that routine exercises, along with prescribed medications, may prevent or delay disability.
8. Advise patient to wear leather- or smooth-soled shoes, but to test the shoes to make sure the soles are not too slippery. Rubber- or crepe-soled shoes grip floors and may cause falls.
9. Encourage patient not to hurry or rush, because this may result in falls. A slow gait and an inability to get to the bathroom fast enough may cause incontinence. Encourage men to keep a urinal at bedside; a bedside commode may be helpful for women.
10. For other interventions, see **Risk for trauma** in "General Care of Patients with Neurologic Disorders," p. 187.

Health-seeking behaviors: Methods for overcoming difficulty initiating movement

Desired outcome: After instruction, patient demonstrates measures that enhance his or her ability to initiate desired movement.

1. Instruct patient that rocking from side to side may help initiate leg movement. Marching in place a few steps before resuming forward motion also may be helpful. Other measures that may help patient become "unglued" are relaxing back on the heels and raising the toes; tapping the hip of the leg to be moved; bending at the knees and straightening up; or raising the arms in a sudden, short motion. If patient's feet remain "glued" to the floor, suggest that he or she think of something else for a few moments and then try again.
2. Teach patients this method for getting out of a chair: slide to the edge of the seat and place the hands on the arm supports; bend forward slightly and move the feet back; then, rhythmically rock back and forth in the chair a few times before trying to get up. Advise patients to use chairs with a back and arms and to buy elevated toilet seats or to install sidebars in the bathroom to assist with rising and to help prevent falls.
3. Teach patient measures that may help with getting out of bed: rocking to a sitting position, placing a block under legs at head of bed to elevate HOB, and tying a rope to the foot of the bed so that patient can pull himself or herself up.
4. "Freezing" can fluctuate with stress or patient's emotional state. Teach patients and significant others to recognize situations that can cause freezing and to plan to avoid them. For example, attempting two movements simultaneously (e.g., trying to change direction quickly while walking) can cause freezing; teach patient to break actions into separate components and to do one thing at a time. Dis-

tracting environmental, visual, or auditory stimuli also can cause freezing. Doorways, narrow passages, or a change in the floor's color, texture, or slope can pose problems for many patients.

Knowledge deficit: Side effects of and precautionary measures for taking antiparkinson medications

Desired outcome: After instruction and before hospital discharge, patient and significant others verbalize knowledge about the side effects of and necessary precautionary measures for taking antiparkinson medications.

N O T E :   Teach patient and significant others to report adverse side effects promptly, because many side effects are dose related and can be controlled by adjusting the dosage.

SIDE EFFECTS COMMON TO MOST ANTIPARKINSON MEDICATIONS

1. Stress the importance of taking medication on schedule and not forgetting a dose. Missing a dose may adversely affect mobility. Patient and physician can adjust the dose schedule so that the medication peaks at mealtime or times when patient needs mobility most.

2. Teach patient to take medications with meals to reduce the potential for nausea and stomach upset. Encourage patient with anorexia to eat frequent, small, nutritious snacks and meals.

3. Advise patients to counteract orthostatic hypotension by making position changes slowly and in stages. Teach patient to dangle legs a few minutes before standing. Antiembolism hose may help some patients. Encourage men patients to urinate from a sitting rather than standing position if possible. Report dizziness to physician.

4. To ease dry mouth and maintain the integrity of the oral mucous membrane, teach patient to use sugarless chewing gum or hard candy, frequent mouth rinses with water, or artificial saliva products.

5. Advise patient to report any urinary hesitancy or incontinence because this may signal urinary retention. Individuals taking anticholinergics may find that voiding before taking the medication relieves this problem. See "Urinary Retention," p. 99, for additional measures.

6. Constipation is a common problem with these medications. For interventions, see **Constipation,** p. 409, in Appendix One, "Caring for Patients on Prolonged Bed Rest."

7. Many of these drugs can cause or aggravate mental status changes (e.g., confusion, mental slowness or dullness) and even agitation, paranoia, and hallucinations. Teach patient to report these signs to physician promptly for possible dosage adjustment.

8. For patient with blurred vision, orient to surroundings, identify yourself when entering the room, keep walkways unobstructed, and encourage patient to ask for assistance when ambulating.

SIDE EFFECTS SPECIFIC TO LEVODOPA

1. Teach patient to avoid vitamin preparations or fortified cereals that contain pyridoxine (vitamin B_6), which reduces the effectiveness of levodopa. The physician may limit patient's intake of foods

high in pyridoxine (e.g., wheat germ, whole grain cereals, legumes, liver).

2. Teach patient that a diet high in protein may interfere with the effectiveness of levodopa. Although the diet should meet the RDA for protein (i.e., 0.8 g/kg body weight), the patient should avoid eating excessive amounts of meat, eggs, dairy products, and legumes. If possible, virtually all protein should be eaten at the evening meal to minimize interaction with levodopa.

3. Instruct patient to report muscle twitching or spasmodic winking because these are early signs of overdose.

4. Abnormal involuntary movements such as facial grimacing and tongue protusion signal that an adjustment in dose may be needed. The physician may prescribe a reduced dose, redistribution throughout the day, or a medically supervised drug holiday.

5. Explain signs and symptoms of parkinsonian crisis (i.e., sudden and severe increase in bradykinesia, muscle rigidity, and tremors). Emphasize the need for immediate medical intervention with this crisis, because respiratory and cardiac support may be necessary. Teach patient that to avoid this crisis, it is necessary to take levodopa as scheduled and not to stop the medication abruptly. Teach significant others what to do if parkinsonian crisis occurs; that is, to keep patient in a quiet, calm environment with subdued lighting until medical help arrives.

6. Explain the signs of the on-off response (i.e., patient relatively mobile one minute and completely immobile the next) and the importance of seeking medical intervention should they occur. Titrating the dose, spacing the doses differently, using sustained-release forms of levodopa, and combining levodopa with other antiparkinson medications may be prescribed to counter the on-off effect. If these interventions are ineffective, a medically supervised drug holiday may be prescribed.

7. Monitor for behavioral changes. Levodopa can cause severe depression with suicidal overtones, which should be reported immediately. The physician may prescribe a dose reduction or, if this is ineffective, a medically supervised drug holiday.

8. Explain that patient's medication may cause dark-colored urine and sweat.

9. Caution patient to avoid alcohol because it impairs levodopa's effectiveness.

10. Explain the importance of medical follow-up while taking this drug to monitor for such problems as increased intraocular pressure and changes in glucose control.

SIDE EFFECTS SPECIFIC TO AMANTADINE

1. Teach patient that taking this drug earlier in the day may prevent insomnia.

2. Teach patient and significant others to monitor for and report any SOB, peripheral edema, significant weight gain, or change in mental status because these often signal congestive heart failure.

3. Instruct patient not to stop taking this medication abruptly because doing so may precipitate parkinsonian crisis.
4. A diffuse, rose-colored mottling of the skin, usually confined to the lower extremities, may develop. The condition may subside with continued therapy and disappears in a few weeks to months after the drug is discontinued. Exposure to cold or standing may make the color more prominent. Teach patient to report this condition if it occurs, but reassure him or her that the condition is more cosmetic than serious.
5. Patients with a history of seizures may have an increase in the number of seizures. Instruct patient to monitor and promptly report to physician a loss of seizure control.
6. Caution patient to avoid alcohol and CNS depressants because these agents potentiate the effects of amantadine.
7. Explain that most side effects of amantadine are dose related.

SIDE EFFECTS SPECIFIC TO DOPAMINE AGONISTS
1. Caution patient to avoid alcohol when taking this medication because he or she will experience less tolerance.
2. Bromocriptine can cause digital vasospasm. Teach patient to avoid exposure to cold and to report the onset of finger or toe pallor.

SIDE EFFECTS SPECIFIC TO ANTICHOLINERGIC MEDICATIONS
1. Teach patient that this medication may reduce perspiration. Explain that patient should avoid strenuous exercise and keep cool during the summer to avoid heat stroke.
2. Teach patient not to stop taking this medication abruptly because doing so can result in parkinsonian crisis.
3. Teach patient to monitor for tachycardia or palpitation and to report either condition.

SIDE EFFECTS SPECIFIC TO SELEGILINE HYDROCHLORIDE (ELDEPRYL)
1. Stress the importance of taking this medication only in the prescribed dosage. Selegiline is a selective MAO type B inhibitor, and in the recommended dosage of ≤10 mg/day does not cause the hypertensive crisis that can occur when tyramine-containing foods (e.g., cheese, red wine, beer, and yogurt) are eaten. Dosages >10 mg/day may result in hypertension if these foods are eaten. Usually, dietary modifications to reduce intake of tyramine-containing foods are recommended, but they are not imperative.
2. Avoiding meperidine and other opioids is suggested. At recommended doses, no drug interactions have been noted. However, fatal drug interactions have occurred with patients taking other nonselective MAO inhibitors and could conceivably occur if higher than recommended doses were taken.
3. Teach patient that taking the drug earlier in the day may prevent insomnia.

Health-seeking behaviors: Facial and tongue exercises that enhance verbal communication and help prevent choking

Desired outcome: After the demonstration and within the 24 h before hospital discharge, patient demonstrates facial and tongue exercises and states the rationale for their use.

1. Explain to patient that special exercises can help strengthen and control facial and tongue muscles, which in turn will improve verbal communication and help prevent choking. Emphasize that routine exercises of the facial and tongue muscles, along with the prescribed medications, may prevent or delay disability.

2. Teach patient the following exercises, and have patient return the demonstration: hold a sound for 5 sec, sing the scale, read aloud, recite the alphabet, count, and extend the tongue and try to touch the chin, nose, and cheek. Encourage patient to practice increasing voice volume, to vary voice pitch and inflection, and to exaggerate facial motion and articulation. Advise patient to practice making faces in front of a mirror.

3. Provide a written handout that lists and describes the preceding exercises. Encourage patient to perform them hourly while awake.

4. Teach patient the importance of stating feelings verbally because monotone speech and lack of facial expression impede nonverbal communication.

Knowledge deficit: Adrenal brain graft surgery

Desired outcome: Before procedure, patient verbalizes accurate information about adrenal brain graft surgery.

1. Determine patient's level of understanding of the procedure. As indicated, explain that the surgery involves grafting one of patient's own adrenal medullary glands to the caudate nucleus of the brain. The medullary portion of the adrenal gland produces dopamine for the peripheral nervous system. When grafted, the adrenal medullary gland may continue to produce dopamine in the CNS, thereby reducing or eliminating the symptoms of Parkinson's disease or the need for medication. The graft involves three surgeries: (1) stereotaxic localization of the caudate nucleus, (2) craniotomy, and (3) laparotomy to obtain the adrenal gland, which is positioned atop the kidney.

2. Explain that patient may have to undergo laboratory tests and CT scan to determine if both adrenal glands are normal because the unharvested gland will have to compensate for both.

3. Also explain that patient may undergo cerebral blood flow tests (see discussions of "Digital Subtraction Angiography," p. 208, and "Cerebral Angiography," p. 209) to evaluate perfusion of brain tissue and thus ensure adequate oxygenation and nutrients for healing. The patient also may require several lumbar punctures to obtain cerebrospinal fluid (CSF) for testing levels of monoamine, a metabolite of dopamine. Comparing serial postoperative values to baseline values gives an indication of graft viability.

4. Teach patient how to splint the laparotomy site to reduce pain. Inform patient that the wound will be monitored at scheduled intervals for signs of bleeding. A purple coloration of the flank may signal retroperitoneal hematoma.

5. Patient will be monitored after surgery for endocrine effects that signal nonfunctioning of the remaining adrenal gland, including hy-

poglycemia, hyperkalemia, and hypervolemia. Teach patient to report headache, irritability, weakness, thirst, nausea, anorexia, or intractable abdominal pain.

6. For additional interventions, see "Brain Tumors" for **Knowledge deficit:** Craniotomy procedure, p. 161.

See "General Care of Patients with Neurologic Disorders" for **Impaired corneal tissue integrity,** p. 189; **Altered nutrition,** p. 190; **Risk for fluid volume deficit,** p. 191; **Risk for aspiration,** p. 192; **Self-care deficit,** p. 193; **Impaired verbal communication,** p. 195; **Constipation,** p. 196; **Impaired swallowing,** p. 201; and **Knowledge deficit:** Neurologic diagnostic tests, p. 205.

For patients with varying degrees of immobility, refer to p. 390, related nursing diagnoses in "Pressure Ulcers," and Appendix One, "Caring for Patients on Prolonged Bed Rest," p. 413.

For patients undergoing surgery, see Appendix One, "Caring for Preoperative and Postoperative Patients," p. 395.

Also see Appendix One, "Caring for Patients with Cancer and Other Life-Disrupting Illnesses," p. 450, for psychosocial nursing diagnoses and interventions for patients and significant others as appropriate.

PATIENT-FAMILY TEACHING
AND DISCHARGE PLANNING

Give patient and significant others verbal and written information about the following:

1. Referrals to community resources, such as local and national Parkinson's Society chapters, public health nurse, Visiting Nurse Association, community support groups, social workers, psychologic therapy, dietitian, vocational rehabilitation agency, home health agencies, and extended and skilled care facilities. Provide these addresses and phone numbers: American Parkinson Disease Association, 60 Bay Street, Staten Island, NY 10301 *phone:* (212)-732-9550 or (800)-223-APDA; United Parkinson's Foundation, 833 West Washington Blvd., Chicago, IL 60607 *phone:* (312)-733-1893; Parkinson's Disease Foundation, Inc., 710 West 168th Street, New York, NY 10032 *phone:* (212)-923-4700 or (800)-457-6676; and the National Parkinson Foundation, Inc., 1501 NW 9th Avenue, Miami, FL 33136 *in Florida:* (800)-433-7022, *all other states:* (800)-327-4545.

2. Related safety measures for patients with bradykinesis, muscle rigidity, and tremors.

3. Emphasis that disability may be prevented or delayed through exercises and medications.

4. Techniques for unlocking a position (see p. 126).

5. Evaluation of home environment and tips for preventing accidents in the home.

6. Measures to prevent or lessen postural hypotension.

7. Signs and symptoms of parkinsonian crisis (see p. 128) and the need for immediate medical attention.
8. For other interventions, see Patient-Family Teaching and Discharge Planning (third through tenth entries) in "Multiple Sclerosis," p. 116.

Alzheimer's Disease

NURSING DIAGNOSES AND INTERVENTIONS

Risk for trauma related to lack of awareness of environmental hazards secondary to cognitive deficit

Desired outcomes: Patient is free of symptoms of physical trauma. At least 24 h before hospital discharge, significant others identify and plan to eliminate or control potentially dangerous factors in patient's home environment.

1. Orient patient to new surroundings. Reorient as needed. Keep necessary items, including water, telephone, and call light, within easy reach. Assess patient's ability to use these items. Keep bed in its lowest position. Side rail position (up or down) will vary with patient. Patient may be at risk of falling from climbing over side rails.
2. Maintain an uncluttered environment to minimize risk of environmental confusion and tripping. Ensure adequate lighting to help prevent falls in the dark.
3. Prevent exposure to hot food or equipment that can burn the skin. Discourage use of heating pads. Check temperature of heating device and bathwater before patient is exposed to them.
4. Encourage patient to use low-heeled, nonskid shoes for walking. Teach use of wide-based gait to give unsteady patients a broader base of support. Assess patient for ataxia, and assist with walking as necessary. Use gestures or turn patient's body in the direction he or she is to go. Canes and walkers may be too complicated for patients with Alzheimer's disease.
5. Request that significant others assist with watching restless patients. Provide attendant care if necessary. Avoid restraining patient because this usually increases agitation. If restraints must be used, reassure patient that he or she is not being punished, that you are trying to help him or her regain control, and that the restraints will be removed when the staff is certain the patient will not cause self-injury. **Note:** For many people with Alzheimer's disease, walking reduces agitation.
6. Check patient at frequent intervals. If necessary, move patient closer to nursing station, away from stairways or unit exits, or seat patient in a chair at nursing station. Consider obtaining a picture of patient to assist in a search if necessary.
7. Watch for nonverbal clues of pain or distress (e.g., restlessness, wincing, wrinkled brow, cautious breathing, rapid or shallow breathing, poor appetite, crying). Report significant findings.
8. Try to make tubes as unobtrusive as possible to prevent removal. Place IV tubing high on dominant arm. Dress patient in long-sleeved gown with a cuff, with IV tubing going up the arm and out

the neck. Place binders over dressing to help prevent picking. Position hand splints to eliminate pincer grasp.

SUGGESTIONS FOR HOME SAFETY

1. Encourage significant others to evaluate home environment carefully for potential safety hazards. Caution them to remove harmful objects (e.g., matches and scissors) from bedside and to store medications and chemicals (e.g., insect spray, cleaning supplies, lighter fluid) in locked cabinets to prevent accidental ingestion because these patients tend to put objects in their mouths. Remove plants that are toxic, plastic fruit, and toiletries because patient may attempt to eat them. The temperature of the home hot water heater should be turned down to prevent accidental scalding. Lock up hazardous power tools, lawn mowers, or kitchen appliances. Place gates or guardrails on porches as needed. Safety plugs should be placed in electrical outlets. Handrails and grab bars also may be helpful. Remind significant others to check the house carefully before leaving because patient may leave the stove on or water running. It may be necessary to remove knobs from stove burners and the oven.

2. Advise significant others to dress these individuals according to the physical environment and individual need. These patients may not know or be able to communicate whether they are too cold or too warm.

3. Advise significant others to keep patient's home environment simple and familiar. Rearranging furniture can increase patient's confusion and the potential for falls. Encourage use of nightlights in patient's home.

4. If patient tends to wander, encourage significant others to have an identification bracelet made with patient's name, phone number, and diagnosis. An identifying label can be sewn into clothes. Alert neighbors and local police to call if they notice patient wandering. Keep a good current picture of patient available to help in searching in case he or she becomes lost. Covering door handles with cloth hangings or pictures may be sufficient to prevent patient from exiting. Locks on doors to keep patient inside may be necessary but should not require a key, because this may hamper escape in case of fire. Door or exit alarms can be installed on home doors. Daily walks or exercise tends to reduce wandering.

5. Caution significant others that patients who are disoriented should be allowed to smoke only while being observed. Advise them to get a smoke detector and take control of matches.

6. Advise significant others that patient should be restricted from driving. Document advisement. Significant others can inform the state automobile licensing bureau about the need for retesting to take the burden of restriction off the family. Suggest that significant others hide car keys or disable the car if necessary to prevent patient from driving.

Altered nutrition: Less than body requirements, related to decreased intake secondary to cognitive and motor deficit and to increased nutritional needs secondary to constant pacing and restlessness

Desired outcome: Patient maintains baseline body weight.

1. Because patient may not eat food that does not look familiar or is on hospital plates, request that significant others assist with menu planning or bring in meals and dishes patient recognizes. These patients often are overwhelmed with choices and need help with menu selection.
2. When patient can no longer handle a fork, knife, and spoon, cut up food for patient and/or provide finger foods.
3. For patient who is in constant motion, provide small snacks around the clock and a high-calorie diet unless contraindicated.
4. Try to limit the number of foods on the plate or serve foods in courses, because too many foods can be overwhelming for patient.
5. If patient clenches teeth and refuses to eat, stimulate oral suck reflex by stroking the cheeks or stimulating the mouth with a spoon. Use patient's forgetfulness to advantage by taking a short break from feeding and returning in a few moments, when patient may be more receptive.
6. Provide privacy. Accept eating with hands and whimsical food mixtures. Tolerate spills without scolding, and obtain nonspill cups when needed. Be creative. A punch card or ticket that allows patient to "pay for the meal" may persuade some to eat.
7. For other interventions, see **Altered nutrition** in "General Care of Patients with Neurologic Disorders," p. 190.

Impaired environmental interpretation syndrome related to chronic confusional state secondary to degeneration of neuronal functioning

Desired outcome: After intervention and on an ongoing basis, patient interacts appropriately with environment.

1. Monitor for and record short-term memory deficit. Once a level of comprehension has been determined, avoid repeatedly asking if patient knows who and where he or she is and what time it is because this may cause frustration and agitation. At frequent intervals, orient patient to reality, time, and place in the following ways: call patient by name; keep clocks and calendars in the room; inform patient of the day and time; correct patient gently; minimize disturbing noise; ensure adequate lighting to prevent shadows; request that significant others bring in familiar objects and family pictures; speak with patient about his or her interests, both present and past; allow patient to reminisce; ensure that staff members show name tags and identify themselves; explain upcoming events; set up regular schedules for hygiene, eating, and waste elimination.
2. Approach patient in a calm, slow, relaxed, nonthreatening, friendly manner. Treat patient with dignity and respect. Remain calm and patient when repeating questions. Be nonjudgmental and objective, even when confronted with inappropriate behavior.
3. Keep patient's personal belongings where they can be used and seen.
4. Evaluate patient's cognitive impairment for any relation to medication use (e.g., such as sedatives or tranquilizers). If found, consult physician.

5. Provide a quiet, calm, pleasant environment. Simple, minimally decorated rooms are best. Patient may not recognize himself or herself in a mirror. Cover or remove artwork and mirrors if patient misinterprets images (e.g., wallpaper patterns may be disturbing to some patients). Turning off public address system in patient's room may prevent patient stimulation and misinterpretation of sound.

6. Provide stimulation that patient can handle. Soft music may be appropriate, but television might be too overwhelming because the images change quickly and may be misperceived.

7. Limit visitors as appropriate because crowds and complex social interaction often are beyond patient's ability to tolerate.

8. Check to ensure that individuals who need eyeglasses or hearing aids wear them as appropriate. Eyeglasses should be clean and have a current prescription; hearing aids should be functioning.

9. If patient becomes agitated, reduce environmental stimuli. Use a soft, reassuring voice and gentle touch. Avoid quick, unexpected movements.

Impaired environmental interpretation syndrome (urinating in inappropriate places) related to cognitive deficit

Desired outcome: Patient habitually urinates in toilet stool (commode).

1. Make sure patient knows location of bathroom. If possible, locate patient within sight of bathroom, ensure a clear path, and provide adequate light at night. Take patient to bathroom q1-2h; avoid a sense of hurry. Restrict fluids in the evenings to minimize the risk of enuresis.

2. Identify bathroom door with a picture of a toilet to help patient locate bathroom.

3. Assess for nonverbal clues (e.g., restlessness, holding himself or herself), which can signal the need to void.

4. As appropriate, provide disposable underpants. Indwelling and external catheters may increase confusion. Men may be able to accept condom catheters to help manage incontinence.

5. Incontinence may signal a UTI. Investigate cause of incontinence to see whether it is treatable.

6. After patient has voided, assess him or her for cleanliness and dryness of perianal area; intervene accordingly to help ensure skin integrity.

Impaired environmental interpretation syndrome (defecating in inappropriate places) related to inability to find bathroom or decreased awareness or loss of sphincter control secondary to cognitive deficit

Desired outcome: After intervention, patient has no or fewer episodes of defecating in inappropriate places.

1. Show patient location of bathroom. Identify bathroom door with a picture of a toilet to help patient locate bathroom.

2. Assess patient's normal bowel habits. Take patient to bathroom at the time of day patient normally has a bowel movement (e.g., after meals).

Neurologic

3. Evaluate patient for nonverbal indications of the need to eliminate wastes (e.g., restlessness, picking at clothes, facial expressions or grunting sounds indicative of bearing down, passing of flatus).

4. As appropriate, provide disposable underpants.

5. After bowel elimination, assess patient for cleanliness of perianal area to maintain skin integrity. Patient may forget to wipe perianal area or may only partly clean the area.

6. For other suggestions, see **Constipation,** p. 196, and Appendix One, "Caring for Patients on Prolonged Bed Rest."

Self-care deficit related to memory loss and coordination problems secondary to cognitive and motor deficits

Desired outcome: Patient's physical needs are met by himself or herself, staff, or significant others.

1. Provide care for totally dependent patients, and assist those who are not totally dependent. Allow ample time to perform activities, encouraging patient's independence. Ask patient to perform only one task at a time; go through each step separately. Do not hurry patient. Involve significant others with care activities if they wish to be involved. Ask them when patient normally bathes at home, and establish this as part of a daily routine. Provide a consistent care giver. Use simple visual and verbal cues and gestures for self-care.

2. Place a stool in the shower if sitting will enhance self-care. Use a hand-held shower head to prevent water from hitting patient's head, which can be frightening.

3. To facilitate dressing and undressing, encourage significant others or patient to buy shoes without laces and clothing that is loose-fitting or has snaps, Velcro closures, or elastic waistbands. Offer clothing items one at a time, sequentially. Allow agitated patients for whom hygiene is not a problem to sleep in their shoes and clothes, and attempt a clothing change later.

4. Provide a commode chair or elevated toilet seat as needed.

5. If patient becomes combative or agitated, postpone ADLs and try again a short time later; patient may forget reason for resistance.

Impaired verbal communication related to aphasia and altered sensory reception, transmission, and integration secondary to cognitive deficits

Desired outcome: After intervention, patient communicates needs to staff, follows instructions, and answers questions.

1. Provide a supportive, relaxed environment for patients unable to form words or sentences or unable to speak clearly or appropriately. Acknowledge patient's frustration about inability to communicate. Maintain a calm, positive attitude; eliminate distracting noises, such as radio or television. Observe for nonverbal communication cues, such as gestures. Consider pain as a possible cause of restlessness, moaning, guarding, and yelling; provide analgesia as needed. Avoid meperidine, if possible, because of its common side effect of restlessness. Anticipate patient's needs.

2. Explain activities in short, easily understood sentences. Use simple gestures, point to objects, or use demonstration if possible. When giving directions, be sure to break tasks into small, understandable

units, using simple terms. Ask patient to do only one task at a time. Give patient time to accomplish one task before progressing to the next.

3. Be sure that you have the patient's attention. Repeat patient's name, or gently touch patient to get his or her attention. Use touch to communicate if patient is receptive to it. Speak slowly and calmly, using a clear, low-pitched voice. Use short, simple words and sentences, but speak as though patient understands you. Ask only one question at a time, and formulate questions that can be answered by "yes" or "no." Wait for a response. If patient does not respond (i.e., after 15 sec), repeat question again, exactly as before, to help patient mentally process question.

4. Listen to and include patient in conversation.

Anxiety related to actual or perceived threats or changes (e.g., from bewildering hospital environment and numerous tests and procedures)

Desired outcome: Within 1 h of intervention, patient's anxiety is absent or reduced, as evidenced by HR ≤100 bpm, RR ≤20 breaths/min with normal depth and pattern, and an absence of or decrease in irritability and restlessness.

1. Remain calm with patient. Use slow, deliberate gestures. Patients with Alzheimer's disease frequently mirror the emotions of others. Use a low, soothing voice and gentle touch. Tone of voice often is more important than actual words used.

2. Provide time for patient to verbalize feelings of fear, concern, and anxiety. Listen with regard. Patients with Alzheimer's disease often have trouble finding the correct words and may not be able to string more than a few words together. Provide calm, realistic reassurance, and stay with patient during periods of acute anxiety.

3. To help reduce anxiety and establish rapport, provide patient with a consistent care giver. Avoid changing patient's room.

4. Patients who still have reading capability may find reassurance with notes, orienting signs, or lists of names, phone numbers, or activities (e.g., the phone numbers of significant others or a note reminder of the reason they are in the hospital); these may reassure them that they are not lost or abandoned.

5. Encourage significant others to bring in familiar items.

6. Permit patient to hoard inanimate objects because this may provide a sense of security. Enable patients to keep personal belongings (e.g., purses or wallets) in bed with them.

7. Help find misplaced items. Label drawers and belongings.

8. Refrain from forcing activities or giving patient too many choices.

9. Encourage ambulation. Often, walking helps reduce anxiety and agitation.

10. Encourage unlimited visiting hours for familiar significant others.

11. Encourage patient to avoid caffeine, which has a stimulating effect.

Risk for violence related to irritability, frustration, and disorientation secondary to degeneration of cognitive thinking

Desired outcome: Patient demonstrates control of his or her behavior with absence of violence.

1. Ask care giver how patient usually acts when tired or overwhelmed, and ask what care giver does to calm patient. Document this information.

2. Monitor patient for signs of increasing anxiety, fright, or panic (e.g., inability to verbalize feelings, suspiciousness of others, fear of others or self, irritability, agitation), which can precede a violent act.

3. Encourage verbalization of feelings rather than suppression because frustration can lead to violence. Praise efforts at self-control.

4. Try to identify what is immediately distressing patient (e.g., full bladder, catheter, pain), and attempt to remedy it. Respond to the emotion. Respond to patient's questions in simple, concrete replies that relate directly to patient's questions, frustrations, or anger. Avoid making promises that cannot reasonably be kept. Do not confront or argue with patient and become authoritarian. If the situation cannot be remedied by calming patient, use distraction and try to defuse the situation by redirecting attention away from the source of irritation. Talk about other topics, and vary the topics periodically. Provide diversional activities, offer juice, or walk with patient until agitation has lessened. A request for patient's help (e.g., with folding and unfolding towels, making a bed) may promote calm behavior by returning a sense of mastery or control.

5. Remain calm and keep gestures slow and deliberate. Keep your hands open and below your waist where they can be seen. Approach patient slowly in a confident, relaxed, open manner. Avoid sudden changes or surprises. Keep your voice low and soft, and smile. Humor and gentle laughter may help change patient's mood. Some patients may respond positively to gentle touch.

6. Reduce environmental stimuli, including people entering room. Provide a private room if possible. Reduce noise level by turning television down or off.

7. Do not give routine care when patient is upset or agitated. Leave the room briefly, and return when patient is calmer and more approachable. If patient cannot be left alone, sit quietly with no talking except gentle reassurance. Use patient's forgetfulness to your advantage.

8. If patient is not combative unless approached, simply supervise from a safe distance. If you must approach patient, do so from the side rather than face to face. Stand off to one side, and maintain a distance of at least one arm's length from patient.

9. If patient is upset or agitated, avoid turning your back on patient. Avoid cornering patient or being cornered. Think of escape routes for yourself, and be alert for potential weapons patient may use. Get help; protect yourself.

10. Never attempt to deal with a physically aggressive patient by yourself. If other interventions fail, use physical or chemical restraints as necessary for your own or patient's safety.

11. Document signs and symptoms of violent behavior, precipitating factor, time of onset, duration, and successful interventions. Prevent further episodes by controlling precipitating stressors (e.g., controlling pain, simplifying schedule, limiting visitors).

Sleep pattern disturbance related to restlessness and disorientation secondary to cognitive deficits

Desired outcome: After intervention, patient sleeps at least 6 h per night or an amount of time appropriate for patient.

1. Space activities with quiet periods so that patient does not become excessively tired and require a daytime nap.
2. Prevent patients from falling asleep during the day through such measures as periodic short walks, planned activities, and keeping them upright as much as possible. **Note:** If patient does nap during the day but also sleeps well at night, there is no need to impose a specific sleep schedule.
3. Patients who nap should do so in an easy chair, if possible, rather than in bed. The easy chair may serve as a cue that their sleep is just a nap.
4. Avoid continuous use of restraints, because they often increase agitation and limit patient's ability to rest.
5. Adhere to regular bedtime schedules and rituals, such as a bedtime snack. Keep room lighted until patient is ready for sleep. Provide soft music and tell patient it is time for sleep.
6. Administer tranquilizers and sedatives as prescribed to facilitate sleep.
7. Avoid turning on overhead light at night, which may cue patient to think it is time to get up.

Altered family processes related to situational crisis (illness of family member)

Desired outcome: Within the 24 h before hospital discharge, significant others verbalize knowledge of measures that will assist with coping with care of patient after hospital discharge.

1. Encourage significant others to interpret patient's behavior as a reflection of the disease process rather than a willful act. Advise them that generally another illness, surgery, or disease process will exaggerate patient's disorientation. Once these problems have been corrected, patient usually returns to his or her previous cognitive level.
2. Encourage patient's major care giver to have other significant others or hired help take care of patient regularly so that he or she can have scheduled respites. A neighbor looking in or a home health aide on a part-time, overnight, or live-in basis is another option. Local day care programs also are useful. If patient is a veteran, he or she may be eligible for some respite programs offered by the Veterans Administration. Advise care giver that some home health agencies or day care programs have sliding payment scales for their services. Refer family to community sources that supply equipment for home use. Encourage use of other support services (e.g., homemakers, choreworkers, home-delivered food, volunteer drivers). Support significant others in asking for help.
3. If significant other is unaccustomed to handling finances, refer him or her to a place where help with financial management is available. Patients with Alzheimer's disease often lose the ability to manage finances and balance checkbooks and may give away money inappropriately. Eventually patient's checkbook and credit

Neurologic

cards will have to be taken away. Phone use may require monitoring because these patients cannot differentiate between local and long-distance calls. As appropriate, suggest that significant others post important phone numbers and secure long-distance numbers to help prevent excessively high phone bills.

4. Encourage early financial planning, and suggest professional financial counseling. Families should locate and identify patient's various assets, sources of income, and liabilities and make arrangements for their security and daily management.

5. Encourage early family legal planning and consultation. This is especially important because an individual must have mental capacity and competence to sign documents. Legal planning may involve wills, inter vivos trusts, subpayee assignment for Social Security, traditional and durable power of attorney, guardianship, and conservatorship. Advise family that some free legal services are available to the elderly in most areas.

6. Explain to significant others that if patient refuses medication or is unable to swallow pills, obtaining a liquid form of the drug or crushing pills and mixing them with soft food may help.

7. Some individuals with this disease go through a phase in which, because of increased motor activity and lessening social inhibitions, they have increased sexual demands. This may result in increased sexual encounters. Be sure the family is aware that this is a symptom of the disease process. Furthermore, the patient eventually will lose the ability to be intimate and tender. Sex will become a mindless act. Mates may feel rejected, frustrated, humiliated, or repulsed. Suggest that professional counseling be obtained to assist patient's spouse or loved one in dealing with these feelings. Suggest that gentle dissuasion or distraction may be effective with these patients. Remind patient that certain public behavior is unacceptable.

8. Encourage care givers to maintain their own friendships and attend social functions. The patient's embarrassing behavior and the demands of giving care can lead to withdrawal from society.

9. Encourage significant others to focus on specific problems as they occur and to establish priorities. Help them develop a plan of care and a schedule of daily activities.

10. Encourage professional counseling and support so that significant others can work through such feelings as anger, guilt, embarrassment, and depression and develop effective coping strategies and mechanisms. Each new and subtle loss of patient function brings another round of grieving. Decisions about institutionalization and the extent of health care measures also are emotionally difficult. Behavior such as hoarding, unjust accusations, angry outbursts, and clinging can precipitate burnout in the care giver. Care givers and significant others must be reassessed continually for their ability to care for the patient at home.

11. Encourage participation in local or national support groups, such as the Alzheimer's Disease and Related Disorders Association (ADRDA) (see "Patient-Family Teaching and Discharge Planning" for address and phone numbers).

12. For other interventions, see **Altered family processes** in Appendix One, "Caring for Patients with Cancer and Other Life-Disrupting Illnesses," p. 463.

For patients experiencing seizures, see "Seizure Disorders," p. 179. See "General Care of Patients with Neurologic Disorders" for **Risk for fluid volume deficit,** p. 191, **Risk for aspiration,** p. 192, **Impaired swallowing,** p. 201, and **Knowledge deficit:** Neurologic diagnostic tests, p. 205.

For patients experiencing varying degrees of immobility, see related nursing diagnoses in "Pressure Ulcers," p. 390, and Appendix One, "Caring for Patients on Prolonged Bed Rest," p. 413.

Also see Appendix One, "Caring for Patients with Cancer and Other Life-Disrupting Illnesses," p. 450, for psychosocial nursing diagnoses for patients and significant others, as appropriate.

PATIENT-FAMILY TEACHING AND DISCHARGE PLANNING

The degree and scope of discharge teaching and planning depend on the severity of the patient's condition. Give patient and significant others verbal and written information about the following, as appropriate:

1. Referrals to community resources, local and national Alzheimer's disease chapters, public health nurse, Visiting Nurse Association, community support groups, social workers, psychologic therapy, home health agencies, and extended and skilled care facilities. Provide the address and phone numbers of the Alzheimer's Disease and Related Disorders Association, 919 North Michigan Avenue, Suite 1000, Chicago, IL 60611 *phone:* (800)-272-3900 or (312)-335-8700, and "Help Line" (708)-933-1000.
2. Safety measures for preventing injury relative to cognitive deficits.
3. Measures that assist in reorienting and communicating with patient in view of cognitive deficits.
4. Importance of scheduled respites and involvement in support groups for significant others.
5. Medications, including drug name, purpose, dosage, schedule, precautions, drug/drug and food/drug interactions, and potential side effects.
6. Exercises that promote muscle strength and mobility; measures for preventing contractures and skin breakdown; transfer techniques and proper body mechanics; and use of assistive devices, if appropriate.
7. Techniques for dealing with incontinence; indications of constipation or infection; implementation of bowel and bladder training programs; and indwelling catheter care, if appropriate.
8. Indications of upper respiratory infection and measures that prevent regurgitation, aspiration, and infection.
9. Techniques for encouraging adequate food and fluid intake and performance of ADLs.
10. Importance of seeking financial and legal counseling.

SECTION THREE: TRAUMATIC DISORDERS OF THE NERVOUS SYSTEM

Spinal Cord Injury

NURSING DIAGNOSES AND INTERVENTIONS

Dysreflexia (or risk for same) related to exaggerated, unopposed autonomic response to noxious stimuli for individuals with spinal cord injury at or above T8

NOTE: Autonomic dysreflexia (AD) is most commonly seen in patients with injuries at or above T6, but cases have been reported in patients with injuries as low as T8.

Desired outcomes: On an ongoing basis, patient is free of symptoms of AD, as evidenced by BP within patient's baseline range, HR 60-100 bpm, and absence of headache and other clinical indicators of AD. After instruction, patient and significant others verbalize factors that cause AD, treatment and prevention, and when immediate emergency treatment is indicated.

1. Monitor for indicators of AD, including hypertension (>20 mm Hg above baseline but may go as high as 240-300/150 mm Hg), pounding headache, bradycardia, blurred vision, nausea, nasal congestion, flushing and sweating above level of injury, and piloerection (goose bumps) or pallor below level of injury.
2. If AD is suspected, raise HOB immediately to 90 degrees or help patient into sitting position to lower BP.
3. Call for someone to notify physician; stay with patient and try to find and ameliorate the noxious stimulus. Speed is essential. Monitor BP q3-5min during hypertensive episode. Remain calm and supportive of patient and significant others.
4. Assess the following sites for causes, and implement measures for removing the noxious stimulus.

Bladder (most likely cause): Distention, UTI, calculus and other obstructions, bladder spasms, catheterization, and bladder irrigations performed too quickly or with too cold a liquid.

- Do not use Credé's method for a distended bladder.
- Catheterize patient (ideally using anesthetic jelly) if there is a possibility or question of bladder distention. Consult physician *stat.*
- If a catheter is already in place, check tubing for kinks and lower drainage bag. For obstruction (e.g., sediment in tubing), irrigate catheter as indicated, using no more than 30 ml of normal saline. If catheter patency is uncertain, recatheterize patient using anesthetic jelly.
- If bladder is not distended, check for signs of UTI and/or urinary calculi (cloudy urine, hematuria, positive laboratory or x-ray results).

Obtain urine specimen for culture and sensitivity studies as indicated.

Bowel (second most likely cause): Constipation, impaction, insertion of suppository or enema, and rectal examination.

- Do not attempt rectal examination without first anesthetizing rectal sphincter with anesthetic jelly.
- Use large amounts of anesthetic jelly in anus and rectum before disimpacting bowel to remove potential stimulus. Allow 5 min for anesthetic jelly to work (as manifested by a falling BP) before disimpacting.

Skin: Pressure, infection, injury, heat, pain, or cold.

- Loosen clothing and remove antiembolism hose, leg bandages, abdominal binder, or constrictive sheets as appropriate.
- For men, check for pressure source on penis or testicles and remove pressure, if present.
- Check skin surface below level of injury. Monitor for pressure area or sore, infection, laceration, rash, sunburn, ingrown toenail, or infected area. If indicated, apply a topical anesthetic.
- Observe for and remove the source of heat or cold (e.g., ice pack or heating pad).

Additional causes: Surgical manipulation, sexual activity, menstruation, and labor.

- Administer antihypertensive agents (e.g., hydralazine, diazoxide, or nifedipine) as prescribed.
- Upon resolution of the crisis, answer patient's and significant others' questions about AD. Discuss signs and symptoms, treatment, and methods of prevention. Encourage patient to wear a Medic-Alert bracelet or tag.

N O T E :   Prevention is the best way to deal with AD. A good bowel regimen and skin integrity program are key factors in preventing the noxious stimuli that constipation or pressure areas may cause. Loosen clothing, bed sheets, and constricting bands; turn patient off side to relieve other possible sources of pressure. Keep bed free of sharp objects and wrinkles. Adhere to turning schedules. Measures should be instituted to reduce the potential for UTI and urinary calculi, and the patient should be taught self-inspection of skin and urinary catheter, as well as the importance of using anesthetic jelly for catheterization and disimpaction.

Constipation or fecal impaction related to immobility and decreased peristalsis, atonic bowel, and loss of sensation and voluntary sphincter control secondary to sensorimotor deficit

Desired outcome: Patient has bowel movements that are soft and formed q2-3days or within preinjury pattern.

1. During acute phase of spinal shock, assess patient's bowel function by auscultating for bowel sounds, inspecting for abdominal distention, and monitoring for nausea, vomiting, and fecal impaction.

Consult physician about significant findings. If fecal impaction is present, gentle manual removal or a small cleansing enema may be prescribed. Because the atonic intestine distends easily, administer small-volume enemas only. Avoid long-term use of enemas.

2. Lesions above the conus medullaris (located at the lower two levels of the thoracic region, where the cord begins to taper) generally leave the S3, S4, and S5 spinal cord nerve segments intact. If this spinal reflex arc is intact, the patient will have an upper motor neuron (UMN) bowel and will be capable of stimulating (training) reflex evacuation of the bowel. Lesions below the conus medullaris (T12) may injure the S3, S4, and S5 nerve segments, disrupting the reflex arc and producing a lower motor neuron (LMN) flaccid bowel. A flaccid bowel usually is managed with increased intraabdominal pressure techniques, manual disimpaction, and small-volume enemas.

3. For the UMN reflex bowel, once bowel activity returns, teach patient to attempt bowel movement 30 min after a meal or warm drink. This regimen will allow patient's gastrocolic and duodenocolic mass peristalsis reflexes to assist with evacuation. Increasing intraabdominal pressure by bearing down, bending forward, or applying manual pressure to the abdomen also will help promote bowel evacuation. Abdominal belts may be used if the patient is unable to strain at stool. A prescribed, medicated suppository also may be used if necessary. If allowed, provide a bedside commode rather than a bedpan. Check patient's ability to maintain balance on a commode.

C A U T I O N :   For patients with injuries at T8 or above, promote use of stool softeners and high-fiber diet. Use suppositories and enemas only when essential and with extreme caution because they can precipitate AD. Use anesthetic jelly liberally when performing a rectal examination or inserting a suppository or enema.

---

4. For patients with hand mobility (who are not at risk for AD), teach technique for suppository insertion and digital stimulation of the anus to promote reflex bowel evacuation. For digital stimulation, insert finger and gently rotate in a circular motion for about 30 sec (or longer) until internal sphincter relaxes. Stop if sphincter spasms are felt or if signs of AD occur. Repeat q10min several times until adequate evacuation occurs. Suppository inserters and rectal stimulation devices are available for patients with limited hand mobility.

5. For other interventions, see **Constipation** in Appendix One, "Caring for Patients on Prolonged Bed Rest," p. 420.

Ineffective airway clearance related to neuromuscular paralysis/weakness or restriction of chest expansion secondary to halo vest obstruction

Desired outcome: After intervention, patient has a clear airway, as evidenced by RR 12-20 breaths/min with normal depth and pattern (eupnea) and absence of adventitious breath sounds.

1. Monitor ventilation capability by checking vital capacity, tidal volume, and pulmonary function tests. Monitor serial ABG values and/or pulse oximetry readings. If vital capacity is less than 1 L or if patient exhibits signs of hypoxia (Pao_2 <80 mm Hg, tachycardia,

increased restlessness, mental dullness, cyanosis), notify physician immediately.

2. Monitor for ascending cord edema, which may be signaled by increasing difficulty with secretions, coughing, respiratory difficulties, bradycardia, fluctuating BP, and increased motor and sensory losses at a higher level than baseline findings. Monitor for loss of previous ability to bend arms at elbows (C5-6) or shrug shoulders (C3-4). If these are noted, consult physician immediately.

3. Maintain patent airway. Keep patient's head in neutral position and suction as necessary. Use jaw thrust technique to open airway. Be aware that suctioning may cause severe bradycardia in a patient with AD. If indicated, prepare patient for tracheostomy, endotracheal intubation, and/or mechanical ventilation to support respiratory function. If appropriate, arrange for a transfer to ICU for continuous monitoring.

4. If patient is wearing halo vest traction, assess respiratory status at least q4h. Ensure that vest is not restricting chest expansion. Teach patient use of incentive spirometry. Be alert for indicators of pulmonary embolus (PE): SOB, hemoptysis, tachycardia, and diminished breath sounds. Pain may or may not be present with PE, depending on level of SCI. Sudden shoulder pain may be referred pain from PE.

5. If patient's cough is ineffective, implement the following technique, known as "assisted coughing": Place palm of the hand under patient's diaphragm (below xiphoid process and above navel). As the patient exhales forcibly, push up into diaphragm to assist in producing a more forceful cough. Assisted cough may be contraindicated in patients with spinal instability.

6. Feed patients in Stryker frames or Foster beds in prone position to minimize the potential for aspiration. Raise stable patients in halo traction to high Fowler's position if it is not contraindicated.

7. For additional interventions, see **Risk for aspiration,** p. 192, in "General Care of Patients with Neurologic Disorders."

Risk for disuse syndrome related to paralysis, immobilization, or spasticity secondary to SCI

Desired outcomes: After stabilization of the injury, patient exhibits complete ROM of all joints. By time of discharge, patient demonstrates measures that enhance mobility, reduce spasms, and prevent complications.

1. Once the injury is stabilized, assist patient with position changes. For example, a prone position, if not contraindicated, helps prevent sacral decubiti and hip contractures. Assist patient into this position on a regular schedule.

2. For patients with spasticity, use hand splints or cones to assist with maintaining a functional grasp.

3. To help prevent foot contractures for patients with spasticity, it may be helpful to fit patient with splints or high-top tennis shoes that are cut off at the toes so that each shoe ends just proximal to the metatarsal head. These shoes help keep the feet dorsiflexed but prevent contact of the balls of the feet with a hard surface, which can cause

spasticity. Avoid footboards for these patients because the hard surface may trigger spasticity and promote plantarflexion.

4. Teach patient that some of the factors that trigger spasms include cold, anxiety, fatigue, emotional distress, infections, bowel or bladder distention, ulcers, pain, tight clothing, and lying too long in one position. Controlling these factors may reduce the number of spasms experienced.

5. Teach patients with spasticity proper positioning, ROM, and daily sustained stretching exercises. Steady, continuous, directional stretching once or twice a day is especially important because it may decrease the amount of spasticity for several hours. Cooling and icing techniques, heat, vibration therapy, and transcutaneous electrical nerve stimulation (TENS) of the spastic muscles also may be helpful.

6. Because tactile stimulation may trigger spasms, touch by care givers should be limited. When touch is necessary, it should be done in a firm, gentle, steady manner. Avoid jarring patient, which also can stimulate spasm.

7. For additional interventions, see **Risk for disuse syndrome** in Appendix One, "Caring for Patients on Prolonged Bed Rest," p. 416.

Risk for injury related to incorrect neck position, irritation of cranial nerves, impaired lateral vision secondary to presence of halo vest traction, and lack of access for external cardiac compression

Desired outcome: At time of discharge (and during use of halo traction), patient exhibits no adverse changes in motor, sensory, or cranial nerve function and is free of symptoms of injury caused by impaired vision.

1. Assess position of patient's neck to the body. Alert physician to presence of flexion or hyperextension. Assess any difficulty with swallowing because this may signal improper positioning of neck and chin. Keep a torque screwdriver in a secure place so that physician can readily adjust tension on bars to return patient's neck position to neutral.

2. Evaluate degree of sensation and movement of upper extremities, and assess cranial nerve function. Changes in cranial nerve function can occur if cranial pins compress or irritate a nerve. Consult physician about sudden changes in motor, sensory, or cranial nerve function (e.g., weakness, paresthesia, ptosis, difficulty chewing or swallowing). Jaw pain may occur when chewing is attempted, and this needs to be differentiated from cranial nerve problems. Soft foods cut into small pieces will help jaw pain.

3. Assess pins, bolts, and vest structure for looseness. Clicking sounds may signal a loose pin. Never use superstructure of halo traction in turning or moving patient. Consult physician if pins or vest becomes loose or dislodged. Stabilize patient's head as necessary.

4. Instruct patient to avoid pulling clothes over the top of the halo apparatus because this may loosen pins. Patient instead should step into and pull clothes up over feet and legs. Advise patient to buy strapless bras, tube tops, or clothes that are several sizes

larger, or to modify neck openings (e.g., with Velcro closures, ties).

5. Avoid loosening a buckle without physician's directive. Buckle holes should be marked so that they are always cinched correctly to the appropriate snugness.

6. If patient is ambulatory, teach him or her how to survey environment while walking, either by using a mirror or by turning the eyes to their extreme lateral positions. A cane may help determine the height of curbs and detect unseen objects or uneven walking surfaces. Explain that trunk flexibility is limited, and achieving balance can be difficult because of the top-heavy weight of the vest. Ambulating with a walker initially may help patient learn to adjust. Abdominal- and back-strengthening exercises may aid balance and walking. Advise patient to walk only in low-heeled shoes. Extra space allowance may be needed when passing through doorways and to avoid bumping into objects.

7. Teach patient that bending over can be hazardous because of top-heaviness. A shower chair that rolls usually can fit over a toilet seat, providing an extra 3-6 in in height. Slip-on shoes should be worn and assistive devices used to reach or pick up objects.

8. To get out of bed, teach patients to roll onto their side at the edge of the bed and then drop their legs over the side of the bed while pushing up their trunk sideways.

9. For getting into a car, recommend backing into the car seat with the body bent forward. Caution patient against driving because of his or her limited field of vision.

10. Teach patient that a high table will help bring objects into view and that a swivel chair at home will permit easier visualization of the environment.

11. Explain that patient will need the assistance of another person to shampoo hair safely. Shampooing a short haircut is easiest, and hair should be blown dry, because toweling the hair may loosen pins.

12. Ensure that an open-end wrench is taped to the halo vest so that the bolts can be released and the vest removed promptly if external cardiac compression is needed. One type of halo vest permits the anterior vest to be lifted up after release of two side belts. Teach significant others how to release vest in an emergency.

Risk for impaired skin integrity and/or **Impaired tissue integrity (or risk for same)** related to altered circulation and mechanical factors secondary to presence of halo vest traction or tongs

Desired outcome: At time of discharge (and thereafter), patient's skin is clear and unbroken; tissue underlying and surrounding halo vest blanches appropriately.

1. Inspect skin around vest edges for erythema and other signs of irritation. Massage nonerythematous areas routinely to promote circulation and help prevent breakdown. Teach skin inspection, which may require use of a mirror, a flashlight, or another person. Teach patient to alert medical personnel if breakdown, sensitive spots, odor, dirty vest liner, or loose pins are present.

2. Investigate complaints of discomfort or uncomfortable fit. A finger should be able to fit between the vest and the patient's skin. Weight loss or gain can affect the fit. Pad vest as needed until it can be properly adjusted or trimmed by physician. Protect vest from moisture and soiling. Be alert for foul odor from in and around cast openings, which can signal pressure necrosis beneath vest.

3. Instruct patient in and assist with body position changes q2h. Support vest while patient is in bed. Use pads to prevent pressure on prominent body areas such as the forehead or shoulder. Use a small pillow under the head for comfort at sleep time.

4. Skin care should include cleansing with soap and warm water. Usually, releasing one vest belt at a time is allowed for washing. Avoid use of lotion and powder, which can cake under vest. Rub unbroken skin with alcohol to toughen skin. Replace soiled linens promptly. Patient's perspiration may be dried with a blow dryer on a cool setting.

5. If a rash appears, patient may be allergic to vest's lining. A synthetic liner, knitted body stockinette, or T-shirt may correct this problem.

6. Provide oral care. A flexible disposable straw can be used both to sip clear water for rinsing teeth and to expel rinse water into a sink or basin.

7. In the event of skin breakdown, keep patient's skin clean, dry, and covered with a transparent dressing. Consult physician and orthotist accordingly because skin breakdown requires a brace adjustment.

8. Place rubber corks over tips of the halo device to diminish annoying sound vibrations if apparatus is bumped and to prevent lacerations from possible sharp edges.

9. Check tong placement. If slippage has occurred, immobilize patient's head with a sandbag and consult physician. Pain may signal erosion of bone and displacement into muscle. Check drainage for CSF (see p. 155). Ensure that traction weights are hanging freely.

10. Provide analgesia as needed for mild headache and discomfort.

11. For a discussion of pin care, see "Fractures," p. 324, for **Knowledge deficit:** Function of external fixation, pin care, and signs and symptoms of pin site infection.

Urinary retention or reflex incontinence related to neurologic impairment (spasticity or flaccidity occurring with SCI)

Desired outcomes: Patient has urinary output without incontinence. Patient empties bladder with residual volumes of <50 ml by time of discharge. After instruction, patient demonstrates triggering mechanism and gains some control over voiding.

N O T E : Bladder dysfunction is complicated and should be assessed by cystometric testing to determine the best type of bladder program. Lesions above the conus medullaris (located at the lower two levels of the thoracic region where the cord begins to taper) generally leave the

S2, S3, and S4 spinal cord nerve segments intact. If this spinal reflex arc is intact, the patient will have a UMN-involved bladder, resulting in a spastic bladder. This bladder has tone and occasional bladder contractions and periodically empties on its own, resulting in reflex incontinence. The UMN-involved bladder is "trainable" with techniques that stimulate reflex voiding. Lesions below the conus medullaris (T12) may injure the S2, S3, and S4 nerve segments, which will disrupt the reflex arc, causing an LMN-involved flaccid bladder. This bladder has no tone and will distend until it overflows, resulting in overflow incontinence.

GENERAL GUIDELINES FOR INDIVIDUALS WITH BLADDER DYSFUNCTION

1. Initially patient will have an indwelling urinary catheter or scheduled intermittent catheterizations. If intermittent catheterization is used and episodes of incontinence occur or more than 500 ml urine is obtained, catheterize patient more often.
2. Teach patient and significant others the procedure for intermittent catheterization, care of indwelling catheters, and indicators of UTI (e.g., fever, cloudy and/or foul-smelling urine, malaise, anorexia, restlessness, incontinence).
3. Habit/bladder scheduling program consists of gradually increasing the time between catheterizations or periodically clamping indwelling catheters. The goal is a gradual increase in bladder tone. When the bladder can hold 300-400 ml of urine, measures to stimulate voiding are attempted.
4. Make sure patient takes fluids at even intervals throughout the day. Restrict fluids before bedtime to prevent nighttime incontinence. Alcohol and caffeine-containing foods and beverages (e.g., cola, chocolate, coffee, tea) have a diuretic effect and may cause incontinence. In addition, caffeine-containing products may increase bladder spasms and reflex incontinence.
5. Patients using bladder-emptying techniques should void at least q3h. To obtain the postvoid residual urine, catheterize patient after an attempt to empty the bladder. Residual amounts >100 ml usually indicate the need for a return to a scheduled intermittent catheterization program.

GUIDELINES FOR PATIENTS WITH UMN-INVOLVED SPASTIC REFLEX BLADDER

1. Explain to these patients that eventually they may be able to empty the bladder automatically and so may not require catheterization.
2. Teach patient techniques that stimulate the voiding reflex, such as tapping the suprapubic area with the fingers, gently pulling the pubic hair, digitally stretching the anal sphincter, stroking the glans penis, stroking the inner thigh, or lightly punching the abdominal area just proximal to the inguinal ligaments. Perform the selected technique for 2-3 min or until a good urine stream has started. Wait 1 min before trying another stimulation technique.
   - *Bladder tapping:* Position self in a half-sitting position. Tapping is performed over the suprapubic area, and patient may shift the

site of stimulation within that area to find the most effective spot. Tapping is performed rapidly (7-8 times/sec) with one hand for approximately 50 single taps. Continue tapping until a good stream starts. When the stream stops, wait about 1 min and repeat tapping until the bladder is empty. One or two tapping attempts without response indicates that no more urine will be expelled.

- *Anal stretch technique (contraindicated in individuals with lesions at T8 or above because of the potential for AD):* Position self on commode or toilet. Lean forward on the thighs and insert one or two lubricated fingers into the anus to the anal sphincter. Spread the anal sphincter gently by spreading the fingers apart or pulling in a posterior direction. Maintain the stretching position, take a deep breath, and hold breath while bearing down to void. Relax and repeat until the bladder is empty.

3. Teach patient with abdominal muscle control to bear down using Valsalva's maneuver when attempting to trigger voiding.
4. Be aware that stimulating the reflex trigger zones accidentally may result in incontinence.
5. Baclofen may be prescribed, inasmuch as it tends to promote more complete emptying of the bladder by reducing the tone of the external urinary sphincter.

GUIDELINES FOR PATIENTS WITH LMN-INVOLVED FLACCID BLADDERS

1. Increasing intraabdominal pressure can overcome sphincter pressure, which may empty the bladder. This may be contraindicated, however, depending on the risk of ureteral reflux.
2. Explain that occasionally these patients may be able to empty their bladders manually well enough to avoid catheterization. Need for catheterization can be determined by checking residual urine volume.
3. Teach patient bladder-emptying techniques, such as straining or Valsalva's maneuver, to increase intraabdominal pressure. If Credé's method is prescribed, teach patient the following technique: Place the ulnar surface of the hand horizontally along the umbilicus; while bearing down with the abdominal muscles, press the hand downward and toward the bladder in a kneading motion until urination is initiated; continue 30 sec or until urination ceases. For both of these techniques, wait a few minutes and repeat the procedure to ensure complete emptying of the bladder.
4. If patient's bladder cannot be trained to empty completely, intermittent catheterization or external collection devices usually are indicated, and patient may be a candidate for an artificial inflatable sphincter device or urinary diversion.
5. See related discussions in "Urinary Incontinence," p. 94, "Urinary Retention," p. 99, and "Neurogenic Bladder," p. 101.

Altered cardiopulmonary and cerebral tissue perfusion related to relative hypovolemia secondary to decreased vasomotor tone with SCI

Desired outcomes: By at least the 24 h before hospital discharge (or as soon as vasomotor tone improves), patient has adequate cardiopulmonary and cerebral tissue perfusion, as evidenced by systolic BP $\geq$90 mm Hg and orientation to time, place, and person. For at least 48 h before hospital discharge, patient is free of dysrhythmias.

1. Monitor patient for hypotension (drop in systolic BP >20 mm Hg, systolic BP <90 mm Hg), lightheadedness, dizziness, fainting, and confusion.
2. Monitor HR and rhythm. Sinus tachycardia/bradycardia may develop because of impaired sympathetic innervation or unopposed vagal stimulation. Document dysrhythmias.
3. Monitor I&O. Give prescribed IV fluids cautiously because impaired vascular tone can make patient sensitive to small increases in circulating volume. Intravascular volume expanders or vasopressors may be required for hypotension.
4. Implement measures that prevent episodes of decreased cardiac output due to postural hypotension:
   - Change position slowly.
   - Perform ROM exercises q2h to prevent venous pooling.
   - Prevent patient's legs from crossing, especially when in a dependent position.
   - Patients with SCI at higher levels, especially above T6, may require abdominal binders in addition to antiembolic hose because these individuals are prone to more severe hypotensive reactions, even with minor changes, such as raising the HOB.
   - Work with the physical therapist (PT) to implement a gradual sitting program that will help patient progress from a supine to an upright position. The goal is to increase patient's ability to sit upright while avoiding adverse effects such as hypertension, dizziness, and fainting. This may include a bed that can rotate gradually from a horizontal position to a vertical position or a chair that has multiple positions progressing from flat to sitting.
5. For additional information, see **Altered cerebral tissue perfusion** in Appendix One, "Caring for Patients on Prolonged Bed Rest," p. 419.

Altered peripheral and cardiopulmonary tissue perfusion related to interrupted blood flow (venous stasis) with corresponding risk of thrombophlebitis and pulmonary emboli secondary to immobility and decreased vasomotor tone

Desired outcome: For at least the 24 h before hospital discharge and thereafter, patient has adequate peripheral and cardiopulmonary tissue perfusion, as evidenced by absence of heat, erythema, and swelling in calves and thighs; HR $\leq$100 bpm; RR $\leq$20 breaths/min with normal depth and pattern (eupnea); and Pao$_2$ $\geq$80 mm Hg.

1. Monitor for indicators of thrombophlebitis: erythema, warmth, decreased pulses, and swelling in calves or thighs. Measure calves and thighs daily while patient is supine or before activity, and monitor for increased circumference. An increase of $\geq$2 cm in one day is significant. The presence of pain or tenderness depends on the level of SCI. Consult physician about significant findings.
2. Protect patient's legs from injury during transfers and turning. Avoid IM injections in the legs, and do not massage them.

3. Provide ROM to legs qid. If not contraindicated, place patient in Trendelenburg position for 15 min q2h to promote venous drainage.

4. Monitor for indicators of pulmonary emboli: tachycardia, SOB, hemoptysis, decrease in Pao_2, and decreased or adventitious breath sounds. Presence of pain depends on level of injury. Consult physician about significant findings.

5. For other interventions, see **Altered peripheral tissue perfusion** in Appendix One, "Caring for Patients on Prolonged Bed Rest," p. 418.

Sexual dysfunction related to altered body function secondary to SCI

Desired outcome: Within the 24 h before hospital discharge, patient discusses concerns about sexuality and verbalizes knowledge of alternative methods of sexual expression, and over time expresses acceptance of changes in sexual functioning.

1. Evaluate your own feelings about sexuality. Refer patient to someone (e.g., knowledgeable staff member, professional sexual therapy counselor) who can address patient's sexual concerns if you are uncomfortable discussing these issues with patient.

2. Provide a supportive environment that gives patient permission to have and express sexual concerns. Sexuality can be discussed as it relates to an erection that occurs during a bath or to objective findings noted during a physical assessment. Elicit patient's knowledge, concerns, and questions. Expect acting-out behavior related to patient's sexuality. This is a normal response to patient's anxiety about his or her sexual response and prognosis.

3. Provide limited information about normal sexual response and changes caused by SCI. Sexual functioning may be different but still possible with SCI. The general rule for men is the higher the lesion, the greater the chance of retaining the ability to have an erection but with less chance to ejaculate. For example, 25% of male SCI patients can attain erections permitting coitus, but less than 10% of paraplegics (SCIs resulting in paralysis of the lower limbs) are able to ejaculate. Women may have problems with lubrication and transient loss of ovulation. Ovulation usually returns, and women can become pregnant and deliver vaginally. However, uterine contractions of labor in women with an SCI lesion at T8 or above may cause AD. Provide information about birth control and oral contraception for women who desire it. Oral contraceptives may be contraindicated because of the risk of thrombophlebitis. For those who desire it, provide information about alternate means of parenting (e.g., adoption, artificial insemination, sperm recovery).

4. Sexual activity may seem impossible to the SCI patient. Specific suggestions that may provide gratification include oral-genital sex, digital stimulation, cuddling, mutual masturbation, anal eroticism, and massage. Specific suggestions for managing common problems include reducing fluid intake 2-3 h before sexual encounter, emptying the bladder and bowels (if necessary) before a sexual encounter, (for men) folding back indwelling catheter along the penis and holding it in place with a condom, (for women) taping the catheter to the abdomen and leaving it in place, taking a warm bath before

sexual activity to reduce spasticity, planning sexual activity for a time of day in which both partners are rested, experimenting with a variety of positions, and applying topical anesthetics to areas that are hypersensitive to touch. Explain that water-soluble lubricants are useful, if needed, but that petroleum-based lubricants can cause UTI and should be avoided. Adductor spasms in women may pose a barrier but can be overcome if a rear entry is acceptable. Penile implants may be an option for some men. If AD occurs during sexual activity, suggest that patient consult physician about preventive measures (e.g., taking a ganglionic blocking agent before having sexual intercourse or applying a topical anesthetic).

5. Nurses may not be able to answer all the patient's concerns and questions. When this occurs, acknowledge patient's concerns and refer to someone with more expertise.

6. Suggest that patient's partner be included in discussion about sexual concerns. Explaining the physical condition caused by the SCI and preparing the partner for scars, lack of muscle tone, atrophy, and the presence of a catheter are important and provide the partner with an opportunity to discuss sexual concerns as well.

7. For additional interventions, see **Altered sexuality pattern** in Appendix One, "Caring for Patients on Prolonged Bed Rest," p. 422.

See "Renal Calculi," p. 67, and "Ureteral Calculi," p. 87, for nursing diagnoses for the prevention and treatment of renal or ureteral calculi.

See "Multiple Sclerosis" for **Knowledge deficit:** Precautions and potential side effects of prescribed medications, p. 114.

See "General Care of Patients with Neurologic Disorders" for **Risk for trauma,** p. 187; **Risk for injury,** p. 189; **Altered nutrition:** Less than body requirements, p. 190; **Risk for fluid volume deficit,** p. 191; **Self-care deficit,** p. 193; **Pain** p. 201; **Altered body temperature,** p. 204; and **Knowledge deficit:** Neurologic diagnostic tests, p. 205.

Also see "Peptic Ulcers," p. 239, for related nursing diagnoses and interventions. For patients with varying degrees of immobility, see related nursing diagnoses and interventions in "Pressure Ulcers," p. 390, and Appendix One, "Caring for Patients on Prolonged Bed Rest," p. 413.

For individuals undergoing surgery, see Appendix One, "Caring for Preoperative and Postoperative Patients," p. 395.

For psychosocial nursing diagnoses, see Appendix One, "Caring for Patients with Cancer and Other Life-Disrupting Illnesses," p. 450, as appropriate.

PATIENT-FAMILY TEACHING
AND DISCHARGE PLANNING

Give patient and significant others verbal and written information about the following:

1. Spinal cord functioning and the effects trauma has on how the body works.

2. Referrals to community resources, such as public health nurse, Visiting Nurse Association, community support groups, social workers,

psychologic therapy, vocational rehabilitation agency, home health agencies, and extended and skilled care facilities. As appropriate, provide these addresses: Information Center for Individuals with Disabilities, Fort Point Place, 1st Floor, 27-43 Wormwood Street, Boston, MA 02110-1606 *phone:* (617)-727-5540; the National Spinal Cord Injury Association, 545 Concord Avenue, Suite 29, Cambridge, MA 02138 *phone:* (617)-935-2722; and the American Paralysis Association, 500 Morris Avenue, Springfield, NJ 07081 *in New Jersey:* (201)-379-2690, *all other states:* (800)-225-0292; the Spinal Cord Injury Hotline: (800)-526-3456.

3. Safety measures relative to decreased sensation, motor deficits, and orthostatic hypotension, as well as the symptoms, preventive measures, and interventions for AD.
4. Use and care of a brace or immobilizer as appropriate.
5. What patient can expect if transferred to a rehabilitation center.
6. Techniques and devices for performing ADLs, including bathing, grooming, turning, feeding, and other self-care activities to patient's maximum potential. Patient may need a home accessibility evaluation as well as driving evaluation and training.
7. Indicators of urinary calculi, and dietary measures to prevent them. (see p. 67 and p. 87).
8. Indicators of deep vein thrombosis, and measures to prevent it (see p. 61).
9. For additional information, see teaching and discharge planning interventions (entries 4 through 10 only) in "Multiple Sclerosis," p. 116, as appropriate.

Head Injury

NURSING DIAGNOSES AND INTERVENTIONS

Knowledge deficit: Caretaker's responsibilities for observing patient sent home with a concussion
Desired outcomes: After instruction, caretaker verbalizes knowledge about observation regimen. Caretaker returns patient to hospital if neurologic deficits are noted.
If patient goes home for observation, provide caretaker with the following verbal and written instructions:

1. Do not give patient anything stronger than acetaminophen to relieve headache. Aspirin usually is contraindicated because it can prolong bleeding if it occurs.
2. Assess patient at least hourly for the first 24 h as follows: Awaken patient; ask patient's name, location, and caretaker's name; monitor for twitching or seizure activity. Return patient to hospital immediately if he or she becomes increasingly difficult to awaken; cannot answer questions appropriately; cannot answer at all; becomes confused, restless, or agitated; develops slurred speech; develops twitching or seizures; develops or reports worsening headache or nausea and vomiting; has visual disturbances (e.g., blurred or double vision), develops weakness, numbness, or clumsiness, or has

difficulty walking; has clear or bloody drainage from the nose or ear; or develops a stiff neck.

3. Ensure that patient rests and eats lightly for the first day or so after the concussion or until he or she feels well. Over the next 2-3 days, patient should avoid alcohol, driving, contact sports, swimming, using power tools, and taking medication for headache or nausea without calling the physician.

4. Inform patient and significant others that some individuals may have a postconcussion syndrome in which they continue to have headaches, dizziness, or lethargy for several weeks or months. Patient also may experience sleep disturbance, difficulty concentrating, poor memory, irritability, emotional lability, and difficulty with judgment or abstract thinking. Explain the importance of reporting these problems to the physician.

Risk for infection related to inadequate primary defenses secondary to basilar skull fractures, penetrating or open head injuries, or surgical wounds

Desired outcomes: Patient is free of symptoms of infection, as evidenced by normothermia, stable or improving LOC, and absence of headache, photophobia, or neck stiffness. Patient verbalizes knowledge about signs and symptoms of infection and the importance of reporting them promptly.

1. Monitor injury site or surgical wounds for indicators of infection (e.g., persistent erythema, warmth, pain, hardness, and purulent drainage). Consult physician about significant findings.

2. Be alert for indicators of meningitis or encephalitis (fever, chills, malaise, back stiffness and pain, nuchal rigidity, photophobia, seizures, ataxia, sensorimotor deficits), which can occur after a penetrating, open head injury or cerebral surgical wound.

3. When examining scalp lacerations and assessing for foreign bodies or palpable fractures, wear sterile gloves and follow aseptic technique. Cleanse area gently, and cover scalp wounds with sterile dressings.

4. Document drainage and its amount, color, and odor. If patient has clear or bloody drainage from the nose, throat, or ears, notify physician of findings and assume that patient has a dural tear with CSF leakage until proven otherwise. Complaints of a salty taste or swallowing frequently may signal CSF dripping down the back of the throat. Bending forward may produce nasal drainage that can be tested for CSF. Inspect dressing and pillowcases for a halo ring, which may indicate CSF drainage. Clear drainage may be tested with a glucose reagent strip. Drainage also may be sent to the laboratory for testing for chloride. The presence of glucose and chloride (the amount of CSF Cl is > serum Cl) in nonsanguineous drainage indicates that drainage is CSF rather than mucus or saliva.

5. If CSF leakage occurs, do not clean the ears or nose unless prescribed by physician. Place a sterile pad over affected ear or under the nose to catch drainage, but do not pack them. Position patient so that fluid can drain. Change dressings when they become damp,

using aseptic technique. Instruct patient to keep his or her hands and fingers away from site of CSF leakage. Mittens or hand restraints may be necessary if patient is unable to comply.

6. Avoid excessive movement. If not contraindicated, place patient on bed rest with HOB up.
7. With CSF leakage or possible basilar fracture, avoid nasal suction to prevent introduction of bacteria into the nervous system. Instruct patient to avoid Valsalva's maneuver, straining with a bowel movement, and vigorous coughing, which may tear the dura and increase CSF flow. Patient also should not blow the nose, sneeze, or sniff in nasal drainage.
8. If patient is intubated, the tube for gastric decompression may be placed orally rather than nasally. If nasogastric (NG) tube is placed nasally, the physician usually performs the intubation. Check placement of tube, preferably by x-ray, before applying suction. NG tubes have been known to enter the fracture site and curl up into patient's cranial vault during insertion attempts. Visually check back of patient's throat for NG tube to help confirm placement.
9. Individuals with basilar skull fractures generally are placed flat in bed on complete bed rest. This position helps reduce pressure and the amount of CSF draining from a dural tear. Patients are prescribed antibiotics to prevent infection and are observed for healing and sealing of the dural tear within 7-10 days.
10. Teach patient to report any indicators of infection promptly.

Risk for disuse syndrome related to prescribed immobility and/or decreased LOC
Desired outcome: Patient has full ROM of all joints.
1. For patients at risk of increased intracranial pressure (IICP), perform passive ROM exercises rather than allow active or assisted ROM exercises, which can increase intraabdominal or intrathoracic pressure and thus ICP. For the same reason, avoid using the prone position.
2. Once the risk of IICP is no longer significant, additional measures to enhance mobility and strength may be implemented. For discussion, see **Risk for activity intolerance,** p. 413, and **Risk for disuse syndrome,** p. 416, in Appendix One, "Caring for Patients on Prolonged Bed Rest."
3. See Table 4-1 for interventions for patients with varying responses to stimuli.

Pain related to headaches secondary to head injury
Desired outcome: Within 1 h of intervention, patient's subjective perception of pain decreases, as documented by a pain scale.
1. Monitor and document the duration and character of patient's pain, rating it on a scale of 0 (no pain) to 10 (worst pain).
2. Administer analgesics as prescribed. Patients with head injuries generally do not have much pain, and the pain usually is relieved by analgesics such as acetaminophen. Sometimes codeine is prescribed, but as a rule, other narcotics are contraindicated because they can mask neurologic indicators of IICP and cause respiratory depression.

Table 4-1   Cognitive rehabilitation goals

Level	Response	Goal/Intervention
I II III	None Generalized Localized	*Goal:* Provide sensory input to elicit responses of increased quality, frequency, duration, and variety. *Intervention:* Give brief but frequent stimulation sessions and present stimuli in an organized manner, focusing on one sensory channel at a time, for example: *Visual:* Intermittent television, family pictures, bright objects *Auditory:* Tape recordings of family or favorite song, talking to patient, intermittent TV or radio *Olfactory:* Favorite perfume, shaving lotion, coffee, lemon, orange *Cutaneous:* Touch or rub skin with different textures such as velvet, ice bag, warm cloth *Movement:* Turn, ROM exercises, up in chair *Oral:* Oral care, lemon swabs, ice, sugar on tongue, peppermint, chocolate
IV	Confused, agitated	*Goal:* Reduce agitation and increase awareness of environment; this stage usually lasts 2-4 wk. *Interventions:* Remove offending devices (e.g., NG tube, restraints), if possible. Do not demand that patient follow through with task. Provide human contact unless this increases agitation. Provide a quiet, controlled environment. Use a calm, soft voice and manner around patient.
V VI	Confused, inappropriate Confused, appropriate	*Goal:* Reduce confusion and incorporate improved cognitive abilities into functional activity. *Interventions:* Begin each interaction with introduction, orientation, and interaction purpose. List and number daily activities in the sequence in which they will be done throughout the day. Maintain a consistent environment. Provide memory aids (e.g., calendar, clock). Use gentle repetition, which aids learning. Provide supervision and structure. Reorient as needed.

Neurologic

Table 4-1   Cognitive rehabilitation goals—cont'd

Level	Response	Goal/Intervention
VII	Automatic, appropriate	*Goal:* Integrate increased cognitive function into functional community activities with minimal
VIII	Purposeful	structuring.
		Interventions: Enable practicing of activities.
		Reduce supervision and environmental structure.
		Help patient plan adaptation of ADLs and home living skills to home environment.

Adapted from Rancho Los Amigos Hospital, Inc, Levels of Cognitive Functioning (scale based on behavioral descriptions or responses to stimuli).

3. For additional interventions, see **Pain,** p. 201, in "General Care of Patients with Neurologic Disorders."

Fluid volume excess related to compromised regulatory mechanisms with increased ADH and increased renal resorption secondary to syndrome of inappropriate antidiuretic hormone (SIADH)

Desired outcome: By hospital discharge (or within 3 days of injury), patient is normovolemic, as evidenced by stable weight, balanced I&O, urinary output ≥30 ml/h, urine specific gravity 1.010-1.030, BP within patient's baseline limits, absence of fingerprint edema over sternum, and orientation to time, place, and person.

1. Monitor I&O, VS, urine specific gravity, and electrolyte and serum osmolarity studies; weigh patient daily. Sudden, significant weight gain; urine output <500 ml/24 h; intake greater than output; urine specific gravity >1.030; and hypertension occur with SIADH. SIADH also creates a dilutional hyponatremia; be alert for serum sodium levels <137 mEq/L, serum osmolality <280 mOsm/kg, low BUN, and increased urine sodium and osmolality. Consult physician about significant changes.

2. Monitor patient for changes in orientation and LOC (e.g., apprehension, irritability, confusion), incoordination, headache, anorexia, muscle cramps, and fatigue. These are mild symptoms of SIADH. As SIADH progresses, expect nausea, vomiting, and abdominal cramps. Symptoms of severe SIADH include weakness, lethargy, confusion, muscle twitching, and seizure. Expect seizure activity when serum sodium level drops below 118 mEq/L; a level ≤115 mEq/L may result in loss of reflexes, coma, and death. Consult physician about significant findings. See "Syndrome of Inappropriate Antidiuretic Hormone," p. 215, for more information.

3. Monitor patient for symptoms of IICP, and institute measures to prevent it (see **Decreased adaptive capacity:** Intracranial, in "General Care of Patients with Neurologic Disorders," p. 197.

4. Assess for fingerprint edema over sternum, which reflects cellular edema. Because fluid is not retained in the interstitium with SIADH, peripheral edema will not necessarily occur.

5. Maintain fluid restriction as prescribed. Depending on serum sodium value, fluids may be restricted to an amount as low as 500 ml/24 h. Remove water or ice chips from bedside. Hypotonic solutions such as D_5W usually are contraindicated, because they are converted to free H_2O.

6. As appropriate, provide measured ice chips and frequent mouth care for thirst.

7. Administer hypertonic saline (3%) as prescribed.

8. As prescribed, give furosemide (Lasix) to promote diuresis; demeclocycline (Declomycin), which acts as an ADH inhibitor; and lithium, which interferes with the action of aldosterone.

9. Ensure that HOB is elevated ≤10-20 degrees to promote venous return and left atrial filling pressure, thereby reducing release of ADH.

10. Institute seizure precautions (see "Seizure Disorders," p. 179).

   If patient has urinary incontinence or retention, or neurogenic bladder, see Chapter 3, "Renal-Urinary Disorders," for related discussions. **Caution:** Credé's method and other measures that can increase intraabdominal and intrathoracic pressure are contraindicated for patients at risk of IICP.

See "Alzheimer's Disease" for **Impaired environmental interpretation syndrome,** p. 135, and **Risk for violence,** p. 137.

See "Brain Tumors" for **Knowledge deficit:** Ventricular shunt procedure, p. 160, and **Knowledge deficit:** Craniotomy procedure, p. 161.

See "Cerebrovascular Accident" for **Impaired physical mobility,** p. 171; **Sensory/perceptual alterations,** p. 172; and **Impaired verbal communication,** p. 174.

See "Seizure Disorders," p. 179, for seizure-related nursing diagnoses.

See "General Care of Patients with Neurologic Disorders" for **Risk for trauma,** p. 187; **Risk for injury,** p. 189; **Impaired corneal tissue integrity,** p. 189; **Altered nutrition,** p. 190; **Risk for fluid volume deficit,** p. 191; **Risk for aspiration,** p. 192; **Self-care deficit,** p. 193; **Constipation,** p. 196; **Decreased adaptive capacity:** Intracranial, p. 197; **Sensory/perceptual alterations,** p. 200; **Impaired swallowing,** p. 201; **Altered body temperature,** p. 204, and **Knowledge deficit:** Neurologic diagnostic tests, p. 205.

For patients with diabetes insipidus, see nursing diagnoses in "Diabetes Insipidus," p. 212.

For patients with SIADH, see "Syndrome of Inappropriate Antidiuretic Hormone," p. 215.

For patients undergoing surgery, see Appendix One, "Caring for Preoperative and Postoperative Patients," p. 395.

For patients with varying degrees of immobility, see related nursing diagnoses in "Pressure Ulcers," p. 390, and Appendix One, "Caring for Patients on Prolonged Bed Rest," p. 413.

See Appendix One, "Caring for Patients with Cancer and Other Life-Disrupting Illnesses," p. 450, for appropriate psychosocial diagnoses and interventions.

Neurologic

PATIENT-FAMILY TEACHING
AND DISCHARGE PLANNING

A patient with a head injury can have varying degrees of neurologic deficit, ranging from mild to severe. As indicated by patient's condition and prognosis, give patient and significant others verbal and written information about the following:

1. Referrals to community resources, such as cognitive retraining specialist, head injury rehabilitation centers, Visiting Nurse Association, community support groups, social workers, psychologic therapy, vocational rehabilitation agency, home health agencies, and extended and skilled care facilities. In addition, provide this address: National Head Injury Foundation, 1776 Massachusetts Avenue NW, Suite 100, Washington, DC 20036 *phone:* (202)-296-6443 or (800)-444-6443.

2. Safety measures related to decreased sensation, visual disturbances, motor deficits, and seizure activity.

3. Measures that promote communication in cases of aphasia.

4. Wound care and indicators of infection.

5. Measures for dealing with cognitive or behavioral problems. As appropriate, include home evaluation for safety. Caution significant others that an individual's personality can change drastically after head injury. Patient may demonstrate inappropriate social behavior, inappropriate affect, hallucination, delusion, and altered sleep pattern.

6. If patient suffered a concussion, a description of problems that may occur at home and would require prompt medical attention (see **Knowledge deficit,** p. 154).

7. For other information, see teaching and discharge planning interventions (entries 4-10 only) in "Multiple Sclerosis," p. 116, as appropriate.

SECTION FOUR: NERVOUS SYSTEM TUMORS

Brain Tumors

NURSING DIAGNOSES AND INTERVENTIONS

Knowledge deficit: Ventricular shunt procedure
Desired outcome: After explanation, patient verbalizes accurate information about ventricular shunt procedure, including presurgical and postsurgical care.

1. Determine patient's understanding of procedure after physician's explanation, including purpose, risks, and anticipated benefits or outcome. Intervene accordingly.

2. Explain that the procedure is performed to enable drainage of CSF when flow is obstructed (e.g., by a tumor or blood). Shunt types vary but can extend from the lateral ventricle of the brain to one of the following: subarachnoid space of the spinal canal, right atrium of the heart, a large vein, or the peritoneal cavity.
3. Explain that it is important to avoid lying on insertion site after procedure to avoid putting pressure on shunt mechanism. The head and neck are kept in alignment to prevent kinking and compression of shunt catheter. Explain that shunt site will be monitored for redness, tenderness, bulging, or fluid collection, and swelling will be assessed along shunt's course.
4. If shunt has a valve for controlling CSF drainage or reflux, explain that the valve will be pumped or compressed a certain number of times at prescribed intervals to flush system of exudate and prevent plugging. Explain that the valve, which usually is located behind or above the ear and is approximately the diameter of a fingertip, can be felt to empty and then refill.
5. Reassure patient and significant others that before hospital discharge, specific instructions will be given about shunt care, recognition of shunt site infection and malfunction, and steps to take should they occur. Teach signs and symptoms of IICP (i.e., headache, change in LOC, such as drowsiness, lethargy, irritability, personality changes), which can signal shunt malfunctioning.
6. For additional interventions, see **Risk for infection,** p. 155, in "Head Injury" and this nursing diagnosis in Appendix One, "Caring for Preoperative and Postoperative Patients," p. 408.

Knowledge deficit: Craniotomy procedure

Desired outcome: After explanation, patient verbalizes accurate understanding of craniotomy procedure, including presurgical and postsurgical care.

1. After physician's explanation of procedure, determine patient's level of understanding of the purpose, risks, and anticipated benefits or outcome. Intervene accordingly or reinforce physician's explanation as appropriate.
2. Explain that a craniotomy is a surgical opening into the skull to remove a hematoma or tumor, repair a ruptured aneurysm, or apply arterial clips, or to wrap the involved vessel to prevent future rupture. As appropriate, explain that bone flap may be left open postoperatively to accommodate cerebral edema and prevent compression. When the bone is removed, the procedure is called a craniectomy.
3. Explain that before surgery, antiseptic shampoos may be given and patient may be started on corticosteroids such as dexamethasone and antiepilepsy drugs. Explain that a baseline neurologic assessment will provide a basis for comparison with postoperative neurologic checks.
4. During the immediate postoperative period, patient is in ICU. Explain the following considerations and interventions that are likely to occur.
   ■ Assessment of VS and neurologic status at least hourly. Patient will be asked to perform a variety of assessment measures, in-

cluding squeezing tester's hand, moving extremities, extending the tongue, and answering questions. Emphasize the importance of performing these tasks to the best of patient's ability.

■ Changes in body image that can occur because of loss of hair, presence of a head dressing, and the potential for and expected duration of facial edema.

■ Possible need for respiratory and airway support, including oxygen, intubation, or ventilation. Typically patients are on a cardiac monitor for 24-48 h because dysrhythmias are not unusual after posterior fossa surgery or when blood is in the CSF.

■ Presence of large head dressing and drains, which will be inspected periodically for bleeding or CSF leakage. Stress the importance of not pulling or tugging on dressing or drains.

■ NPO status for the first 36-48 h because of the risk of vomiting and choking. Explain that once fluids are allowed, they usually are limited to minimize cerebral edema.

■ Periorbital swelling, which usually occurs within 24-48 h of supratentorial surgery. Explain that this can be relieved by applying cold or warm compresses around the eyes. Having HOB up with patient lying on nonoperative side also may help reduce edema.

■ Insertion of indwelling urinary catheter to enable accurate measurement of I&O and to monitor for problems such as diabetes insipidus.

■ Measurement of core temperature (e.g., rectal, tympanic, bladder) at frequent intervals. Rectal probe or bladder catheter temperature probe may be used for continuous monitoring. Oral temperatures are not taken during period cognitive function is decreased.

5. Teach patient that postsurgical positioning is a key factor during recovery.

■ *Supratentorial craniotomy:* Patient is maintained with HOB elevated to 30 degrees or as prescribed. Patient will be assisted with turning and usually will be kept off the operative site, especially if lesion was large. Head and neck will be kept in good alignment.

■ *Infratentorial craniotomy* (for cerebellar or brainstem surgery): HOB is kept flat or as prescribed. Because pressure usually is kept off operative site, especially with a craniectomy, these patients are kept off their backs for 48 h. In posterior fossa surgery, the supporting neck muscles are altered. Log-roll patient to alternate sides, keeping head in good alignment. A soft cervical collar may be used to prevent anterior or lateral angulation of the neck. A small pillow may be used for comfort.

6. Explain that bed rest will be enforced immediately after surgery.

7. Teach patients undergoing infratentorial surgery that they are likely to experience the following:

■ Dizziness and hypotension, necessitating a longer period of bed rest.

■ Nausea, which should be reported so that antiemetics (e.g., metoclopramide or trimethobenzamide) can be given.

- Cranial nerve edema, which might result in swallowing difficulties, extraocular movements, or nystagmus, any of which should be reported promptly.

8. Teach patient the following precautions for preventing increased intraabdominal and intrathoracic pressure, which can cause IICP:
   - Exhaling when being turned.
   - Not straining at stool.
   - Not moving self in bed; rather, letting staff members do all moving.
   - Importance of deep breathing and avoiding coughing and sneezing. If coughing and sneezing are unavoidable, they must be done with an open mouth to minimize pressure buildup.
   - Avoiding hip flexion and lying prone.
   - For additional precautions against IICP, see **Decreased adaptive capacity:** Intracranial, p. 197.

9. Teach patient that precautions are taken for seizures (see **Risk for trauma** related to oral, musculoskeletal, and airway vulnerability secondary to seizure activity, p. 179).

10. Teach patient about wound care and indicators of infection. Generally, a surgical cap is worn after head dressing is removed. Patient must not scratch wound or sutures and must keep incision dry. After sutures are removed, the hair can be shampooed, but patient should be careful not to scrub around suture line. Patient should not use a hair dryer until hair has regrown (incision line usually is distal to normal hair line and will not be apparent when hair regrows). For more information, see **Risk for infection,** p. 155, in "Head Injury."

11. Explain that patients undergoing excision of an acoustic neuroma may have nausea, hearing loss, facial weakness or paralysis, diminished or absent blinking, eye dryness, tinnitus, vertigo, headache, and occasionally swallowing, throat, and voice problems. Nausea and dizziness can be profound problems after surgery. Provide prescribed antiemetics, and turn and move patient slowly. Speak to patient on unaffected side for best hearing, and place telephone and call light on that side of the bed. Contralateral routing of signal hearing aids may improve hearing by directing sound from deaf ear to hearing ear *via* a tiny microphone and transmitter. Background music or other "white noise" may mask tinnitus. Patient's awareness of tinnitus eventually should diminish. Balance exercises and walking with assistance will start the process of compensation by the functioning vestibular system.

12. For additional interventions, see this nursing diagnosis in Appendix One, "Caring for Preoperative and Postoperative Patients," p. 395.

If patient has urinary incontinence or retention, or neurogenic bladder, see Chapter 3, "Renal-Urinary Disorders," for related discussions.

See "Alzheimer's Disease" for **Impaired environmental interpretation syndrome,** p. 134, and **Risk for violence,** p. 137.

See "Head Injury" for **Risk for disuse syndrome**, p. 156. If patient has SIADH, also see **Fluid volume excess**, p. 158.

See "Cerebrovascular Accident" for **Impaired verbal communication**, p. 174; **Impaired physical mobility**, p. 171; and **Sensory/perceptual alterations**, p. 172.

See "Seizure Disorders," p. 179, for nursing diagnoses related to seizures.

See "General Care of Patients with Neurologic Disorders," p. 187, for related diagnoses.

For patients with diabetes insipidus, see related nursing diagnoses in "Diabetes Insipidus," p. 212.

For patients with SIADH, see "Syndrome of Inappropriate Antidiuretic Hormone," p. 215.

For patients with a pituitary tumor, see related nursing diagnoses in "Pituitary and Hypothalamic Tumors," p. 213.

For patients with varying degrees of immobility, see related nursing diagnoses in "Pressure Ulcers," p. 390, and Appendix One, "Caring for Patients on Prolonged Bed Rest," p. 413.

See Appendix One, "Caring for Preoperative and Postoperative Patients," p. 395, and "Caring for Patients with Cancer and Other Life-Disrupting Illnesses," p. 450, as appropriate.

PATIENT-FAMILY TEACHING AND DISCHARGE PLANNING

Give patient and significant others verbal and written information about the following as appropriate:

1. Safety measures specific to sensory deficits, motor deficits, incoordination, cognitive deficits, and seizures.
2. Measures to promote communication in cases of aphasia.
3. Appropriate referrals to community resources, such as public health nurse, Visiting Nurse Association, community support groups, social workers, psychologic therapy, vocational rehabilitation agency, home health agencies, and extended and skilled care facilities. In addition, provide these addresses and phone numbers: the American Cancer Society, 1599 Clifton Road NE, Atlanta, GA 30329 *phone:* (404)-320-3333 or (800)-ACS-2345; and the National Cancer Institute Information Service, *phone:* (800)-422-6237. The American Brain Tumor Association has set up local support groups and will try to assist brain tumor patients and their families. The association's address is 2720 River Road, Des Plaines, IL 60018 *phone:* (800)-886-2282. Provide this address for acoustic neuroma patients: Acoustic Neuroma Association, P.O. Box 12402, Atlanta, GA 30355 *phone:* (404)-237-8023.
4. Care of postoperative or postprocedural wounds and indicators of infection.
5. Potential side effects and precautions for patients undergoing radiation therapy.

6. Medications, including drug name, purpose, dosage, schedule, precautions, drug/drug and food/drug interactions, and potential side effects, especially for chemotherapeutic agents.
7. Exercises that promote muscle strength and mobility, measures for preventing contractures and skin breakdown, transfer techniques and proper body mechanics, use of assistive devices, and other measures that promote independence with ADLs.
8. Measures for relieving pain, nausea, or other discomfort.
9. Indications of constipation, urinary retention, or urinary tract infection; implementation of bowel and bladder training programs; and, if appropriate, care of indwelling catheters.
10. Indications of upper respiratory infections, and measures to prevent regurgitation, aspiration, and respiratory infection.
11. Importance of follow-up care, including visits to physician, PT, OT, speech therapy, psychologic counseling, and laboratory monitoring for side effects of radiation therapy or chemotherapy.
12. First aid measures for seizures.
13. Causes of IICP and measures to prevent it.
14. Care of ventricular shunt, if present. Include specific instructions for shunt care, information about how to identify shunt infection or malfunction, and steps to take should it develop.
15. Measures that assist with reorientation and dealing with behavioral or cognitive problems, as well as communicating with patient in view of cognitive deficits.

Spinal Cord Tumors

NURSING DIAGNOSES AND INTERVENTIONS

Pain (acute or chronic) related to tissue compression secondary to tumor growth

Desired outcomes: Within 1 h of intervention, patient's subjective perception of pain decreases, as documented by a pain scale. Objective indicators, such as grimacing, are absent or diminished.

N O T E : Symptoms of primary tumors usually develop slowly, whereas those of metastatic tumors develop rapidly. Intense localized pain generally is the first symptom, with localized tenderness over the spine.

---

1. Assess character and degree of patient's pain, using a pain scale. Rate pain from 0 (no pain) to 10 (worst pain). Pain may signal the need for immediate medical treatment (e.g., corticosteroids, radiation therapy, decompressive laminectomy) to help prevent or minimize neurologic deficits that may be permanently disabling. Have patient alert staff members or physician to the following: backache; sensations of heaviness or weakness in the arms or legs; any incoordination; loss of sensations of light touch, pain, and temperature; incontinence or difficulty urinating or defecating; and sexual impotence.

2. Advise patient that moving slowly with good body alignment may help minimize pain. A soft cervical collar may help neck alignment.
3. Suggest that keeping knees and hips slightly flexed when in bed helps reduce pain by preventing traction on nerve roots caused by full extension of spinal cord.
4. Inform patient that sneezing and straining can cause pain.
5. For other interventions, see **Pain** in "General Care of Patients with Neurologic Disorders," p. 201.

If patient has urinary incontinence or retention, or neurogenic bladder, see related discussions in Chapter 3, "Renal-Urinary Disorders."

See "Spinal Cord Injury," p. 142, for nursing diagnoses and interventions related to the care of patients with spinal cord disorders.

See "General Care of Patients with Neurologic Disorders" for **Knowledge deficit:** Neurologic diagnostic tests, p. 205.

See "Pressure Ulcers," p. 390, and Appendix One, "Caring for Patients on Prolonged Bed Rest," p. 413, for nursing diagnoses and interventions for immobilized patients.

Also see Appendix One, "Caring for Preoperative and Postoperative Patients," p. 395, and "Caring for Patients with Cancer and Other Life-Disrupting Illnesses," p. 450.

PATIENT-FAMILY TEACHING AND DISCHARGE PLANNING

Give patient and significant others verbal and written information about the following:
1. Safety measures relative to sensorimotor deficits.
2. For more information, see entries 3-11 in "Brain Tumors," p. 164.

SECTION FIVE: VASCULAR DISORDERS OF THE NERVOUS SYSTEM

Cerebral Aneurysm

NURSING DIAGNOSES AND INTERVENTIONS

The following nursing diagnoses relate primarily to the patient whose aneurysm is graded 1-3. If patient's aneurysm is graded 4-5, see nursing diagnoses in "Cerebrovascular Accident," p. 170, for patient care.

Grading: Individuals with aneurysms are graded according to the severity of the bleeding or injury:

- *Grade 1:* Patient alert with no neurologic deficit; slight neck stiffness; minimal headache, if present.
- *Grade 2:* Patient alert with mild to severe headache; presence of stiff neck; may have minimal neurologic deficit, such as third cranial nerve palsies.

- *Grade 3*: Patient drowsy or confused; presence of stiff neck; may have mild focal neurologic deficits.
- *Grade 4*: Patient stuporous, semicomatose; presence of stiff neck; may have neurologic deficits, such as hemiparesis.
- *Grade 5*: Patient comatose and posturing.

Knowledge deficit: Aneurysms and the potential for rebleeding, rupture, or vasospasm

Desired outcome: After instruction, patient verbalizes knowledge about potential for rebleeding or vasospasm, measures to prevent their occurrence, and symptoms to report to the health care staff.

1. Assess patient for sensorimotor deficits (e.g., decreased or absent vision, impaired temperature and pain sensation, unsteady gait, weakness, or paralysis). Document baseline neurologic and physical assessments so that changes in patient's status are detected promptly. Teach patient and significant others these indicators, and explain the importance of reporting them to staff promptly.

2. Teach these patients the importance of reducing activity level to avoid rebleeding or rupture. Strict bed rest may be prescribed. Emphasize the necessity of allowing others to help them with moving, ADLs, and passive ROM, even though they may feel capable of self-care. Explain that the number and frequency of visitors will be limited, and that individuals whose presence is stressful to the patient should not be allowed to visit. The telephone will be removed from the room, and television, radio, and reading may be restricted or limited to programs and books that are not overstimulating. The room will be darkened to promote rest, and sedatives and tranquilizers may be offered. Caffeine and other stimulants may be restricted, as well as nicotine, which can increase the risk of vasospasm.

3. Teach patient measures to prevent a sudden increase in ICP.
   - Avoid coughing and sneezing; if they are unavoidable, do them with an open mouth.
   - Exhale when being turned.
   - Avoid straining with bowel movements.
   - Avoid extreme hip flexion or lying prone.
   - Avoid moving self up in bed because this requires a pushing movement. Do not grip, push, or pull on side rails or push feet against mattress or foot of bed. Request help from staff member for all moving and turning movements.

4. Explain that HOB may be maintained at 30 degrees, and patient may be asked to keep head and neck in good alignment to promote venous return to the heart and reduce cerebral congestion and ICP.

5. Explain that patient may be given a high-fiber diet and stool softeners to promote bowel elimination without straining.

6. Describe, as appropriate, the following preventive measures: corticosteroids to prevent or reduce cerebral edema, antiepilepsy medications to prevent seizures, antihypertensive medications to keep BP within defined parameters, and a low-sodium, low-cholesterol diet to help control BP.

7. Teach patient to avoid taking aspirin or aspirin-containing products, which increase the risk of hemorrhage.

Knowledge deficit: Effects of aminocaproic acid drug therapy
Desired outcome: After instruction, patient verbalizes knowledge about side effects of aminocaproic therapy, measures to prevent complications from drug therapy, and signs and symptoms that should be reported immediately to health care staff.

1. Teach patients taking aminocaproic acid therapy the indicators of pulmonary embolus, including SOB, chest pain (especially that which increases with inspiration), and blood-tinged sputum, as well as indicators of deep vein thrombosis (e.g., calf pain or tenderness; increased heat, swelling, or redness of the leg). Stress the importance of notifying staff immediately if these signs develop. Encourage patient to wear antiembolism hose.

2. Monitor patient's IV site for signs of phlebitis. Instruct patient to report any tenderness or swelling at site.

3. Alert patient to potential for loose stools, frequent stools (more than 3/day), cramps, and weakness with aminocaproic acid therapy. Instruct patient to report these problems promptly because if the diarrhea is a side effect of oral aminocaproic therapy, the physician may switch patient to IV medication.

4. Inform patients that because the drug may cause postural hypotension, they should make position changes very slowly and in stages. Faintness or dizziness should be reported promptly.

5. Instruct patient to report any muscle weakness, muscle pain, sweating, fever, or myoglobinuria (reddish-brown urine) because these may be signs of myopathy caused by this drug therapy.

6. Teach patient to report nausea, tinnitus, nasal stuffiness, or fatigue, which are other side effects of aminocaproic drug therapy.

Ineffective airway clearance (or risk for same) related to imposed inactivity secondary to risk of aneurysm rupture or bleeding
Desired outcomes: After intervention, patient's lungs are clear upon auscultation. Secretions are thin and clear, and patient remains normothermic.

1. Assess patient for increased SOB or change in rate or depth of respirations. Auscultate lung fields for breath sounds, noting crackles, rhonchi, or diminished sounds. Assess for fever, purulent sputum, and cyanosis. Monitor patient's ABG values for hypoxemia (Pao_2 <80 mm Hg) or hypercapnia ($Paco_2$ >45 mm Hg). Consult physician about significant findings.

2. Encourage patient to breathe deeply and change positions q2h to help expand lungs. Instruct patient to avoid coughing or sneezing because these activities increase intraabdominal and intrathoracic pressure, which in turn increases ICP and the risk of aneurysm rupture. Explain that if sneezing is unavoidable, it should be done with an open mouth.

3. Maintain patient on oxygen as prescribed.

4. Help patient with incentive spirometry, if prescribed.

Risk for disuse syndrome related to prescribed immobilization secondary to risk of aneurysm rupture or rebleeding
Desired outcome: Patient exhibits complete ROM.

1. To maintain joint mobility, perform passive ROM exercises during period of activity restriction. Even if patient feels well enough to

perform assisted or active ROM, these activities are contraindicated because they increase ICP and the risk of rupture or rebleeding. Explain to patient the rationale for activity limitation.
2. Maintain joint alignment, and support joints and extremities with pillows, trochanter rolls, sandbags, and other positioning devices.
3. When patient is no longer on bed rest and activity restriction, additional strengthening and conditioning exercises may be necessary to counteract the effects of prolonged bed rest. In addition, patient may have residual neurologic deficits that require gait training or use of assistive devices to promote mobility. Obtain a physical therapy or occupational therapy referral as appropriate. For additional interventions, see **Risk for disuse syndrome** in Appendix One, "Caring for Patients on Prolonged Bed Rest," p. 416.

Self-care deficit related to imposed activity restrictions secondary to risk of aneurysm rupture or rebleeding
Desired outcome: Patient's care activities are performed for him or her during period of strict bed rest.
1. During period of strict bed rest and activity restriction, perform care activities, even for patients who do not show signs of neurologic deficit. Explain the reason for patient's activity restriction.
2. If patient has bathroom privileges, provide a commode as appropriate and assist patient with transferring as necessary.

As appropriate, see "Head Injury" for **Fluid volume excess** related to SIADH, p. 158.

For surgical patients, see "Brain Tumors" for **Knowledge deficit:** Ventricular shunt procedure, p. 160. See "Cerebrovascular Accident" for **Knowledge deficit:** Cerebral artery bypass surgery, p. 176. As appropriate, see "Seizure Disorders," p. 179, for related nursing diagnoses.

See "General Care of Patients with Neurologic Disorders" for **Risk for fluid volume deficit,** p. 191; **Constipation,** p. 196; **Decreased adaptive capacity:** Intracranial, p. 197; **Pain,** p. 201; and **Knowledge deficit:** Neurologic diagnostic tests, p. 205.

As appropriate, see "Diabetes Insipidus" for **Altered protection** related to side effects of vasopressin, p. 212.

For patients with varying degrees of immobility, see "Pressure Ulcers," p. 390, and Appendix One, "Caring for Patients on Prolonged Bed Rest," p. 413.

Also see Appendix One, "Caring for Patients with Cancer and Other Life-Disrupting Illnesses," p. 450, as appropriate, for psychosocial interventions.

PATIENT-FAMILY TEACHING AND DISCHARGE PLANNING

Give patient and significant others verbal and written information about the following:
1. Wound care and indicators of wound infection for patients who have undergone surgery.

2. Importance of avoiding strenuous physical activity. Consult physician about restrictions and limitations on activities, and instruct patient accordingly.
3. If prescribed, a diet low in sodium (see Table 1-4, p. 18, for a list of high-sodium foods to avoid) and low in cholesterol (see Table 2-3, p. 28, for guidelines) to control hypertension and atherosclerosis.
4. Medications, including drug name, purpose, dosage, schedule, precautions, drug/drug and food/drug interactions, and potential side effects.
5. Signs and symptoms of rupture and rebleeding; patient is at risk for these for 6 mo after initial episode of bleeding.
6. Care of ventricular shunt, if present. Instructions should include indicators of shunt infection and steps to take in the event of shunt infection or malfunction.

In Addition

7. See teaching and discharge planning section in "Cerebrovascular Accident," p. 179, for additional interventions for patients who have residual neurologic deficits.

Cerebrovascular Accident

NURSING DIAGNOSES AND INTERVENTIONS

Unilateral neglect related to disturbed perceptual ability secondary to neurologic insult

Desired outcome: After intervention, patient scans environment and responds to stimuli on affected side.

1. Assess patient's ability to: recognize objects to right or left of his or her visual midline; perceive body parts as his or her own; perceive pain, touch, and temperature sensations; judge distances; orient self to changes in environment; differentiate left from right; maintain posture sense; and identify objects by sight, hearing, or touch. Document specific deficits.
2. Neglect of and inattention to stimuli on affected side occur more often with right hemisphere injury. Neglect cannot be totally explained on the basis of loss of physical senses (e.g., both ears are used in hearing, but with auditory neglect, patient may ignore conversation or noises that occur on affected side). Assess patient for neglect of affected side as follows:
    - *Visual neglect:* Patient does not turn his or her head to see all parts of an object (e.g., may read only half of a page or eat from only one side of plate). When patient exhibits signs of visual neglect, continue to place objects necessary for ADLs and call light on unaffected side and approach patient from that side, but gradually increase stimuli on affected side (e.g., while communicating with patient, physically move across her or his visual boundary and stand on that side to shift patient's attention to neglected side; encourage patient to turn his or her head past midline and scan entire environment. Place patient's food on neglected side, and encourage patient to look to neglected side and name food before eating. Place a bright red tape or ribbon on af-

fected side, and encourage patient to scan and find it). Continuously clue patient to environment. Initially place patient's unaffected side toward most active part of room, but as compensation occurs, reverse this. As patient begins to compensate, place additional items out of his or her visual field.

- *Self-neglect:* Patient does not perceive his or her arm or leg as being a part of the body. For example, when combing or brushing the hair, patient attends to only one (unaffected) side of the head. Inadequate self-care and injury may occur. Encourage patients to touch or massage and look at their affected sides and make a conscious effort to care for neglected body parts; also, check them for proper position to prevent contractures and skin breakdown. To enhance patient's self-recognition, periodically refer to patient's body parts on neglected side. When patient is in bed or up in a chair, provide safety measures, such as side rails and restraints, to prevent patient from attempting to get up, which can occur because of unawareness of affected side. Teach patient to use unaffected arm to perform ROM exercises on affected side. Integrate patient's neglected arm into activities. Position arm on bedside table or wheelchair lap board with hand or arm past midline, where patient can see it. Teach patient to attend to affected side first when performing ADLs, consciously look for affected side, monitor its position, and check for exposure to sharp objects and irritants. Provide a mirror so that patients can watch themselves shave or brush their teeth and hair. Instruct patient to take precautions with hot or cold items or when around moving machinery. Teach the use of an arm sling to support affected arm when patient is out of bed and when in bed to elevate affected arm. Stand on patient's affected side when ambulating with patient.
- *Auditory neglect:* Patient ignores individuals who approach and speak from his or her affected side, but communicates with those who approach or speak from unaffected side. To stimulate patient's attention to affected side, move across auditory boundary while speaking, and continue speaking from patient's neglected side to bring patient's attention to that area.

3. Arrange environment to maximize performance of ADLs by keeping necessary objects, such as call light, on patient's unaffected side. If possible, move bed so that patient's unaffected side faces the largest section of the room. Approach and speak to patient from unaffected side. If you must approach affected side, announce yourself to avoid startling patient. Perform activities on unaffected side unless you are specifically attempting to stimulate neglected side. After attempting to stimulate neglected side, return to patient's unaffected side for activities and communication. Inform significant others about patient's deficit and compensatory interventions.

Impaired physical mobility related to neuromuscular impairment with limited use of upper and/or lower limbs secondary to cerebrovascular accident (CVA)

Desired outcome: By at least the 24 h before hospital discharge, patient and significant others demonstrate techniques that promote ambulation and transferring.

1. Teach patient methods for turning and moving, using stronger extremity to move weaker extremity. For example, to move affected leg in bed or when changing from a lying to a sitting position, slide unaffected foot under affected ankle to lift, support, and bring affected leg along in desired movement.

2. Encourage patient to make a conscious attempt to look at extremities and check position before moving. Remind patient to make a conscious effort to lift and then extend foot when ambulating.

3. Instruct patient with impaired sense of balance to compensate by leaning toward stronger side. (The tendency is to lean toward the weaker or paralyzed side.) As necessary, remind patient to keep body weight forward over feet when standing.

4. Protect impaired arms with a sling, to support arm and shoulder when patient is up and to help maintain anatomic position. Position patient in correct alignment and provide a pillow or lap board for support. Encourage active/passive ROM to improve muscle tone. Avoid pulling on patient's shoulders or arms. Use a transfer belt or turn sheet. Monitor for subluxation of shoulder (e.g., shoulder pain and tenderness, swelling, decreased ROM, altered appearance).

5. General principles when transferring include:
   - Encourage weight-bearing on patient's stronger side.
   - Instruct patient to pivot on stronger side and use stronger arm for support.
   - Teach patient that transferring toward unaffected side generally is easiest and safest.
   - Instruct patient to place unaffected side closest to bed or chair he or she wishes to transfer to.
   - Explain that when transferring, the affected leg should be under patient with the foot flat on the ground.
   - Position a braced chair or locked wheelchair close to patient's stronger side. If patient requires assistance from staff member, teach patient not to support himself or herself by pulling on or placing hands around assistant's neck. Staff members should use their own knees and feet to brace the feet and knees of patients who are very weak.

6. Obtain PT and OT referrals as appropriate. Reinforce special mobilization techniques (e.g., Bobath, proprioceptive neuromuscular facilitation [PNF]) per patient's individualized rehabilitation program. These techniques may vary from the above general principles (e.g., Bobath focuses on use of affected side in mobility training).

Sensory/perceptual alterations related to altered sensory reception, transmission, and/or integration secondary to neurologic damage

Desired outcome: After intervention, patient interacts appropriately with his or her environment and shows no evidence of injury caused by sensory/perceptual deficit.

1. Patients who have a dominant (left) hemisphere injury usually have normal awareness of their body and spatial orientation despite possible lack of or decreased pain sensation and position sense and vi-

sual field deficit on right side of the body. These patients may need reminders to scan their environment but usually do not exhibit unilateral neglect. They tend to be slow, cautious, and disorganized when approaching an unfamiliar problem and benefit from frequent, accurate, and immediate feedback on their performance. Because of a short attention span and impaired logical reasoning, patient is easily distracted, so give short, simple messages or questions and step-by-step directions. Since patient may have poor abstract thinking, keep conversation on a concrete level (e.g., say "water," not "fluid," "leg," not "limb"). These patients may have difficulty recognizing items by touch and benefit from touching them (e.g., washcloth, comb) and having caretaker name them.

2. Patients with nondominant (right) hemisphere injury also may have decreased pain sensation, pain sense, and visual field deficit, but typically are unaware of or deny their deficits or lost abilities. They tend to be impulsive and too quick with movements. Typically, they have impaired judgment about what they can or cannot do and often overestimate their abilities. Encourage these patients to slow down and check each step or task as it is completed. These individuals are at risk for burns, bruises, cuts, and falls and may need to be restrained from attempting unsafe activities. They also are more likely to show unilateral neglect (see **Unilateral neglect,** p. 170). Patient generally retains the ability to think logically, but sees specifics rather than global picture (i.e., can see the trees but not the forest). Be careful what you say because it may be taken literally (e.g., if you say "ate the lion's share," the patient may think that someone literally ate the lion's portion of the meal). Impaired ability to recognize subtle distinctions may occur (e.g., difference between a fork and a spoon may become too subtle to detect).

3. Patients with apraxia are unable to carry out previously learned motor tasks, although they may be able to describe them in detail. Have these patients return your demonstration of the task. They may be able to be talked through a task or may be able to talk themselves through a task step by step.

4. Patients may have visual field deficits in which they can only physically see a portion of the normal visual field. Encourage making a conscious effort to scan the rest of the environment by turning the head from side to side.

5. Patients with nondominant (right) hemisphere injury also may have the following sensory/perceptual alterations:
   - Impaired ability to recognize, associate, or interpret sounds (e.g., voice quality, animal noises, musical pieces, types of instruments): direct patient's attention to a particular sound (e.g., if a cat meows on the television, state that it is the sound a cat makes and point to the cat on the screen).
   - Visual-spatial misperception: for example, patient may underestimate distances and bump into doors, or confuse the inside and outside of an object, such as an article of clothing. (Marking the outer aspects of the shoes "L" and "R" may help in dressing efforts.) These patients may lose their place when reading or add-

ing numbers and thus never complete tasks. They benefit from a structured, consistent environment.

- Difficulty recognizing and associating familiar objects: patients may not recognize dangerous or hazardous objects because they do not know the purpose of the object. Help these individuals with eating, because they may not know the purpose of silverware. Monitor environment for safety hazards and remove unsafe objects (e.g., scissors) from bedside.
- Inability to orient self in space: patients may require a restraint or wheelchair belt for support because they may not know if they are standing, sitting, or leaning.
- Misperception of own body and body parts: patients may not perceive their foot or arm as being a part of their body. Teach them to concentrate on their body parts (e.g., by watching their feet carefully while walking).
- Impaired ability to recognize objects by means of the senses of hearing, vibration, or touch: patients rely more on visual cues; keep their environment simple to reduce sensory overload and enable concentration on visual cues; remove distracting stimuli.

Impaired verbal communication related to aphasia secondary to cerebrovascular insult

Desired outcome: At a minimum of the 24 h before hospital discharge, patient demonstrates improved self-expression and relates decreased frustration with communication.

N O T E : Aphasia, the partial or complete inability to use or comprehend language and symbols, may occur with dominant (left) hemisphere damage. It is not the result of impaired hearing or intelligence. There are many different types of aphasia. Generally, the patient has a combination of types, which vary in severity. *Receptive aphasia* (e.g., Wernicke's or sensory aphasia) is characterized by inability to recognize or comprehend spoken words. It is as if a foreign language were being spoken or the patient had word deafness. The patient often is good at responding to nonverbal cues. *Expressive aphasia* (e.g., Broca's or motor aphasia) is characterized by difficulty expressing words or naming objects. Gestures, groans, swearing, or nonsense words may be used.

---

1. Evaluate nature and severity of patient's aphasia. When doing so, avoid giving nonverbal cues. Assess patient's ability to point or look toward a specific object, follow simple directions, understand yes or no questions, understand complex questions, repeat both simple and complex words, repeat sentences, name objects that are shown, demonstrate or relate the purpose or action of the object, fulfill written requests, write requests, and read. When evaluating patient for aphasia, be aware that patient may be responding to nonverbal cues and may understand less than you think. Document this assessment with simple descriptions and specific examples of patient's aphasia symptoms. Use it as the basis for a communication plan.
2. Obtain a referral to a speech therapist or pathologist as needed. Provide therapist with a list of words that would enhance patient's

independence and/or care. In addition, ask for tips that will help improve communication with patient.

3. When communicating with patient, try to reduce distractions in environment, such as television or others' conversations. Because fatigue affects a person's ability to communicate, try to ensure that patient is well rested.

4. Communicate with patient as much as possible. General principles for patients who may not recognize or comprehend the spoken word include: face patient and establish eye contact; speak slowly and clearly; give patient time to process your communication and answer; keep messages short and simple; stay with one clearly defined subject; avoid questions with multiple choices, but rather phrase questions so that they can be answered "yes" or "no"; and use the same words each time you repeat a statement or question (e.g., "pill" versus "medication," "bathroom versus "toilet"). If patient does not understand after repetition, try different words. Use gestures, facial expressions, and pantomime to supplement and reinforce your message. Give short, simple directions, and repeat as needed to ensure understanding. Use concrete terms (e.g., "water" instead of "fluid," "leg" instead of "limb").

5. When helping patients regain use of symbolic language, start with nouns first and progress to more complex statements as indicated, using verbs, pronouns, and adjectives. For continuity, keep a record at bedside of words to be used (e.g., "pill" rather than "medication").

6. Treat patient as an adult. It is not necessary to raise the volume of your voice unless patient is hard of hearing. Be respectful.

7. When patients have difficulty expressing words or naming objects, encourage them to repeat words after you for practice in verbal expression. Begin with simple words such as "yes" or "no" and progress to others, such as "cup." Progress to more complex statements as indicated. Listen and respond to patient's communication efforts; otherwise patient may give up. Praise accomplishments. Be prepared for labile emotions because these patients become frustrated and emotional when faced with their impaired speech.

8. When improvement is noted, let patient complete your sentence (e.g., "This is a _____"). Keep a list of words patient can say, and add to list as appropriate. Use this list when forming questions patient can answer. Do not finish patient's sentences.

9. Patients who have lost the ability to monitor their verbal output may not produce sensible language but may think they are making sense and may not understand why others do not comprehend or respond appropriately to them. Avoid labeling patient "belligerent" or "confused" when the problem is aphasia and frustration. Listen for errors in conversation and provide feedback.

10. Patients who have lost the ability to recognize number symbols or relationships will have difficulty understanding the concept of time or telling time. Avoid instructing patient to "wait 5 minutes" because this may not be meaningful.

11. Give practice in receiving word images by pointing to an object and clearly stating its name. Watch signals patient gives you.

Neurologic

12. Patients with nondominant (right) hemisphere damage often have no difficulty speaking; however, they may use excessive detail, give irrelevant information, and go off on a tangent. Bring patient back to the subject by saying, "Let's go back to what we were talking about."

13. Provide a supportive, relaxed environment for patients who cannot form words or sentences or speak clearly or appropriately. If patient makes an error, do not criticize patient's effort, but rather compliment it by saying, "That was a good try." Do not react negatively to patient's emotional displays. Address and acknowledge patient's frustration over inability to communicate. Maintain a calm, positive attitude. If you do not understand patient, say so. Ask patient to repeat unclear words, ask for more clues, ask patient to use another word, or have patient point to object. Observe for nonverbal cues and anticipate patient's needs. Allow time to listen if patient speaks slowly. To validate patient's message, repeat or rephrase it aloud.

14. Ensure that call light is available and patient knows how to use it.

15. Dysarthria can complicate aphasia. For additional interventions for patients with dysarthria, see **Impaired verbal communication** in "General Care of Patients with Neurologic Disorders," p. 195.

Knowledge deficit: Cerebral artery bypass surgery

Desired outcome: Before procedure, patient verbalizes understanding of surgical procedure, including the purpose, risks, and anticipated benefits or outcome.

1. After physician has explained cerebral artery bypass surgery to patient, determine patient's level of understanding. Reinforce information or clarify as indicated.

2. As indicated, explain that cerebral artery bypass surgery connects an extracranial vessel to an intracranial vessel to bypass an obstruction and increase blood flow to the brain.

3. Describe the following postoperative interventions, which may occur in the ICU during the immediate postoperative period:

   - VS and neurologic status checks are performed at least hourly: Patient will be asked to squeeze examiner's hands, move extremities, answer questions, and extend the tongue. Emphasize the importance of performing these activities to the best of patient's ability and reporting any numbness, tingling, or weakness. Neurologic deficits, especially differences on either side of the body or face or indicators of IICP, will be reported to physician.

   - BP will be monitored frequently, and patient may require vasoactive medications to keep BP within prescribed parameters. Hypertension can cause bypass stretching and bleeding, with loss of anastomosis and graft. Hypotension may promote thrombosis, with loss of graft.

   - Strict bed rest usually is enforced for 24-48 h.

   - For patients with bypass surgery involving the temporal artery, preventing impaired perfusion to the temporal area graft site is a key consideration. HOB probably will be elevated 30 degrees, and the head, neck, and body will be kept in good alignment to prevent neck flexion or hyperextension. It is critical that no pressure be put on graft site. Explain that patient will be positioned away from operative side. Dressings will be kept loose to prevent constriction of graft site. Patient can expect elastic bands on nasal cannulas or O_2 masks to be taped to face to ensure that they do not constrict the head, neck, and graft. Eyeglasses are contraindicated unless the earpiece on the operative side is removed. These precautions with eyeglasses and other constrictive gear usually apply for 3 mo after surgery.

- Head dressing will be checked at frequent intervals for drainage and tightness. The scalp may swell after surgery, causing dressing to tighten. Dressing should be loose enough to slip a finger beneath. Instruct patient to report any burning sensation on the scalp, which may indicate ischemia.
- Graft patency will be assessed periodically, either by palpation or by using a Doppler probe on the temporal pulse.
- Patient can expect anticoagulant and/or antiplatelet therapy for 3-6 mo after procedure.
- Precautions are taken against IICP (see "General Care of Patients with Neurologic Disorders" for **Decreased adaptive capacity:** Intracranial, p. 197. Teach these precautions to patient and significant others.

4. For additional interventions, see this nursing diagnosis in Appendix One, "Caring for Preoperative and Postoperative Patients," p. 395.

Knowledge deficit: Carotid endarterectomy procedure

Desired outcome: Before surgery, patient verbalizes understanding of procedure, including the purpose, risks, expected benefits or outcome, and postsurgical care.

1. After physician has explained procedure to patient, determine patient's level of understanding and reinforce or clarify information as needed.
2. As indicated, explain that carotid endarterectomy is the removal of plaque in the obstructed artery to increase blood supply to the brain.
3. Describe the following postsurgical assessments, which will occur in the ICU during the immediate postsurgical period.
   - Monitoring of VS and neurologic status at least hourly. Explain that the patient may be asked to swallow, move the tongue, smile, speak, and shrug shoulders to determine facial drooping, tongue weakness, hoarseness, dysphagia, shoulder weakness, or loss of facial sensation, which are signs of cranial nerve impairment. The cranial nerves can be stretched during surgery, which may cause edema and leave a temporary deficit. Patient should report any numbness, tingling, or weakness, which may indicate occlusion of the carotid. In addition, the superficial temporal and facial pulses will be palpated for strength, quality, and symmetry to evaluate the patency of the external carotid artery.
   - Periodic assessment of the neck for edema, hematoma, bleeding, or tracheal deviation. Explain that patient should report immediately any respiratory distress, difficulty managing secretions, or sensation of neck tightness. Explain that neck symmetry will be

checked, including the back, for hematoma posterior to incision and tracheal deviation from midline, which would signal swelling that may obstruct airway. Additional oxygen most likely will be supplied even without respiratory distress or airway compromise because manipulation of the carotid sinus may cause temporary loss of normal physiologic response to hypoxia.

- BP may be checked often because temporary carotid sinus dysfunction may cause BP problems (usually hypertension). Patient may need vasoactive drugs that will keep BP within a specified range and maintain cerebral perfusion while preventing disruption of graft or sutures.
- HOB must be kept in prescribed position (flat or elevated), and patient generally is positioned off the operative side.
- A drain may be left in place in the neck for a few days, and patient may have a leg incision if graft was taken from leg's saphenous vein. Wound drain suction will be maintained. An ice pack may be prescribed prn to reduce swelling.
- Teach patient to support head and neck with hands during position changes to prevent turning or hyperextension.
- Anticoagulant/antiplatelet therapy (e.g., aspirin, warfarin) usually is instituted for 3-6 mo after procedure.

4. For additional interventions, see this nursing diagnosis in Appendix One, "Caring for Preoperative and Postoperative Patients," p. 395.

See "Pulmonary Embolus" for **Altered protection** related to risk of prolonged bleeding or hemorrhage secondary to anticoagulant therapy, p. 7.

See "Renal-Urinary Disorders" for related diagnoses for incontinence, urinary retention, and neurogenic bladder. **Caution:** Credé's method and other interventions that increase intrathoracic or intraabdominal pressure are contraindicated until the risk of IICP is no longer a factor.

See "Alzheimer's Disease" for **Impaired environmental interpretation syndrome,** p. 134. See "Head Injury" for **Risk for disuse syndrome** related to prolonged inactivity, p. 156, and **Fluid volume excess** (related to SIADH), p. 158.

For patients undergoing surgery, see "Brain Tumors" for **Knowledge deficit:** Craniotomy procedure, p. 161.

See "Seizure Disorders," p. 179, for related nursing diagnoses.

See "General Care of Patients with Neurologic Disorders" for **Risk for trauma,** p. 187; **Risk for injury,** p. 189; **Impaired corneal tissue integrity,** p. 189; **Altered nutrition,** p. 190; **Risk for fluid volume deficit,** p. 191; **Risk for aspiration,** p. 192; **Self-care deficit,** p. 193; **Constipation,** p. 196; **Decreased adaptive capacity:** Intracranial, p. 197; **Sensory/perceptual alterations** (visual), p. 200; **Impaired swallowing,** p. 201; and **Knowledge deficit:** Neurologic diagnostic tests, p. 205.

See "Diabetes Insipidus," p. 212, for patients who have or are at risk of this disorder.

See "Pressure Ulcers," p. 390, and Appendix One, "Caring for Patients on Prolonged Bed Rest," p. 413, for nursing diagnoses and interventions related to immobility. Adjust interventions accordingly if patient has IICP or is at risk for this problem. See Appendix One, "Caring for Patients with Cancer and Other Life-Disrupting Illnesses," p. 450, for appropriate psychosocial nursing diagnoses.

PATIENT-FAMILY TEACHING AND DISCHARGE PLANNING

Give patient and significant others verbal and written information about the following:

1. Importance of minimizing or treating these risk factors: diabetes mellitus, hypertension, diet high in cholesterol and sodium, obesity, inactivity, smoking, prolonged bed rest, and stressful life-style.
2. Interventions that increase effective communication in cases involving aphasia or dysarthria.
3. Referrals to the following organizations, as appropriate: public health nurse, Visiting Nurse Association, psychologic therapy, vocational rehabilitation agency, home health agencies, and extended and skilled care facilities. Also provide these addresses and phone numbers: the National Stroke Association, 300 East Hampden Avenue, Suite 240, Englewood, CO 80110-2654 *phone:* (303)-762-9922 or (800)-787-6537. Pamphlets are available from the National Institute of Neurological Disorders and Stroke (NINDS), Box 5801, Bethesda, MD 20892 *phone:* (800)-352-9424.
4. For other information, see teaching and discharge planning (entries 3 through 10 only) in "Multiple Sclerosis," p. 116.

SECTION SIX: SEIZURE DISORDERS

NURSING DIAGNOSES AND INTERVENTIONS

Risk for trauma related to oral, musculoskeletal, and airway vulnerability secondary to seizure activity
Desired outcomes: Patient exhibits no signs of oral or musculoskeletal tissue injury or airway compromise after the seizure. Before hospital discharge, patient's significant others verbalize knowledge of actions necessary during seizure activity.

Seizure Precautions

1. Pad side rails with blankets or pillows. Keep side rails up and the bed in its lowest position when the patient is in bed. Keep bed, wheelchair, or stretcher brakes locked.
2. Tape a soft rubber oral airway to the bedside. Remove wooden tongue depressors (if used, they may splinter). Keep suction and oxygen equipment readily available. Consider a heparin lock for IV access for high-risk patient.
3. Avoid using glass or other breakable oral thermometers when taking

patient's temperature. If only breakable thermometers are available, take temperature *via* axillary or rectal route.

4. Caution patients to lie down and push the call button if they experience a prodromal or aural warning. Encourage patient to empty the mouth of dentures or foreign objects. Keep call light within reach.

5. Do not allow unsupervised smoking.

6. Evaluate need for and provide protective headgear as indicated.

DURING THE SEIZURE

1. Remain with patient. Observe for, record, and report type, duration, and characteristics of seizure activity and any postseizure response. This should include, as appropriate, precipitating event, aura, initial location and progression, automatisms, type and duration of movement, changes in LOC, eye movement (e.g., deviation, nystagmus), pupil size and reaction, bowel and bladder incontinence, head deviation, tongue deviation, or teeth clenching.

2. Prevent or break the fall, and ease patient to the floor if the seizure occurs while patient is out of bed. Keep patient in bed if the seizure occurs while there, and lower HOB to a flat position.

3. If the patient's jaws are clenched, do not force an object between the teeth, because this can break teeth or lacerate oral mucous membrane. If able to do so safely and without damage to oral tissue, insert an airway. Tongue depressors should not be used, because they may splinter. A rolled washcloth may be used as an alternative. Never put your fingers in the patient's mouth.

4. Protect patient's head from injury during seizure activity. A towel folded flat may be used to cushion the head from striking the ground. Be sure the head's position does not occlude the airway. Remove from the environment objects (e.g., chairs) that the patient may strike. Pad the floors to protect the patient's arms and legs. Remove patient's glasses.

5. Do not restrain patient but rather guide the patient's movements gently to prevent injury.

6. Roll patient into a side-lying position to promote drainage of secretions and maintain a patent airway. Use the head tilt, chin lift maneuver. Provide O_2 and suction as needed.

7. Loosen tight clothing.

8. Maintain patient's privacy. Clear nonessential people out of the room.

9. Administer antiepilepsy drugs as prescribed.

AFTER THE SEIZURE

1. Reassure and reorient patient. Check neurologic status and VS; ask patient if an aura preceded the seizure activity. Record this information and postictal characteristics.

2. Provide a quiet, calm environment because sounds and stimuli can be confusing to the awakening patient. Keep talk simple and to a minimum. Speak slowly and with pauses between sentences. Repeating may be necessary. Use room light that is behind, not above,

patient to prevent additional seizures and for patient comfort. Do not offer food or drink until patient is fully awake.

3. Check patient's tongue for lacerations and body for injuries. Monitor urine for red or cola color, which may signal rhabdomyolysis or myoglobinuria from muscle damage. Monitor for the presence of weakness or paralysis, dysphasia, or visual disturbances.

4. Check blood fingerstick glucose and obtain serum lab tests as prescribed. Administer antiepilepsy medication as prescribed.

5. Monitor for status epilepticus (i.e., state of continuous or rapidly recurring seizures in which the individual does not completely recover baseline neurologic functioning). This condition is life-threatening and can cause cerebral anoxia and edema, aspiration, hyperthermia, and exhaustion. Notify physician immediately.

6. Provide significant others with verbal and written information for the preceding interventions.

Impaired tissue integrity (or risk for same) related to chemical irritation from IV phenytoin administration

Desired outcome: Patient's tissue surrounding IV site remains undamaged, as evidenced by absence of swelling, discoloration, discomfort, and blistering.

1. If possible, avoid administering IV phenytoin through an insertion site in the wrist, hand, or foot. Ideally, IV phenytoin is administered through a central line. If a central line is not present, administer drug through largest-gauge needle possible.

2. Monitor insertion site for inflammation or infiltration before administering drug. Check for line patency periodically during administration. Stop injection immediately if any indicators of infiltration or inflammation develop.

3. Flush line with 0.9% sodium chloride solution before and after giving drug to reduce likelihood of irritation and prevent precipitation. Flush with enough solution to clear line and tubing completely. Do not mix phenytoin with other medications. Phenytoin will precipitate in the presence of D_5W.

4. Administer drug undiluted and at a rate ≤ 50 mg/min. More rapid administration will irritate the vein and also can cause hypotension, apnea, and cardiac dysrhythmias. For older adult or a person with cardiovascular disease, a slower rate of 25 mg/min is recommended.

5. After administration, inspect insertion site often, for several hours. Monitor for swelling or discoloration. Instruct patient to report any pain at the site.

6. Report any swelling or discoloration to physician, and remove vascular access device. Monitor for worsening discoloration, blistering, edema, or tissue sloughing. To control swelling, elevate patient's arm above chest and, if prescribed, wrap arm in warm compresses. Check circulation, sensation, and movement in affected arm and hand, and report significant findings. Protect blisters with sterile dressing.

Knowledge deficit: Life-threatening environmental factors and preventive measures for seizures

Desired outcomes: Before hospital discharge, patient verbalizes accurate information about measures that may prevent seizures and environmental factors that can be life-threatening in the event of a seizure. Patient exhibits health care measures that reflect this knowledge.

1. Assess patient's knowledge of measures that can prevent seizures and environmental hazards that can be life-threatening with seizure activity. Provide or clarify information as indicated.

2. Advise patient to check into state regulations about driving. Most states require 1-3 seizure-free years before an individual can obtain a driver's license.

3. Caution patient to refrain from operating heavy or dangerous equipment, swimming, and possibly even bathing in a tub until he or she is seizure free for the amount of time specified by physician. Teach patient never to swim alone, regardless of how long he or she has been seizure free. Caution patient to swim only in shallow water and in the company of a strong swimmer, to make rescue easier if a seizure occurs.

4. Advise patient to turn the temperature of hot water heaters down to prevent scalding if a seizure occurs in the shower.

5. Encourage stress management, progressive relaxation techniques, and diaphragmatic respiratory training to control emotional stress and hyperventilation, which often trigger seizures.

6. Advise patient that some activities (e.g., climbing, bicycle riding) require careful risk-benefit evaluation.

7. Encourage vocational assessment and counseling. Patient's epilepsy may place others at risk in some occupations, such as bus driver or airline pilot.

8. Advise women patients that seizure activity may change (increase or decrease) during menses or pregnancy. Tonic-clonic seizures have caused fetal death. Antiepilepsy drugs are associated with birth defects; however, 90% of women have normal pregnancies and normal children. Provide birth control information if requested.

9. Teach patient that use of stimulants (e.g., caffeine) and depressants (e.g., alcohol) should be avoided. Withdrawal from stimulants and depressants can increase the likelihood of seizures.

10. Teach patient that getting rest, avoiding physical and emotional stress, and maintaining a nutritious diet may help prevent seizure activity. Meals should be spaced throughout the day to prevent hypoglycemia. Overhydration may precipitate seizure activity. If stimuli such as flashing lights or loud music appear to trigger seizures, advise patient to avoid environments that are likely to have these stimuli. Poorly adjusted TVs may trigger seizures and should be fixed.

11. Encourage individuals who have seizures that occur without warning to avoid chewing gum or sucking on lozenges, which may be aspirated during a seizure.

12. Encourage patient to wear a Medic-Alert bracelet or similar identification or to carry a medical information card.

Knowledge deficit: Purpose, precautions, and side effects of antiepilepsy medications

Desired outcome: Before hospital discharge, patient verbalizes accurate information about prescribed antiepilepsy medication.

1. Stress the importance of taking prescribed medication regularly and on schedule and of not discontinuing medication without physician's guidance. Explain that missing a scheduled dose can precipitate a seizure several days later. Stress that abrupt withdrawal of any antiepilepsy medication can precipitate seizures and that discontinuing these medications is the most common cause of status epilepticus. Assist patients in finding methods to help them remember to take medication and monitor their drug supply to avoid running out. Drugs may be necessary for the rest of the patient's life. Medications cannot be taken prn, and lack of seizures does not mean the drug is unnecessary. Explain the concept of drug half-lives and steady blood levels.

2. Reinforce prescribed instructions for drug dosage.

3. Stress the importance of informing physician about side effects and keeping appointments for periodic laboratory work, which determines whether blood levels are therapeutic and assesses for side effects. Many antiepilepsy medications can cause blood dyscrasias or liver damage. Teach patient to report immediately any bruising, bleeding, or jaundice. Vitamin D, vitamin K, and folic acid supplements may be prescribed.

4. Explain that antiepilepsy medications may make people drowsy. Advise patient to avoid activities that require alertness until his or her CNS response to medication has been determined.

5. Nausea and vomiting are common side effects of most antiepilepsy medications. Teach patient to take drug with food or large amounts of liquid to minimize gastric upset. Patients taking valproic acid (Depakote) should not chew medication because it may irritate oral mucous membrane. Also advise patients taking valproic acid that this drug may produce a false-positive test result for urine ketones, and that any change in vision should be reported immediately, because it may signal ocular toxicity.

6. Instruct patient to notify physician if a significant weight gain or loss occurs because it may necessitate a change in dosage or scheduling.

7. Teach patient to avoid alcoholic beverages and OTC medications containing alcohol. Chronic alcohol use stimulates the body to metabolize phenytoin (Dilantin) more quickly, lowering the seizure threshold because of the decrease in plasma phenytoin levels. Patients taking phenobarbital (Luminal) or primidone (Mysoline) should avoid alcohol, which potentiates CNS-depressant effects. Anticonvulsant agents are potentiated or inhibited by many other drugs, including aspirin and antihistamines, and may affect potency of other medications as well. Caution patient to avoid OTC medications.

8. Other side effects common to antiepilepsy medications are ataxia, diplopia, nystagmus, and dizziness. Instruct patient to report these symptoms.

9. Teach patients who take carbamazepine (Tegretol) or ethosuximide (Zarontin) to report immediately fever, mouth ulcers, sore throat,

bruising, or bleeding.

10. Advise patients taking phenytoin that this drug can cause gingival hypertrophy. Patient should perform frequent oral hygiene with gum massage and gentle flossing and brush teeth 3-4 ×/day with a soft toothbrush. These patients also should report immediately any measles-like rash.

11. Caution patients taking phenytoin that there are two types of this drug. Dilantin Kapseal is absorbed more slowly and is longer acting. It is important not to confuse this extended-release phenytoin with prompt-release phenytoin. Doing so may cause dangerous underdose or overdose. Generic phenytoin should not be substituted for Dilantin Kapseal.

Noncompliance with therapy related to denial of illness or perceived negative consequences of treatment regimen secondary to social stigma, negative side effects of antiepilepsy medications, or difficulty with making necessary life-style change

Desired outcome: Before hospital discharge, patient verbalizes knowledge about disease process and treatment plan, acknowledges consequences of continued noncompliant behavior, explains experience that caused patient to alter prescribed behavior, describes appropriate treatment of side effects or appropriate alternatives, and exhibits health care measures that reflect this knowledge, following an agreed-on plan of care.

1. Assess patient's understanding of disease process, medical management, and treatment plan. Explain or clarify information as indicated.

2. Assess for causes of noncompliance (e.g., medication side effects, or difficulty making significant life-style changes or following medication schedule).

3. Ensure awareness that stopping medications can be life-threatening (e.g., status epilepticus). Explain drug half-life and the concept of a steady blood level. Intermittent medication use may be informal experimentation or an effort to gain control. Explain the importance of physician's guidance if medication is stopped for any reason.

4. Evaluate patient's perception of his or her vulnerability to disease process, and be alert for signs of denial of illness. In addition, evaluate patient's perception of effectiveness or noneffectiveness of treatment. Stress the importance of expressing feelings.

5. Determine if a value, cultural, or spiritual conflict is causing noncompliance. Confront myths and stigmas. Provide realistic assessment of risks and counter misconceptions.

6. Discuss methods of dealing with common problems (e.g., obtaining insurance, job or workplace discrimination).

7. Assess patient's support systems. Determine whether a family disruption pattern (whether or not caused by patient's illness) is making compliance difficult and "not worth it."

8. After reason for noncompliance is found, intervene accordingly to ensure compliance. If it appears that changing the medical treatment plan (e.g., in scheduling medications) may promote compliance, discuss this possibility with physician. Provide patient with informa-

tion about interventions that can minimize drug side effects (e.g., taking drug with food or large amounts of liquid to minimize gastric distress).
9. Encourage involvement with support systems such as local epilepsy centers and national organizations.

See "General Care of Patients with Neurologic Disorders" for **Knowledge deficit:** Neurologic diagnostic tests, p. 205.

See Appendix One, "Caring for Patients with Cancer and Other Life-Disrupting Illnesses" for **Body image disturbance,** p. 459, **Ineffective individual coping,** p. 455, and **Altered family processes,** p. 463.

PATIENT-FAMILY TEACHING AND DISCHARGE PLANNING

Give patient and significant others verbal and written information about the following:
1. Reinforcement of knowledge of disease process, pathophysiology, symptoms, and precipitating or aggravating factors.
2. Medications, including drug name, purpose, dosage, schedule, precautions, drug/drug and food/drug interactions, and potential side effects. Table 4-2 presents the common antiepilepsy drugs.
3. Importance of follow-up care and keeping medical appointments. Stress that use of antiepilepsy drugs requires periodic monitoring of blood levels to ensure therapeutic dosage, as well as assessment for side effects. Instruct patient to keep emergency numbers for contacting physician.
4. An uncomplicated convulsive seizure in an individual known to have epilepsy is not necessarily a medical emergency. On average, these people can continue about their business after a rest period. An ambulance should be called or medical attention sought if the seizure happens in water; if there is any question about the seizure's having been caused by epilepsy; if the individual is injured, pregnant, or diabetic; if the seizure lasts longer than 5 min; if a second seizure starts; or if consciousness does not begin to return.
5. Environmental factors that can be life-threatening in the event of a seizure, measures that may help prevent seizures, and safety interventions during seizures. Review state and local laws that apply to individuals with seizure disorders.
6. Employment or vocational counseling as needed. Discuss the need to avoid overprotection and to maintain, as possible, normal work and recreation.
7. Risks of antiepilepsy drugs during pregnancy. Provide birth control information or genetic counseling referral as requested.

IN ADDITION
8. Provide this address and phone number as appropriate: Epilepsy Foundation of America, 4351 Garden City Drive, Suite 406, Landover, MD 20785 *phone:* (301)-459-3700 and (800)-332-1000.

Table 4-2   Common antiepilepsy drugs

Name	Side Effects	Precautions
phenytoin (Dilantin)	Drowsiness, gingival hypertrophy, nausea, vomiting, increased body hair, rash, or blood dyscrasias. Signs of overdose include nystagmus, ataxia, slurred speech, confusion, and diplopia.	Ensure frequent oral hygiene, gum massage, and gentle flossing. Take drug with food or large amounts of liquid to reduce gastric upset. Periodic blood counts are necessary. Call physician if rash or jaundice appears. Vitamin K may be given to pregnant women 1 mo before and during delivery to prevent neonatal hemorrhage. If prescribed, supplement with vitamins K and D and folic acid.
carbamazepine (Tegretol)	Blood dyscrasias, ataxia, rash, nystagmus, diplopia, nausea, vomiting, liver damage, drowsiness, and dizziness.	Check CBC frequently. Patient should report fever, mouth ulcers, sore throat, bruising, or bleeding immediately. Take drug with food. Liver and renal function tests should be performed periodically. Report jaundice to physician.
ethosuximide (Zarontin)	Gastric distress, nausea, vomiting, dizziness, drowsiness, aplastic anemia, vaginal bleeding.	Take with food or large amounts of fluid. Follow-up laboratory studies are important for detecting anemia. Patient should immediately report fever, mouth ulcers, sore throat, bruising, and bleeding.
valproic acid (Depakote)	Sedation, dizziness, nausea, vomiting, anorexia, liver damage, transient alopecia, ataxia, and thrombocytopenia. Any visual change may signal ocular toxicity.	Do not chew; this may irritate mucous membranes. Take with food to prevent gastric upset. Patient should report any bleeding, bruising, or visual change immediately. Monitor liver function studies *via* periodic laboratory tests. This drug can cause false-positive test result for ketones in the urine.

Table 4-2   Common antiepilepsy drugs—cont'd

Name	Side Effects	Precautions
phenobarbital (Luminal)	Drowsiness, lethargy, dizziness, nausea, vomiting, constipation, ataxia, anemia, mild rash, depression.	Do not stop abruptly; this may cause withdrawal seizures. Avoid alcohol, which would potentiate CNS-depressant effects. Vitamin D supplements usually are advised. Take with foods to prevent stomach upset. Vitamin K usually is given to pregnant women 1 mo before and during labor to prevent neonatal hemorrhage.
primidone (Mysoline)	Drowsiness; emotional changes, including depression and irritability; anemia; rash; nausea; vomiting; and impotence. Incoordination, slurred speech, and blurred vision may be early signs of overdose.	Do not stop abruptly; this may cause withdrawal seizures. Take with food or large amounts of fluid. See information with phenobarbital above regarding avoiding alcohol and taking vitamin K.

SECTION SEVEN: GENERAL CARE OF PATIENTS WITH NEUROLOGIC DISORDERS

NURSING DIAGNOSES AND INTERVENTIONS

Risk for trauma related to unsteady gait secondary to sensorimotor deficit

Desired outcomes: Patient is free of trauma caused by gait unsteadiness. Before hospital discharge, patient demonstrates proficiency with assistive devices, if appropriate.

1. Evaluate patient's gait, and assess for motor deficits (e.g., weakness, tremors, spasticity, or paralysis). Document baseline neurologic and physical assessments so that changes in status can be detected promptly.
2. To minimize the risk of injury, assist patient as needed when unsteady gait, weakness, or paralysis is noted. Instruct patient to ask

or call for assistance with ambulation. Check frequently on patients who may forget to call for assistance. Stand on patient's weak side to assist with balance and support. Use transfer belt for safety. Instruct patient to use stronger side for gripping railing when stair climbing.

3. Orient patient to new surroundings. Keep necessary items (including water, snacks, telephone, and call light) within easy reach, and assess patient's ability to use these items. Patient who is very weak or partly paralyzed may require a tap bell instead of a call light.

4. Maintain an uncluttered environment with unobstructed walkways to minimize the risk of tripping. Ensure adequate lighting at night (e.g., a night light) to help prevent falls in the dark. In addition, keep side rails up and bed in its lowest position with bed brakes on. Encourage patient to use any needed hearing aids and corrective lenses when ambulating.

5. For unsteady, weak, or partly paralyzed patient, encourage use of low-heel, nonskid shoes for walking. Teach patient to use a wide-based gait to provide a broader base of support. Instruct patient to note foot placement when ambulating or transferring to ensure that the foot is flat and in a position of support. Teach, reinforce, and encourage use of assistive device (e.g., cane, walker, or crutches) that provides added stability. Teach exercises that strengthen arm and shoulder muscles for using walkers and crutches. Teach safe use of transfer or sliding boards. Teach patients in wheelchairs how and when to lock and unlock the wheels. Demonstrate how to secure and support weak or paralyzed arms to prevent subluxation and injury from falling into wheelchair spokes or wheels. Patients with poor sitting balance may need a seat or chest belt, H-straps for leg positioning, and a wheelchair with an antitip device.

6. Teach patients to maintain a sitting position for a few minutes before assuming a standing position for ambulating; this gives patients time to get their feet flat and under them for balance and minimizes any dizziness from rapid position changes.

7. Monitor spasticity and antispasmodic drugs and their effect on physical function. Uncontrolled or severe spasms may cause falls; mild to moderate spasms can be useful in ADLs and transfers if patient learns to control and trigger them.

8. Review with patient and significant others potential safety needs at home, such as safety appliances (wall, bath, and toilet handrails; elevated toilet seat; nonslip surface in tub or shower). Loose rugs should be removed to prevent slipping and falling. Temperatures on hot water heaters should be turned down to prevent scalding in case of a fall in the shower or tub. In the home, furniture may need to be moved to create clear, safe pathways that avoid sharp corners on furniture, glass cabinets, or large windows that patient may fall against. Strategically placed additional lighting also may be needed. The edges of steps may need to be marked with a strip of bright-colored tape to provide sufficient contrast so that edges can be more easily recognized and safely negotiated. Beds should be modified to prevent rolling. Activity should be balanced with rest periods, be-

cause fatigue tends to increase unsteadiness and the potential for falls.
9. Seek referral by physical therapist (PT) as appropriate.

Risk for injury related to impaired pain, touch, and temperature sensations secondary to sensory deficit or decreased LOC

Desired outcomes: Patient is free of symptoms of injury caused by impaired pain, touch, and temperature sensations. Before hospital discharge, patient and significant others identify factors that increase the potential for injury.

1. Assess patient for indicators of sensory deficits (e.g., decreased or absent vision, impaired temperature and pain sensation). Document baseline neurologic and physical assessments so that changes in status can be detected promptly.
2. Protect patient from exposure to hot food or equipment that can burn the skin. Avoid use of heating pads.
3. Always check the temperature of heating devices and bathwater before patient uses them. Teach patient and significant others about these precautions.
4. Inspect patient's skin bid for irritation. Teach coherent patient to perform self-inspection, and provide a mirror for inspecting posterior aspects of the body. Skin should be kept soft and pliable with emollient lotion.
5. Teach patient to check placement of limbs with altered sensation to ensure that they are safely supported, and to avoid placing ankles directly on top of each other. Pad wheelchair seat, and teach patient to change position q15-30min by lifting himself or herself and shifting position side to side and forward to backward. Encourage frequent turning while in bed and, if tolerated and not contraindicated, periodic movement into prone position. Have patient lift, not drag, himself or herself during transfers to prevent shearing damage.
6. Give injections in muscles with tone for better absorption and less risk of sterile abscess formation. Avoid injecting ≥ 1 ml into a flaccid muscle.

Impaired corneal tissue integrity related to irritation secondary to diminished blink reflex or inability to close the eyes

Desired outcome: Patient's corneas remain clear and intact.

1. Normally, blinking occurs q5-6sec. If patient has a diminished blink reflex and/or is stuporous or comatose, assess the eyes for irritation or foreign objects. Instill eye drops or apply ointment prescribed to prevent corneal irritation. Instruct coherent patients to make a conscious effort to blink the eyes several times a minute to help prevent corneal irritation. Indicators of such irritation include red, itchy, teary, scratchy, or painful eyes; a sensation of having something in the eye; scleral edema; blurred vision; or mucus discharge. Apply eye patches or warm, sterile compresses over closed eyes for relief.
2. For patient who cannot close the eyes completely, use caution in applying an eye shield or taping the eyes shut. Semiconscious patients may open their eyes underneath and injure the corneas. Also consider use of moisture chambers (plastic eye bubble), protective glasses, soft contacts, or humidifiers.

3. Teach patient to avoid exposing eyes to irritants such as talc or baby powder, wind, cold air, smoke, dust, sand, or bright sunlight. Instruct patient not to rub eyes; restrain patients who may be incoherent.

Altered nutrition: Less than body requirements, related to inability to ingest food secondary to chewing and swallowing deficits, fatigue, weakness, paresis, paralysis, visual neglect, or decreased LOC

Desired outcome: Patient has adequate nutrition, as evidenced by maintenance of or return to baseline body weight by hospital discharge.

1. Assess patient's alertness, ability to cough, and swallow and gag reflexes before all meals. Keep suction equipment at bedside if indicated.

2. Assess patient for type of diet that can be eaten safely. Request soft, semisolid, or chopped foods as indicated. Although a pureed diet may be needed eventually, this type of food can be unappealing to many people and may have a negative impact on patient's self-concept.

3. To help patient focus on eating, reduce other stimuli in the room (e.g., turn off the TV or radio). Minimize conversation and other disruptions, such as phone calls.

4. Provide analgesics, if appropriate, before meals so that patient is comfortable and can concentrate on eating.

5. Evaluate patient's food preferences and offer small, frequent servings of nutritious food. Encourage significant others to bring in patient's favorite foods if they are not contraindicated. Plan mealtimes for times when patient is rested; use a warming tray or microwave oven to keep food warm and appetizing until patient can eat.

6. Provide oral care before feeding to enhance patient's ability to taste. Clean and insert dentures before each meal.

7. Encourage liquid nutritional supplements, and try different methods to make them more palatable (e.g., making a milkshake, serving it over ice, or diluting it with carbonated beverages).

8. Cut up foods, unwrap silverware, and otherwise "set up" food tray so that patients with a weak or paralyzed arm can manage the tray one-handed.

9. For patient with visual neglect, place food within patient's unaffected visual field and return during the meal to make sure she or he has eaten from both sides of the plate. Turn the plate around so that any remaining food is in patient's visual field.

10. Feed or assist very weak or paralyzed patients. If not contraindicated, position patient in a chair or elevate HOB as high as possible. Ensure that patient's head is flexed slightly forward to close airway. Begin with small amounts of food. Do not hurry patient. Be sure that each bite is completely swallowed before giving another.

11. If appropriate, provide assistive devices (e.g., built-up utensil handles, broad-handled spoons, spill-proof cups, rocker knife for cutting, wrist or hand splints with clamps to hold utensils, stabilized plates, sectionalized plates) and other devices that promote

self-feeding and independence. Encourage eating of finger foods to promote independence and oral intake.

12. Provide materials for oral hygiene after meals to minimize risk of aspiration of food particles. Good oral hygiene also helps maintain integrity of mucous membranes to minimize risk of stomatitis, which may prevent adequate oral intake. Provide oral care for patients unable to do so for themselves.

13. Document assessment of patient's appetite. Weigh patient regularly (at least weekly) to assess for loss or gain. If indicated, consult physician about possible need for high-protein or high-calorie supplements. Obtain dietetic consultation. Patients unable to obtain adequate nutrition by eating may need enteral or parenteral nutrition. For additional information, see "Providing Nutritional Support," p. 378.

14. For weak, debilitated, or partly paralyzed patient, assess support systems, such as family or friends, who can assist patient with meals. Consider referral to an organization that will deliver a daily meal to patient's home.

15. If appropriate for patient's diagnosis (e.g., multiple sclerosis) consider referral to a speech pathologist for exercises that enhance the ability to swallow.

16. For patients with visual problems, assess their ability to see their food. Identify utensils and food, and describe their location. Arrange foods in an established pattern to promote independence.

17. For patients with chewing or swallowing difficulties, see interventions with **Impaired swallowing,** p. 201.

Risk for fluid volume deficit related to facial and throat muscle weakness, depressed gag or cough reflex, impaired swallowing, or decreased LOC

Desired outcome: Patient is normovolemic, as evidenced by balanced I&O, stable weight, good skin turgor, moist mucous membranes, BP within patient's normal range, HR $\leq$100 bpm, normothermia, and urinary output $\geq$30 ml/h.

1. Assess patient's gag reflex, alertness, and ability to cough and swallow before offering fluids. Keep suction equipment at bedside if indicated.

2. Monitor I&O to assess for fluid volume imbalance. Involve patient or significant others with keeping fluid intake records. Ensure that weight is measured daily if patient is at risk for sudden fluid shifts or imbalances. Patients with neurologic deficits may have great difficulty attaining adequate fluid intake. Alert physician to a significant I&O imbalance, which may signal the need for enteral or IV therapy to prevent dehydration.

3. Assess for and teach patient and significant others the indicators of dehydration: thirst, poor skin turgor, decreased BP, increased pulse rate, dry skin and mucous membranes, increased body temperature, concentrated urine, and decreased urinary output. Advise them that conditions such as fever or diarrhea increase fluid loss and place patient at increased risk of dehydration.

Neurologic

4. Evaluate patient's fluid type and temperature preferences, and offer fluids q1-2h. For nonrestricted patients, encourage a fluid intake of at least 2-3 L/day.

5. Feed or assist very weak or paralyzed patients. If not contraindicated, assist patient into high Fowler's position to facilitate oral fluid intake. Instruct patient to flex the head slightly forward, which closes the airway and helps prevent aspiration. Begin with small amounts of liquid. Instruct patient to sip rather than gulp fluids. Do not hurry patient.

6. Provide periods of rest to prevent fatigue, which can contribute to decreased oral intake. Provide oral care as needed to enhance taste perception and prevent stomatitis, which may reduce oral intake.

7. If appropriate, provide assistive devices (spill-proof cups, straws), which promote independence. Teach patient with hemiparalysis or paresis to tilt the head toward the unaffected side to facilitate intake. An individual who is paralyzed (e.g., with spinal cord injury) may be able to drink independently by means of extra-long tubing or straw connected to a water pitcher.

8. For patients at risk for IICP, maintain fluid restrictions.

9. For patients with chewing or swallowing difficulties, see interventions with **Impaired swallowing,** p. 201.

Risk for aspiration related to facial and throat muscle weakness, depressed gag or cough reflex, impaired swallowing, or decreased LOC

Desired outcomes: Patient is free of signs of aspiration, as evidenced by RR 12-20 breaths/min with normal depth and pattern (eupnea), normal color, normal breath sounds, normothermia, and absence of adventitious breath sounds. After instruction, patient or significant others relate measures that prevent aspiration.

1. Monitor patient for dyspnea, pallor, restlessness, diaphoresis, and a change in rate or depth of respirations. Auscultate lung fields for breath sounds. Note crackles, rhonchi, or wheezes and diminished breath sounds. Assess effectiveness of patient's cough and quality, amount, and color of sputum. Measure body temperature q4h. Often, a low-grade fever (≤38° C [100° F]) indicates a need for aggressive pulmonary hygiene.

2. Teach patient to breathe deeply and cough, and assist with repositioning at least q2h. If not contraindicated, maintain patient in side-lying position with HOB elevated. **Caution:** Instruct patients at risk of IICP not to cough, because it increases intraabdominal and intrathoracic pressure, which in turn increase ICP. Explain that if sneezing is unavoidable, it should be done with an open mouth to minimize the increase in ICP.

3. Assess swallow and gag reflexes. If poor or absent, withhold oral fluids and foods, and consult physician about possible need for IV therapy or enteral or parenteral nutrition. Maintain adequate hydration to keep secretions thin.

4. Keep HOB elevated after meals, or assist patient into right side-lying position to minimize potential for regurgitation and aspiration. Provide small, frequent meals. Consult physician for an upper GI stimulant (e.g., metoclopramide) to reduce potential for regurgita-

tion. Provide oral hygiene after meals to prevent aspiration of food particles.
5. For patients not at risk for IICP, assist with prescribed postural drainage, chest physiotherapy, and IPPB. Provide incentive spirometry as indicated.
6. Keep O_2 and suction apparatus available as indicated. Assess patient frequently for obstructive material or secretions in throat or mouth; suction as needed. Anticipate need for an artificial airway if secretions cannot be cleared. Teach significant others the Heimlich maneuver.

Self-care deficit related to spasticity, tremors, weakness, paresis, paralysis, or decreasing LOC secondary to sensorimotor deficits

Desired outcome: At least 24 h before hospital discharge, patient performs care activities independently and demonstrates ability to use adaptive devices for successful completion of ADLs. (Totally dependent patients express satisfaction with activities that are completed for them.)

1. Assess patient's ability to perform ADLs.
2. As appropriate, demonstrate use of adaptive devices (e.g., long- or broad-handled combs, brushes, and eating utensils; nonspill cups; stabilized plates), all of which may assist patient in maintaining independent care. A flexor-hinge splint or universal cuff may aid in brushing teeth and combing hair.
3. Set short-range, realistic goals with patient to reduce frustration and improve learning. Acknowledge progress, and encourage continued effort and involvement (e.g., in selection of meals, clothing).
4. Provide care for totally dependent patient, and assist those who are not totally dependent according to degree of disability. Encourage patient to perform self-care to his or her maximum ability, as defined by patient. Encourage autonomy. Allow sufficient time for patient to perform task; do not hurry patient. Involve significant others with care activity if they are comfortable with doing so. Ask for patient's help in planning schedules. Supervise activity until patient can safely perform task without help.
5. To improve mobility, encourage use of electronically controlled chair and other technical advances (e.g., environmental control system) that may allow independent operation of electronic devices such as lights, radio, door openers, and window shade openers.
6. Provide privacy and a nondistracting environment. Place patient's belongings within reach. Set out items needed to complete self-care tasks in the order they are to be used. Apply any needed adaptive devices (e.g., hand splints).
7. Encourage patient to wear any prescribed corrective eye lenses or hearing aids.
8. Provide analgesics to relieve pain, which can hinder self-care activity.
9. Provide a rest period before self-care activity, or plan activity for a time when patient is rested, because fatigue alters self-care ability.

10. To facilitate dressing and undressing, encourage patient or significant others to buy shoes without laces, long-handled shoe horns,
loose-fitting clothing, wide-legged pants, and clothing with front
fasteners, zipper pulls, or Velcro closures. Avoid items with small
buttons or tight buttonholes. Lay out clothing in the order it will be
put on.

11. Place stool in shower if sitting down will enhance self-care with
bathing. Bathrooms should have nonslip mats and grab bars for
safety. Hand-held shower spray, long-handled bath sponge, or a
washer mitt with a pocket that holds soap may promote autonomy.

12. Provide a commode chair or elevated toilet seat or urinal if it will
facilitate self-care with elimination. Teach self-transfer techniques
that will enable patient to get to commode or toilet. Keep call light
within patient's reach. Instruct patient to call as early as possible
so that staff will have time to respond and patient will not have to
rush because of urgency. Offer toileting reminders q2h, after
meals, and before bedtime.

13. Some patients may have difficulty with perineal care after elimination. For many patients with limited hand or arm mobility, a long-
handled reacher that can hold tissues or washcloth may help patient maintain independence with perineal care.

14. For patient with hemiparesis or hemiparalysis, teach use of
stronger or unaffected hand and arm for dressing, eating, bathing,
and grooming. Instruct patient to dress weaker side first.

15. For patients with visual field deficit, avoid placing items on blind
side. Encourage these patients to scan environment for needed
items by turning the head.

16. Obtain a referral by occupational therapist (OT) if indicated to determine best method for performing activity.

17. Individuals with cognitive defects need simple visual or verbal
cues, increased gesture use, demonstration, reminders of next step,
and gentle repetition. Provide a consistent care giver and ADL routine.

18. If indicated, teach patient self-catheterization, or teach technique to
care giver. At-home intermittent catheterization usually is done
with clean, not sterile, technique and equipment. Catheter is
washed after use in warm, soapy water, rinsed, and place in a clean
plastic sack. Crusted catheters are soaked in a solution made up of
half distilled vinegar and half water. Teach patient to monitor for
and notify health professional of cloudy, foul-smelling, or bloody
urine; urine with sediment; chills or fever; pain in lower back or
abdomen; or red or swollen urethral meatus.

19. Discuss, as appropriate, changing home environment to improve
ADLs and independence (e.g., with extended sinks, lower closet
hooks, wheelchair-accessible shower, modified telephones, lowered mirrors, and lever door handles that operate with reduced
hand pressure).

20. Listen and provide opportunities for patient to express himself or
herself, and communicate that it is normal to have negative feelings about changes in autonomy. Discuss with health care team

ways to provide consistent, positive encouragement and strategies that progressively increase independence.

Self-care deficit (oral hygiene) related to sensorimotor deficit or decreased LOC

Desired outcome: Before hospital discharge, patient or significant other demonstrates ability to perform patient's oral care.

1. Assess patient's ability to perform mouth care. Identify performance barriers (e.g., sensorimotor or cognitive deficits).
2. If patient has decreased LOC or is at risk for aspiration, remove dentures and store them in a water-filled denture cup.
3. If patient cannot perform mouth care, clean teeth, tongue, and mouth at least 2 × per day with a soft-bristled toothbrush and nonabrasive toothpaste. If patient is unconscious or at risk for aspiration, turn him or her to side-lying position. Swab mouth and teeth with sponge-tipped applicator or gauze pad moistened with mouthwash solution described earlier, and irrigate mouth with a syringe. If patient cannot self-manage secretions, use only a small amount of liquid at a time, using a suction catheter or Yankauer tonsil suction catheter to remove secretions; this regimen should be performed at least q4h. As appropriate, teach procedure to significant others.
4. For patients with physical disabilities, the following toothbrush adaptations can be made:
   - *For patients with limited hand mobility:* Enlarge toothbrush handle by covering it with a sponge hair roller or aluminum foil, attaching with an elastic band; or by attaching a bicycle handle grip with plaster of Paris.
   - *For patients with limited arm mobility:* Extend toothbrush handle by overlapping another handle or rod over it and taping them together.

Impaired verbal communication related to facial/throat muscle weakness, intubation, or tracheostomy

Desired outcome: After intervention, patient communicates effectively, either verbally or nonverbally, and reports less frustration with communication.

1. Assess patient's ability to speak, read, write, and comprehend.
2. If appropriate, obtain referral to a speech therapist or pathologist to assist patient in strengthening muscles used in speech. Encourage patient to perform exercises that increase ability to control facial muscles and tongue. These exercises may include holding a sound for 5 sec, singing the scale, reading aloud, and extending the tongue to try to touch the chin, nose, or cheek.
3. Provide a supportive, relaxed environment for patients unable to form words or sentences or unable to speak clearly or appropriately. Acknowledge patient's frustration over inability to communicate, and explain that patience is needed for both patient and caregiver. Maintain a calm, positive, reassuring attitude. Continue to use normal volume when speaking to patient unless patient's hearing is impaired. Maintain eye contact to promote focus. Provide enough time for patient to articulate. Ask patient to repeat unclear words. Observe for nonverbal cues; watch patient's lips

closely. Do not interrupt or finish sentences. Anticipate needs, and phrase questions to allow simple answers such as "yes" or "no." Provide continuity of care to reduce patient's frustration.

4. Provide alternative methods of communication if patient cannot speak (e.g., language board, alphabet cards, flash cards, or pad and pencil). Other alternatives are systems that use eye blinks or hand squeezes, bell signal taps, or gestures (e.g., hand signals, head nods, pantomime, or pointing). Use communication board for urgent situations. Document method of communication used.

5. If patient's voice is weak and difficult to hear, reduce environmental noise to enhance listener's ability to hear words. Suggest that patient take a deep breath before speaking; provide a voice amplifier if appropriate for patient. Encourage patients to organize thoughts and plan what they will say before speaking and to express ideas in short, simple phrases or sentences. Remind patient to speak slowly, exaggerate pronunciation, and use facial expressions.

6. If patient has swallowing difficulties that result in accumulation of saliva, suction mouth to promote clearer speech.

7. For a patient with muscle rigidity or spasm, massage facial and neck muscles before he or she attempts to communicate.

8. If patient has a tracheostomy, ensure that a tap bell is within reach. Reassure patients with a temporary tracheostomy that they will regain the ability to speak. For patients with permanent tracheostomy, discuss learning alternate communication systems, such as sign language or esophageal speech. Fenestrated tubes or covering opening of tracheostomy tube with a finger allows speech.

9. Establish a method of calling for assistance, and ensure that patient knows how to use it. Keep calling device where patient can activate it (e.g., place call bell on unparalyzed side). Depending on the deficit, use a tap bell for weak patients, a pillow pad call light (triggered by arm or head movement), or a sip and puff device (triggered by mouth).

10. If patient can write, encourage him or her to keep a diary or write letters as a means of ventilating feelings and expressing concerns. If patient has a weak writing arm, evaluate for need of a splint that will enable patient to hold a pen or pencil. Felt-tip markers also are useful, because they require minimal pressure for writing.

Constipation related to inability to chew and swallow a high-roughage diet, side effects of medications, immobility, and spinal cord involvement

Desired outcome: Within 2-3 days of intervention, patient passes soft, formed stools and maintains his or her normal bowel pattern.

1. Although a high-roughage diet is ideal for patient who is immobilized or on prolonged bed rest, the individual with chewing and swallowing difficulties may be unable to consume such a diet. For these patients, consuming a serving or two of cooked fruit or cooked bran cereal each day may be effective. Otherwise, encourage use of natural fiber laxatives such as psyllium (e.g., Metamucil).

2. A bowel elimination program may include: setting a regular time of day for attempting a bowel movement, preferably 30 min after eat-

ing a meal or drinking a hot beverage; using a commode instead of a bedpan for easier elimination; using a medicated suppository 15-30 min before a scheduled attempt; bearing down by contracting abdominal muscles or applying manual pressure to abdomen to help increase intraabdominal pressure; and drinking 4 oz of prune juice nightly. Abdominal and pelvic exercise may be included in patient's morning and evening routine. Keep a call bell within patient's reach. Assess patient's sitting balance to ensure safety while up on commode. **Caution:** SCI patients with involvement at T8 and above should use *extreme* caution if use of an enema or suppository is unavoidable because either can precipitate life-threatening autonomic dysreflexia (AD). Liberal application of anesthetic jelly into the rectum should precede use of enemas or suppositories. In addition, instruct patient at risk of IICP not to bear down with bowel movements because this action can cause increased intraabdominal pressure, which in turn increases ICP.

3. If indicated by patient's diagnosis (e.g., MS), provide instructions for digital stimulation of anus to promote reflex bowel evacuation. **Caution:** This intervention is contraindicated for SCI patients with involvement at T8 or above because it can precipitate life-threatening AD.

4. For other interventions, see **Constipation,** p. 420, in Appendix One, "Caring for Patients on Prolonged Bed Rest."

Decreased adaptive capacity: Intracranial (risk of IICP and herniation), related to positional factors, increased intrathoracic or intraabdominal pressure, fluid volume excess, hyperthermia, or discomfort

Desired outcome: Patient is free of symptoms of IICP and herniation, as evidenced by stable or improving score on Glasgow Coma Scale (Table 4-3); stable or improving sensorimotor functioning; BP within patient's normal range; HR 60-100 bpm; pulse pressure 30-40 mm Hg (the difference between the systolic and diastolic readings); orientation to time, place, and person; normal vision; bilaterally equal and normoreactive pupils; RR 12-20 breaths/min with normal depth and pattern (eupnea); normal gag, corneal, and swallowing reflexes; and absence of headache, nausea, nuchal rigidity, posturing, and seizure activity.

N O T E : ICP is the pressure exerted by brain tissue, CSF, and cerebral blood volume within the rigid, unyielding skull. An increase in any one of these components without a corresponding decrease in another will increase ICP. Normal ICP is 0-15 mm Hg; IICP is >15 mm Hg. Cerebral perfusion pressure (CPP) is the difference between systemic arterial pressure and ICP. As ICP rises, CPP may fall. Normal CPP is 80-100 mm Hg. If CPP falls below 60 mm Hg, irreversible ischemia occurs. When CPP falls to 0, cerebral blood flow ceases. Cerebral edema and IICP usually peak 2-3 days after an injury and then decline over 1-2 wk.

1. Monitor for and report any of the following indicators of IICP or impending or occurring herniation:
   - *Early indicators of IICP:* Declining score on Glasgow Coma Scale, alterations in LOC ranging from irritability, restlessness,

Table 4-3   Glasgow Coma Scale

Response	Rating	Score
Best eye-opening response (Record *C* if eyes closed because of swelling.)	Spontaneously	4
	To speech	3
	To pain	2
	No response	1
Best motor response (Record best upper limb response to painful stimuli.)	Obeys verbal command	6
	Localizes pain	5
	Flexion—withdrawal	4
	Flexion—abnormal	3
	Extension—abnormal	2
	No response	1
Best verbal response (Record *E* if endotracheal tube is in place, or *T* if tracheostomy tube is in place.)	Conversation—oriented × 3	5
	Conversation—confused	4
	Speech—inappropriate	3
	Sounds—incomprehensible	2
	No response	1
Total score:	15 = normal	
	13-15 = minor head injury	
	9-12 = moderate head injury	
	3-8 = severe head injury	
	≤7 = coma	
	3 = deep coma or brain death	

and confusion to lethargy; possible onset or worsening of headache; beginning pupillary dysfunction (e.g., sluggishness); visual disturbances (e.g., diplopia, blurred vision); onset of or increase in sensorimotor changes or deficits (e.g., weakness); onset of or worsening of nausea. **Note:** The single most important indicator of early IICP is a change in LOC.

■ *Late indicators of IICP* (generally related to brainstem compression and disruption of cranial nerves and vital centers): Continuing decline in score on Glasgow Coma Scale; continued deterioration in LOC, leading to stupor and coma; projectile vomiting; hemiplegia; posturing; widening pulse pressure, decreased HR, and increased systolic BP; Cheyne-Stokes breathing or other respiratory irregularity; pupillary changes (e.g., inequality, dilatation, nonreactivity to light); papilledema; and impaired brainstem reflexes (corneal, gag, swallowing).

■ *Brain herniation:* Deep coma; fixed, dilated pupils (first unilateral and then bilateral); posturing progressing to bilateral flaccidity; lost brainstem reflexes; continuing deterioration in VS and respirations.

2. If changes occur, prepare for possible transfer of patient to ICU. Insertion of ICP sensors for continuous ICP monitoring, CSF ven-

tricular drainage, intubation, mechanical ventilation, neuromuscular blocking, or barbiturate coma therapy may be necessary.

3. For patients at risk for IICP, preventing hypoxia and CO_2 retention is essential for preventing vasodilatation of cerebral arteries. Preventive measures include ensuring a patent airway, delivering O_2 as prescribed, hyperventilating ("sighing" or bagging) patient before suctioning, and limiting suctioning to 10-15 sec. Reduce $Paco_2$ *via* hyperventilation by instructing conscious patients to take deep breaths on their own or by providing manual or machine hyperventilation when patient is intubated or has a tracheostomy. Monitor patient's ABG or pulse oximetry values.

4. Promote venous blood return to the heart to reduce cerebral congestion by keeping HOB elevated at 15-30 degrees (unless otherwise directed); maintaining head and neck alignment to avoid hyperextension, flexion, or rotation; ensuring that tracheostomy and endotracheostomy ties or O_2 tubing does not compress jugular vein; and avoiding Trendelenburg's position for any reason. Ensure that pillows under patient's head are flat so that the head is in a neutral rather than flexed position.

5. Take precautions against increased intraabdominal and intrathoracic pressure in the following ways: Teach patient to exhale when turning. Provide passive ROM exercises rather than allow active or assistive exercises. Administer prescribed stool softeners or laxatives to prevent straining at stool; avoid enemas and suppositories, because they can cause straining. Instruct patient not to move himself or herself in bed because it requires a pushing movement; allow only passive turning; use a pull sheet. Instruct patient to avoid pushing or pulling against side rails or foot board. Avoid foot boards; use high-top tennis shoes instead. Assist patient with sitting up and turning. Instruct patient to avoid coughing and sneezing or, if unavoidable, to cough or sneeze with an open mouth; provide antitussive for cough as prescribed and antiemetic for vomiting. Instruct patient to avoid hip flexion (increases intraabdominal pressure). Do not place patient in prone position, and avoid using restraints (straining against them increases ICP). Rather than have patient perform Valsalva's maneuver to prevent an air embolism during insertion of a central venous catheter, physician should use a syringe to aspirate air from catheter lumen.

6. Help reduce cerebral congestion by enforcing fluid limitations as prescribed, typically <1,500 ml/day. Administer IV fluids with a control device to prevent fluid overload. Keep accurate I&O records. When administering additional IV fluids (e.g., IV drugs) avoid using D_5W because its hypotonicity can increase cerebral edema.

7. Because fever increases metabolic requirements (10% for each 1° C) and aggravates hypoxia, help maintain patient's body temperature within normal limits by giving prescribed antipyretics, regulating temperature of environment, limiting use of blankets, keeping patient's trunk warm to prevent shivering, and administering tepid sponge baths or using hypothermia blanket to reduce fever.

When using a hypothermia blanket, wrapping patient's extremities in a blanket may prevent shivering. If prescribed, administer chlorpromazine to prevent shivering, which would increase ICP.

8. Administer prescribed osmotic and loop diuretics to reduce cerebral edema and produce a state of dehydration. Administer glucocorticosteroids to reduce edema and inflammation. Administer BP medications as prescribed to keep BP within prescribed limits, which will promote optimal cerebral blood flow without increasing cerebral edema. Because pain can increase BP and consequently ICP, administer prescribed analgesics promptly and as necessary. Barbiturates and narcotics usually are contraindicated because they may mask the signs of IICP and cause respiratory depression.

9. Administer antiepilepsy drugs as prescribed to prevent or control seizures, which would increase cerebral metabolism, hypoxia, and CO_2 retention, thereby increasing cerebral edema and ICP.

10. Monitor bladder drainage tubes for obstruction or kinks because a distended bladder can increase ICP.

11. Provide a quiet, soothing environment. Control noise and other environmental stimuli. Speak softly, use a gentle touch, and avoid jarring the bed. Try to limit painful procedures; avoid tension on tubes (e.g., urinary catheter); and consider limiting pain-stimulation testing. Avoid unnecessary touch (e.g., leave BP cuff in place for frequent VS); and talk softly, explaining procedures before touching to avoid startling patient. Try to avoid situations in which patient may become emotionally upset. Do not say anything in patient's presence that you would not say if he or she were awake. Family discussions should take place outside the room. Limit visitors as necessary. Encourage significant others to speak quietly to patient because hearing a familiar voice may promote relaxation and reduce ICP. Listening to soft favorite music with earphones also may reduce ICP.

12. Because multiple procedures and nursing care activities can increase ICP by increasing discomfort and anxiety, individualize care to ensure rest periods and optimal spacing of activities. Rousing patients from sleep has been shown to increase ICP. Plan activities and treatments accordingly so that patient can sleep undisturbed as often as possible.

Sensory/perceptual alterations (visual) related to diplopia
Desired outcome: Following intervention, patient verbalizes that his or her vision has improved.

1. Assess patient for diplopia.
2. If patient has diplopia, provide eye patch, or eyeglasses with a frosted lens, which is a temporary means of eliminating this condition. Alternate eye patch q4h.
3. Orient patient to his or her environment as needed.
4. Advise patient of availability of "talking books" (tapes) and large-type reading materials.
5. Place a sign over patient's bed that indicates his or her visual impairment.

6. Teach patient that depth perception will be altered, and how to use visual cues and scanning.

Pain related to spasms, headache, and photophobia secondary to neurologic dysfunction

Desired outcomes: Within 1 h of intervention, patient's subjective perception of discomfort decreases, as documented by a pain scale. Objective indicators, such as grimacing, are absent or diminished.

1. Assess characteristics (e.g., quality, severity, location, onset, duration, precipitating factors) of patient's pain or spasms. Devise a pain scale with patient, and document discomfort on a scale of 0 (no pain) to 10 (worst pain).

2. Respond immediately to patient's complaints of pain. Administer analgesics and antispasmodics as prescribed. Consider scheduling doses of analgesia. Document effectiveness of medication, using the pain scale. Monitor for untoward effects. Consult physician if dosage or interval change seems necessary. Teach patient and significant others about the importance of timing pain medication so that it is taken before pain becomes too severe and before major moves.

3. Teach patient about the relationship between anxiety and pain, as well as other factors that enhance pain and spasms (e.g., staying in one position for too long, fatigue, chilling).

4. Instruct patient and significant others in the use of nonpharmacologic pain management techniques: repositioning; ROM; supporting painful extremity or part; back rubs, massage, warm baths, and other tactile distraction; auditory distraction (e.g., listening to soothing music); visual distraction (e.g., television); heat applications (e.g., warm blankets or moist compresses); cold applications (e.g., ice massage); guided imagery; breathing exercises; relaxation tapes and techniques; biofeedback; and a transcutaneous electrical nerve stimulation (TENS) device, as appropriate. See **Health-seeking behaviors:** Relaxation technique effective for stress reduction, p. 27.

5. Encourage rest periods to facilitate sleep and relaxation. Fatigue tends to exacerbate pain. Pain may result in fatigue, which in turn may cause exaggerated pain and further exhaustion. Try to provide uninterrupted sleep at night.

6. If patient has photophobia, provide quiet, dark environment. Close door and curtains; avoid artificial lights whenever possible.

7. Pain in SCI patient often is poorly localized and may be referred. Intrascapular area pain may be from the stomach, duodenum, or gallbladder. Umbilical pain may be from the appendix. Testicular or inner thigh pain may be from the kidneys (e.g., pyelonephritis). Evaluate patient for signs of infection or inflammatory process (e.g., tachycardia, restlessness, urinary incontinence when it was previously controlled, fever).

8. If patient's current pain varies significantly from previous episodes of pain, or if interventions are ineffective, consult physician.

Impaired swallowing related to decreased or absent gag reflex, decreased strength or excursion of muscles involved in mastication, perceptual impairment, or facial paralysis

Desired outcome: Before oral foods and fluids are reintroduced, patient exhibits ability to swallow safely.

1. Assess patient for factors that affect ability to swallow safely: LOC, gag and cough reflexes, and strength and symmetry of tongue, lip, and facial muscles. Monitor for signs of impaired swallowing: regurgitation of food and fluid through nares, drooling, food oozing from lips, and food trapped in buccal spaces. Development of a weak or hoarse voice during or after eating may signal potential for impaired swallowing. Check swallow reflex by first asking patient to swallow his or her own saliva. If larynx elevates with attempt (a sign that swallow reflex is intact), ask patient to swallow 3-5 ml of plain water. Document your findings.

C A U T I O N :   The cough reflex must be present for the patient to relearn swallowing safely.

---

2. Obtain a referral to a speech therapist for patients with a swallowing dysfunction. The act of swallowing is complex, and interventions vary according to the phase of swallowing that is dysfunctional. Video fluoroscopy may be used to evaluate swallowing. Encourage patient to practice any prescribed exercises (e.g., tongue and jaw ROM).

3. Enteral or parenteral nutrition may be necessary for patient who cannot chew or swallow effectively or safely. Alert physician to your findings. Be aware that an NG tube may desensitize patient and impair reflexive response to food bolus stimulus, thereby hindering the ability to relearn to swallow.

4. Keep suction equipment and a manual resuscitation bag with face mask at patient's bedside. Suction secretions in patient's mouth as necessary.

5. Ensure that patient is alert and responsive to verbal stimuli before attempting to swallow. Drowsy, inattentive, or fatigued patients have difficulty cooperating and are at risk of aspirating. To help minimize fatigue, provide a rest period before meals or swallowing attempts.

6. Initial swallowing attempts should be made with plain water (see above) because of the risk of aspiration. Progressively add easy to swallow food and liquids as patient's ability to swallow improves. Determine which foods and liquids are easiest for patient to swallow. Generally, semisolid foods of medium consistency (e.g., puddings, hot cereals, and casseroles) tend to be easiest to swallow. Thicker liquids, such as nectars, tend to be better tolerated than thin liquids. Adding gravy or sauce to dry foods often facilitates swallowing. Sticky, mucus-producing foods (e.g., peanut butter, chocolate, milk) often are restricted or limited.

7. To help patient focus on swallowing, reduce stimuli in the room (e.g., turn off television, lower radio volume, minimize conversation, limit disruption from phone calls). Caution patient not to talk while eating.

8. Most patients swallow best in an upright position. Sitting in a straight-backed chair with feet on the floor is ideal. If patient must remain in bed, use high Fowler's position if possible. Support shoulders and neck with pillows. Ensure that the head is erect and flexed forward slightly, with the chin at midline and pointing toward the chest, to promote movement of food and fluid into esophagus and minimize the risk of its going into the airway. Stroking the neck lightly may help some patients swallow. Maintain patient in an upright position for at least 30-60 min after eating to prevent regurgitation and aspiration.

9. Teach patient to break down the act of chewing and swallowing. Encourage him or her to concentrate and take adequate time. Talk patient through the following steps:
   - Take small bites or sips.
   - Place food on the tongue.
   - Use the tongue to transfer food so that it is directly under the teeth on the unaffected side of the mouth.
   - Chew the food thoroughly.
   - Move the food to the middle of the tongue and hold it there.
   - Flex the neck and tuck the chin against the chest.
   - Hold the breath and think about swallowing.
   - Without breathing, raise the tongue to the roof of the mouth and swallow.
   - Swallow several times if necessary.
   - When the mouth is empty, raise the chin and clear the throat or cough purposefully once or twice.

10. Start with small amounts of food or liquid. Feed slowly. Ensure that each previous bite has been swallowed. Check mouth for pockets of food. After every few bites of solid food, provide a liquid to help clear the mouth. Avoid using a syringe because the force of the fluid, if sprayed, may cause aspiration.

11. Teach patient with food pockets in buccal spaces to periodically sweep the mouth with the tongue or finger or to clean these areas with a napkin.

12. For patients who have a weak or paralyzed side, teach them to place food on the side of the face they can control. Tilting the head toward the stronger side allows gravity to help keep food or liquid on the side of the mouth they can manipulate. Some patients may find that rotating the head to the weak side will close the damaged side of the pharynx and facilitate more effective swallowing.

13. Patients with loss of oral sensation may be unable to identify foods or fluids that are too hot or too cold by their tongue or oral mucosa, potentially resulting in tissue injury. Serve only warm or cool foods to these individuals. Verbal cues and use of a mirror may help ensure that these patients keep their mouths clear after swallowing.

14. Patients with a rigid tongue (e.g., who have parkinsonism) have difficulty getting the tongue to move the bolus of food into the pharynx for swallowing. Encourage repeated swallowing attempts to facilitate movement of food. Evaluate patient's swallowing abil-

Neurologic

ity at different times of the day. Reschedule mealtimes to times of
the day when patient has improved swallowing or, as appropriate,
discuss with physician the possibility of changing the schedule of
patient's antiparkinson medication.

15. If decreased salivation is contributing to patient's swallowing difficulties, perform one of the following before feeding to stimulate
salivation: swab patient's mouth with a lemon-glycerine sponge;
have patient suck on a tart-flavored hard candy, dill pickle, or
lemon slice; teach patient to move the tongue in a circular motion
against inside of the cheek; or use artificial saliva. Moisten food
with melted butter, broth or other soup, or gravy. Dip dry foods
such as toast into coffee or other liquid to soften them. Rinse patient's mouth as needed to remove particles and lubricate the
mouth. Investigate medications patient is taking for the potential
side effect of decreased salivation.

16. Tablets or capsules may be swallowed more easily when added to
foods such as puddings or ice cream. Crushed tablets or opened
capsules also mix easily into these types of foods. However, check
with pharmacist to ensure that crushing a tablet or opening a capsule does not adversely affect its absorption or duration.

17. Teach significant others the Heimlich (abdominal thrust) maneuver
so that they can intervene in the event of choking.

Altered body temperature related to illness or trauma affecting
temperature regulation and inability or decreased ability to perspire,
shiver, or vasoconstrict

Desired outcome: After intervention, patient is normothermic with
core temperatures between 36.5° and 37.8° C (97.8° and 100° F).

N O T E :   Infection and hypothalamic dysfunction due to cerebral insult (trauma, edema) are two common causes of hyperthermia. Rapid
development of spinal lesions (e.g., in SCI) breaks the connection between the hypothalamus and the sympathetic nervous system (SNS),
resulting in inability to adapt to the environmental temperature. In spinal cord shock, temperatures tend to lower toward the ambient temperature. Inability to vasoconstrict and shiver makes heat conservation
difficult; inability to perspire prevents normal cooling.

---

1. Monitor rectal, tympanic, or bladder core temperature q4h or, if patient is in spinal shock, q2h. Observe for signs of hypothermia: impaired ability to think, disorientation, confusion, drowsiness, apathy,
and reduced HR and RR. Monitor for complaints of being too cold,
goose bumps, and cool skin (in SCI patients, above level of injury).
Observe for signs of hyperthermia: flushed face, malaise, rash,
respiratory distress, tachycardia, weakness, headache, and irritability. Monitor for complaints of being too warm, sweating, or hot and
dry skin (in SCI patients, above level of injury). Observe for signs
of dehydration: parched mouth, furrowed tongue, dry lips, poor skin
turgor, decreased urine output, and weak, fast pulse.

2. *For hyperthermia:* Maintain a cool room temperature (20° C [68°
F]). Provide a fan or air-conditioning to prevent overheating. Remove excess bedding, and cover patient with a thin sheet. Give

tepid sponge baths. Place cool, wet cloths at patient's head, neck, axillae, and groin. Administer antipyretic agent as prescribed. Use a padded hypothermia blanket. Provide cool drinks. Evaluate for potential infectious cause.

3. *For hypothermia:* Increase environmental temperature. Protect patient from drafts. Provide warm drinks, extra blankets, and warming (hyperthermia) blanket as needed.

4. Keep feverish patient dry. Change bed linens after diaphoresis. Provide careful skin care when patient is on a hypothermia or hyperthermia blanket. Maintain adequate hydration. Consider insensible water loss from fever, which may affect total hydration, when measuring I&O. Increase caloric intake because of increased metabolic needs. Remember that steroids may mask fever or infection.

Knowledge deficit: Neurologic tests (EEG, positron emission tomography [PET], MRI, CT, lumbar puncture [LP], myelography, digital subtraction angiography [DSA], cerebral angiography, oculoplethysmography, electromyography [EMG], nerve conduction velocity [NCV], and evoked potentials [EP])

Desired outcome: After explanation and before procedure, patient verbalizes understanding of prescribed diagnostic test, including purpose, risks, anticipated benefits, and expectations for patient before, during, and after test.

1. After physician has explained the diagnostic study to the patient, reinforce or clarify information as indicated. Adjust and simplify information to level patient can understand and repeat several times, as appropriate to the patient's cognitive dysfunction.

2. If an EEG has been prescribed, explain that this test indicates the amount of brain activity present and may reveal abnormal patterns of electrical activity, particularly with such stimuli as flashing lights or hyperventilation. Explain that an EEG may be performed while patient is either asleep or awake and sometimes by telemetry. Cooperation is important, and the test may take 40-60 min. Alert EEG staff to medications patient is taking. In addition, discuss the following as appropriate:

   ▪ *Before the test:* Antiepilepsy medications, sedatives, and tranquilizers may be withheld 24-48 h before the test. Patient's hair should be thoroughly washed and dried, but sprays, creams, and oils must be avoided. If a sleep EEG has been prescribed, patient will need to stay awake the night before the test. Patient usually is allowed a normal diet the morning of the test to prevent hypoglycemia, but caffeine-containing foods (e.g., chocolate) and beverages (e.g., coffee, tea, colas) are restricted.

   ▪ *During the test:* Small electrode patches are attached to patient's head. Reassure patient that he or she will not receive any electric shocks. Patient may be asked to watch flashing lights or to hyperventilate to elicit electrical activity patterns in the brain.

   ▪ *After the test:* Patient's hair will be washed or acetone swabs will be provided to remove paste used for attaching electrodes. Medications probably will be reinstated at this time. If needle electrodes were used, do not wash hair for 24 h.

Neurologic

3. If PET has been prescribed, explain that this test may locate areas of cerebral glucose metabolism that correspond to the seizure-causing focus; distinguish tumor tissue from normal tissue by identifying abnormal metabolic activity of the tumor tissue; or identify areas of ischemia or low metabolism (e.g., Alzheimer's disease). In addition, discuss the following as appropriate.

   ■ *Before the test:* Procedure is contraindicated for pregnancy. Alcohol, caffeine, and tobacco may be restricted for 24 h to prevent skewing of test results. Because the test is based on tissue glucose metabolism, patient should eat a meal 3-4 h before the test. If patient has diabetes mellitus, physician may give special instructions about insulin administration because insulin alters glucose metabolism. Generally, patient will be allowed to take insulin before the pretest meal.

   ■ *During the test:* Explain that the test takes 60-90 min and the patient is required to be still during that time. Tranquilizers are contraindicated because they alter glucose metabolism.

   ■ *After the test:* Encourage fluids if not contraindicated.

4. If MRI has been prescribed, explain that this test may reveal biochemical changes caused by hypoxia, necrosis, or degenerative disease, or by a mass (e.g., tumor, hemorrhage, tissue shift, or hydrocephalus). This test also may show structural lesions that may be responsible for symptoms such as seizures. MRI is more useful than CT scanning in evaluating pituitary tumors, acoustic neuromas, posterior fossa tumors, spinal cord tumors and trauma, demyelinating disease, cerebral atrophy, and situations in which patient is allergic to contrast medium. In addition, discuss the following as appropriate.

   ■ *Before the test:* Confirm with patients that they do not have a pacemaker, surgical aneurysm clip, prosthetic heart valve, or umbrella filter for emboli and are not pregnant. Explain that MRI is contraindicated during pregnancy and can deactivate pacemakers, and that the strong magnetic field can move ferrous metal aneurysm clips and valve and umbrella filters within the body, putting patient at obvious risk. The presence of these internal items makes patient ineligible for MRI. MRI also is not used on critically ill or unstable patients because it is impossible to monitor cardiac rhythm and VS inside the scanner. Patient must be able to cope with confined spaces and lie motionless throughout the 15-90-min test. A soft humming sound and on-off pulses will be heard. The physician may prescribe a sedative. Patient should void before the test and remove such items as jewelry, hair clips, clothing with metal fasteners, and glasses before entering the scanner.

5. If a CT scan has been prescribed, explain that the test may detect masses caused by tumors, hemorrhage, tissue shift, or hydrocephalus. Serial scans may be performed to determine a tumor's response to therapy or detect a resolution or increase in a hemorrhage. CT scanning is more useful than MRI in evaluating acute trauma or hemorrhage, supratentorial enhancing tumors, and hy-

drocephalus; in predicting vasospasm; and when patient has a pacemaker or internal ferrous metal objects or is uncooperative. If contrast agents are not used, there are no known complications from CT scans. If a contrast agent is used, discuss the following with patient as indicated.

- *Before the test:* Allergies to iodine or iodine-containing substances such as shellfish or contrast medium must be reported to the physician. Food and fluids may be restricted 4 h before the test. Remove hair pins. The test usually lasts 15-30 min, and patient can expect to hear a clicking noise as the machine moves. Patient must lie still, and sedation may be prescribed.

- *During the test:* A warm, flushed feeling or burning sensation is normal and may be felt with administration of the dye. Patient also may experience a salty taste with dye injection, nausea, vomiting, or a headache during or after the test. Patient may be asked to take and hold several deep breaths during scanning.

- *After the test:* If not contraindicated, fluids are increased to ensure elimination of contrast dye *via* the kidneys. Patient will be monitored for hives, rash, and itching, which may be delayed allergic reactions to the dye.

6. If an LP has been prescribed, explain that it is performed to remove a sample of CSF for analysis and to determine CSF pressure. Typically, the CSF is evaluated for microorganisms, blood cells, and tumor markers and undergoes chemical analysis. Skin or bone infection at the puncture site is a contraindication. This procedure is performed with great caution when IICP is a factor because of the risk of herniation. An uncooperative patient, severe degenerative joint disease, or anticoagulant therapy also may preclude the procedure. Discuss the following as indicated.

- *Before the test:* Reassure patient that the needle will not enter the spinal cord. Explain that patient should empty bladder at this time.

- *During the test:* Patient will be assisted into a side-lying position, with the chin tucked into the chest and the knees drawn up to the abdomen. This position curves the spine and widens the intervertebral space for easier insertion of the spinal needle. Patient must lie still during the procedure, and a nurse will assist patient with maintaining the position. Patient should breathe normally during the test. There may be a short burning sensation when the local anesthetic is injected and some local, transient pain when the spinal needle is inserted. Patient should report any pain or sensations that continue after or differ from these expected discomforts. Patient will be monitored for discomfort, elevated HR, pallor, and clammy skin during the procedure.

- *After the test:* Patient will remain in bed with HOB flat or raised slightly for a prescribed period, usually no more than 8 h; he or she may turn from side to side during this time and should drink a large amount of fluids unless contraindicated. These measures help prevent or minimize any postprocedural headache, which is the most common adverse effect of LP. Patient should report any headache to the nurse so that analgesia, if prescribed, can be administered. The nurse will check LP site periodically for redness, swelling, and drainage. The nurse also will check VS and neurologic status. Patient should report any neck stiffness, pain, numbness, or weakness.

7. If myelography has been prescribed, explain that it is performed when other diagnostic tests are inconclusive, to delineate or rule out blockage or disruption of the spinal cord. Radiopaque dye is injected into the subarachnoid space of the spine by means of a lumbar or cervical puncture. Discuss the following with patient as indicated.

   - *Before the test:* Allergies or sensitivity to iodine, shellfish, and contrast medium; history of medications that could lower seizure threshold (e.g., phenothiazines, tricyclic antidepressants, amphetamines) and epilepsy medication must be reported to radiologist. Foods and fluids usually are withheld 4-8 h before the test.

   - *During the test:* Patient may feel transient burning when the contrast dye is injected and a salty taste, headache, or nausea after injection. With oil-based dyes, the table will tilt to facilitate flow of contrast dye to different parts of the spinal canal. With water-based dyes, patient will need to sit quietly to allow controlled upward dispersion of the dye. Patient may feel some discomfort during the procedure due to needle insertion, positions used, and removal of contrast dye (oil-based dyes) at the end of the procedure. Explain the importance of lying quietly during the 60-min procedure.

   - *After the test:* VS and neurologic status will be monitored at frequent intervals. Patient should report any increased deficit from pretest status, chills, fever, neck stiffness, and redness or swelling at the puncture site. Headache, nausea, and vomiting are common side effects and should be reported so that comfort measures can be taken. Nonrestricted patients should drink extra fluids to replace CSF lost during the test. The following positions may be used:
     - –If an oil-based dye was used (e.g., isophendylate): patient must remain flat 6-24 h or as prescribed.
     - –If a water-based dye was used (e.g., metrizamide): HOB will be elevated to 60 degrees for 8 h to minimize irritation to cranial nerves and structures; seizures, hallucination, depression, confusion, speech problems, chest pain, and dysrhythmias may occur if metrizamide reaches cranial vault.

8. If DSA has been prescribed, explain that it is performed to help visualize cerebral blood flow and detect vascular abnormalities such as stenosis, aneurysm, and hematoma. Patients are expected to lie still for the 30-60-min procedure and hold their breath on command. This test is considered safer than angiography. Vein injection carries no risk of embolus and can be done on an outpatient basis. Vein injection (versus arterial injection) requires more dye and carries an increased risk of kidney damage. This test consists

of two scans: one scan without contrast and the other with. The two images are then digitally subtracted from one another. Also discuss the following as indicated.

- *Before the test:* Patient will be assessed for good cardiac output to disperse the dye and good kidney function to excrete the dye. Allergies to iodine, shellfish, or radiopaque dye must be reported to the physician. Food and fluids usually are withheld 3-4 h before the procedure, although clear liquids sometimes are allowed. Patient may feel transient discomfort with insertion of the needle or catheter, as well as a headache, warm sensation, or metallic taste when the dye is injected.

- *After the test:* Patient will be required to drink large amounts of fluid, if not contraindicated, to promote excretion of the dye by the kidneys. Nurses will check venipuncture site for redness and swelling. If an arterial route was used for injection, see the discussion of cerebral angiography that follows.

9. If cerebral angiography has been prescribed, explain that it allows visualization of the cerebral vasculature after injection of a contrast medium and determines the site, structure, and size of an aneurysm or arteriovenous malformation, the presence of vasospasm, and the site of rupture or obstructed blood flow. It also may show an abnormal perfusion pattern, which suggests the presence of a tumor. Severe kidney, liver, or thyroid disease may contraindicate this test. Also discuss the following as indicated.

- *Before the test:* Allergies to iodine, shellfish, or radiopaque dyes must be reported to the physician. Foods and fluids are withheld for 8-10 h or as prescribed. Local anesthetic is used at the puncture site. Patient will feel a warm or burning sensation when the dye is administered and will have a transient headache or metallic taste in the mouth. The proposed site may be shaved. If the femoral approach is used, pedal pulses will be checked and their location marked. If the carotid approach is used, the patient's neck circumference will be measured, marked, and recorded. Baseline neurologic status is checked and recorded for postprocedural comparison so that small changes can be detected early. Dentures and eyeglasses usually are removed.

- *After the test:* Patient will be on strict bed rest for 6-24 h, followed by a specified period of "bathroom privileges only." Patient's VS and pulse quality will be checked frequently. Patient should notify staff if signs of reaction to the dye occur: respiratory distress, lightheadedness (hypotension), hives, or itching. Fluids will be encouraged to eliminate dye and prevent kidney damage. The puncture site will be checked frequently for bleeding or hematoma. Patient should not be alarmed if bleeding occurs. Manual pressure will be maintained until bleeding stops. A pressure dressing may then be applied, and the physician consulted. The quality of distal pulses and the temperature, color, and sensation in the extremity will be monitored at frequent intervals. Weakening pulses, pallor, coolness, or cyanosis may signal thrombus formation and artery obstruction.

Neurologic

–If the femoral approach was used, patient should keep the leg straight for the prescribed amount of time (usually 6-12 h) to minimize the risk of bleeding. Patient will use a bedpan or urinal and eat on his or her side during this time.

–If the brachial approach was used, patient's arm will be immobilized for 6-12 h or as prescribed. A sign will be posted over patient's bed that cautions against measuring BP or drawing blood in this arm.

–If the carotid artery was the puncture site, patient should report any difficulty swallowing or breathing or any weakness or numbness. The neck will be checked for increasing circumference or tracheal displacement, which may signal hematoma formation. Changes in LOC or neurologic deficits may indicate thrombus formation and arterial obstruction.

10. If oculoplethysmography has been prescribed, explain that it will help detect carotid occlusive disease and aid in its evaluation by indirect measurement of blood flow in the ophthalmic artery, which is the first major branch of the internal carotid artery. Also discuss the following as indicated.

   ■ *Before the test:* A history of recent eye surgery (within 6 mo), retinal detachment, or lens implantation, allergic reaction to local anesthetics, and current anticoagulant therapy should be reported to the physician. Contact lenses will be removed. Patients with glaucoma may take their usual eye medication. Anesthetic drops are instilled, and patient's eyes may burn slightly for a short time after instillation.

   ■ *During the test:* Small eye cups that resemble contact lenses are placed on the corneas, and suction is applied. Patient must be able to lie very still and resist blinking, because constant blinking or nystagmus may cause an artifact, making the results difficult to interpret.

   ■ *After the test:* Patient should not rub the eyes for at least 2 h, because they are susceptible to corneal abrasion from the local anesthetic. Patient should report symptoms of corneal abrasion, including pain and photophobia. As the eye drops wear off, patient probably will experience mild burning but should report severe burning. Patients who wear contact lenses should leave them out for 2 h to allow anesthetic eye drops to wear off. A darkened room and sterile normal saline may sooth irritated eyes. A conjunctival hemorrhage may occur but will fade with time.

11. EMG and NCV studies usually are performed together to diagnose and differentiate between peripheral nerve and muscle disorders.

   ■ *Before the test:* Bleeding disorders or extensive skin infection may contraindicate the test. Explain that patient's cooperation will be necessary during the 20-30-min test.

   ■ *During the test:* Patient will feel some discomfort as small needles are inserted into muscle. The muscle will twitch when electrical stimulus is applied, but this is not painful.

   ■ *After the test:* Needle sites will be monitored for hematomas or inflammation.

12. EPs measure changes in the brain's electrical activity in response to sensory stimulation. The hair should be washed before the procedure to remove oil and lotions. The hair is washed again after the procedure to remove the electrode paste. Also discuss the following:

   ■ *Visual evoked response:* Cooperation is needed. Electrodes are placed over the occipital region. Prescription glasses should be worn. Patterned and flashing lights will provide retinal stimulation. This test is good for diagnosing optic neuritis with MS.

   ■ *Somatosensory evoked response:* Peripheral nerve responses in upper or lower extremities help evaluate spinal cord function, sensory dysfunction with MS, and nerve root compression.

   ■ *Brainstem auditory evoked responses:* Used to evaluate brainstem functioning. Auditory stimulation *via* headphone is provided. A series of clicks will be heard, varying in rate, intensity, and duration. This test does not require patient's cooperation. It can help diagnose brainstem lesion in MS, acoustic neuroma, brainstem lesions related to coma, and hearing loss. It also may be used to monitor cranial nerve VIII for surgical injury.

13. After teaching, evaluate patient's understanding of diagnostic test.

Endocrine Disorders 5

SECTION ONE: DISORDERS OF THE PITUITARY GLAND

Diabetes Insipidus

NURSING DIAGNOSES AND INTERVENTIONS

Fluid volume deficit related to active loss secondary to polyuria

Desired outcomes: Within 7 days of onset of symptoms, patient becomes normovolemic, as evidenced by stable weight, balanced I&O, good skin turgor, moist tongue and oral mucous membrane, BP ≥90/60 mm Hg (or within patient's normal range), HR ≤100 bpm, and CVP 2-6 mm Hg (or 5-12 cm H_2O).

1. Monitor I&O and VS closely; weigh daily. Be alert for evidence of hypovolemia: weight loss, inadequate fluid intake to balance output, thirst, poor skin turgor, furrowed tongue, hypotension, and tachycardia. If possible, monitor CVP for evidence of hypotension. Consult physician if any of the following occurs: (1) urinary output >200 ml in each of 2 consecutive hours, (2) urinary output >500 ml in any 2-h period, or (3) urine specific gravity <1.002.
2. Provide unrestricted fluids. Keep water pitcher full and within easy reach of patient. Explain the importance of consuming as much fluid as can be tolerated.
3. Administer vasopressin and antidiuretic agents (or thiazide diuretic for patients with nephrogenic diabetes insipidus [DI]) as prescribed.
4. For unconscious patients, administer IV fluids as prescribed. Unless otherwise directed, for every 1 ml of urine output, deliver 1 ml of IV fluid.

Altered protection related to potential for side effects of vasopressin

Desired outcomes: Optimally, patient verbalizes orientation to time, place, and person and is free of signs of injury caused by side effects of vasopressin. By hospital discharge, patient and/or significant others, as appropriate, demonstrate administration of coronary artery vasodilators.

1. Monitor VS and report significant changes (e.g., systolic BP elevated >20 mm Hg over baseline systolic BP, or HR increased >20 bpm over baseline HR).

2. Be alert for indicators of water intoxication: changes in LOC, confusion, weight gain, headache, convulsions, and coma. If these develop, stop medication, restrict fluids, and consult physician. Institute safety measures accordingly, and reorient patient as needed.
3. For older adult or persons with vascular disease, keep prescribed coronary artery vasodilators (i.e., nitroglycerin) at bedside for use if angina occurs. Teach patient and significant others how to administer these medications.

PATIENT-FAMILY TEACHING AND DISCHARGE PLANNING

Give patient and significant others verbal and written information about the following:
1. Importance of continued medical follow-up; confirm date and time of next appointment.
2. Indicators that require medical attention (e.g., signs of dehydration or water intoxication).

Pituitary and Hypothalamic Tumors

NURSING DIAGNOSES AND INTERVENTIONS

Altered protection related to potential for increased intracranial pressure (IICP), DI, cerebrospinal fluid (CSF) leakage, hemorrhage, and infection secondary to transsphenoidal hypophysectomy
Desired outcomes: Optimally, patient verbalizes orientation to time, place, and person and is free of indicators of injury caused by complications of transsphenoidal hypophysectomy. Immediately after instruction, patient and significant others verbalize understanding of the importance of patient avoiding Valsalva-type maneuvers; can describe the signs and symptoms of IICP, DI, and infection; and verbalize the importance of notifying staff of postnasal drip or excessive swallowing.
1. Be alert for indicators of IICP: change in LOC, sluggish or unequal pupils, changes in respiratory rate or pattern. Monitor for decreased vision, eye muscle weakness, abnormal extraocular eye movement, double vision, and airway obstruction. Report significant findings to physician. A change in vision may necessitate a CT scan.
2. Measure I&O hourly for 24 h, and monitor urine specific gravity q1-2h. Report an output >200 ml/h for 2 consecutive hours or a total of 500 ml/h. Specific gravity <1.007 is found with DI. Monitor weight daily for evidence of loss. Explain signs of DI (see p. 212). DI can occur as a result of edema caused by manipulation of the pituitary stalk and usually is transitory.
3. Inspect nasal packing frequently for frank bleeding or CSF leakage. Note number of times mustache dressing is changed. Nasal packing usually is removed in about 3-4 days. Test *nonsanguineous* drainage for CSF fluid using a glucose reagent strip. If drainage contains CSF, test result will be positive for glucose. Monitor patient for

complaints of postnasal drip or excessive swallowing, which may signal CSF drainage down the back of patient's throat. **Caution:** Because the presence of CSF represents a serious breach in the integrity of the cranium, elevate HOB to minimize potential for bacteria entering the brain, and immediately report any suspicious drainage.

4. Elevate HOB 30 degrees to reduce ICP and swelling. Dexamethasone may be prescribed to reduce cerebral swelling.

5. Explain to patient that coughing, sneezing, and other Valsalva-type maneuvers must be avoided, because these actions can stress the operative site and increase ICP, causing CSF leakage. Teach patient to cough or sneeze with an open mouth if either is unavoidable. Remind patient that nose blowing should be avoided until nasal mucosa has healed (about 1 mo). Advise patient about the importance of mouth breathing and the possibility of having a soft nasal airway. If indicated, obtain a prescription for a mild cathartic or stool softener to prevent straining with bowel movements.

6. To avoid disturbing the integrity of the operative site, do not allow patient to brush his or her teeth. Provide mouthwash (e.g., hydrogen peroxide diluted with water to half strength) and sponge-tipped applicator for oral hygiene. Monitor for extreme erythema or swelling at suture line. Remind patient that front teeth should not be brushed until incision has healed (about 10 days). Advise patient that diet will be liquid initially but quickly will progress to soft.

7. Patient may have periorbital edema, headache, and tenderness over sinuses for 2-3 days, which may be eased by applying cold compresses to the eyes. The transsphenoidal donor site for fat or muscle packing usually is taken from the thigh or abdomen, and patient should expect a small dressing there. Advise patient that the sense of smell usually returns in 2-3 wk.

8. Be alert for and teach patient the following signs and symptoms of infection, which require medical attention: fever, nuchal rigidity, headache, and photophobia.

Sexual dysfunction related to physiologic changes secondary to abnormal hormone levels

Desired outcome: As appropriate, patient reports satisfying sexual activity within 1 mo of hospital discharge.

1. Encourage patient to express feelings of anger and frustration and to communicate feelings to significant other.

2. If appropriate, suggest alternatives to sexual intercourse for pleasuring partner and self.

3. Administer testosterone or estrogens as prescribed.

4. Support physician's referral, or suggest referral for psychotherapy related to loss of libido, sterility, impotence, or loss of self-esteem.

See Appendix One for nursing diagnoses and interventions in "Caring for Preoperative and Postoperative Patients," p. 395.

PATIENT-FAMILY TEACHING AND DISCHARGE PLANNING

Give patient and significant others verbal and written information about the following:

1. Medications, including drug name, purpose, dosage, schedule, precautions, drug/drug and food/drug interactions, and potential side effects. Reinforce that after hypophysectomy, patient will undergo lifetime hormone replacement therapy.
2. Relationship between hormone levels and stress. Advise patient to seek medical help during times of emotional or physical stress so that drug dosages can be adjusted accordingly.
3. Measures for maximizing coping mechanisms to deal with stress (e.g., relaxation tapes, meditation, diversional activities). See **Health-seeking behaviors:** Relaxation technique effective for stress reduction, p. 27.
4. Importance of continued medical follow-up; confirm time and date of next appointment.
5. Indicators of *adrenal hormone excess:* weight gain, easy bruising, muscle weakness, moon face, thirst, polyuria; *adrenal hormone insufficiency:* weight loss, easy fatigue, abdominal pain; *hypothyroidism:* weight gain, anorexia, apathy, slowed mentation, intolerance of cold; and *hyperthyroidism:* tachycardia, diaphoresis, heat intolerance. All of these signs and symptoms require medical attention.
6. For patients who require permanent vasopressin replacement therapy, the importance of obtaining a Medic-Alert bracelet and identification card outlining diagnosis and emergency treatment.

PATIENTS FOUND TO BE ACROMEGALIC DURING HOSPITALIZATION FOR ANOTHER ILLNESS

1. Role of growth hormone (GH) excess in the development of hyperglycemia, diabetes mellitus, arthralgia, osteoarthritis, cardiac enlargement, headaches, sexual/reproductive dysfunction, dental problems, and changes in physical appearance.
2. Anatomy and physiology of the pituitary gland and hypothalamus, along with changes effected by pituitary tumors.
3. Management of pituitary tumors, including medical and surgical treatments.

Syndrome of Inappropriate Antidiuretic Hormone

NURSING DIAGNOSES AND INTERVENTIONS

Fluid volume excess related to compromised regulatory mechanisms resulting in increased serum antidiuretic hormone (ADH) level, renal water reabsorption, and renal sodium (Na^+) excretion

Desired outcome: Patient becomes normovolemic (and normonatremic) within 7 days of onset of symptoms, as evidenced by orientation to time, place, and person; intake that approximates output

Endocrine

plus insensible losses; stable weight; CVP 2-6 mm Hg; BP within patient's normal range; and HR 60-100 bpm.

1. Assess LOC, VS, and I&O at least q4h; weigh patient daily. Be alert for decreasing LOC, elevated BP and CVP, urine output <30 ml/h, and weight gain. Promptly report significant findings or changes to physician.

2. Monitor laboratory results, including those for serum Na^+, urine and serum osmolality, and urine specific gravity. Be alert for decreased serum Na^+ and plasma osmolality, urine osmolality elevated disproportionately in relation to plasma osmolality, and increased urine Na^+. *Normal values:* urine specific gravity: 1.010-1.020; serum Na^+: 137-147 mEq/L; urine osmolality: 300-1090 mOsm/kg; serum osmolality: 280-300 mOsm/kg. Consult physician about significant findings.

3. Maintain fluid restriction as prescribed. Explain the need for this treatment to patient and significant others. Do not keep water or ice chips at the bedside. Ensure precise delivery of fluid administered intravenously by using a monitoring device.

4. Elevate HOB no more than 10-20 degrees to enhance venous return and thus reduce ADH release.

5. Administer demeclocycline, lithium, furosemide, or bumetanide as prescribed; carefully observe and document patient's response.

6. Administer hypertonic NaCl as prescribed. Rate of administration usually is based on serial serum Na^+ levels. To minimize the risk of hypernatremia, make sure that specimens for laboratory tests are drawn on time and that results are reported to physician promptly.

7. Institute seizure precautions to prevent injury to patient in the event of seizure: padded side rails; supplemental oxygen; oral airway at bedside; side rails up at all times when staff member is not present.

See "Diabetic Ketoacidosis" for **Risk for injury** related to altered cerebral function, p. 226. If patient has undergone a transsphenoidal hypophysectomy, see "Pituitary and Hypothalamic Tumors" for **Altered protection** related to risk of IICP, DI, CSF leakage, hemorrhage, and infection, p. 213.

PATIENT-FAMILY TEACHING
AND DISCHARGE PLANNING

Give patient and significant others verbal and written information about the following:

1. Importance of complying with fluid restriction for prescribed period. Help patient plan permitted fluid intake (e.g., by saving liquids for social and recreational situations).

2. How to safely enrich the diet with sodium and potassium salts, especially if continuous use of a diuretic is prescribed.

3. Weighing patient daily, as an indicator of hydration status.

4. Indicators of water intoxication and hyponatremia: altered LOC, fa-

tigue, headache, nausea, vomiting, and anorexia—any of which should be reported promptly to patient's physician.

5. Medications, including drug name, purpose, dosage, schedule, precautions, drug/drug and food/drug interactions, and potential side effects.

6. Importance of continued medical follow-up: confirm date and time of next appointment.

7. Procedure for obtaining a Medic-Alert bracelet or card with patient's diagnosis on it.

SECTION TWO: DIABETES MELLITUS

General Discussion

NURSING DIAGNOSES AND INTERVENTIONS

Altered peripheral, cardiopulmonary, renal, cerebral, and GI tissue perfusion (or risk for same) related to interrupted blood flow secondary to development and progression of macroangiopathy and microangiopathy

Desired outcome: Optimally, patient has adequate tissue perfusion, as evidenced by warmth, sensation, brisk capillary refill time (<2 sec), and peripheral pulses >2+ on a 0-4+ scale in the extremities; BP within his or her optimal range; urinary output ≥30 ml/h; baseline vision; good appetite; and absence of nausea and vomiting.

1. Compliance with the therapeutic regimen is essential for promoting optimal tissue perfusion. Check blood glucose before meals and at bedtime. Encourage patient to perform regular home blood glucose monitoring. Urine testing is less reliable and should not be used by patients with reduced renal function.

2. Hypertension is a common complication of diabetes. Careful control of BP is critical in preventing or limiting the development of heart disease, retinopathy, or nephropathy. Check BP q4h. Consult physician about values outside patient's normal range. Administer antihypertensive agents as prescribed, and document response.

3. Patients may experience decreased sensation in extremities because of peripheral neuropathy. In addition to sensation, assess capillary refill, temperature, peripheral pulses, and color. Protect patients with impaired peripheral perfusion from injury caused by sharp objects or heat (e.g., do not use heating pads). Teach patient to prevent venous stasis by avoiding pressure at the back of the knees (e.g., by not crossing the legs or "gatching" the bed under the knees), and avoiding constricting garments on extremities and lower body. For additional information, see **Impaired tissue integrity,** p. 218.

4. Provide a safe environment for patients with diminished eyesight caused by diabetic retinopathy. Orient patient to the location of such items as water, tissues, glasses, and call light.

5. Approximately half of all people with type I diabetes mellitus (DM) develop chronic renal failure (CRF) and end-stage renal disease.

Monitor patients for changes in renal function (e.g., increases in blood urea nitrogen [BUN] [>20 mg/dl] and creatinine [>1.5 mg/dl] and altered urine output). Proteinuria (protein >8 mg/dl in a random sample of urine) is an early indicator of developing CRF. Individuals with DM and reduced renal function are at significant risk for dehydration or for developing acute renal failure (ARF) after exposure to contrast medium. Observe these patients for indicators of ARF. (See "Acute Renal Failure," p. 73, and "Chronic Renal Failure," p. 77, for more information.) Insulin doses will decrease as renal function decreases.

6. Be alert for indicators of hypoglycemia: changes in mentation, apprehension, erratic behavior, trembling, slurred speech, staggering gait, seizure activity. Treat hypoglycemia as prescribed.

IN ADDITION

7. Individuals with DM may experience several problems resulting from autonomic neuropathy, such as the following:

   - *Orthostatic hypotension:* Assist patients when getting up suddenly or after prolonged recumbency. Check BP while patient is lying down, sitting, and then standing to document presence of orthostatic hypotension. Alert physician to significant findings.

   - *Impaired gastric emptying with nausea, vomiting, and diarrhea:* Administer metoclopramide or cisapride before meals, if prescribed. Keep a record of all stools. Nausea, vomiting, and anorexia can signal developing uremia in patients with progressive renal failure.

   - *Neurogenic bladder:* Encourage patient to void q3-4h during the day, using manual pressure (Credé's method) if necessary. Intermittent catheterization may be necessary in severe cases. Avoid use of indwelling urinary catheters because of the high risk of infection. For additional information, see "Neurogenic Bladder," p. 101.

Risk for infection related to chronic disease process (e.g., hyperglycemia, neurogenic bladder, poor circulation)

Desired outcome: Patient is asymptomatic for infection, as evidenced by normothermia, negative cultures, and WBC ≤11,000/µl.

N O T E : Infection is the most common cause of diabetic ketoacidosis (DKA).

---

1. Monitor temperature q4h. Alert physician to elevations.
2. Maintain meticulous sterile technique when changing dressings, performing invasive procedures, or manipulating indwelling catheters.
3. Monitor for indicators of infection (see Table 2-5, p. 39).
4. Consult physician about obtaining culture specimens for blood, sputum, and urine during temperature spikes, or for wounds that produce purulent drainage.

Impaired tissue integrity (or risk for same) related to altered circulation and sensation secondary to peripheral neuropathy and vascular pathology

Desired outcomes: Patient's lower extremity tissue remains intact. Within the 24 h before hospital discharge, patient verbalizes and demonstrates knowledge of proper foot care.

1. Assess integrity of the skin and evaluate reflexes of lower extremities by checking knee and ankle deep tendon reflexes, proprioceptive sensations, and vibration sensation (using a tuning fork on the medial malleolus). If sensations are impaired, anticipate patient's inability to respond appropriately to harmful stimuli. Monitor peripheral pulses, comparing quality bilaterally. Be alert for pulses $\leq 2+$ on a $0\text{-}4+$ scale.

2. Use foot cradle on bed, space boots for ulcerated heels, elbow protectors, and a pressure-relief mattress to prevent pressure points and promote patient's comfort.

3. To alleviate acute discomfort yet prevent hemostasis, minimize patient's activities and incorporate progressive passive and active exercises into daily routine. Discourage extended rest periods in the same position.

4. Teach patient the following steps for foot care:
   - Wash feet daily with mild soap and warm water; check water temperature with water thermometer or elbow.
   - Inspect feet daily for erythema or trauma, using mirrors as necessary for adequate vision.
   - Alternate between at least two pairs of properly fitted shoes to avoid potential for pressure points that can occur by wearing one pair only.
   - Prevent infection from moisture or dirt by changing socks or stockings daily and wearing cotton or wool blends.
   - Use gentle moisturizers to soften dry skin, avoiding areas between the toes.
   - Prevent ingrown toenails by cutting toenails straight across after softening them during bath. File nails with an emery board.
   - Do not self-treat corns or calluses; visit podiatrist regularly.
   - Attend to any foot injury immediately, and seek medical attention to avoid potential complication.
   - Do not go barefoot indoors or outdoors.

Knowledge deficit: Proper insulin administration and dietary precautions for promoting normoglycemia

Desired outcome: Within the 24 h before hospital discharge, patient verbalizes and demonstrates knowledge of proper insulin administration and prescribed dietary regimen.

1. Teach patient to check expiration date on insulin vial and to avoid using outdated insulin. Also teach patient proper storage of insulin and the importance of avoiding temperature extremes.

2. Explain that intermediate- and long-acting insulins require mixing (contraindicated for intermediate/rapid types). Demonstrate rolling insulin vial between palms to mix contents. Caution patient that vigorous shaking produces air bubbles, which can interfere with accurate dose measurement.

3. Explain that insulin should be injected 30 min before mealtime.

Endocrine

4. Explain that either changing the type of insulin or withholding a dose may be required for the following: when fasting for studies or surgery, when not eating because of nausea and vomiting, or when hypoglycemic. Remind patient that stress from illness or infection can increase insulin requirements (or necessitate insulin therapy for one who normally is controlled with oral hypoglycemics), and that increased exercise requires additional food intake to prevent hypoglycemia when no change is made in insulin dosage. Adjustments are always individually based and require clarification with patient's physician.

5. Provide patient with a chart depicting rotation of injection sites. Explain that injection sites should be at least 1 in apart.

6. Explain the importance of inserting the needle perpendicular to the skin rather than at an angle, to ensure deep SC administration of insulin. Very thin people may use a 45-degree angle.

7. Ensure that patient understands and demonstrates the technique and timing for home monitoring of blood glucose using a commercial kit, which provides ongoing data reflecting the degree of control and may identify necessary changes in diet and medication before severe metabolic changes occur. This test also allows for patient's self-control and psychologic security.

8. Caution patient about the importance of following a diet that is low in fat and high in water-soluble fiber as an effective means of controlling blood fats, especially cholesterol and triglycerides. Stress that diet is the sole method of control for many individuals with type II DM. Adequate nutrition and controlled calories are essential to maintaining normoglycemia in these people.

As appropriate, see "Atherosclerotic Arterial Occlusive Disease," p. 56, and "Amputation," p. 328. Also see Appendix One, "Caring for Patients with Cancer and Other Life-Disrupting Illnesses," for psychosocial nursing diagnoses and interventions, p. 450.

PATIENT-FAMILY TEACHING AND DISCHARGE PLANNING

Give patient and significant others verbal and written information about the following:

1. Importance of carrying a diabetic identification card and wearing a Medic-Alert bracelet or necklace.

2. Recognizing warning signs of both hyperglycemia and hypoglycemia, treatment, and factors that contribute to both conditions. Remind patient that stress from illness or infection can increase insulin requirements (or necessitate insulin therapy for one who normally is controlled with oral hypoglycemics), and that increased exercise requires additional food intake to prevent hypoglycemia when no change is made in insulin dosage under normoglycemic conditions. Blood glucose >250 mg/dl at the beginning of exercise will make exercise a stressor that elevates the glucose level rather than decreasing it.

3. Drugs that potentiate **hyperglycemia:** estrogens, corticosteroids, thyroid preparations, diuretics, phenytoin, glucagon, and drugs that contain sugar (e.g., cough syrup). Drugs that potentiate **hypoglycemia:** salicylates, sulfonamides, tetracyclines, methyldopa, anabolic steroids, acetaminophen, MAO inhibitors, ethanol, haloperidol, and marijuana. Propranolol and other beta-adrenergic agents mask the signs of and inhibit recovery from hypoglycemia.

4. Home monitoring of blood glucose using commercial kits and possibly daily urine testing for glucose and ketones, which provide ongoing data reflecting the degree of control and may identify necessary changes in diet and medication before severe metabolic changes occur. These tests also give patient a sense of self-control and psychologic security. Stress the need for careful control of blood glucose as a means of reducing the risk or minimizing long-term complications of DM.

5. Importance of daily exercise, maintaining a normal body weight, and yearly medical evaluation. Explain that exercise is as important as diet in treating DM. It lowers blood glucose, helps maintain normal cholesterol levels, and increases circulation. These effects increase the body's ability to metabolize glucose and help reduce the therapeutic dosage of insulin for most patients. Stress that each exercise program must be individualized (especially for type I diabetics) and implemented consistently. Patient should be given a complete physical examination and encouraged to incorporate acceptable exercise activities into his or her daily routine.

6. Low-fat, high-fiber diet as an effective means of controlling blood fats, especially cholesterol and triglycerides. Stress that diet is the sole method of control for many individuals with type II DM. Adequate nutrition and calorie control are essential to maintaining normoglycemia in these individuals.

7. Necessity for individuals with type I DM to use ^{100}U syringes with ^{100}U insulin. Various *types/sources* of insulin (beef, pork, biosynthetic) should not be mixed. When mixing various *acting* insulins, draw up regular first, followed by intermediate- or long-acting insulin.

8. Availability of syringe magnifiers that can be used for patients with poor visual acuity. Other products that aid in safe, accurate filling of syringes are also available.

9. Necessity of rotating injection sites and injecting insulin at room temperature. Provide chart showing possible injection sites, and describe system for rotating sites. Complications related to insulin injections (lipodystrophy, insulin resistance, allergic reactions) should be discussed thoroughly.

10. Importance of meticulous skin, wound, and foot care.

11. Importance of annual eye examination for early detection and treatment of retinopathy.

12. Importance of regular dental checkups because periodontal disease poses a major problem for individuals with DM. The mouth often is the primary site of origin for low-grade infections.

Endocrine

In Addition

13. Explain the importance of inserting the needle perpendicular to the skin rather than at an angle, to ensure deep SC administration of insulin. Individuals who are very thin may use a 45-degree angle.

14. For any supplemental medications used, patient should be taught the drug name, purpose, dosage, schedule, precautions, drug/drug and food/drug interactions, and potential side effects.

15. Assist patient with identifying available resources for ongoing assistance and information, including nurses, dietitian, patient's physician, and other individuals with DM in the patient care unit. Other resources include the local chapter of the American Diabetes Association and the local library for free access to current materials on diabetes. The following are addresses of journals available to patients:

   - *Diabetes 95,* American Diabetes Association Subscription Department, 1660 Duke Street, Alexandria, VA 22314.
   - *Diabetes Forecast,* American Diabetes Association Membership Center, Box 2055, Harlan, IA 51593-0238.
   - *Diabetes in the News,* Ames Center for Diabetes Education, Miles Inc, Box 3105, Elkhart, IN 46515.
   - *Diabetes Self-Management,* Box 51125, Boulder, CO 80321-1125.
   - *Health-O-Gram,* SugarFree Center, 13725 Burbank Blvd, Van Nuys, CA 91401.
   - *Living Well with Diabetes,* Diabetes Center, 13911 Ridgedale Drive, Suite 250, Minnetonka, MN 55343.
   - *Diabetes Interview,* 3715 Balboa Street, San Francisco, CA 94121.

16. Review applicable sections of Table 5-1 or Table 5-2 with patient.

Diabetic Ketoacidosis

NURSING DIAGNOSES AND INTERVENTIONS

Fluid volume deficit related to failure of regulatory mechanisms or decreased circulating volume secondary to hyperglycemia with osmotic diuresis

Desired outcome: Within 10 h of treatment, patient becomes normovolemic, as evidenced by BP $\geq$90/60 mm Hg (or within patient's normal range); HR 60-100 bpm; CVP 2-6 mm Hg (5-12 cm H_2O); good skin turgor; moist, pink mucous membranes; balanced I&O; and urinary output $\geq$30 ml/h.

1. Monitor VS q15min until stable for 1 h. Consult physician promptly about the following: HR >120 bpm, BP <90/60 mm Hg or decreased $\geq$20 mm Hg below baseline, and CVP <2 mm Hg (or <5 cm H_2O).

2. Monitor patient for physical indicators of dehydration: poor skin turgor; dry mucous membranes; soft, sunken eyeballs; tachycardia; orthostatic hypotension.

Table 5-1   Sulfonylurea oral hypoglycemic agents

Drug Dose (mg)	Usual Dose (mg)/Administration	Maximum Dose (mg)	Duration of Action (h)
acetohexamide (Dymelor)	250-1,500/single or divided	1,500	12-24
chlorpropamide (Diabinese)	100-500/single	750	60
glibornuride	12.5-75/single or divided	100	12-24
glipizide (Glucotrol)	5-25/single or divided	40	10-24
glyburide (Micronase, Glynase, DiaBeta)	1.25-10/single or divided	20	12-24
tolazamide (Tolinase)	100-750/single or divided	1,000	12-24
tolbutamide (Orinase)	500-2,000/divided	3,000	12-24

Table 5-2 Types of insulin*

Insulin Type	Examples	Onset of Action (h)/SC Injection	Peak Action (h)	Duration (h)	Mixture Compatibilities
Rapid-Acting					
Regular	crystalline zinc insulin injection	½-1	2-4	4-8	All
Semilente	prompt insulin zinc suspension	1-1½	5-10	12-16	Lente
Intermediate-Acting					
NPH	isophane insulin suspension	1-1½	4-12	20-24	Regular
Lente	insulin zinc suspension	1-2½	7-16	20-24	Regular, Semilente
Long-Acting					
Ultralente	extended insulin zinc suspension	4-8	14-24	>36	Regular, Semilente
Intermediate/Rapid					
70% NPH/30% regular	isophane insulin suspension, insulin injection	½-1	4-8	20-24	Premixed; do not mix
50% NPH/50% regular	isophane insulin suspension, insulin injection	½-1	2-4	18-24	Premixed; do not mix

*Source may be beef or pork, pancreatic extracts, or biosynthetic human insulin preparations.

3. Weigh patient daily, and measure I&O accurately. Decreasing urinary output may signal diminishing intravascular fluid volume or impending renal failure. Report to physician urine output <30 ml/h for 2 consecutive hours.

4. Administer IV fluids as prescribed to ensure adequate rehydration. Be alert for indicators of fluid overload, which can occur with rapid infusion of fluids: jugular vein distention, dyspnea, crackles, CVP >6 mm Hg (>12 cm H_2O).

5. Administer insulin as prescribed to correct or stabilize existing hyperglycemia. Be aware that when added to IV solutions, insulin may be absorbed by the container and plastic tubing. Before initiating treatment, flush tubing with 50 ml of insulin-containing IV solution to ensure that maximum adsorption of insulin by container and tubing has occurred before patient use.

6. Monitor laboratory results for abnormalities. Serum potassium (K^+) should decline until it reaches normal levels. Promptly report to physician serum K^+ level <3.5 mEq/L. Serum sodium (Na^+) will increase gradually with appropriate IV saline replacement.

7. Observe for clinical manifestations of electrolyte, glucose, and acid-base imbalances associated with DKA as follows:
   - *Hyperkalemia:* Lethargy, nausea, hyperactive bowel sounds with diarrhea, numbness or tingling in extremities, muscle weakness.
   - *Hypokalemia:* Muscle weakness, hypotension, anorexia, drowsiness, hypoactive bowel sounds.
   - *Hyponatremia:* Headache, malaise, muscle weakness, abdominal cramps, nausea, seizures, coma.
   - *Hypophosphatemia:* Muscle weakness, progressive encephalopathy possibly leading to coma.
   - *Hypomagnesemia:* Anorexia, nausea, vomiting, lethargy, weakness, personality changes, tetany, tremor or muscle fasciculations, seizures, confusion progressing to coma.
   - *Hypochloremia:* Hypertonicity of muscles, tetany, depressed respirations.
   - *Hypoglycemia:* Headache, impaired mentation, agitation, dizziness, nausea, pallor, tremors, tachycardia, diaphoresis.
   - *Metabolic acidosis:* Lassitude, nausea, vomiting, Kussmaul's respirations, lethargy progressing to coma.

Risk for infection related to inadequate secondary defenses (suppressed inflammatory response) secondary to protein depletion

Desired outcome: Patient is free of infection, as evidenced by normothermia, HR ≤100 bpm, BP within patient's normal range, WBC count ≤11,000/µl, and negative culture results.

1. Monitor patient for evidence of infection. Monitor laboratory results for increased WBC count, and culture purulent drainage as prescribed.

2. Ensure good handwashing technique when caring for patient.

3. Because patient is at increased risk of bacterial infection, use of invasive lines should be limited. Peripheral IV sites should be rotated q48-72h, depending on agency policy. Central lines should be discontinued as soon as feasible, and when in place should be handled

carefully. Schedule dressing changes according to agency policy, and inspect site for signs of local infection: erythema, swelling, purulent drainage. Document presence of any of these indicators, and consult physician.
4. Provide good skin care to maintain skin integrity. Use a pressure-relief mattress on the bed to help prevent skin breakdown. Air circulation beds are recommended for severe skin breakdown.
5. Use meticulous aseptic technique when caring for or inserting indwelling catheters, to minimize the risk of bacterial entry *via* these sites. **Note:** Because of the increased risk of infection, limit use of indwelling urethral catheters to patients who cannot void in a bedpan, or when continuous assessment of urine output is essential.
6. To help prevent pulmonary infection, provide incentive spirometry and encourage its use, along with deep-breathing and coughing exercises, qh while patient is awake.

Risk for injury related to altered cerebral function secondary to dehydration or cerebral edema associated with diabetic ketoacidosis (DKA)

Desired outcome: Patient verbalizes orientation to time, place, and person; normal breath sounds are auscultated over airway; and oral cavity and musculoskeletal system are intact and free of injury.
1. Monitor patient's orientation, LOC, and respiratory status, especially airway patency, at frequent intervals. Keep an appropriately sized oral airway, manual resuscitator and mask, and supplemental oxygen at bedside.
2. Reduce the likelihood of injury due to falls by maintaining bed in lowest position, keeping side rails up at all times, and using soft restraints as necessary.
3. Insert gastric tube in comatose patients, as prescribed, to reduce the likelihood of aspiration. Attach gastric tube to low, intermittent suction, and assess patency q4h.
4. Elevate HOB to 45 degrees to minimize risk of aspiration.
5. Initiate seizure precautions. For details, see "Seizure Disorders," p. 179.

Altered peripheral tissue perfusion (or risk for same) related to interrupted venous or arterial flow secondary to increased blood viscosity, increased platelet aggregation and adhesiveness, and patient's immobility

Desired outcomes: Optimally, patient has adequate peripheral perfusion, as evidenced by peripheral pulses >2+ on a 0-4+ scale; warm skin; brisk capillary refill (<2 sec); and absence of swelling, bluish discoloration, erythema, and discomfort in calves and thighs. Alternatively, if signs of altered peripheral tissue perfusion occur, they are detected and reported promptly.
1. Monitor Hct. Normal values are 40%-54% for men and 37%-47% for women. With proper fluid replacement, results should return to normal within 24-48 h. Assess for falling BUN as an indicator of improved tissue perfusion and renal function. Normal BUN is 6-20 mg/dl.

2. Assess peripheral pulses q2-4h. Immediately report to physician any decrease in amplitude or absence of pulses.
3. Be alert for indicators of deep vein thrombosis: erythema, pain, tenderness, warmth, swelling, or bluish discoloration or prominence of superficial veins in extremities, especially lower extremities. Arterial thrombosis may produce cyanosis with delayed capillary refill, mottling, and coolness of extremity. Report significant findings to physician immediately.
4. Assist with active or passive ROM exercises to all extremities q4h to increase blood flow to the tissues.
5. Apply antiembolic hose, Ace wraps, or pneumatic alternating pressure stockings to lower extremities as prescribed to aid in prevention of thrombosis.

Knowledge deficit: Cause, prevention, and treatment of DKA

Desired outcome: Within the 24 h before hospital discharge, patient verbalizes understanding of cause, prevention, and treatment of DKA.

1. Determine patient's knowledge about DKA and its treatment. As needed, explain the disease process of diabetes mellitus (DM) and DKA and the common early symptoms of worsening hyperglycemia: polyuria; polydipsia; polyphagia; dry, flushed skin; and increased irritability (see Table 5-3).
2. Stress the importance of maintaining a regular diet, exercise, and insulin regimen for optimal control of serum glucose and prevention of adverse physical effects of DM, such as peripheral neuropathies and increased atherosclerosis.
3. Explain the importance of testing urine ketone and blood glucose levels consistently and increasing the frequency of assessment during episodes of illness, injury, and stress. Blood glucose >200 mg/dl and large amounts of urine ketones should be reported to the physician so that the insulin dosage can be increased. As indicated, review testing procedure with patient. Caution patient that DKA requires professional medical management and cannot be self-treated.
4. Teach patient that insulin must be taken every day and that lifetime insulin therapy is necessary to achieve control of blood glucose. Explain that insulin is administered 1-4 ×/day as prescribed and that it may require adjustment during periods of illness or stress.
5. Remind patient of the importance of maintaining an adequate oral fluid intake during illness. Anorexia or nausea may limit food intake, but patient should make every effort to continue fluid intake.
6. Teach patient the indicators of *insulin excess (hypoglycemia),* such as dizziness, impaired mentation, irritability, pallor, and tremors; and *insulin deficiency (hyperglycemia),* such as increased polyuria and polydipsia and dry, flushed skin. Teach patient the importance of receiving prompt treatment if any of these indicators occurs.
7. Explain the importance of dietary changes as prescribed by physician. Typically patient is put on a fixed-calorie diet from the American Diabetes Association (ADA) composed of 60% carbohydrates, 20%-30% fats, and 12%-20% proteins. Explain that fats

Endocrine

Table 5-3 Comparison of diabetic ketoacidosis (DKA), hyperosmolar hyperglycemic nonketotic syndrome (HHNK), and hypoglycemia

	DKA	HHNK	Hypoglycemia
Type of diabetes	Usually type I (IDDM)	Usually type II (NIDDM)	
Signs, symptoms/ physical assessment	**Note:** Symptoms are a result mainly of hyperglycemia, intracellular hypoglycemia, hypotension or impending hypovolemic shock, and fluid-electrolyte imbalance with possible acid-base imbalance		**Note:** Symptoms result from intracellular hypoglycemia and hypotension/impending "insulin" shock (vasogenic)
Neurologic	Altered LOC (confusion, lethargy, irritability, coma); strokelike symptoms (unilateral/bilateral weakness, paralysis, numbness, paresthesia); fatigue	Same as DKA; also possible seizures and tremors	Tremors, trembling, shaking, confusion, apprehension, erratic behavior; may be same as DKA
Respiratory	Deep, rapid Kussmaul's respirations	Shallow, rapid (tachypneic) breathing	Usually rapid (tachypneic) breathing
Cardiovascular	Tachycardia, hypotension, ECG changes	Same as DKA	Same as DKA, possibly with diaphoresis
Metabolic/GI/ endocrine	Polyuria, polyphagia, polydipsia, fruity "acetone" breath, abdominal pain, weight loss, fatigue, generalized weakness, nausea, vomiting	Polyuria, polyphagia, polydipsia, fatigue, generalized weakness, nausea, vomiting	Hunger, nausea, eructation

Integumentary	Dry, flushed skin; poor turgor; dry mucous membranes	Same as DKA	Cool, clammy, pale skin
VS monitoring	BP: low (>20% below normal) HR: >100 bpm CVP: <2 mm Hg (<5 cm H_2O) Temperature: normal	BP: low (>20% below normal) HR: >100 bpm CVP: <2 mm Hg (<5 cm H_2O) Temperature: possibly elevated	BP: normal to low HR: >100 bpm CVP: usually unchanged
Diagnostic tests/laboratory values	Values reflect dehydration/metabolic acidosis (ketosis) secondary to hyperglycemia, abnormal lipolysis, and osmotic diuresis; fluid loss ≥6.5 L	Values reflect dehydration secondary to hyperglycemia, osmotic diuresis, and possible lactic acidosis from hypoperfusion; fluid loss ≥9 L	Values reflect hypoglycemia, possibly with vasodilatation owing to insulin shock
Hgb/Hct	Elevated	Same as DKA	Unchanged to slightly decreased
Serum BUN/creatinine	Elevated	Same as DKA	Normal
Serum electrolytes	Initially elevated, then decreased	Same as DKA	Usually unchanged
Serum glucose	250-800 mg/dl (+ ketones)	800-2000 mg/dl (− ketones)	15-50 mg/dl
ABGs	pH 6.8-7.3; HCO_3^- 12-20 mEq/L; CO_2 15-25 mEq/L	pH 7.3-7.5; HCO_3^- 20-26 mEq/L; CO_2 30-40 mEq/L	pH 7.3-7.5; HCO_3^- 20-26 mEq/L; CO_2 30-40 mEq/L
Serum osmolality	300-350 mOsm/L	>350 mOsm/L	<280 mOsm/L

Continued.

Endocrine

Table 5-3 Comparison of diabetic ketoacidosis (DKA), hyperosmolar hyperglycemic nonketotic syndrome (HHNK), and hypoglycemia—cont'd

	DKA	HHNK	Hypoglycemia
Urine glucose/acetone	Positive/positive	Positive/negative	Negative/negative
Onset	Hours to days	Same as DKA	Minutes to hours
History/risk factors for development of crisis	Undiagnosed DM, infections, acute pancreatitis, uremia, insulin resistance	Undiagnosed DM; infections, especially gram negative; acromegaly; Cushing's syndrome; thyrotoxicosis, acute pancreatitis, hyperalimentation; pancreatic carcinoma; cranial trauma/subdural hematoma; uremia, hemodialysis, peritoneal dialysis; burns, heat stroke; pneumonia, MI, CVA	Excessive dose of insulin; excessive dose of sulfonylureas/oral hypoglycemic agents; skipping meals; too much exercise with controlled blood glucose without extra food intake
	Medications: digitalis intoxication; omission/reduction of insulin dosage; failure to increase insulin to compensate for stress of infections, injury, emotional problems, or surgery	*Medications:* loop and thiazide diuretics (i.e., hydrochlorothiazide, chlorthalidone, furosemide); diazoxide; glucocorticoids (i.e., hydrocortisone, dexamethasone); propranolol (Inderal); phenytoin (Dilantin); sodium bicarbonate	*Medications:* insulin, sulfonylureas (see Table 5-1)
Mortality rate	≤10%	10%-25%	<0.1%

CVA, Cerebrovascular accident; *DM,* diabetes mellitus; *IDDM,* insulin-dependent diabetes mellitus; *MI,* myocardial infarction; *NIDDM,* non-insulin-dependent diabetes mellitus.

should be polyunsaturated and proteins chosen from low-fat sources. Teach patient the importance of eating three meals a day at regularly scheduled times and a bedtime snack.

8. Explain the causes for adjustments in insulin dosage: (1) increased or decreased food intake; (2) any physical (e.g., exercise) or emotional stress. Teach patient that exercise and emotional stress increase release of glucose from the liver, which may increase insulin demand. Instruct patient to monitor blood glucose and urine ketones closely during periods of increased emotional stress and of increased or decreased exercise and to adjust insulin dosage accordingly.

9. Explain that persons with diabetes are susceptible to infection and that preventive measures (e.g., good hygiene and meticulous daily foot care) are necessary to prevent infection. Stress the importance of avoiding exposure to communicable diseases, and explain that the following indicators of infection require prompt medical treatment: fever, chills, increased HR, diaphoresis, nausea, vomiting. In addition, teach patient and significant others to be alert to wounds or cuts that do not heal, burning or pain on urination, and a productive cough.

10. Instruct patient to implement the following therapy if he or she becomes ill for any reason:

    ■ Do not alter insulin or sulfonylurea dosage unless physician has prescribed a supplemental regimen to be implemented by individuals with type I DM for hyperglycemia secondary to illness.
    ■ Perform blood glucose monitoring and urine ketone checks q3h, and promptly report to physician glucose >300 mg/dl and positive ketones.
    ■ Eat small, frequent meals of soft, easily digestible, nourishing foods if regular meals are not tolerated.
    ■ Maintain adequate hydration, particularly if diarrhea, vomiting, or fever is persistent.
    ■ Use a balance of regular sodas or juices and water to ensure adequate calories yet prevent hyperosmolality due to sugars in the beverages.
    ■ Report any of the above conditions to physician to gain further insight into treatment and prevention of dehydration.

11. Provide the address of the ADA for pamphlets and magazines related to the disease, its complications, and appropriate treatment: American Diabetes Association, Inc., 18 East 48th Street, New York, NY 10017.

Also see psychosocial nursing diagnoses and interventions in Appendix One, "Caring for Patients with Cancer and Other Life-Disrupting Illnesses," p. 450.

PATIENT-FAMILY TEACHING AND DISCHARGE PLANNING

See **Knowledge deficit:** Cause, prevention, and treatment of DKA, above.

Endocrine

Hyperosmolar Hyperglycemic Nonketotic Syndrome

NURSING DIAGNOSES AND INTERVENTIONS

Knowledge deficit: Causes, prevention, and treatment of hyperosmolar hyperglycemic nonketotic syndrome (HHNK)

Desired outcome: Within the 24 h before hospital discharge, patient verbalizes understanding of the causes, prevention, and treatment of HHNK

1. Determine patient's understanding of HHNK and its treatment. Allow patient to express fears and feelings about diagnosis; correct any misconceptions. As needed, explain disease process of DM and HHNK and the common early symptoms of worsening diabetes: polyuria; polydipsia; polyphagia; dry, flushed skin; increased irritability. Review Table 5-3.

2. Teach the importance of testing urine acetone and blood glucose levels qid or as prescribed before meals and at bedtime. Explain that blood glucose >200 mg/dl should be reported to physician so that the insulin dosage can be increased. As indicated, review testing procedure with patient.

3. Stress the importance of dietary changes as prescribed by physician. Typically the person with type II DM is obese and will be on a reduced-calorie diet with fixed amounts of carbohydrate, fat, and protein. Explain that fats should be polyunsaturated and proteins chosen from low-fat sources. Teach patient the importance of eating three meals a day at regularly scheduled times and a bedtime snack. Explain that an increase or decrease in food intake will require an adjustment in insulin dosage. Provide a referral to a dietitian as needed.

4. Caution patient about the importance of taking oral hypoglycemic agents as prescribed. In addition, explain that exogenous insulin may be required during periods of physical and emotional stress and that blood glucose levels should be monitored closely during these times.

5. For patients with type II DM, explain the benefits of regular exercise for maintaining blood glucose levels. Exercise increases insulin effectiveness and reduces serum triglyceride and cholesterol levels, thus also reducing the risk of atherosclerosis. Aerobic exercises (e.g., walking, swimming) are most effective in lowering blood glucose levels. Caution patient always to monitor blood glucose level before exercise. A level >250 mg/dl indicates abnormal metabolism. Under this circumstance exercise would be a stressor, resulting in further elevation of blood glucose.

6. Explain the need for measures to prevent infection, such as good hygiene and meticulous daily foot care. Stress the importance of avoiding exposure to communicable diseases. Explain that the following indicators of infection require prompt medical treatment: fever, chills, tachycardia, diaphoresis, and nausea and vomiting. In ad-

dition, teach patient and significant others to be alert for wounds or cuts that do not heal, burning or pain with urination, and a cough that produces sputum.
7. Provide booklets or pamphlets from the American Diabetes Association or pharmaceutical companies about diabetes and appropriate treatment.

See "Seizure Disorders" for **Risk for trauma** related to musculoskeletal, oral, and airway vulnerability secondary to seizure activity, p. 179. See "Diabetic Ketoacidosis" for **Fluid volume deficit,** p. 222; **Risk for infection,** p. 225; and **Altered peripheral tissue perfusion,** p. 226. For psychosocial nursing diagnoses and interventions, see Appendix One, "Caring for Patients with Cancer and Other Life-Disrupting Illnesses," p. 450.

PATIENT-FAMILY TEACHING AND DISCHARGE PLANNING

See above nursing diagnoses and interventions.

Hypoglycemia

NURSING DIAGNOSES AND INTERVENTIONS

Altered protection related to potential for brain damage or death secondary to hypoglycemia
Desired outcome: Within 10-30 min of intervention, patient is alert and verbalizes orientation to time, place, and person.

C A U T I O N : Hypoglycemia requires immediate intervention because, if severe, it can lead to brain damage and death. When the cause of coma in a person with diabetes mellitus (DM) is unknown, immediately draw a blood sample for evaluation of glucose and prepare to administer IV D_{50}.

1. Administer a fast-acting carbohydrate: 2-3 tsp sugar; 4-6 oz fruit juice or nondiet soda; or 6-10 Life-Savers candies (or 2-4 commercially manufactured glucose tablets). Consult physician if patient is incoherent, unresponsive, or incapable of taking carbohydrates by mouth. If any of these indicators occur, an IV access is required; prepare to administer prescribed 50 ml D_{50} by IV push. Consciousness should be restored within 10 min.
2. Using an appropriate reagent strip, continue to monitor blood glucose levels q30-60min to identify recurrence of hypoglycemia.
3. Once patient is alert, question him or her about most recent food intake. Any situation preventing food intake (e.g., nausea, vomiting, dislike of hospital food related to cultural preferences, fasting for a scheduled test) should be determined and addressed immediately.
4. If food intake has been adequate, consult physician about reducing patient's daily dose of antihyperglycemic medication.

N O T E :   Sometimes hypoglycemia leads to rebound hyperglycemia (Somogyi phenomenon). If hypoglycemia goes undetected, the rebound hyperglycemia may be inappropriately treated with increased insulin. Suspect Somogyi phenomenon if wide fluctuations in blood glucose occur over several hours. Consult physician if these changes are observed or if patient is experiencing nocturnal hypoglycemia.

Altered protection related to neurosensory alterations with risk of seizures secondary to hypoglycemia
Desired outcome: Within 4 h of event, patient verbalizes orientation to time, place, and person and is free of signs of trauma caused by seizures or altered LOC. Alternatively, if patient experiences a seizure, it is detected, reported, and treated promptly.

1. Monitor LOC at frequent intervals. Anticipate seizure potential with severe hypoglycemia and have airway, protective padding, and suction equipment at bedside. Keep all side rails raised.
2. Notify physician of any seizure activity; do not leave patient unattended if a seizure occurs.
3. Place call light within patient's reach, and have patient demonstrate its proper use every shift. If patient is unable to use call light properly, assess at least q30min. If necessary, consider moving patient to a room next to the nurses' station for close monitoring.
4. Keep all potentially harmful objects (knives, forks, hot beverages) out of patient's reach.
5. If necessary to prevent patient from wandering and causing self-injury, obtain a prescription for soft restraints. Explain these safety precautions to patient and significant others.
6. For other information, see "Seizure Disorders," p. 179.

Knowledge deficit: Disease process, diagnostic testing, indicators of hypoglycemia, and therapeutic regimen
Desired outcome: Within the 24 h before hospital discharge, patient verbalizes knowledge about DM, including testing and management, indicators of hypoglycemia, and therapeutic regimen.

1. Assess patient's knowledge about DM, including diagnostic testing and management. Provide information or clarify as appropriate.
2. Review indicators and immediate interventions for hypoglycemia (review Table 5-3).
3. Evaluate current diet for adequate nutritional requirements, caloric content, and patient satisfaction. Assist patient in making acceptable and realistic changes. Consider patient's activity level and need for changes to achieve normoglycemia. Refer patient and significant others to dietitian as needed.
4. Review with patient the onset, peak action, and duration of hypoglycemic medication. Advise patient to avoid drugs that contribute to hypoglycemia (salicylates, sulfonamides, methyldopa, anabolic steroids, acetaminophen, ethanol, haloperidol, marijuana).
5. Stress the importance of testing blood glucose when symptoms of hypoglycemia occur.
6. Explain that injecting insulin into a site that is about to be exercised heavily (e.g., a jogger's thigh) results in quicker absorption of the insulin and possibly hypoglycemia.

7. Inform patient that a change in the type of medication may require a change in dosage to prevent hypoglycemia. Caution patient about the importance of following prescription directions precisely.
Also see "General Discussion," p. 217.

PATIENT-FAMILY TEACHING
AND DISCHARGE PLANNING

See **Knowledge deficit,** above. Also see interventions in "Diabetes Mellitus," p. 217, for general care guidelines.

Gastrointestinal Disorders

6

SECTION ONE: DISORDERS OF THE ESOPHAGUS

Hiatal Hernia and Reflux Esophagitis

NURSING DIAGNOSES AND INTERVENTIONS

Knowledge deficit: Disease process and treatment for hiatal hernia and reflux esophagitis
Desired outcome: Within the 24 h before hospital discharge, patient verbalizes knowledge about the cause of and therapeutic regimen for hiatal hernia and reflux esophagitis.

N O T E :   The cornerstone for many patients with reflux is a change in life-style.

---

1. Assess patient's knowledge about the disorder, its treatment, and the methods used to prevent symptoms and their complications. Provide instructions as appropriate.
2. Explain methods of dietary management: eating a low-fat, high-protein diet; eating small, frequent meals; eating slowly; chewing well to avoid reflux; avoiding extremely hot or cold foods; limiting stimulants of gastric acid (e.g., alcohol, caffeine, chocolate, spices, fruit juices, and nicotine); and losing weight, if appropriate.
3. Advise patient to drink water after eating to cleanse the esophagus of residual food, which can irritate the esophageal lining.
4. Explain alterations in body positions and activities: avoiding the supine position for 2-3 h after eating; sleeping on the right side with HOB elevated on 4- to 10-in blocks to promote gastric emptying; and avoiding bending, coughing, lifting heavy objects, straining with bowel movements, strenuous exercise, and clothing that is too tight around the waist.
5. Stress the importance of the pharmacologic regimen: antacids after meals; histamine H_2-receptor blockers regularly, even if symptoms resolve; and sucralfate 3-4 ×/day, 1 h after antacids are taken.

Pain, nausea, and feeling of fullness related to gastrocsophageal reflux and increased intraabdominal pressure

Desired outcomes: Within 1 h of intervention, patient's subjective perception of discomfort decreases, as documented by a pain scale. Objective indicators, such as grimacing, are absent or diminished.

1. Assess and document amount and character of discomfort. Devise a pain scale with patient, rating discomfort from 0 (no pain) to 10 (worst pain).
2. Administer medications as prescribed. Document their effectiveness, using pain scale.
3. Encourage patient to follow dietary and activity restrictions.
4. If prescribed, insert NG tube and connect it to suction to reduce pressure on the diaphragm and relieve vomiting.
5. Determine whether a position change would improve symptoms (e.g., raise HOB or have patient turn from side to side).
6. For additional information, see this nursing diagnosis in Appendix One, p. 396.

PATIENTS WITH A FUNDOPLICATION

Ineffective breathing pattern related to guarding secondary to pain of thoracic incision or chest tube insertion

Desired outcome: Within 1 h of intervention, patient's RR is 12-20 breaths/min with normal depth and pattern (eupnea).

1. If a thoracic rather than an abdominal approach was used, chest tubes may be present. Assess insertion site and suction apparatus for integrity, patency, function, and character of drainage. Tape all chest tube insertion sites. **Caution:** Be alert for indications of a pneumothorax: dyspnea, cyanosis, sharp chest pain. (See "Pneumothorax/Hemothorax," p. 10, for care of the patient with a chest tube.)
2. Encourage and assist patient with coughing, deep breathing, incentive spirometry, and turning q2-4h, and note quality of breath sounds, cough, and sputum.
3. Facilitate coughing and deep breathing by teaching patient how to splint incision with hands or pillow.
4. To enhance compliance with postoperative routine, medicate patient about ½ h before major moves, such as ambulation and turning. If patient-controlled analgesia (PCA) is available, advise its use accordingly. Be aware that narcotics may depress respirations.
5. Reassure patient that sutures will not break and tubes will not fall out with coughing and deep breathing.

Altered protection related to risk of obstruction, recurring reflux, esophageal tear, or perforation, which can occur secondary to surgery

Desired outcomes: Patient is free of GI complications, as evidenced by bowel sounds 24-72 h after surgery; bowel movements 48-72 h after surgery; soft, nondistended abdomen; absence of reflux and severe midsternal pain; ease of swallowing and burping; BP, RR, and HR within patient's baseline limits; and normothermia.

1. Assess abdomen for distention, tenderness, and bowel sounds; document all findings. Bowel sounds normally reappear within 24-72 h and bowel movements within 48-72 h after surgery.
2. Instruct patient to report reflux, a symptom that should *not* be present after fundoplication and that may signal that the surgical

wraparound is too loose. Also have patient alert you to difficulty with swallowing or burping, which could indicate a wraparound that is too tight and may lead to obstruction.

3. Patient will have an NG tube after surgery, which often remains in place until the esophagus has healed. Assess for patency immediately after surgery, qh for 6 h, and then q2-3h for 24 h. Generally the surgeon prescribes a specific irrigating solution; if one has not been prescribed, check for patency by instilling 10 ml of normal saline and aspirating the same amount. Do not leave the tube connected to low intermittent suction unless specifically prescribed because this may lead to ulceration. If suction is prescribed, check settings q8h: low is ≤20 cm suction. **Caution:** Do not attempt to replace or manipulate NG tube because esophageal perforation can occur. It may be necessary to restrain the hands of patients who attempt to remove or reposition the tube.

4. Take measures to reduce intraabdominal pressure, which may cause disruption of the suture line: control nausea and vomiting; prohibit use of straws, which can cause aerophagia; and introduce food and fluids gradually and in small amounts because the stomach's storage capacity will be reduced. When fluids are allowed, administer them in amounts <60 ml/h, and be alert to indicators of esophageal tear (see following).

5. An esophageal tear or perforation can be a complication of surgery. Be alert for and report these indicators: severe midsternal pain, a drop in BP, increases in TPR.

6. Teach patient the signs and symptoms of potential complications, and stress the importance of reporting them to staff promptly if they occur.

See "Providing Nutritional Support," p. 378, for information on administering tube feedings. See Appendix One for nursing diagnoses and interventions in "Caring for Preoperative and Postoperative Patients," p. 395.

PATIENT-FAMILY TEACHING AND DISCHARGE PLANNING

Give patient and significant others verbal and written information about the following:

1. Importance of dietary management and activity restrictions (see **Knowledge deficit,** p. 236).
2. Medications, including drug name, purpose, dosage, schedule, precautions, drug/drug and food/drug interactions, and potential side effects.
3. Indicators that hernia or reflux has recurred (which happens only rarely after surgery): dysphagia, hematemesis, increased pain.
4. Importance of follow-up care; confirm date and time of next medical appointment.
5. Care of incision, including dressing changes. Ensure that patient can verbalize indicators of infection (increasing pain, local warmth, fever, purulent drainage, swelling, foul odor).
6. Procedure for enteral feedings and care of tubes, if appropriate.

SECTION TWO: DISORDERS OF THE STOMACH AND INTESTINES

Peptic Ulcers

NURSING DIAGNOSES AND INTERVENTIONS

Pain related to gastric or duodenal lesions secondary to increased secretions

Desired outcomes: Within 24 h of admission, patient's subjective perception of pain abates, as documented by a pain scale; upon hospital discharge, pain is absent. Objective indicators, such as grimacing, are absent or diminished.

1. Assess for and document pain: severity, character, location, duration, precipitating factors, methods of relief. Devise a pain scale with patient, rating discomfort from 0 (no pain) to 10 (worst pain).
2. Administer histamine H$_2$-receptor blockers, sucralfate, and other medications as prescribed (Table 6-1). If antacids are administered *via* NG tube, use a 14-Fr tube or larger because antacids often plug smaller feeding tubes. Flush tube thoroughly after use. Rate degree of relief obtained, using pain scale.
3. Advise patient to avoid irritating foods and drugs, especially those associated with symptoms.
4. Instruct patient to eat three balanced meals a day and to avoid bedtime snacks.
5. Offer nonpharmacologic methods of pain control (e.g., distraction, back rub, massage, guided imagery). See Table A-6, p. 403.
6. Help patient prevent or control anxiety by teaching self-help measures and encouraging expression of feelings.
7. Encourage patient to use stress-reduction techniques. See **Health-seeking behaviors:** Relaxation technique effective for stress reduction, p. 27.

Altered protection related to potential for bleeding, obstruction, and perforation secondary to ulcerative process

Desired outcome: Patient is free of signs and symptoms of bleeding, obstruction, perforation, and peritonitis, as evidenced by negative results on tests for occult blood; passage of stool and flatus; soft, nondistended abdomen; good appetite; and normothermia.

1. Assess for indicators of bleeding (e.g., hematemesis, melena). Check all stools for occult blood. Consult physician about positive findings. Be alert for these values:
   Men: Hct: <40%; Hgb: <14 g/dl
   Women: Hct: <37%; Hgb: <12 g/dl.
2. If indicated, insert gastric tube to evacuate blood from stomach and to administer gastric lavage as prescribed. Do not use gastric tubes in patients who have or are suspected of having esophageal varices.

Gastrointestinal

Table 6-1 Peptic ulcer medications

	Anticholinergics (e.g., atropine, propantheline)	Antacids (e.g., Maalox, Mylanta, Riopan)	Sucralfate (Carafate)	H₂-blockers (e.g., cimetidine, ranitidine, famotidine, nizatidine)	Misoprostol (Cytotec)	Omeprazole (Prilosec)
Mechanism of action	Block secretion of acid	Neutralize acid	Coats mucosa	Block secretion of acid	Enhances mucosal protection; reduces acid secretion	Inhibits proton pump
Relative efficacy	+	++	++	++	++	+++
Drug interactions	Few	Many	Some	Many with cimetidine; some with others	Few	Some
Comments	Many side effects; not first-line therapy; not for gastric ulcers	Inconvenient; magnesium-containing type causes diarrhea; aluminum-containing type causes constipation. Usually given prn for pain	Give 30 min before meal or hs	Single daily dose often given hs. Cimetidine may cause impotence and other undesired effects with long-term use	Used for NSAID-induced ulcers; causes diarrhea. May cause abortion; do not give to pregnant patients	Very potent; may completely inhibit secretion of gastric acid; not for long-term use

3. Monitor and note indicators of obstruction: abdominal pain, distention, anorexia, nausea, vomiting, inability to pass stool or flatus. For more information, see "Obstructive Processes" in this chapter.

4. Be alert for indicators of perforation and peritonitis: sudden or severe abdominal pain, distention, and abdominal rigidity; fever; nausea; vomiting. Consult physician immediately about significant findings. See "Peritonitis" in this chapter for more information.

5. Teach patient the signs and symptoms of GI complications and the importance of reporting them promptly to a health care provider if they occur.

Impaired tissue integrity related to exposure to chemical irritants (gastric acid and pepsin)

Desired outcomes: Throughout hospital stay, patient complies with medical recommendations for treating peptic ulcer; within the 24 h before hospital discharge, patient verbalizes knowledge of necessary life-style changes. Gastric and duodenal mucosal tissues heal and remain intact, as evidenced by absence of or diminished pain and absence of bleeding.

1. Encourage patient to avoid foods that seem to cause pain or increase acid secretion; this response is highly individual.

2. Instruct patient to avoid foods and drugs associated with increased acidity and GI erosion: coffee, caffeine, alcohol, aspirin, ibuprofen and other NSAIDs.

3. If applicable, recommend strategies to help patient quit smoking.

4. Stress the importance of taking medications at prescribed intervals, not just for symptomatic pain relief.

5. If applicable, refer patient to community resources and support groups to help him or her quit smoking and drinking.

Pain, abdominal fullness, weakness, and diaphoresis after meals related to postgastrectomy dumping syndrome

Desired outcome: Within the 24 h before hospital discharge, patient verbalizes measures to prevent discomfort and has no discomfort after meals.

1. Advise patient to avoid meals high in carbohydrates, which precipitate an osmotic pull of fluids into the GI tract and contribute to symptoms.

2. Instruct patient to avoid fibrous foods and to chew all food thoroughly.

3. Advise patient to avoid drinking liquids with meals and to lie down after eating to discourage the rapid gastric emptying that occurs with dumping syndrome.

If patient has a gastric obstruction, see "Obstructive Processes" in this chapter. Also see Appendix One for nursing diagnoses and interventions in "Caring for Preoperative and Postoperative Patients," p. 395.

PATIENT-FAMILY TEACHING
AND DISCHARGE PLANNING

Give patient and significant others verbal and written information about the following:

1. Importance of following the prescribed diet to facilitate ulcer healing, prevent exacerbation or recurrence, or control postsurgical dumping syndrome. If appropriate, arrange a consultation with a dietitian.
2. Medications, including drug name, purpose, dosage, schedule, precautions, drug/drug and food/drug interactions, and potential side effects (see Table 6-1).
3. Signs and symptoms of exacerbation and recurrence, and potential complications.
4. Care of the incision line and dressing change technique, as necessary. Teach patient the signs of wound infection: persistent redness, swelling, purulent drainage, local warmth, fever, foul odor.
5. Role of life-style changes in preventing exacerbation or recurrence of ulcer, including quitting smoking and reducing stress (see **Health-seeking behaviors:** Relaxation technique effective for stress reduction, p. 27); reducing or eliminating consumption of alcohol; and avoiding irritating foods and drugs. If applicable, explain to patient that histamine H_2-receptor blockers are more effective in individuals who do not smoke.
6. Referral to a health care specialist for help with stress reduction, as necessary.
7. Referrals to community support groups, such as Alcoholics Anonymous.

Obstructive Processes

NURSING DIAGNOSES AND INTERVENTIONS

Pain, nausea, and distention related to obstructive process or malfunction of gastric or intestinal drainage tube
Desired outcomes: Within 8 h of admission, patient's perception of discomfort abates, as documented by a pain scale; by hospital discharge, discomfort has been eliminated. Objective indicators, such as grimacing, are absent or diminished.
1. Assess degree of discomfort. Devise a pain scale with patient, rating discomfort from 0 (no discomfort) to 10 (worst discomfort). Be alert for characteristics of pain, vomiting, and distention, depending on type of obstructive process (see Table 6-2).
2. Implement comfort measures to relieve pain: distraction, back rub, conversation, relaxation therapy. See **Health-seeking behaviors:** Relaxation technique effective for stress reduction, p. 27.
3. Administer prescribed analgesics and antiemetics as indicated. **Note:** Do not administer narcotic analgesics until surgical evaluation has been completed. Assess and document degree of relief obtained, using pain scale. Remember that opioid analgesics contribute to intestinal hypomotility.
4. Maintain patency and proper functioning of gastric or intestinal tube:
   - Maintain connection to low intermittent suction or as prescribed.
   - Irrigate tube with 30 ml of normal saline prn or as prescribed.

Table 6-2   Assessment of patients with obstructive processes

	Small Bowel Obstruction	Large Bowel Obstruction	Paralytic Ileus
Pain*	Severe, episodic	Moderate, more continuous	Not prominent
Vomiting	Occurs early; may be projectile	Occurs late; feculent (with incompetent duodenal valve)	Not prominent
Abdominal distention	Occurs late	Pronounced	Present
Passage of stool/flatus	None, except with partial obstruction of large bowel, with which "pencil" stools may be passed		

*With obstruction caused by intestinal strangulation, pain is always severe and is accompanied by vomiting and a distended, rigid, tender abdomen.

- Keep gastric tube properly positioned in stomach by securing it with tape or other adhesive.
- Avoid occlusion of vent side of sump suction tubes because this may result in vacuum occlusion of the tube and excessive suction to gastric mucosa.
- Advance intestinal tube slowly, 2-3 in at a time or as prescribed, until it reaches the desired location. Putting patient in various positions (right side-lying, supine, left side-lying) may facilitate passage of the tube. Do not tape the tube to patient's skin until it reaches the desired location.

5. Keep HOB elevated 30-45 degrees as permitted, to promote comfort and facilitate ventilation. A slightly Trendelenburg, right side-lying position may reduce gas pains in patients with paralytic ileus.
6. Encourage turning in bed and activity as permitted to promote peristalsis.
7. Provide oral care at frequent intervals. Frequent brushing of the teeth and rinsing of the mouth alleviates dryness. Provide lubricant for lips.
8. To alleviate discomfort caused by tube: provide mouth rinses at frequent intervals for pharyngeal discomfort; also, apply water-soluble lubricant to naris and, as prescribed, use a viscous topical anesthetic for naris and back of throat.

Risk for fluid volume deficit related to *excessive loss* secondary to obstructive process and subsequent vomiting or gastric decompression of large volumes of GI fluids; and *decreased intake* secondary to fluid restrictions

Desired outcome: Patient is normovolemic, as evidenced by good skin turgor, moist mucous membranes, urinary output ≥30 ml/h, stable weight, HR ≤100 bpm, absence of orthostatic systolic BP changes, and absence of thirst.

1. Ensure precise measurement and documentation of fluid I&O. Weigh patient daily.
2. Take special note of amount and character of GI aspirate. Check GI aspirate for electrolyte loss or pH as prescribed.
3. Administer appropriate IV fluids at prescribed rate. Replace volume of GI fluids aspirated by suction, if prescribed.
4. Measure abdominal girth q8h.
5. For other interventions, see this nursing diagnosis in Appendix One, p. 406.

For nursing diagnoses and interventions for delivery of enteral and parenteral nutrition, see "Providing Nutritional Support," p. 378. If surgery was performed, see Appendix One, "Caring for Preoperative and Postoperative Patients," p. 395.

PATIENT-FAMILY TEACHING AND DISCHARGE PLANNING

Give patient and significant others verbal and written information about the following:
1. Specific disease process that precipitated the obstruction and ways to prevent recurrence, such as compliance with prescribed therapies.
2. Symptoms of recurring obstruction to report to physician.
3. Medications, including drug name, purpose, dosage, schedule, precautions, drug/drug and food/drug interactions, and potential side effects.

Hernia

NURSING DIAGNOSES AND INTERVENTIONS

Pain (especially with straining) related to hernia condition or surgical intervention

Desired outcomes: Within 1 h of intervention, patient's subjective perception of discomfort decreases, as documented by a pain scale. Objective indicators, such as grimacing, are absent or diminished.
1. Assess and document pain: severity, character, location, duration, precipitating factors, and methods of relief. Devise a pain scale with patient, rating discomfort from 0 (no pain) to 10 (worst pain). Report severe, persistent pain, which can signal complications.
2. Advise patient to avoid straining, stretching, coughing, and heavy lifting. Teach patient to splint incision with the hands or a pillow during coughing episodes; this is especially important during the early postoperative period and for up to 6 wk after surgery.
3. Teach patient how to use a truss, if prescribed, and advise its use as much as possible, especially when out of bed. **Note:** Put on truss before patient gets out of bed.
4. Apply or teach patient application of scrotal support or ice packs, which often are prescribed to limit edema and control pain after inguinal hernia repair.
5. Administer prescribed analgesics as indicated, especially before postoperative activities. Use comfort measures as well: distraction,

verbal interaction to enhance expression of feelings and reduce anxiety, back rubs, and stress-reduction techniques, such as relaxation exercises. Document degree of relief obtained, using pain scale.

6. For additional information, see this nursing diagnosis in Appendix One, p. 396.

Urinary retention (or risk for same) related to pain, trauma, and use of anesthetic during lower abdominal surgery

Desired outcomes: Within 8-10 h of surgery, patient voids without difficulty. Urine output is ≥100 ml for each voiding and is adequate (approximately 1,000-1,500 ml) over a 24-h period.

1. Assess for and document suprapubic distention or patient's reports of being unable to void.

2. Monitor urinary output. Document and report frequent voidings of <100 ml at a time.

3. Facilitate voiding by implementing interventions in "Urinary Retention," p. 99.

Knowledge deficit: Potential for GI complications associated with presence of a hernia, and measures that can prevent their occurrence

Desired outcome: After instruction, patient verbalizes knowledge about signs and symptoms of GI complications and complies with prescribed measures for prevention.

1. Teach patient to be alert for and report severe, persistent pain; nausea and vomiting; fever; and abdominal distention, which can herald the onset of bowel incarceration or strangulation.

2. Encourage patient to comply with medical regimen: use of a truss or other support and avoiding straining, stretching, constipation, and heavy lifting.

3. Teach patient to consume a high-residue diet or to take dietary fiber supplements to prevent constipation. Encourage intake of at least 2-3 L/day of fluids to promote soft consistency of stools.

4. Teach patient proper body mechanics for moving and lifting.

Altered sexual function may occur in men after repair of an inguinal hernia because of vascular disruption. See nursing diagnoses **Body image disturbance, Altered sexuality patterns,** and **Sexual dysfunction,** as appropriate, in other sections of this book. Also see Appendix One for nursing diagnoses and interventions in "Caring for Preoperative and Postoperative Patients," p. 395.

PATIENT-FAMILY TEACHING
AND DISCHARGE PLANNING

Give patient and significant others verbal and written information about the following:

1. Care of incision and dressing change technique, if appropriate. Teach patient the signs of infection at incision site, which require medical intervention: fever, persistent redness, swelling, local warmth, tenderness, purulent drainage, foul odor.

2. Symptoms of hernia recurrence and postsurgical complications.

3. Postsurgical activity limitations as directed: usually heavy lifting (>10 lb) and straining are contraindicated for about 6 wk. Antici-

pate return to work in 2 wk for office workers and 6 wk for heavy laborers.
■ Importance of proper body mechanics to prevent recurrence, especially when lifting and moving.
■ Preventing constipation and straining at stools (e.g., by eating a high-residue diet [see Table 6-3] and using laxatives when needed.)
■ Medications, including drug name, purpose, dosage, schedule, drug/drug and food/drug interactions, and potential side effects.

Peritonitis

NURSING DIAGNOSES AND INTERVENTIONS

Pain, abdominal distention, and nausea related to inflammatory process, fever, and tissue damage
Desired outcomes: Within 1 h of intervention, patient's subjective perception of pain decreases, as documented by a pain scale. Objective indicators, such as grimacing and abdominal guarding, are absent or diminished.
1. Assess and document character and severity of discomfort q1-2h. Devise a pain scale with patient, rating discomfort from 0 (no pain) to 10 (worst pain).

Table 6-3   Guidelines for low-residue, high-residue, and gluten-free diets

Low-Residue Diet	High-Residue Diet
Encourage intake of enriched/refined breads and cereals; rice and pasta dishes	Encourage intake of fruits, vegetables, large amounts of fluid, whole grain breads and cereals
Avoid fruits, vegetables, whole wheat products (cereals and breads)	Avoid highly refined cereals and pasta (e.g., white rice, white bread, spaghetti noodles, and ice cream)

Gluten-Free Diet	
Avoid cereals and bakery goods made from wheat, malt, barley, rye, and oats. Also avoid the following if they contain any of the above grain products: coffee substitutes, sauces, commercially prepared luncheon meats, gravies, noodles, macaroni, spaghetti, flour tortillas, crackers, cakes, cookies, pastries, puddings, commercial ice cream, and alcoholic beverages	Use the following (if allowed): rice, corn, eggs, potatoes; breads made from rice flours, cornmeal, soybean flour, gluten-free wheat starch, and potato starch; cereals made from corn or rice (grits, corn meal mush, cooked Cream of Rice, puffed rice, rice flakes); pasta made from rice or corn flour; homemade ice cream; tapioca pudding

2. After diagnosis has been made, administer narcotics, analgesics, and sedatives as prescribed to promote comfort and rest. Document relief obtained, using pain scale.
3. Keep patient on bed rest to minimize pain, which can be aggravated by activity; provide a restful, quiet environment.
4. Keep patient in a position of comfort, usually semi-Fowler's position.
5. Explain all procedures to patient to help minimize anxiety, which can exacerbate discomfort.
6. Offer mouth care and lip moisturizers at frequent intervals to help relieve discomfort and nausea from continuous or intermittent suction, dehydration, and NPO status.

Ineffective breathing pattern related to decreased depth of respirations secondary to guarding with abdominal pain or distention

Desired outcomes: Patient has an effective breathing pattern, as evidenced by absence of adventitious breath sounds, Pao_2 $\geq$80 mm Hg, oxygen saturation $\geq$95%, BP $\geq$90/60 mm Hg (or within patient's baseline range), HR $\leq$100 bpm, and orientation to time, place, and person. Eupnea occurs within 1 h of pain-relieving intervention.

1. Monitor ABG results and be alert for indicators of hypoxemia (low O_2 saturation and Pao_2) and for the following clinical signs: hypotension, tachycardia, hyperventilation, restlessness, CNS depression, and possibly cyanosis.
2. Auscultate lung fields to assess ventilation and detect pulmonary complications. Note and document adventitious breath sounds.
3. Keep patient in semi-Fowler's or high Fowler's position to aid respiratory effort; encourage deep breathing to promote oxygenation.
4. Administer oxygen as prescribed.

Altered protection related to potential for worsening/recurring peritonitis or development of septic shock secondary to inflammatory process

Desired outcome: Patient is free of symptoms of worsening/recurring peritonitis or septic shock, as evidenced by normothermia, BP $\geq$90/60 mm Hg (or within patient's normal range), HR $\leq$100 bpm, eupnea, urinary output $\geq$30 ml/h, CVP 2-6 mm Hg (5-12 cm H_2O), decreasing abdominal girth, and minimal tenderness to palpation.

1. Assess abdomen q1-2h during acute phase and q4h once patient's condition has stabilized. Monitor for increasing distention by measuring abdominal girth, and auscultate bowel sounds to assess motility. Bowel sounds often are frequent during the beginning phase of peritonitis but are absent with paralytic ileus. *Lightly* palpate abdomen for evidence of increasing rigidity or tenderness, which indicates progression of the disease. If patient experiences more pain upon removal of your hand, rebound tenderness is present. Consult physician about significant findings.
2. If prescribed, insert gastric tube and connect it to suction to prevent or reduce distention.
3. Monitor VS at least q2h, more often if patient's condition is unstable. Be alert for signs of septic shock: increased temperature;

hypotension; tachycardia; shallow, rapid respirations; urine output <30 ml/h; CVP <2 mm Hg (or <5 cm H_2O). In the early (warm) stage of shock, the skin usually is warm, pink, and dry secondary to peripheral venous pooling, and BP and CVP begin to drop. In the late (cold) stage of shock, the extremities become pale and cool because of decreasing tissue perfusion.

4. Administer antibiotics as prescribed.
5. Monitor CBC for leukocytosis, which signals infection, and hemoconcentration (increased Hct and Hgb), which occurs with a decline in plasma volume. Normal values are:
   Men: WBCs: 4,500-11,000/μl; Hgb: 14-18 g/dl; Hct: 40%-54%.
   Women: WBCs: 4,500-11,000/μl; Hgb: 12-16 g/dl; Hct: 37%-47%.
   With peritonitis, the WBC count usually is >20,000/μl.
   Consult physician about significant findings.
6. Maintain sterile technique with dressing changes and all invasive procedures.
7. Teach patient the signs and symptoms of recurring peritonitis and the importance of reporting them promptly if they occur: fever, chills, vomiting, abdominal pain and distention.

Altered nutrition: Less than body requirements, related to vomiting and intestinal suctioning
Desired outcome: By a minimum of 24 h before hospital discharge, patient has adequate nutrition, as evidenced by stable weight, balanced or positive nitrogen state, and serum albumin 3.5-5.5 g/dl.
1. Keep patient NPO as prescribed during acute phase of disorder. If patient has an ileus, an NG tube will be inserted to decompress the abdomen. Reintroduce oral fluids gradually once motility has returned, as evidenced by bowel sounds, decreased distention, and passage of flatus.
2. As prescribed, support patient with peripheral parenteral nutrition (PPN) or TPN, depending on duration of acute phase (usually by day 3).
3. Administer replacement fluids, electrolytes, and vitamins as prescribed.

See "Providing Nutritional Support," p. 378, for interventions for patients receiving enteral or parenteral feeding.

See Appendix One for nursing diagnoses and interventions in "Caring for Preoperative and Postoperative Patients," p. 395. Also in Appendix One, see "Caring for Patients on Prolonged Bed Rest" for **Risk for activity intolerance,** p. 413, and **Risk for disuse syndrome,** p. 416.

PATIENT-FAMILY TEACHING
AND DISCHARGE PLANNING

Give patient and significant others verbal and written information about the following:
1. Medications, including drug name, purpose, dosage, schedule, precautions, drug/drug and food/drug interactions, and potential side effects.

2. Activity alterations as prescribed by physician, such as avoiding heavy lifting (>10 lb), resting after periods of fatigue, getting maximum amounts of rest, and gradually increasing activities to tolerance.

3. Notifying physician of indicators of recurrence: fever, chills, abdominal pain, vomiting, abdominal distention.

4. If patient has undergone surgery, indicators of wound infection: fever, pain, chills, incisional swelling, persistent erythema, purulent drainage.

5. Importance of follow-up medical care; confirm date and time of next medical appointment.

Appendicitis

NURSING DIAGNOSES AND INTERVENTIONS

Risk for infection related to inadequate primary defenses (risk of rupture, peritonitis, and abscess formation) secondary to inflammatory process

Desired outcomes: Patient is free of infection, as evidenced by normothermia; HR ≤100 bpm; BP ≥90/60 mm Hg; RR 12-20 breaths/min with normal depth and pattern (eupnea); soft, nondistended abdomen; and bowel sounds 5-34/min in each abdominal quadrant. After instruction, patient verbalizes the rationale for not administering enemas or laxatives preoperatively and enemas postoperatively and complies with therapeutic regimen.

1. Assess and document quality, location, and duration of pain. Be alert for pain that becomes accentuated and generalized or for recurrent vomiting, and note whether patient assumes side-lying or supine position with flexed knees. Any of these signs can signal worsening appendicitis, which can lead to rupture. Be alert for pain that worsens and then disappears—a signal that rupture may have occurred.

2. Monitor VS for elevated temperature, increased pulse rate, hypotension, and shallow/rapid respirations; assess abdomen for rigidity, distention, and decreased or absent bowel sounds, any of which can occur with rupture. Consult physician about significant findings.

3. Caution patient about the danger of preoperative self-treatment with enemas and laxatives because they increase peristalsis, which increases the risk of perforation. If constipation occurs postoperatively, physician may prescribe laxatives/stool softeners hs after the third day. Remind patient that enemas should be avoided until approved by physician (usually several weeks after surgery).

4. Teach patient about postoperative incisional care, as well as care of drains if patient is to be discharged with them.

5. Provide instructions about prescribed antibiotics if patient is to be discharged with them.

6. See "Peritonitis" in this chapter for more information.

Pain and nausea related to inflammatory process

Desired outcomes: Within 1-2 h of pain-relieving intervention, patient's subjective perception of pain decreases, as documented by a pain scale. Objective indicators, such as grimacing, are absent or diminished.

1. Assess and document quality, location, and duration of pain. Devise a pain scale with patient, rating discomfort from 0 (no pain) to 10 (worst pain). Be aware of the characteristics of discomfort during the following stages of appendicitis:
   - *Early stage:*   Abdominal pain (either epigastric or umbilical) that may be vague and diffuse; nausea and vomiting; fever; sensitivity over appendix area.
   - *Intermediate (acute) stage:*   Pain that shifts from the epigastrium to the RLQ at McBurney's point (approximately 2 in from the anterior superior iliac spine on a line drawn from the umbilicus) and that is aggravated by walking or coughing. Pain may be accompanied by a sensation of constipation ("gas stoppage" sensation). Anorexia, malaise, occasional diarrhea, and diminished peristalsis also can occur.
   - *Acute appendicitis with perforation:*   Increasing, generalized pain; recurrence of vomiting; increasing abdominal rigidity.
2. Medicate patient with antiemetics, sedatives, and analgesics as prescribed; evaluate and document patient's response, using pain scale.
3. Keep patient NPO before surgery; after surgery, nausea and vomiting usually disappear. If prescribed, insert gastric tube for decompression.
4. Teach technique for slow, diaphragmatic breathing to reduce stress and help relax tense muscles.
5. Help position patient for optimal comfort. Many patients find comfort in a side-lying position with the knees bent, whereas others find relief when supine with pillows under the knees. Avoid pressure on the popliteal area.

See Appendix One for nursing diagnoses and interventions in "Caring for Preoperative and Postoperative Patients," p. 395.

PATIENT-FAMILY TEACHING AND DISCHARGE PLANNING

Give patient and significant others verbal and written information about the following:

1. Medications, including drug name, purpose, dosage, schedule, precautions, drug/drug and food/drug interactions, and potential side effects.
2. Care of incision, including dressing changes and bathing restrictions, if appropriate.
3. Indicators of infection: fever, chills, incisional pain, redness, swelling, and purulent drainage.
4. Postsurgical activity precautions: avoiding lifting heavy objects (>10 lb) for the first 6 wk or as directed, being alert for and resting after symptoms of fatigue, getting maximum rest, gradually increasing activities to tolerance.

5. Importance of avoiding enemas for the first few postoperative weeks. Caution patient about the need to check with physician before having an enema.

SECTION THREE: INTESTINAL NEOPLASMS AND INFLAMMATORY PROCESSES

Diverticulosis/Diverticulitis

NURSING DIAGNOSES AND INTERVENTIONS

For diverticulitis treated with an emergency diverting temporary colostomy: see "Fecal Diversions" for **Risk for impaired peristomal skin integrity** *and* **Impaired stomal tissue integrity (or risk for same)**, p. 260; **Bowel incontinence**, p. 262; and **Body image disturbance**, p. 263. See Appendix One for nursing diagnoses and interventions in "Caring for Preoperative and Postoperative Patients," p. 395, and "Caring for Patients with Cancer and Other Life-Disrupting Illnesses," p. 450.

PATIENT-FAMILY TEACHING AND DISCHARGE PLANNING

Give patient and significant others verbal and written information about the following:

1. Medications, including drug name, purpose, dosage, schedule, precautions, drug/drug and food/drug interactions, and potential side effects.
2. Signs and symptoms that require medical attention: fever; nausea or vomiting; cloudy or malodorous urine; diarrhea or constipation; change in stoma color from the normal bright, shiny red; peristomal skin irritation; and incisional pain, drainage, swelling, or redness.
3. Importance of a normal diet that includes all four food groups (meat, eggs, and fish; fruits and vegetables; milk and cheese; cereal and breads) and drinking adequate fluids (at least 2-3 L/day). Also teach patient to add fiber to his or her diet in the form of fruits and vegetables, and whole grain cereals with the addition of bran in the form of 100% bran cereal or 2 Tbsp/day of coarse, unprocessed bran that can be taken with milk or juice or sprinkled over cereal. Because bran initially may cause abdominal distention and excessive flatus, instruct patient to begin with 1 Tbsp/day and increase gradually. Caution patient to avoid nuts, berries, and foods with seeds.
4. Gradual resumption of ADLs, excluding heavy lifting (>10 lb), pushing, or pulling for 6 wk to prevent development of incisional herniation.
5. Care of incision, dressing changes, and permission to take baths or showers once sutures and drains are removed.

6. Care of stoma and peristomal skin; use of ostomy skin barriers, pouches, and accessory equipment; and method for obtaining supplies.
7. Referral to community resources: enterostomal therapy (ET) nurse, home health care agency, and the United Ostomy Association.
8. Importance of follow-up care with physician or ET nurse; confirm date and time of next appointment.

Colorectal Cancer

NURSING DIAGNOSES AND INTERVENTIONS

Health-seeking behaviors: Recommendations for follow-up diagnostic care after a colon resection or polypectomy for malignant polyps
Desired outcome: Before hospital discharge, patient verbalizes accurate information about recommendations for follow-up diagnostic care.

Patients Who Have Had Colorectal Cancer Resections

1. Teach patient that colonoscopy is recommended 6-12 mo after surgery, followed by yearly colonoscopy for 2 consecutive years; if the aforementioned are negative, colonoscopy or ACBaE plus proctosigmoidoscopy is performed q3yr.
2. Explain that fecal occult blood testing is performed every year.
3. Remind patient that serum carcinoembryonic antigen (CEA) levels are measured at regular intervals (3 × at 6-mo intervals, then 5 × at yearly intervals).

Postpolypectomy Patients with Malignant Polyps

1. Teach patient that a colonoscopy is performed within 6 mo of polypectomy; if this second examination is negative, colonoscopy is performed q2yr. However, if the second examination is positive, colonoscopy is performed at yearly intervals until negative, and then done at 2-yr intervals.
2. Explain that fecal occult blood testing is performed between colonoscopies.

See "Fecal Diversions" for **Risk for impaired peristomal skin integrity** *and* **Impaired stomal tissue integrity (or risk for same),** p. 260; **Bowel incontinence,** p. 262; **Body image disturbance,** p. 263; and **Knowledge deficit:** Colostomy irrigation procedure, p. 264.

See Appendix One for nursing diagnoses and interventions in "Caring for Preoperative and Postoperative Patients," p. 395, and "Caring for Patients with Cancer and Other Life-Disrupting Illnesses," p. 423.

PATIENT-FAMILY TEACHING
AND DISCHARGE PLANNING

Give patient and significant others verbal and written information about the following:

1. Medications, including drug name, purpose, dosage, schedule, precautions, drug/drug and food/drug interactions, and potential side effects.
2. Signs and symptoms that require medical attention: fever, nausea, vomiting, diarrhea, constipation.
3. If patient has an intestinal stoma, the importance of reporting a change in stoma color from the normal bright, shiny red; peristomal skin irritation; and incisional pain, drainage, swelling, or redness.
4. Importance of a normal diet that includes all four food groups (meat, eggs, and fish; fruits and vegetables; milk and cheese; cereal and breads) and drinking adequate fluids (at least 2-3 L/day).
5. Enteral or parenteral feeding instructions if patient is on supplement diet or is NPO.
6. Gradual resumption of ADLs, excluding heavy lifting (>10 lb), pushing, or pulling for 6 wk to prevent incisional herniation.
7. Care of incision and perianal wounds, including dressing changes, and bathing once sutures and drains are removed. Sitz baths may be recommended for perianal wound.
8. If patient has a stoma, care of stoma and peristomal skin; use of ostomy skin barriers, pouches, and accessory equipment; and method for obtaining supplies.
9. Referral to community resources, including home health care agency, American Cancer Society, and if appropriate, ET nurse and the United Ostomy Association.
10. Importance of follow-up care with physician (or ET nurse if appropriate); confirm date and time of next appointment.
11. Recommendations for follow-up diagnostic care after colon resection or polypectomy: see **Health-seeking behaviors,** p. 252.

Ulcerative Colitis

NURSING DIAGNOSES AND INTERVENTIONS

Fluid volume deficit related to active loss secondary to diarrhea and GI bleeding or hemorrhage

Desired outcome: Within 24 h of admission, patient is normovolemic, as evidenced by balanced I&O, urine output ≥30 ml/h, good skin turgor, moist mucous membranes, stable weight, BP ≥90/60 mm Hg (or within patient's normal range), and RR 12-20 breaths/min.

1. Monitor I&O, and weigh patient daily. Monitor laboratory values to evaluate fluid, electrolyte, and hematologic status.
   Optimal values: serum potassium (K^+): ≥3.5-5 mEq/L (men and women); also
   Men: Hct: 40%-54%; Hgb: 14-18 g/dl; RBCs: 4.5-6 million/μl
   Women: Hct: 37%-47%; Hgb: 12-16 g/dl; RBCs: 4-5.5 million/μl.
2. Monitor frequency and consistency of stool. Assess for blood, mucus, fat, and undigested food, and document findings.
3. Monitor for indicators of dehydration: thirst, poor skin turgor (may not be a reliable indicator in an older adult), dryness of mucous membranes, fever, concentrated and reduced urinary output.

4. Monitor for signs for hemorrhage: hypotension, increased HR and RR, pallor, diaphoresis, restlessness. Assess stool for quality (e.g., liquid, grossly bloody) and quantity (e.g., mostly blood or mostly stool). Consult physician about significant findings.
5. If patient is acutely ill, maintain parenteral replacement of fluids, electrolytes, and vitamins as prescribed.
6. Administer blood products and iron as prescribed to correct existing anemia and loss caused by hemorrhage.
7. When patient is taking food by mouth, provide bland, high-protein, high-calorie, low-residue diet, as prescribed. Assess tolerance to diet by determining incidence of cramping, diarrhea, and flatulence.

Altered protection related to risk of perforation secondary to deeply inflamed colonic mucosa
Desired outcome: Patient is free of signs of perforation, as evidenced by normothermia; HR 60-100 bpm; RR 12-20 breaths/min with normal depth and pattern (eupnea); normal bowel sounds; absence of abdominal distention, tympany, or rebound tenderness; negative culture results; and orientation to time, place, and person.

N O T E : Patients with severe ulcerative colitis can have markedly elevated WBC counts, $>20,000/\mu l$, occasionally as high as $50,000/\mu l$.

1. Monitor patient for fever, chills, increased HR and RR, diaphoresis, and increased abdominal discomfort, which can occur with perforation of the colon and may result in localized abscess or generalized fecal peritonitis and septicemia. **Note:** Systemic therapy with corticosteroids and antibiotics can mask the development of this complication.
2. Report any evidence of sudden abdominal distention associated with the preceding symptoms because this can signal toxic megacolon. Factors that contribute to the development of this complication are hypokalemia, barium enema examinations, and use of opiates and anticholinergics.
3. If patient's temperature rises suddenly, culture blood and other sites as prescribed. Monitor culture reports, and consult physician promptly about any positive results.
4. Administer antibiotics as prescribed and in a timely fashion.
5. Evaluate patient's orientation and LOC q2-4h.

Pain, abdominal cramping, and nausea related to intestinal inflammatory process
Desired outcomes: Within 4 h of intervention, patient's subjective perception of discomfort decreases, as documented by a pain scale. Objective indicators, such as grimacing, are absent or diminished.

1. Monitor and document characteristics of discomfort, and assess whether it is associated with certain foods or medications or with emotional stress. Devise a pain scale with patient, rating discomfort from 0 (no pain) to 10 (worst pain). Eliminate foods that cause cramping and discomfort.
2. As prescribed, keep patient NPO or on TPN to provide bowel rest.

3. Provide nasal and oral care at frequent intervals to lessen discomfort from NPO status or presence of gastric tube.
4. Keep patient's environment quiet, and plan nursing care to provide maximum periods of rest.
5. Administer sedatives and tranquilizers as prescribed to promote rest and reduce anxiety.
6. Administer hydrophilic colloids, anticholinergics, and antidiarrheal drugs as prescribed to relieve cramping and diarrhea.
7. Document degree of relief obtained, using pain scale.
8. Observe for intensification of symptoms, which can indicate complications. Consult physician about significant findings.

Diarrhea related to inflammatory process of the intestines

Desired outcome: Within 3 days of admission, patient's stools become normal in consistency, and frequency is lessened.

1. Monitor and record amount, frequency, and character of stools.
2. Provide covered bedpan, commode, or bathroom that is easily accessible and ready to use at all times.
3. Empty bedpan and commode to control odor and reduce patient's anxiety and self-consciousness.
4. Administer hydrophilic colloids, anticholinergics, and antidiarrheal drugs as prescribed to reduce fluidity and number of stools.
5. Administer topical corticosteroid preparations and antibiotics *via* retention enema, as prescribed, to relieve local inflammation. If patient has difficulty retaining enema for prescribed amount of time, consult physician about use of corticosteroid foam, which is easier to administer and retain.
6. Monitor serum electrolytes, particularly K^+, for abnormalities. Consult physician about K^+ level <3.5 mEq/L.

Risk for impaired perineal/perianal skin integrity related to persistent diarrhea

Desired outcome: Patient's perineal and perianal skin remains intact, with no erythema.

1. Provide materials for or help patient with cleaning and drying of perineal area after each bowel movement.
2. Apply protective skin care products (e.g., skin preparations, gels, or barrier films) *only* to normal, unbroken skin. Petrolatum emollients, moisture barrier ointments, and vanishing creams also can be used to prevent irritation from frequent liquid stools.
3. Administer hydrophilic colloids, anticholinergics, and antidiarrheal drugs as prescribed to reduce fluidity and number of stools.

See "Fecal Diversions" for **Risk for impaired peristomal skin integrity** *and* **Impaired stomal tissue integrity (or risk for same),** p. 260; **Bowel incontinence,** p. 262, and **Body image disturbance,** p. 263.

If surgery is performed, see Appendix One for nursing diagnoses and interventions in "Caring for Preoperative and Postoperative Patients," p. 395, and "Caring for Patients with Cancer and Other Life-Disrupting Illnesses," p. 450.

PATIENT-FAMILY TEACHING
AND DISCHARGE PLANNING

Give patient and significant others verbal and written information about the following:

1. Medications, including drug name, purpose, dosage, schedule, precautions, drug/drug and food/drug interactions, and potential side effects. **Note:** If patient is undergoing high-dose steroid therapy, caution him or her against abruptly discontinuing the medication, since this can precipitate adrenal crisis. Withdrawal symptoms include weakness, lethargy, restlessness, anorexia, nausea, and muscle tenderness. Instruct patient to notify physician if these symptoms occur.

2. Signs and symptoms that require medical attention: fever, nausea, vomiting, diarrhea or constipation, and any significant change in appearance and frequency of stools, any of which can signal exacerbation of the disease.

3. Dietary management to promote nutritional and fluid maintenance and prevent abdominal cramping, discomfort, and diarrhea.

4. Importance of perineal care after bowel movements.

5. Enteral or parenteral feeding instructions if patient is to supplement diet or is NPO.

6. Referral to community resources, including Crohn's and Colitis Foundation of America.

7. Importance of follow-up medical care, particularly in patients with long-standing disease, since so many of them develop colonic adenocarcinoma.

8. Referral to a mental health specialist if recommended by health care provider.

IN ADDITION (WITH FECAL DIVERSION)

9. Care of incision and dressing changes, and permission to take baths or showers once sutures and drains have been removed.

10. Care of stoma, peristomal/perianal skin, or perineal wound; use of ostomy equipment; and method for obtaining supplies. Sitz baths may be indicated for perineal wound.

11. Medications that are contraindicated (e.g., laxatives) or that may not be well tolerated or absorbed (e.g., antibiotics, enteric-coated tablets, long-acting tablets).

12. Gradual resumption of ADLs, excluding heavy lifting (>10 lb), pushing, or pulling for 6-8 wk to prevent incisional herniation.

13. Referral to community resources, including home health care agency, ET nurse, and local chapter of United Ostomy Association.

14. Importance of reporting signs and symptoms that require medical attention: change in stoma color from the normal bright, shiny red; peristomal or perianal skin irritation; diarrhea, incisional pain, drainage, swelling, or redness; indicators of fluid and electrolyte imbalance; and indicators of mechanical or functional obstruction.

Crohn's Disease

NURSING DIAGNOSES AND INTERVENTIONS

Fluid volume deficit related to active loss secondary to diarrhea or GI fistula

Desired outcomes: Within 24 h of admission, patient is normovolemic, as evidenced by balanced I&O, urinary output $\geq$30 ml/h, BP $\geq$90/60 mm Hg (or within patient's normal range), RR 12-20 breaths/min, stable weight, good skin turgor, and moist mucous membranes. Patient reports that diarrhea is controlled.

1. Monitor I&O, weigh patient daily, and monitor laboratory values to evaluate fluid and electrolyte status. *Optimal values:* potassium (K^+): 3.5-5 mEq/L, sodium (Na^+): 137-147 mEq/L, and chloride (Cl^-): 95-108 mEq/L.
2. Monitor frequency and consistency of stools. Assess for and record blood, mucus, fat, or undigested food in stool.
3. Monitor for indicators of dehydration: thirst; poor skin turgor; dryness of mucous membranes; fever; concentrated, decreased urinary output.
4. Maintain patient on parenteral replacement of fluids, electrolytes, and vitamins as prescribed to promote anabolism and healing.
5. When patient is taking food by mouth, provide bland, high-protein, high-calorie, low-residue diet, as prescribed. Assess tolerance to diet by determining incidence of cramping, diarrhea, and flatulence. Modify diet plan accordingly.

Risk for infection/altered protection related to potential for complications caused by intestinal inflammatory disorder

Desired outcome: Patient is free of indicators of infection and intraabdominal injury, as evidenced by normothermia; HR 60-100 bpm; RR 12-20 breaths/min; normal bowel sounds; absence of abdominal distention, rigidity, or localized pain and tenderness; absence of nausea and vomiting; negative culture results; and orientation to time, place, and person.

1. Monitor patient for indicators of intestinal obstruction, including abdominal rigidity and increased episodes of nausea and vomiting. **Note:** Factors that contribute to the development of this complication are use of opiates and prolonged use of antidiarrheal drugs.
2. Monitor patient for fever, increased RR and HR, chills, diaphoresis, and increased abdominal discomfort, which can occur with intestinal perforation, abscess or fistula formation, or generalized fecal peritonitis and septicemia. **Note:** Systemic therapy with corticosteroids and antibiotics can mask development of these complications.
3. Evaluate patient's orientation and LOC q2-4h.
4. If patient's temperature rises suddenly, obtain cultures of blood, urine, fistulas, or other possible sources of infection, as prescribed. Abscesses or fistulas to the abdominal wall, bladder, or vagina are common in Crohn's disease, as well as abscesses or fistulas to other

loops of small bowel and colon. Monitor culture reports and consult physician promptly about any positive results.

5. If draining fistulas or abscesses are present, change dressings or irrigate tubes or drains as prescribed. Note color, character, and odor of all drainage. Report foul-smelling or abnormal drainage or loss of tube or drain patency.

6. Administer antibiotics as prescribed and in a timely manner.

7. Prevent transmission of potentially infectious organisms by good handwashing before and after caring for patient and by disposing of dressings and drainage using proper infection control technique.

Pain, abdominal cramping, and nausea related to intestinal inflammatory process

Desired outcomes: Within 4 h of intervention, patient's subjective perception of discomfort decreases, as documented by a pain scale. Objective indicators, such as grimacing, are absent or diminished.

1. Monitor and document characteristics of discomfort, and assess whether it is associated with certain foods or emotional stress. Devise a pain scale with patient, rating discomfort from 0 (no discomfort) to 10 (worst discomfort). Eliminate foods that cause cramping and discomfort.

2. As prescribed, keep patient NPO and provide parenteral nutrition to allow bowel to rest.

3. Administer antidiarrheal drugs and analgesics as prescribed to reduce abdominal discomfort.

4. Provide nasal and oral care at frequent intervals to lessen discomfort from NPO status and presence of gastric tube.

5. Administer antiemetics before meals to enhance appetite when nausea is a problem.

6. Document relief obtained, using pain scale.

7. For additional information, see this nursing diagnosis in Appendix One, p. 396.

Diarrhea related to intestinal inflammatory process

Desired outcome: Within 3 days of admission, patient reports a reduction in frequency of stools and a return to more normal stool consistency.

1. If patient is experiencing frequent and urgent passage of loose stools, provide covered bedpan or commode, or be sure bathroom is easily accessible and ready to use at all times.

2. Empty bedpan and commode promptly to control odor and reduce patient's anxiety and self-consciousness.

3. Administer antidiarrheal drugs as prescribed to reduce fluidity and number of stools.

4. If bile salt deficiency (caused by ileal disease or resection) is a contributing factor, administer cholestyramine as prescribed to control diarrhea.

5. Eliminate or reduce fat content in diet, because it can increase diarrhea in individuals with malabsorption syndromes. Also, restrict foods and beverages that can precipitate diarrhea and cramping (e.g., raw vegetables and fruits, whole grain cereals, condiments,

gas-forming foods, alcohol, iced and carbonated beverages and, in lactose-intolerant patients, milk and milk products).

Activity intolerance related to generalized weakness secondary to intestinal inflammatory process

Desired outcome: Patient adheres to prescribed rest regimen and sets appropriate goals for self-care as condition improves (optimally within 3-7 days of admission).

1. Keep patient's environment quiet to facilitate rest.
2. Because adequate rest is necessary to sustain remission, assist patient with ADLs, and plan nursing care to provide maximum rest periods.
3. As prescribed, administer sedatives and tranquilizers to promote rest and reduce anxiety.
4. As patient's physical condition improves, encourage self-care to greatest extent possible, and assist patient with setting realistic, attainable goals.
5. For additional information, see Appendix One for **Risk for activity intolerance,** p. 413.

If surgery is performed, see "Fecal Diversions" for **Risk for impaired peristomal skin integrity** *and* **Impaired stomal tissue integrity (or risk for same),** p. 260; **Bowel incontinence,** p. 262, and **Body image disturbance,** p. 263.

See Appendix One for nursing diagnoses and interventions in "Caring for Preoperative and Postoperative Patients," p. 395, and "Caring for Patients with Cancer and Other Life-Disrupting Illnesses," p. 450.

PATIENT-FAMILY TEACHING
AND DISCHARGE PLANNING

Give patient and significant others verbal and written information about the following:

1. Medications, including drug name, purpose, dosage, schedule, precautions, drug/drug and food/drug interactions, and potential side effects.
2. Signs and symptoms that require medical attention: fever, nausea, vomiting, abdominal discomfort, any significant change in appearance and frequency of stools, passage of stool through vagina, or stool mixed with urine, any of which can signal recurrence or complications of Crohn's disease.
3. Importance of dietary management to promote nutritional and fluid maintenance and prevent abdominal cramping, discomfort, and diarrhea.
4. Importance of perineal/perianal skin care after bowel movements.
5. Importance of balancing activities with rest periods, even during remission, because adequate rest is necessary to sustain remission.
6. Referral to community resources, including the Crohn's and Colitis Foundation of America.
7. Importance of follow-up medical care, including supportive psychotherapy, because of the chronic, progressive nature of Crohn's disease.

In Addition (with Fecal Diversion)

8. Care of incision, dressing changes, and bathing.
9. Care of stoma and peristomal skin, use of ostomy equipment, and method for obtaining supplies.
10. Gradual resumption of ADLs, excluding heavy lifting (>10 lb), pushing, or pulling for 6-8 wk to prevent incisional herniation.
11. Referral to community resources, including home health care agency, ET nurse, and local chapter of United Ostomy Association.
12. Importance of reporting signs and symptoms that require medical attention: change in stoma color from normal bright, shiny red; lesions of stomal mucosa that may indicate recurrence of disease; peristomal skin irritation; diarrhea or constipation; fever; chills; abdominal pain or distention; nausea; vomiting; incisional pain, drainage, swelling, or redness.

Fecal Diversions

NURSING DIAGNOSES AND INTERVENTIONS

Risk for impaired peristomal skin integrity related to exposure to effluent or sensitivity to appliance material; *and*
Impaired stomal tissue integrity (or risk for same) related to improperly fitted appliance, resulting in impaired circulation
Desired outcome: Patient's stomal and peristomal skin and tissue remain intact.

After Colostomy or Conventional Ileostomy (Permanent or Temporary)

1. Apply a pectin, methylcellulose-based, solid-form skin barrier around stoma to protect peristomal skin from contact with stool, which would cause irritation.
   - Cut an opening in skin barrier the exact circumference of stoma, remove release paper, and apply sticky surface directly to peristomal skin.
   - Remove skin barrier and inspect skin q2-3days. Peristomal skin should look like other abdominal skin. Changes such as erythema, erosion, serous drainage, bleeding, or induration signal infection, irritation, or sensitivity to materials placed on the skin and should be documented and reported to the physician because topical medication may be required. Irritating materials should be discontinued, and other materials substituted. Patch test patient's abdominal skin to determine sensitivity to suspected materials.
   - Because stomas become less edematous for some weeks after surgery, the opening in the skin barrier must be recalibrated each time it is changed to ensure that it is always the exact circumference of the stoma and thus prevents contact between stool and skin.
2. Apply a two-piece pouch system or a pouch with access cap so that stoma can be inspected for viability q12-24h. A matured stoma is red with overlying mucus. A nonmatured stoma is red and moist

where the mucous membrane is exposed but can be a darker, mottled, grayish red with a transparent or translucent film of serosa elsewhere.

3. After removing skin barrier and pouch for routine care, clean skin with mild soap and water, rinse well, and dry so that skin retains its normal integrity, and skin barrier and pouch materials adhere well.

4. To maintain a secure pouch seal, empty pouch when it is one-third to one-half full of stool or gas.

AFTER A CONTINENT ILEOSTOMY

1. A catheter is inserted through the stoma and into the continent ileostomy reservoir, and sutured to the peristomal skin. Avoid stress on the suture, and monitor for erythema, induration, drainage, or erosion. Consult physician about significant findings. As prescribed, maintain catheter on low continuous suction or gravity drainage to prevent stress on nipple valve and to maintain reservoir decompression so that suture lines are allowed to heal without stress or tension.

2. Check catheter q2h for patency, and irrigate with 30 ml of sterile saline to prevent obstruction. Consult physician if unable to instill solution, if there are no returns per suction catheter, or if leakage of irrigating solution or reservoir's contents appears around catheter.

3. To prevent irritation of peristomal skin, change 4×4 dressing around stoma q2h or as often as it becomes wet. Drainage will be serosanguineous at first and mixed with mucus. Report frank bleeding to physician.

4. Assess stoma for viability with each dressing change; it should be red, wet, and shiny with mucus. A pale or dark purple to black color or dull appearance can indicate circulatory impairment and should be reported to physician immediately and documented.

AFTER ILEOANAL RESERVOIR

1. Perform routine care for diverting ileostomy (see earlier).

2. After the first stage of the operation, patient may have incontinence of mucus. Maintain perineal/perianal skin integrity by irrigating mucus out of reservoir daily with 60 ml of water, or by gently cleansing area with water and cotton balls or soft tissues. (**Note:** Pouch irrigation to remove mucus rarely is indicated now because of new reservoir configurations that allow spontaneous emptying.) Do not use soap, which can cause itching or irritation. Use a pad at night to absorb mucus.

3. After the second stage of the operation (when ileostomy is taken down), expect patient to have frequency and urgency of defecation.

4. Wash perineal/perianal area with warm water or commercial perianal/perineal cleansing solution, using a squeeze bottle, cotton balls, or soft tissues. Do not use toilet paper because it can cause irritation. If desired, dry area with a hair dryer on a cool setting.

5. Provide sitz baths to promote comfort and help clean perineal/perianal area.

Gastrointestinal

6. Apply protective skin sealants or ointments. Skin sealants should not be used on irritated or eroded skin because of their high alcohol content, which would cause a painful burning sensation.

Bowel incontinence related to disruption of normal function with fecal diversion

Desired outcomes: Within 2-4 days after surgery, patient has bowel sounds and eliminates gas and stool *via* fecal diversion. Within 3 days after teaching begins, patient verbalizes understanding of measures to maintain normal elimination pattern and demonstrates care techniques specific to fecal diversion.

AFTER COLOSTOMY AND CONVENTIONAL ILEOSTOMY (PERMANENT AND TEMPORARY)

1. Empty stool from bottom opening of pouch, and assess quality and quantity of stool to document return of normal bowel function.

2. If colostomy is not eliminating stool after 3-4 days and bowel sounds have returned, gently insert a gloved, lubricated finger into stoma to determine if there is a stricture at the skin or fascial levels; note any stool within reach of examining finger. To stimulate elimination of gas and stool, physician may prescribe colostomy irrigation. (For procedure, see **Knowledge deficit:** Colostomy irrigation procedure, p. 264.)

AFTER CONTINENT ILEOSTOMY

1. Monitor I&O, and record color and consistency of output.

2. Expect aspiration of bright red blood or serosanguineous liquid drainage from continent ileostomy reservoir during early postoperative period.

3. As GI function returns (after 3-4 days), expect drainage to change color from blood-tinged to greenish brown. When ileal output appears, suction is discontinued and reservoir catheter uses gravity drainage.

4. As patient's diet progresses from clear liquids to solid food, ileal output thickens. Check and irrigate catheter q2h and as needed to maintain patency. If patient reports abdominal fullness in the area of the reservoir, along with decreased fecal output, check placement and patency of catheter.

5. When patient is alert and taking food by mouth, teach him or her catheter irrigation procedure, which should be performed q2h; demonstrate how to empty reservoir contents through catheter into toilet.

6. Before hospital discharge, teach patient how to remove and reinsert catheter.

AFTER ILEOANAL RESERVOIR

1. Monitor I&O, observing quantity, quality, and consistency of output from diverting ileostomy and reservoir. Monitor patient for rise in temperature accompanied by perianal pain and discharge of purulent, bloody mucus from drains and anal orifice. Consult physician about significant findings.

2. If drains are present, irrigate as prescribed to maintain patency, minimize stress on suture lines, and reduce incidence of infection.

3. After the first stage of the operation, patient may experience incontinence of mucus. Advise patient to wear a small pad to avoid soiling of outer garments.

4. After the second stage of the operation (when ileostomy is taken down), expect incontinence and 15-20 bowel movements per day with urgency when patient is on a clear-liquid diet. Assist patient with perianal care, and apply protective skin care products. To reduce incontinence at night, the catheter can be placed in the reservoir and connected to a gravity drainage bag.

5. Expect the number of bowel movements to diminish to 6-12/day and the consistency to thicken when patient is on solid foods.

6. Administer hydrophilic colloids and antidiarrheal drugs as prescribed to reduce frequency and fluidity of stools.

7. Provide diet consultation so that patient will be able to avoid foods that cause liquid stools (spinach, raw fruits, highly seasoned foods, green beans, broccoli, prune and grape juice, alcohol) and increase intake of foods that cause thick stools (cheese, ripe bananas, applesauce, creamy peanut butter, gelatin, pasta).

8. Reassure patient that frequency and urgency are temporary and that as reservoir expands and absorbs fluid, bowel movements should become thicker and less frequent.

Body image disturbance related to presence of fecal diversion

Desired outcome: Within 5-7 days after surgery, patient demonstrates actions that reflect beginning of acceptance of fecal diversion and incorporates changes into self-concept, as evidenced by acknowledging body changes, viewing stoma, and participating in care of fecal diversion.

1. Patients with a fecal diversion may express any or all of the following fears: that their physical, social, and work activities will be curtailed significantly; that they will be rejected and will feel isolated and unclean; that everyone will know about their altered pattern of fecal elimination; and that they may lose voluntary control over elimination (many patients see incontinence as a return to infancy).

2. Encourage patient to discuss feelings and fears; clarify any misconceptions. Involve family members in discussions, because they, too, may have anxieties and misconceptions.

3. Provide a calm, quiet environment for patient and significant others to discuss the surgery. Initiate an open, honest discussion. Monitor carefully for and listen closely to expressed or nonverbalized needs because each patient reacts differently to the surgical procedure.

4. Encourage acceptance of fecal diversion by having patient participate in care. Assure patient that education offers a means of control.

5. Assure patient that physical, social, and work activities will not be affected by having a fecal diversion.

6. Expect patient to have fears about sexual acceptance, although these fears usually are not expressed overtly. Concerns center on change in body image; fears about odor and the ostomy appliance interfering with intercourse; conception, pregnancy, and discomfort from

Gastrointestinal

perianal wound and scar in women; and impotence and failure to
ejaculate in men, especially after more radical dissection of the pelvis in a patient with cancer. If you are uncomfortable talking about
sexuality with patients, be aware of these potential concerns and arrange for a consultation with someone who can speak openly and
honestly about these problems.

7. Consult patient's surgeon about a visit by another ostomate. Patients gain reassurance and build positive attitudes by seeing
a healthy, active person who has undergone the same type of surgery.

Knowledge deficit: Colostomy irrigation procedure

Desired outcome: Within 3 days after teaching begins, patient
demonstrates proficiency in procedure for colostomy irrigation.

N O T E :   Teach prescribed colostomy irrigation to patient with permanent descending or sigmoid colostomy. Colostomy irrigation is performed daily or every other day so that wearing a pouch becomes unnecessary. An appropriate candidate is a patient who has one or two
formed stools each day at predictable times (same as normal stool
elimination pattern before illness). In addition, the patient must be able
to manipulate the equipment and remember the technique, and must be
willing to spend approximately 1 hour a day performing the procedure.
It may take 4-6 wk for the patient to be able to successfully regulate
stool elimination with irrigation.

GIVE PATIENT THE FOLLOWING INSTRUCTIONS:

1. Position an irrigating sleeve over the colostomy, and secure it in
place with an adhesive disk or belt.
2. Fill an enema container with 1-1¾ pt (500-1,000 ml) of warm water. Sit down on the toilet, and position the open end of the irrigating sleeve so that it empties into the toilet. Place the enema container so that its bottom surface is at shoulder level.
3. Flush the tubing with some of the water to remove air from the tubing. Then, allow the water to enter the colostomy slowly from the
container through the tubing, which will have either a lubricated
cone attachment or a shield on a lubricated catheter, which keeps
the irrigating water in the colostomy. Hold the cone snugly against
the stoma. It should take 3-5 minutes for the water to enter the colon.
4. After the water has entered the colon, wait 30-40 minutes for it to
be eliminated, along with stool.
5. Remove the irrigation sleeve, and clean and dry the area around the
stoma.
6. Between irrigations, keep a small dressing or security pouch over
the colostomy.

See Appendix One for nursing diagnoses and interventions in "Caring for Preoperative and Postoperative Patients," p. 395, and "Caring
for Patients with Cancer and Other Life-Disrupting Illnesses," p. 450.

PATIENT-FAMILY TEACHING
AND DISCHARGE PLANNING

Give patient and significant others verbal and written information about the following:

1. Medications, including drug name, purpose, dosage, schedule, precautions, drug/drug and food/drug interactions, and potential side effects.
2. Importance of dietary management to promote nutritional and fluid maintenance.
3. Care of incision and dressing changes, and permission to take baths or showers once sutures and drains are removed.
4. Care of stoma and peristomal and perianal skin; use of ostomy equipment; and method for obtaining supplies.
5. Gradual resumption of ADLs, excluding heavy lifting (>10 lb), pushing, or pulling for 6-8 wk to prevent development of incisional herniation.
6. Referral to community resources, including home health care agency, ET nurse, and local chapter of United Ostomy Association.
7. Importance of follow-up care with physician and ET nurse; confirm date and time of next appointment.
8. Importance of reporting signs and symptoms that require medical attention: change in stoma color from the normal bright, shiny red; peristomal or perianal skin irritation; any significant changes in appearance, frequency, and consistency of stools; fever; chills; abdominal pain or distention; incisional pain, drainage, swelling, or redness.

SECTION FOUR: ABDOMINAL TRAUMA

NURSING DIAGNOSES AND INTERVENTIONS

Fluid volume deficit related to active loss secondary to bleeding/hemorrhage

Desired outcomes: Within 4 h of admission or upon definitive repair (e.g., surgery), patient is normovolemic, as evidenced by systolic BP ≥90 mm Hg (or within patient's baseline range); HR 60-100 bpm; CVP 2-6 mm Hg (or 5-12 cm H_2O); urinary output ≥30 ml/h; warm extremities; brisk capillary refill (<2 sec); distal pulses >2+ on a 0-4+ scale; and absence of orthostasis.

1. *Recently injured patient:* Monitor BP qh (or more often with obvious bleeding or unstable VS). Be alert for rising diastolic BP and falling systolic BP. A sudden fall in systolic BP, even if minimal, requires consultation with physician, especially for a trauma patient when the extent of injury is unknown. Most trauma patients are young, and excellent neurovascular compensation results in near-normal BP until large intravascular volume depletion develops.
   Stable postoperative patient: Perform routine VS assessment.

2. Be alert for and report clinical indicators of fluid volume deficit (see Table 6-4).
3. Monitor HR and cardiovascular status qh until patient's condition is stable. Consult physician about sudden increases or decreases in HR, especially if associated with indicators of fluid volume deficit, as noted above.
4. Monitor for physical indicators of fluid volume deficit: diaphoresis, cool extremities, delayed capillary refill (≥ 2 sec), and absent or diminished distal pulses.
5. If patient has evidence of volume depletion or active blood loss, administer prescribed fluids rapidly through one or more large-caliber (16-gauge or larger) IV catheters. **Caution:** Evaluate patency of IV catheters frequently during rapid-volume resuscitation. Monitor patient closely to avoid fluid volume overload and complications such as heart failure (see p. 34) and pulmonary edema (see p. 49).
6. Measure CVP q1-4h if indicated. Be alert for low or decreasing values. Report sudden decreases in CVP, especially if associated with other indicators of fluid volume deficit, as noted above.
7. Measure urinary output q4h (or when patient voids). Be alert for decreasing urinary output and infrequent voidings. In patients with abdominal trauma, low urine output usually reflects inadequate intravascular volume. Before administering diuretics, evaluate patient for fluid volume deficit, as noted above.
8. Estimate ongoing blood loss. Measure all bloody drainage from tubes or catheters, noting drainage color (e.g., coffee-ground, burgundy, bright red). Note the frequency of dressing changes due to saturation with blood to estimate amount of blood loss *via* wound site. Consult physician about significant increases in amount of drainage, especially if bloody.

Pain related to irritation caused by intraperitoneal blood or secretions, actual trauma or surgical incision, and manipulation of organs during surgery

Desired outcomes: Within 4 h of admission, patient's subjective perception of pain decreases, as documented by a pain scale. Objective indicators, such as grimacing, are absent or diminished.

Table 6-4   Indicators of fluid volume deficit

Rising diastolic BP (early)
Falling systolic BP (later)
Tachycardia (>100 bpm)
Tachypnea (>20 breaths/min)
Anxiety (early)
Altered/depressed mental status (later)
Delayed capillary refill (≥ 2 sec)
Cool, pale skin
Low or decreasing CVP
Low urinary output (<30 ml/h)

1. Evaluate patient for preoperative and postoperative pain. Devise a pain scale with patient, rating discomfort from 0 (no pain) to 10 (worst pain). Preoperative pain is expected and is a vital diagnostic aid. The location and character of postoperative pain also are important. Incisional and some visceral pain can be expected, but intense or prolonged pain, especially when accompanied by other peritoneal signs (see Table 6-5), can signal bleeding, bowel infarction, infection, or other complications. Recognize that the autonomic nervous system (ANS) response to pain can complicate assessment of abdominal injury and hypovolemia. For details, see Appendix One for **Pain,** p. 396.

2. Administer narcotics and other analgesics as prescribed. Do not administer analgesics preoperatively until patient has been evaluated thoroughly by a trauma surgeon. Administer postoperatively prescribed analgesics on a continual or regular schedule promptly, with additional analgesia as needed, or provide patient with patient-controlled analgesia (PCA). Analgesics are helpful in relieving pain and aiding in the recovery process by promoting greater ventilatory excursion. Be aware that intoxication often is involved in traumatic events; therefore, victims may be drug or alcohol users, with a higher than average tolerance for narcotics. These same individuals may suffer symptoms of alcohol or narcotic withdrawal that must be recognized and treated. In addition, recognize that narcotic analgesics can reduce GI motility and may delay return to normal bowel function. Document degree of relief obtained, using pain scale.

3. Monitor PCA, if prescribed, and document effectiveness, using pain scale.

4. Supplement analgesics with nonpharmacologic methods (e.g., positioning, back rubs, distraction) to help relieve pain.

Risk for infection related to inadequate primary defenses secondary to disruption of GI tract (particularly of terminal ileum and colon) and traumatically inflicted open wound; related to multiple indwelling catheters and tubes; and related to compromised immune state due to blood loss and metabolic response to trauma

Desired outcome: Patient is free of infection, as evidenced by core or rectal temperature <37.8° C (100° F); HR ≤100 bpm; orientation to time, place, and person; and absence of unusual erythema, warmth, or drainage at surgical incisions or wound sites.

1. Monitor VS for evidence of infection, noting temperature increases

Gastrointestinal

Table 6-5 Signs and symptoms suggestive of peritoneal irritation

Generalized abdominal pain or tenderness
Involuntary guarding of abdomen
Abdominal wall rigidity
Rebound tenderness
Abdominal pain with movement or coughing
Diminished or absent bowel sounds

and associated increases in HR and RR. Consult surgeon about sudden temperature elevations.
2. Evaluate orientation and LOC q8h. Note mental confusion or deterioration from baseline LOC.
3. Ensure patency of all surgically placed tubes or drains. Irrigate or attach to low-pressure suction as prescribed. Promptly report unrelieved loss of tube patency.
4. Evaluate incisions and wound sites for evidence of infection: unusual erythema, warmth, delayed healing, purulent or unusual drainage.
5. Note amount, color, character, and odor of all drainage (Table 6-6). Report foul-smelling or abnormal drainage. Test drainage for pH and blood; compare to expected characteristics.
6. Administer antibiotics in a timely fashion. Reschedule parenteral antibiotics if a dose is delayed for more than 1 h. Recognize that failure to administer antibiotics on schedule may result in inadequate blood levels and treatment failure.
7. As prescribed, administer pneumococcal vaccine in patients with total splenectomy to minimize the risk of postsplenectomy sepsis.

Table 6-6   Characteristics of gastrointestinal drainage

Source	Composition and Usual Character
Mouth and oropharynx	Saliva; thin, clear, watery; pH 7
Stomach	Hydrochloric, gastrin, pepsin, mucus; thin, brownish to greenish; acidic
Pancreas	Enzymes and bicarbonate; thin, watery, yellowish brown; alkaline; usually abundant after surgery
Biliary tract	Bile, including bile salts and electrolytes; bright yellow to brownish green
Duodenum	Digestive enzymes, mucus, products of digestion; thin, bright yellow to light brown, may be greenish; alkaline
Jejunum	Enzymes, mucus, products of digestion; brown; watery with particles
Ileum	Enzymes, mucus, digestive products, greater amounts of bacteria; brown, liquid, feculent
Colon	Digestive products, mucus, large amounts of bacteria; brown to dark brown; semiformed to firm stool
Postoperative (GI surgery)	Initial drainage is expected to contain fresh blood; later drainage is mixed with old blood and then approaches normal composition
Infection	Drainage is cloudy, may be thicker than usual; strong or unusual odor; drain site often is erythematous and warm

8. Administer tetanus immune globulin and tetanus toxoid as prescribed.

9. Change dressings as prescribed, using aseptic technique. Prevent cross-contamination from various wounds by changing one dressing at a time.

10. If patient has or develops evisceration, do not reinsert tissue or organs. Place sterile, saline-soaked gauze over evisceration and cover with a sterile towel until evisceration can be evaluated by the surgeon.

Ineffective breathing pattern related to pain from injury or surgical incision; chemical irritation of blood or bile on pleural tissue; and diaphragmatic elevation due to abdominal distention

Desired outcome: Within 24 h of admission or surgery, patient is eupneic, with RR 12-20 breaths/min and clear breath sounds.

1. Administer supplemental oxygen as prescribed. Monitor and document effectiveness.

2. Administer analgesics at dosage and frequency that relieves pain and associated impaired chest excursion.

3. For additional interventions, see this nursing diagnosis in Appendix One, p. 404, in "Caring for Preoperative and Postoperative Patients."

Altered gastrointestinal (GI) tissue perfusion (or risk for same) related to interrupted blood flow to abdominal viscera secondary to vascular disruption or occlusion, or related to moderate to severe hypovolemia caused by hemorrhage

Desired outcomes: Patient has adequate GI tissue perfusion, as evidenced by normoactive bowel sounds; soft, nondistended abdomen; and return of bowel elimination. Gastric secretions, drainage, and excretions test negative for occult blood.

1. Auscultate for bowel sounds qh for recently injured patients and q8h during recovery phase. Report prolonged or sudden absence of bowel sounds, because this may signal bowel ischemia or infarction. Anticipate absent or diminished bowel sounds for up to 72 h after surgery.

2. Evaluate patient for peritoneal signs (see Table 6-5), which may occur acutely secondary to injury or may not develop until days or weeks later if complications due to slow bleeding or other mechanisms occur.

3. Ensure adequate intravascular volume (see interventions in **Fluid volume deficit**, p. 265).

4. Evaluate laboratory data for evidence of bleeding (e.g., serial Hct) or organ ischemia (e.g., SGPT, SGOT, LDH). Optimal values are Hct >30%; SGOT 5-40 IU/L; SGPT 5-35 IU/L; and LDH 90-200 ImU/ml.

5. Document amount and character of GI secretions, drainage, and excretions. Note changes suggestive of bleeding (frank or occult blood), infection (e.g., increased or purulent drainage), or obstruction (e.g., failure to eliminate flatus or stool within 72 h after surgery).

Risk for impaired skin integrity related to exposure to irritating GI drainage; *and* **Impaired tissue integrity (or risk for same)** related to direct trauma and surgery, catabolic posttraumatic state, and altered circulation

Desired outcome: By hospital discharge, patient exhibits wound healing and skin remains clear and unbroken.

1. Promptly change all dressings that become soiled with drainage or blood.
2. Protect skin surrounding tubes, drains, or fistulas, keeping these areas clean and free of drainage. Gastric and intestinal secretions and drainage are irritating and can lead to skin excoriation. If necessary, apply ointments, skin barriers, or drainage bags to protect surrounding skin. Apply reusable dressing supports (e.g., Montgomery straps) to protect surrounding skin. Consult ostomy nurse for complex or involved cases.
3. Inspect wounds, fistulas, and drain sites for signs of irritation, infection, and ischemia.
4. Identify infected and devitalized tissue. Aid in their removal by irrigation, wound packing, or preparing patient for surgical debridement.
5. Ensure adequate protein and calorie intake for tissue healing (see **Altered nutrition,** below).
6. For more information, see "Managing Wound Care," p. 384.

Altered nutrition: Less than body requirements, related to decreased intake secondary to disruption of GI tract integrity (traumatic or surgical) and increased need secondary to hypermetabolic posttrauma state

Desired outcome: By a minimum of 24 h before hospital discharge, patient has adequate nutrition, as evidenced by maintenance of baseline body weight and positive or balanced nitrogen state.

1. Collaborate with physician, dietitian, and pharmacist to estimate patient's metabolic needs, based on type of injury, activity level, and nutritional status before injury.
2. Consider patient's specific injuries when planning nutrition (e.g., expect patients with hepatic or pancreatic injury to have difficulty with blood sugar regulation; patients with trauma to the upper GI tract may be fed enterally, but feeding tube must be placed distal to injury; disruption of GI tract may require feeding gastrostomy or jejunostomy; patients with major hepatic trauma may have difficulty with protein tolerance).
3. Ensure patency of gastric or intestinal tube to maintain decompression and encourage healing and return of bowel function. Maintain suction as prescribed. Consult surgeon about loss of patency or failure to maintain suction. Do not occlude vent side of sump suction tubes, because this may result in vacuum occlusion of the tube and excessive suction to gastric mucosa. Use caution when irrigating NG or other tubes placed in or near recently sutured organs.
4. Do not start enteral feeding until bowel function returns (i.e., bowel sounds are present, patient feels hungry).
5. Recognize that narcotics reduce GI motility and may contribute to nausea, vomiting, abdominal distention, and ileus. Consider supplemental administration of prescribed nonnarcotic analgesics (e.g., ketorolac).
6. For more information, see "Providing Nutritional Support," p. 378.

Posttrauma response related to life-threatening accident or event resulting in trauma

Desired outcomes: By a minimum of 24 h before hospital discharge, patient verbalizes that psychosocial impact of event has abated, and he or she does not show signs of severe stress reaction (e.g., display of inconsistent affect, suicidal or homicidal behavior, or extreme agitation or depression). Patient cooperates with treatment plan.

N O T E : Many victims of major abdominal trauma sustain life-threatening injury. The patient often is aware of the situation and fears death. Even after the physical condition stabilizes, the patient may have a prolonged or severe reaction triggered by recollection of the trauma.

---

1. Evaluate mental status at systematic intervals. Be alert for indicators of severe stress reaction (e.g., display of affect inconsistent with statements or behavior, suicidal or homicidal statements or actions, extreme agitation or depression, and failure to cooperate with instructions related to care).
2. Consult specialists such as psychologist, psychiatric nurse clinician, or pastoral counselor if patient displays signs of severe stress reaction as described above.
3. Consider organic causes that may contribute to posttraumatic response (e.g., severe pain, alcohol intoxication or withdrawal, electrolyte imbalance, metabolic encephalopathy, or impaired cerebral perfusion).
4. For other psychosocial interventions, see Appendix One, "Caring for Patients with Cancer and Other Life-Disrupting Illnesses," p. 450.

As appropriate, see nursing diagnoses and interventions in "Fecal Diversions," p. 260; "Caring for Preoperative and Postoperative Patients," p. 395; "Caring for Patients on Prolonged Bed Rest," p. 413; and "Caring for Patients with Cancer and Other Life-Disrupting Illnesses," p. 450.

PATIENT-FAMILY TEACHING
AND DISCHARGE PLANNING

Anticipate extended physical and emotional rehabilitation for patient and significant others. Provide verbal and written information about the following:

1. Probable need for emotional care, even for patients who have not required extensive physical rehabilitation. Provide referrals to support groups for trauma patients and family members.
2. Availability of rehabilitation programs, extended care facilities, and home health agencies for patients unable to accomplish self-care upon hospital discharge.
3. If applicable, the availability of community support groups (e.g., Alcoholics Anonymous, Cocaine Anonymous) and of rehabilitation programs for substance abuse. In the period immediately after the traumatic event, the patient and family members are very impres-

Gastrointestinal

sionable; this is an ideal time for the substance abuser to begin addressing the problem.

4. Medications, including drug name, purpose, dosage, schedule, precautions, drug/drug and food/drug interactions, and potential side effects. Encourage patients taking antibiotics to take the medications for the prescribed length of time, even though they may be asymptomatic. If patient received tetanus immunization, ensure that he or she receives a wallet-sized card documenting the immunization.

5. Wound and catheter care. Have patient or care giver describe and demonstrate proper technique before hospital discharge.

6. Importance of seeking medical attention if indicators of infection or bowel obstruction occur (e.g., fever, severe or unusual abdominal pain, nausea, vomiting, unusual drainage from wounds or incisions, or a change in bowel habits).

7. Injury prevention. Immediately after a traumatic injury, patient is especially likely to respond to injury prevention education. Provide instructions on proper wearing of seat belts (across pelvic girdle rather than soft tissue of lower abdomen), safety for infants and children, and other factors suitable for individuals involved.

SECTION FIVE: HEPATIC AND BILIARY DISORDERS

Hepatitis

NURSING DIAGNOSES AND INTERVENTIONS

Fatigue related to reduced metabolic energy production secondary to liver dysfunction, which causes faulty absorption, metabolism, and storage of nutrients

Desired outcome: By a minimum of 24 h before hospital discharge, patient's fatigue has abated, and he or she is regaining energy.

1. Take a diet history to determine food preferences. Encourage significant others to bring in desirable foods, if permitted.

2. Monitor and record intake.

3. Encourage small, frequent feedings and provide emotional support during meals.

4. Obtain prescription for vitamin and mineral supplements, if appropriate.

5. Provide rest periods of at least 90 min before and after activities and treatments.

6. Keep frequently used objects within easy reach.

7. Promote rest and sleep by cutting back on environmental stimuli, providing back massage and relaxation tapes, and conversing with patient in short, simple terms.

8. Administer antacids, antiemetics, antidiarrheal drugs, and cathartics as prescribed to minimize gastric distress and promote absorption of nutrients.

Knowledge deficit: Causes of hepatitis and modes of transmission
Desired outcome: Within the 24 h before hospital discharge, patient verbalizes knowledge of the causes of hepatitis and measures that help prevent transmission.

1. Assess patient's knowledge of disease process, and teach him or her as necessary (see Table 6-7). Make sure patient knows you are not making moral decisions about alcohol or drug use or sexual behavior.
2. Teach patient and significant others the importance of good handwashing and of wearing gloves if contact with feces is possible.
3. If appropriate, advise patients with HAV that crowded living conditions with poor sanitation should be avoided to prevent recurrence.
4. Remind patients with HBV and HCV that they should modify sexual behavior. Explain that blood donation is no longer possible.
5. Advise patients with HBV that their sexual partners should receive HB vaccine.
6. Refer patient to drug treatment programs as necessary.

Risk for impaired skin integrity related to pruritus secondary to hepatic dysfunction
Desired outcome: Patient's skin remains intact.

1. Keep patient's skin moist by using tepid water or emollient baths, avoiding alkaline soap, and applying emollient lotions at frequent intervals.
2. Encourage patient not to scratch skin and to keep nails short and smooth. Suggest patient use knuckles for scratching. Wrap or place gloves on patient's hands (especially comatose patients).
3. Treat any skin lesion promptly to prevent infection.
4. Administer antihistamines as prescribed; observe closely for excessive sedation.
5. Encourage patient to wear loose, soft clothing; provide soft linens (cotton is best).
6. Keep environment cool.
7. Change soiled linen as soon as possible.

Body image disturbance related to presence of jaundice
Desired outcome: Within the 24 h before hospital discharge, patient verbalizes knowledge of measures for enhancing appearance and demonstrates an interest in daily grooming.

1. Encourage patient and significant others to express their feelings and concerns.
2. Encourage patient to maintain daily grooming.
3. Explain that wearing yellow and green intensifies yellow skin tone. Suggest wearing bright reds and blues or black instead.
4. Provide privacy as necessary.
5. For additional information, see this nursing diagnosis in Appendix One, p. 459.

Altered protection related to increased risk of bleeding secondary to reduced absorption of vitamin K
Desired outcome: Patient is free of bleeding, as evidenced by negative test results for occult blood in feces and urine, absence of ecchymotic areas, and absence of bleeding at gums and injection sites.

Text continued on page 278.

Table 6-7 Types and characteristics of viral hepatitis

	Hepatitis A Virus (HAV)	Hepatitis B Virus (HBV)	Hepatitis C Virus (HCV)	Hepatitis D Virus (HDV)	Hepatitis E Virus (HEV)
Likely modes of transmission	Fecal-oral; food-borne most common; parenteral transmission rare; most infectious 2 wk before symptoms appear	Contact with blood or serum; sexual contact; perinatal transmission; often transmitted by chronic carriers; most infectious before symptoms appear and for 4-6 mo after acute infection	Contact with blood or serum; perinatal transmission rare unless mother is HIV infected; often transmitted by chronic carriers; most infectious 1-2 wk before symptoms appear and throughout acute infection	Similar to HBV; can cause infection only if individual already has HBV; blood infectious throughout HDV infection	Fecal-oral; food-borne; water-borne

	HAV	HBV	HCV	HDV	HEV
Population most often affected	Children; individuals living in or traveling to areas with poor sanitation	Injecting drug users; health care and public safety workers exposed to blood; clients and staff of institutions for the developmentally disabled; homosexual men; men and women with multiple heterosexual partners; young children of infected mothers; recipients of certain blood products; hemodialysis patients	Injecting drug users; individuals who received blood products before 1991; potential risk to health care and public safety workers exposed to blood	Injecting drug users; hemophiliacs; recipients of multiple blood transfusions (infects only individuals who already have HBV)	People living in or traveling to parts of Asia, Africa, or Mexico where sanitation is poor
Incubation	2-6 wk	6 wk-6 mo	18-180 days	Varies; not well established	
Serum markers of acute infection	Antibody to HAV (anti-HAV); IgG-class antibody to HAV (IgG anti-HAV) indicates immunity	HBsAg; HBeAg; IgM-class antibody to HBcAg (IgM anti-HBc)	Only test available is antibody to HCV (anti-HCV), which detects chronic but not acute cases	Antibody to HDV (anti-HDV)	

Continued.

Gastrointestinal

Table 6-7 Types and characteristics of viral hepatitis—cont'd

	Hepatitis A Virus (HAV)	Hepatitis B Virus (HBV)	Hepatitis C Virus (HCV)	Hepatitis D Virus (HDV)	Hepatitis E Virus (HEV)
Measures for reducing exposure	Handwashing; good personal hygiene; sanitation; appropriate infection control measures (see Appendix Two, p. 479)	Handwashing; good personal hygiene; appropriate infection control measures (see Appendix Two, p. 479); autoclaving of all nondisposable items; careful handling of needles and sharps; ensuring that needles are not reused and are discarded carefully in special containers	As for HBV	As for HBV	As for HAV

Prophylaxis	Sanitation measures; immunoglobulin before exposure or 1-2 wk after exposure	Screening of donated blood; protective devices for health care providers and immunization for all health care workers who come in contact with blood, as well as for risk groups noted above; use of condoms; HBIG for known exposure to HBsAg-contaminated material; also, CDC recommends routine immunization of all children	Screening of donated blood and protective devices for health care providers; no vaccine exists for HCV	Immunization against HBV	Effectiveness of immunoglobulin manufactured in the United States is not known
Comments	Symptoms usually mild; rarely causes fulminant hepatic failure	HBsAg persists in carrier state; chronic hepatitis may develop; fulminant hepatic failure may result	Carrier state and chronic hepatitis may develop; fulminant hepatic failure may result	Increased risk of serious complications (including fulminant hepatic failure) and death; carrier state and chronic hepatitis may develop	Disease is not endemic in the United States or western Europe

HBcAg, hepatitis B core antigen; *HBeAg*, hepatitis B early antigen; *HBIG*, hepatitis B immunoglobulin; *HBsAg*, hepatitis B surface antigen; *IgG*, immunoglobulin G; *IgM*, immunoglobulin M.

Gastrointestinal

1. Monitor PT levels daily; optimal range is 10.5-13.5 sec.
2. Handle patient gently (e.g., when turning or transferring).
3. Minimize IM injections. Rotate sites, and use small-gauge needles. Apply moderate pressure after injection, but do not massage site. Administer medications orally or intravenously when possible.
4. Observe for ecchymotic areas. Inspect gums, and test urine and feces for blood. Consult physician about significant findings.
5. Advise patient to use electric razor and soft-bristled toothbrush.
6. Administer vitamin K as prescribed.

PATIENT-FAMILY TEACHING AND DISCHARGE PLANNING

Give patient and significant others verbal and written information about the following:
1. Importance of rest and adequate nutrition.
2. Importance of avoiding hepatotoxic agents, including OTC drugs (see Table 6-8).
3. Prescribed medications (e.g., multivitamins), including drug name, purpose, dosage, schedule, precautions, drug/drug and food/drug interactions, and potential side effects.
4. Importance of informing physicians, dentists, and other health care providers about the hepatitis diagnosis.
5. Potential complications: delayed healing, skin injury, and bleeding tendency.
6. Importance of avoiding alcohol during recovery.
7. If applicable, referral to alcohol and/or drug treatment programs.

Cirrhosis

NURSING DIAGNOSES AND INTERVENTIONS

Altered nutrition: Less than body requirements, related to anorexia, nausea, or malabsorption
Desired outcome: Within the 24 h before hospital discharge, patient verbalizes knowledge of foods that are permitted and restricted and develops a 3-day menu that includes or excludes these foods appropriately.
1. Explain dietary restrictions; remember that sodium and fluids are restricted (see Table 1-4, p. 18, for a list of foods high in sodium). Encourage patient to eat foods permitted. If patient's ammonia level rises (*normal:* whole blood: 70-200 μg/dl; plasma: 56-150 μg/dl), protein and foods high in ammonia also will be restricted.
2. Monitor I&O; weigh patient daily.
3. Encourage small, frequent meals to ensure adequate nutrition.
4. Encourage significant others to bring in desirable foods as permitted.
5. Have nourishing foods available to patient at night.
6. Administer vitamin and mineral supplements, as prescribed.
7. Administer the following prescribed medications to alleviate gastric distress: antacids, antiemetics, antidiarrheal drugs, cathartics.

Table 6-8   Drugs that can cause hepatotoxicity

Prescription Drugs
allopurinol
amiodarone
androgenic steroids
carbamazepine
carmustine (BCNU)
chlorpromazine (CPZ)
cyclosporine
dantrolene
diazepam
erythromycin
glucocorticoids
haloperidol
halothane (and related anesthetics)
isoniazid (INH)
ketoconazole
mercaptopurine (6-MP)
methotrexate (MTX)
methyldopa
mitomycin
monoamine oxidase (MAO) inhibitors
oral contraceptives
oxacillin
phenindione
phenylbutazone
phenytoin sodium
rifampin
sulfonamides

Nonprescription Drugs
acetaminophen
alcohol
aspirin and other salicylates
NSAIDs
vitamin A

Gastrointestinal

8. Promote bed rest to reduce metabolic demands on the liver.
9. Provide soft diet if patient has esophageal varices that are not bleeding (patients with bleeding esophageal varices are NPO).
10. Discuss need for feeding supplements and enteral or parenteral nutrition (see "Providing Nutritional Support," p. 378) with physician if appropriate.

Impaired gas exchange related to altered oxygen supply secondary to shallow breathing occurring with ascites or pleural effusion; altered oxygen-carrying capacity of the blood secondary to erythrocytopenia; and possible intrapulmonary shunting.

Desired outcome: Within 24 h of admission, patient has adequate gas exchange, as evidenced by $Paco_2$ ≤45 mm Hg, Pao_2 ≥80 mm Hg, O_2 saturation ≥95%, and RR 12-20 breaths/min with normal depth and pattern (eupnea).

1. If patient complains of dyspnea or orthopnea, help him or her into semi-Fowler's or high Fowler's position to promote gas exchange.
2. Administer oxygen as prescribed.
3. Monitor ABG values and pulse oximetry (O_2 saturation); consult physician about significant findings.
4. Encourage patient to change positions and breathe deeply at frequent intervals to promote gas exchange. If secretions are present, make sure patient coughs frequently.
5. Consult physician about indicators of respiratory infection: spiking temperature, chills, diaphoresis, adventitious breath sounds.
6. Obtain baseline abdominal girth measurement; measure girth daily or every shift. Measure around the same circumferential area each time; mark site with indelible ink. Consult physician about significant findings.

Altered protection related to increased risk of esophageal bleeding secondary to portal hypertension and altered clotting factors

Desired outcomes: Patient is free of esophageal bleeding, as evidenced by BP ≥90/60 mm Hg; HR ≤100 bpm; warm extremities; distal pulses >2+ on a 0-4+ scale; brisk capillary refill (<2 sec); and orientation to time, place, and person.

1. Monitor VS q4h (or more often if VS are outside patient's baseline values). Be alert for hypotension and increased HR, as well as for physical indicators of hypovolemia and hemorrhage: cool extremities, delayed capillary refill, decreased amplitude of distal pulses, decreasing LOC.
2. Teach patient to avoid swallowing foods that are chemically or mechanically irritating and therefore injurious to the esophagus (e.g., rough or spicy foods, hot foods, hot liquids, alcohol).
3. Advise patient to avoid actions that increase intraabdominothoracic pressure (e.g., coughing, sneezing, lifting, or vomiting).
4. Administer stool softeners as prescribed to help prevent straining with defecation.
5. Inspect stools for blood, which would signal bleeding within the GI tract; perform stool occult blood test as indicated.
6. As appropriate, instruct patient about alcohol's role in causing esophageal varices.
7. Monitor PT for abnormality (*normal:* 10.5-13.5 sec), and assess patient for signs of bleeding: altered VS, irritability, air hunger, pallor, weakness, melena, hematemesis.
8. As appropriate, encourage intake of foods rich in vitamin K (e.g., spinach, cabbage, cauliflower, liver) to help reduce PT.
9. As often as possible, avoid invasive procedures, such as giving injections or taking rectal temperatures.
10. Monitor patient undergoing injection sclerotherapy for evidence of perforation: increased HR, decreased BP, pallor, weakness, air hunger. If these signs occur, immediately consult physician. Keep patient NPO and prepare for gastric suction. Administer antibiotics as

prescribed to prevent infection. For more information, see Table 6-9.

Altered protection related to increased risk of neurosensory changes secondary to hepatic coma occurring with cerebral accumulation of ammonia or GI bleeding

Desired outcome: Patient verbalizes orientation to time, place, and person; exhibits intact signature; and is free of symptoms of injury caused by neurosensory changes.

1. Perform a baseline assessment of patient's personality characteristics, LOC, and orientation. Enlist the aid of significant others to help determine slight changes in personality or behavior.
2. Have patient demonstrate his or her signature daily. If writing deteriorates, ammonia levels may be increasing. Be alert for generalized muscle twitching and asterixis (flapping tremor induced by dorsiflexion of wrist and extension of fingers). Report significant findings to physician.
3. Remind patient to avoid protein and foods high in ammonia (e.g., gelatin, onions, strong cheeses). A diseased liver cannot convert ammonia to urea, and the buildup of ammonia adds to the progression of hepatic encephalopathy.
4. Monitor for indicators of GI bleeding, including melena or hematemesis. GI bleeding can precipitate hepatic coma. Promptly consult physician about bleeding, and obtain prescription for cleansing enemas if indicated.
5. Protect patient against injury resulting from confused state (e.g., keep side rails up and bed in lowest position; assist patient with ambulation when need is determined).
6. Use caution when administering sedatives, antihistamines, and other agents that affect the central nervous system. Avoid opiate analgesics and phenothiazines.

Table 6-9   Side effects and complications of esophageal sclerotherapy

Normal Mild Side Effects
Mild retrosternal pain
Transient fever
Diminished breath sounds
Transient dysphagia
Local ulcerations

Serious Side Effects/Complications
Bleeding from remaining varices or ulcers
Stricture formation evidenced by prolonged dysphagia
Perforation evidenced by bleeding, severe pain, or fever
Pulmonary problems, including aspiration pneumonia, pleural effusion, mediastinitis
Bacteremia evidenced by fever, tachycardia, positive results on blood cultures

Gastrointestinal

Fluid volume excess related to compromised regulatory mechanism with sequestration of fluids secondary to portal hypertension and hepatocellular failure

Desired outcome: By a minimum of 24 h before hospital discharge, patient is normovolemic, as evidenced by stable or decreasing abdominal girth, RR 12-20 breaths/min with normal depth and pattern (eupnea), HR ≤100 bpm, edema ≤1+ on a 0-4+ scale, and absence of crackles.

1. Obtain baseline abdominal girth measurement. Place patient in supine position and mark abdomen with indelible ink to ensure serial measurements from the same circumferential site. Measure girth daily or every shift, as appropriate.

2. Monitor I&O and weight. Output should equal or exceed input; weight loss should not exceed 0.23 kg (½ lb) a day. Assess degree of edema, rating it from 1+ (barely detectable) to 4+ (deep, persistent pitting), and document findings.

3. Be alert for clinical indicators of pulmonary edema: dyspnea, basilar crackles that do not clear with coughing, orthopnea, tachypnea.

4. Give frequent mouth care, and provide ice chips to help minimize thirst.

5. Monitor serum sodium (Na^+) and potassium (K^+) values and report abnormalities to physician. *Optimal values:* serum Na^+: 137-147 mEq/L; serum K^+: 3.5-5 mEq/L. Restrict sodium and replace potassium as prescribed.

6. Remind patient to avoid foods that contain sodium (see Table 1-4, p. 18), as well as nonfood items that have sodium (e.g., antacids, baking soda, some mouthwashes).

7. Elevate extremities to reduce peripheral edema. Apply elastic wrap or support stockings as prescribed.

8. Bear in mind that rapid increases in intravascular volume can precipitate variceal hemorrhage in susceptible patients. Monitor for hemorrhage accordingly (see **Altered protection,** above).

9. If a LeVeen peritoneovenous or Denver shunt is in place, teach patient to inhale against resistance, using a blow bottle to facilitate the flow of ascitic fluid through the shunt. Inhaling against resistance raises intraperitoneal pressure sufficiently to allow ascitic fluid to flow through the shunt. Also, provide instructions about the following: importance of life-style changes (e.g., low-sodium diet), forgoing alcohol, practicing breathing exercises, measuring weight and abdominal girth daily, and monitoring I&O and edema.

See "Hepatitis" for **Knowledge deficit:** Causes of hepatitis and modes of transmission, p. 273, and **Body image disturbance,** p. 273.

PATIENT-FAMILY TEACHING
AND DISCHARGE PLANNING

Give patient and significant others verbal and written information about the following:

1. Medications, including drug name, purpose, dosage, schedule, precautions, drug/drug and food/drug interactions, and potential side effects.

2. Dietary restrictions, particularly sodium (see Table 1-4, p. 18, for a list of foods high in sodium), protein, and ammonia.
3. Potential need for life-style changes, including forgoing alcoholic beverages. Stress that giving up alcohol is a major factor in surviving cirrhosis. Include appropriate referrals (e.g., Alcoholics Anonymous, Al-Anon, Al-Ateen). As appropriate, provide referrals to community nursing support agencies.
4. Awareness of hepatotoxic agents (see Table 6-8), especially OTC drugs such as acetaminophen and aspirin.
5. Importance of breathing exercises (see p. 282) when ascites is present.
6. Indicators of variceal bleeding or hemorrhage (vomiting of blood, change in LOC), and the need to inform a health care provider should they occur.

Cholelithiasis and Cholecystitis

NURSING DIAGNOSES AND INTERVENTIONS

Pain, spasms, nausea, and itching related to obstructive or inflammatory process
Desired outcomes: Within 1 h of intervention, patient's subjective perception of discomfort decreases, as documented by a pain scale. Objective indicators, such as grimacing, are absent or diminished.
1. Monitor patient for pain or other discomfort. Devise a pain scale with patient, rating discomfort from 0 (no pain) to 10 (worst pain).
2. Explain to patient that low Fowler's position will minimize pressure in RUQ.
3. Teach patient to avoid fatty and rough or fibrous foods to prevent nausea and spasms.
4. Administer bile salt–binding agent (e.g., cholestyramine) as prescribed for itching.
5. Help control itching by providing cool Alpha-Keri baths and cold water or ice for topical application and using soft linens on the bed.
6. For additional interventions, see **Pain** in Appendix One, p. 396.

Altered protection related to use of T-tube or recurrence of biliary obstruction
Desired outcomes: Patient is free of symptoms of postsurgical perforation, as evidenced by <1,000 ml/day of dark brown drainage (with gradual diminishment) and a soft, nondistended abdomen. Patient is free of symptoms of recurring biliary obstruction, as evidenced by normal skin color, brown stools, and straw-colored urine.
1. Monitor color of skin, sclera, urine, and stool. If obstruction recurs and bile is forced back into the bloodstream, jaundice will be present, the urine will be amber, and stools will be clay colored (clay color is normal if bile is drained *via* the tubes). Brown color should return to stools once bile begins to drain normally into duodenum.
2. When patient returns from surgery, mark T-tube at skin line with a narrow strip of sterile tape to provide a baseline for position assessment.

3. Tape the tube securely to the abdomen with adhesive tape, avoiding any tension on the tube.
4. Note and record the color, amount, odor, and consistency of drainage q2h on the day of surgery and at least every shift thereafter. Initially drainage will be dark brown with small amounts of blood and can amount to 500-1,000 ml/day. Report greater amounts of blood or drainage to physician. Amount should subside gradually as the swelling diminishes in the common duct and drainage into the duodenum normalizes. Typically the tube is removed within 6 days of surgery.
5. Be alert for abdominal distention, rigidity, and complaints of diaphragmatic irritation, along with cessation of or significant decrease in amount of drainage. If these occur, consult physician immediately and anticipate tube replacement with a 14-Fr catheter.
6. When patient ambulates with T-tube, attach a small drainage collection container to distal end, position it in a robe pocket, and ensure that it is below the level of the common duct to prevent reflux.

See "Hepatitis" for **Risk for impaired skin integrity** related to pruritus, p. 273. Also see Appendix One for nursing diagnoses and interventions in "Caring for Preoperative and Postoperative Patients," p. 395.

PATIENT-FAMILY TEACHING AND DISCHARGE PLANNING

Give patient and significant others verbal and written information about the following:
1. Notifying health care provider if the following indicators of recurrent biliary obstruction occur: dark urine, pruritus, jaundice, clay-colored stools. Inform patient that loose stools may occur for several months as the body adjusts to the continuous flow of bile.
2. Medications, including drug name, purpose, dosage, schedule, precautions, drug/drug and food/drug interactions, and potential side effects.
3. Care of dressings and tubes if patient is discharged with them, and monitoring of incision and drain sites for signs of infection (e.g., persistent redness, pain, purulent discharge, swelling, local warmth).
4. For medically managed patients, the importance of maintaining a low-fat diet and eating frequent, small meals.
5. Importance of follow-up care; confirm date and time of next appointment.
6. Forgoing alcoholic beverages during the first 2 mo after surgery to minimize the risk of pancreatic involvement.
7. Postsurgical activity precautions: no lifting of heavy objects (>10 lb) for the first 4-6 wk or as directed; resting after periods of fatigue; getting maximum amounts of rest; and gradually increasing activities to tolerance.

SECTION SIX: PANCREATIC DISORDERS

Pancreatitis

NURSING DIAGNOSES AND INTERVENTIONS

Fluid volume deficit related to active loss secondary to NG suctioning, vomiting, diaphoresis, or pooling of fluids in abdomen and retroperitoneum

Desired outcome: Within 8 h of admission, patient is normovolemic, as evidenced by HR 60-100 bpm, CVP 2-6 mm Hg (5-12 cm H_2O), brisk capillary refill (<2 sec), peripheral pulse amplitude >2+ on a 0-4+ scale, urinary output ≥30 ml/h, and stable weight and abdominal girth measurements.

1. Monitor VS q2-4h, and be alert for falling BP and increasing tachycardia, which can occur with moderate to severe fluid loss.
2. Measure I&O and CVP, if available, q2-4h. Because fluid loss requires immediate replacement to prevent shock and circulatory collapse, be alert for and report I&O imbalances. CVP <2 mm Hg (<5 cm H_2O) can occur with volume-related hypotension. Measure orthostatic VS initially and q8h in patients without CVP catheters. Be alert for decreasing BP and increasing HR on standing, which suggests the need for volume expansion.
3. Administer plasma volume expanders as prescribed. For high volumes, use volume control pump to prevent sudden fluid shifts caused by excessive osmotic pressure, which can result in fluid overload.
4. Administer electrolytes (potassium [K^+], calcium [Ca^{2+}]) as prescribed to prevent cardiac dysrhythmias and tetany.
5. Be alert for indicators of hypocalcemia (e.g., muscle twitching, tetany, irritability), which can occur with electrolyte loss.
6. Monitor values for Hct, Hgb, Ca^{2+}, glucose, BUN, and K^+. *Normal values:* Ca^{2+}: 8.5-10.5 mg/dl (4.3-5.3 mEq/L); glucose: <145 mg/dl (2 h postprandial) and 65-110 mg/dl (fasting); BUN: 6-20 mg/dl; and K^+: 3.5-5 mEq/L. Also
   Men: Hct: 40%-54%; Hgb: 14-18 g/dl;
   Women: Hct: 37%-47%; Hgb: 12-16 g/dl.

Pain related to inflammatory process of the pancreas

Desired outcomes: Within 6 h of intervention, patient's subjective perception of discomfort decreases; within 24 h, it is controlled, as documented by a pain scale. Objective indicators, such as splinting of abdominal muscles, are absent or diminished.

1. Assess for and document degree and character of discomfort. Devise a pain scale with patient, rating discomfort from 0 (no pain) to 10 (worst pain).
2. To minimize pancreatic secretions and pain and to maximize needed rest, ensure that patient maintains bed rest.
3. Maintain NPO status to minimize stimulation of pancreatic secretions.

4. Administer opiate analgesics, histamine H_2-receptor antagonists (Table 6-10), and anticholinergics as prescribed; be alert for patient's response to medications, using pain scale. If analgesia is ineffective, consult physician because patient may require a nerve block or other intervention. Optimally, analgesics are administered *via* patient-controlled pumps. Small, frequent doses of IV opiates are more effective than IM injections. Do not give IM injections to individuals with clotting or bleeding complications or unstable BP.

5. Help patient find a comfortable position. A sitting or supine position with knees flexed often helps relax abdominal muscles.

6. Emphasize nonpharmacologic pain interventions: relaxation techniques, distraction, guided imagery, massage. These methods are especially important for patients who develop chronic pancreatitis and are prone to chemical dependence. See **Health-seeking behaviors:** Relaxation technique effective for stress reduction, p. 27.

7. Pancreatitis can be very painful. Prepare significant others for personality changes and behavioral alterations associated with extreme pain and narcotic analgesia. Family members sometimes misinterpret patient's lethargic or unpleasant disposition and may even blame themselves. Reassure them that these are normal responses to severe pain, and high doses of opiates typically are required to alleviate the pain.

8. Monitor patient's respiratory pattern and LOC closely, because both may be depressed by the large amount of opiate analgesics usually required to control pain. If epidural analgesia is used, monitor patient closely for respiratory compromise. Continuous pulse oximetry can serve as a warning system for decreasing oxygen saturation associated with hypoventilation. **Note:** Narcotic analgesics reduce intestinal motility and delay return of normal bowel function.

9. For additional pain interventions, see **Pain**, p. 396, in Appendix One.

Table 6-10   Histamine H_2-receptor antagonists

Drug	Usual Dosage	Comments
cimetidine (Tagamet)	800-1,200 mg/day*	Reduces hepatic blood flow; inhibits metabolism of some drugs in the liver
ranitidine (Zantac)	150-300 mg/day*	5-12 × more potent than cimetidine; fewer drug interactions than with cimetidine
famotidine (Pepcid)	40-120 mg/day*	30-100 × more potent than cimetidine
nizatidine (Axid)	150-300 mg/day†	

*PO, IM, or IV administration or continuous IV infusion titrated to gastric pH value.
†Available only in oral form.

Impaired gas exchange (or risk for same) related to alveolar capillary membrane changes secondary to atelectasis and pulmonary fluid accumulation

Desired outcome: Patient has adequate gas exchange, as evidenced by RR 12-20 breaths/min with normal depth and pattern (eupnea); oxygen saturation $\geq$95%; orientation to time, place, and person; and breath sounds that are clear and audible throughout lung fields.

1. Monitor and document RR q2-4h as indicated by patient's condition. Note pattern, degree of excursion, and whether patient uses accessory muscles of respiration. Consult physician about significant deviations from baseline.
2. Auscultate both lung fields q4-8h. Note abnormal (crackles, rhonchi, wheezes) or diminished breath sounds.
3. Be alert for early signs of hypoxia (e.g., restlessness, agitation, alterations in mentation).
4. Monitor oxygen saturation by pulse oximetry q8h or as indicated. Monitor ABG results as available. Be alert for decreasing oxygen levels.
5. Administer oxygen as prescribed. Check oxygen delivery system q4-8h.
6. Maintain body position that optimizes ventilation and oxygenation. Elevate HOB $\geq$30 degrees, depending on the patient's comfort. If pleural effusion or other defect is present on one side, position patient with unaffected lung dependent to maximize ventilation/perfusion relationship.
7. Avoid overaggressive fluid resuscitation.

Risk for infection related to tissue destruction with resulting necrosis secondary to release of pancreatic enzymes

Desired outcome: Patient remains free of infection, as evidenced by body temperature <37.8° C (<100° F); negative culture results; HR 60-100 bpm; RR 12-20 breaths/min; BP within patient's normal range; and orientation to time, place, and person.

1. Check patient's temperature q4h for increases. Be aware that hypothermia may precede hyperthermia in some individuals.
2. If patient's temperature rises suddenly, obtain specimens for culture of blood, sputum, urine, wound, drains, and other sites as indicated. Monitor culture reports, and consult physician about positive test results.
3. Evaluate patient's orientation and LOC q4-8h. Consult physician about significant deviations from baseline.
4. Monitor BP, HR, and RR q4h. Be alert for increases in HR and RR associated with temperature elevations.
5. Administer parenteral antibiotics in a timely fashion. Reschedule antibiotics if a dose is delayed for longer than 1 h. Recognize that failure to administer antibiotics on schedule can result in inadequate blood levels and treatment failure.
6. Observe all secretions and drainage for changes in appearance or odor that may signal infection.
7. Prevent transmission of potentially infectious agents by using good handwashing technique before and after caring for patient and by disposing of dressings and drainage carefully.

Altered nutrition: Less than body requirements, related to anorexia, dietary restrictions, and digestive dysfunction

Desired outcomes: Within 24 h of hospital discharge, patient is maintaining baseline body weight and shows a positive or balanced nitrogen state on nitrogen studies.

1. Initiate parenteral nutrition and adjust insulin amounts according to blood glucose levels, as prescribed.

2. Provide oral hygiene at frequent intervals to enhance appetite and minimize nausea.

3. Monitor blood sugar levels for hyperglycemia, and be alert for dysphagia, polydipsia, and polyuria, which occur with a hyperglycemic state. These indicators reflect the need for medical evaluation and intervention to ensure proper metabolism of carbohydrates.

4. When the gastric tube is removed, provide diet as prescribed (e.g., small, high-carbohydrate meals at frequent intervals [6/day] with protein added according to patient's tolerance). Keep diet bland to minimize pancreatic stimulation, and instruct patient to avoid stimulants that increase enzyme secretion (e.g., coffee, tea, alcohol, nicotine).

5. Weigh patient daily to assess gain or loss. Weight loss may signal the need to change the diet or provide enzyme replacement therapy.

6. Note amount and degree of steatorrhea (foamy, foul-smelling stools high in fat content) as an indicator of fat intolerance. As prescribed, administer pancreatic enzyme supplements, which are given before introducing fat into the diet.

7. If prescribed, administer other dietary supplements that support nutrition and caloric intake. These may include products that consist of medium-chain triglycerides (MCTs) such as Isocal or MCT oil. These supplements do not require pancreatic enzymes for absorption.

8. Avoid administering pancreatin with hot foods or drinks, which will deactivate enzyme activity.

9. To help alleviate the bloating, nausea, and cramps some patients experience, provide meals in small feedings throughout the day.

See Appendix One for nursing diagnoses and interventions in "Caring for Preoperative and Postoperative Patients," p. 395.

PATIENT-FAMILY TEACHING
AND DISCHARGE PLANNING

Give patient and significant others verbal and written information about the following:

1. Cause for current episode of pancreatitis, if known, so that recurrence may be avoided.

2. Alcohol consumption, which can cause or exacerbate chronic pancreatitis.

3. Availability of chemical dependency programs to prevent or treat drug dependence, which is a common occurrence with chronic pancreatitis, or to treat alcoholism.

4. Availability of community support groups, such as Alcoholics Anonymous.
5. Diet: frequent, small meals that are high in carbohydrates and protein. Food should be bland until gradual return to normal diet is prescribed. Remind patient to avoid enzyme stimulants (e.g., coffee, tea, nicotine, alcohol).
6. Medications, including drug name, purpose, dosage, schedule, precautions, drug/drug and food/drug interactions, and potential side effects.
7. Signs and symptoms of diabetes mellitus: fatigue, weight loss, polydipsia, polyuria, polyphagia.
8. Necessity of medical follow-up; confirm time and date of next medical appointment.
9. Potential for recurrence of steatorrhea, as evidenced by foamy, foul-smelling stools high in fat content. Steatorrhea can indicate recurrence of disease process or ineffectiveness of drug therapy and should be reported to physician.
10. Weighing daily at home; importance of reporting weight loss to physician.
11. If surgery was performed, the indicators of wound infection: redness, swelling, discharge, fever, pain, local warmth.

Pancreatic Tumors

NURSING DIAGNOSES AND INTERVENTIONS

Risk for fluid volume deficit related to postsurgical hemorrhage (due to vascularity of surgical site or multiple anastomosis sites) or fluid shift to third space (interstitial) compartments

Desired outcome: Patient is normovolemic, as evidenced by BP ≥90/60 mm Hg (or within patient's baseline range), HR ≤100 bpm, RR ≤20 breaths/min with normal depth and pattern (eupnea), good skin turgor, brisk capillary refill (<2 sec), balanced I&O, urinary output ≥30 ml/h, stable weight, and moist mucous membranes.

1. Monitor BP, HR, and RR, and check capillary refill in nail beds at frequent intervals. Tachycardia, hypotension, increased respirations, and slow capillary refill can signal dehydration and hypovolemia, which can lead to shock. Also be alert for cool, clammy skin, which can develop with hemorrhage and a low urinary output (<30-40 ml/h for 2 consecutive hours). Consult physician about significant findings.
2. Administer crystalloids and colloids (e.g., albumin) as prescribed. Large amounts of fluid may be necessary because of fluid sequestration, surgical loss, and loss from incisions or drains. Fluid often is prescribed as a baseline amount with additional amounts according to previous 8-h drainage.
3. Prevent increased pressure on suture lines by keeping all tubes patent and free of kinks. Maintain prescribed suction. Consult physician if loss of patency or failure to maintain suction occurs. *Gently* irrigate NG tube with air or saline q4h or as needed. Keep gravity drains dependent to wound site, and secure all connections with tape.

4. Note and document amount and character of drainage from tubes. Drainage from surgical incision or drains may be profuse. Increasing amounts of fluid from surgical incision or drains can suggest infection or fistula formation. Note amount, consistency, color, and odor, and inform surgeon accordingly. Persistent, bloody drainage that is steady or increasing signals active bleeding. Consult physician about significant findings.

5. Monitor blood study results, including PT, for clotting factor and for Hct and Hgb, which can fall with blood loss.
   Optimal values: PT 11-15 sec (men and women); also
   Men: Hct: 40%-54%; Hgb: 14-18 g/dl
   Women: Hct: 37%-47%; Hgb: 12-16 g/dl.

6. Monitor serum protein levels (normal for a random specimen: 2-8 mg/dl), and be alert for weight gain, which may signal third spacing of fluids. Monitor I&O; note whether intake exceeds output. After surgery most of these patients are protein deficient. Low serum protein alters serum colloid osmotic pressure, resulting in fluid shift from intravascular to interstitial compartments (third spacing of body fluids). **Note:** Intravascular fluid loss can occur despite adequate fluid replacement.

7. Monitor laboratory studies for electrolyte imbalances, especially potassium (K^+) and sodium (Na^+). *Normal:* K^+: 3.5-5 mEq/L; Na^+: 137-147 mEq/L.

Impaired skin integrity (or risk for same) related to wound drainage or pressure on incision
Desired outcome: Patient's skin remains intact and shows good wound healing.

1. Promote adequate drainage from drainage tubes to prevent pressure from fluid collection around wound site. Evaluate proper functioning of wall suction and drains. Do not occlude air port of sump drainage devices, which could result in excessive suction. Protect surrounding skin by using Karaya or other nonirritating adhesive disks and stoma pouches over drain or wound sites. Consult ET nurse or wound specialist as available.

2. Assess and document condition of incision and quality and quantity of wound drainage. Fistula formation is a major complication of pancreaticoduodenectomy (Whipple's procedure); therefore, it is important to monitor periincisional skin carefully for signs of irritation. If irritation occurs or a fistula forms, cover site with a pectin wafer skin barrier (with a fistula, then apply a stoma pouch).

3. Keep patient in semi-Fowler's position to minimize pressure on incision. Use pressure-relief mattress to minimize potential for skin breakdown.

4. When regular diet is resumed after surgery, provide small, frequent meals that are high in protein, vitamins, and calories and low in fat. Administer pancreatic enzyme replacements and insulin, as prescribed, for patient who has had a total pancreatectomy. These interventions also help ensure optimal tissue repair.

5. For more information, see "Managing Wound Care," p. 384.

Pain related to major abdominal surgery

Desired outcomes: Within 1 h of intervention, patient's subjective perception of discomfort decreases, as documented by a pain scale. Objective indicators, such as splinting of abdominal muscles, are absent or diminished.

1. Assess degree and quality of discomfort. Devise a pain scale with patient, rating discomfort from 0 (no pain) to 10 (worst pain).
2. Physical dependence on narcotics is of minimal importance in patients who are terminally ill. Administer analgesics liberally. Document degree of pain relief obtained, using pain scale.
3. Note and report patient's failure to respond to analgesics, because peritonitis and pancreatitis are potential postoperative complications.
4. Because intraabdominal pressure may be a source of discomfort, ensure proper drainage from tubes.
5. For additional pain interventions, see **Pain** in Appendix One, p. 396.

See "Hepatitis" for **Risk for impaired skin integrity** related to pruritus, p. 273, **Body image disturbance** related to jaundice, p. 273, and **Altered protection** related to increased risk of bleeding secondary to decreased vitamin K absorption, p. 273.

See Appendix One for nursing diagnoses and interventions in "Caring for Preoperative and Postoperative Patients," p. 395, and "Caring for Patients with Cancer and Other Life-Disrupting Illnesses," p. 423.

PATIENT-FAMILY TEACHING
AND DISCHARGE PLANNING

Give patient and significant others verbal and written information about the following:

1. For patients who develop diabetes mellitus, a review of insulin action, dosage, and administration; diabetic diet; and signs and symptoms of hyperglycemia and hypoglycemia. See "Diabetes Mellitus," p. 217, for more information.
2. Wound care (e.g., cleansing, dressing changes, care of drains if patient is discharged with them) and indicators of wound infection (e.g., drainage, warmth along incision line, persistent incisional redness, swelling, fever, pain).
3. Medications, including drug name, purpose, dosage, schedule, precautions, drug/drug and food/drug interactions, and potential side effects.
4. Arrangements for community services in home care (e.g., Visiting Nurse Association) or placement in hospice facility.

Hematologic Disorders

7

SECTION ONE: DISORDERS OF COAGULATION

Thrombocytopenia

NURSING DIAGNOSES AND INTERVENTIONS

Altered protection related to increased risk of bleeding secondary to decreased platelet count

Desired outcomes: Patient is free of signs of bleeding, as evidenced by secretions and excretions negative for blood, BP ≥90/60 mm Hg or within patient's baseline range, HR ≤100 bpm, RR 12-20 breaths/min with normal depth and pattern (eupnea), and absence of bruising.

1. Monitor patient for hematuria, melena, epistaxis, hematemesis, or severe ecchymosis. Teach patient to be alert for and report these indicators promptly.
2. When appropriate, protect patient from injury by padding and keeping up side rails.
3. When possible, avoid venipuncture. If performed, apply pressure on site for 5-10 min or until bleeding stops.
4. Avoid IM injections. If performed, use small-gauge needle when possible.
5. Monitor platelet count daily; optimal range is 150,000-400,000/μl.
6. Advise patient to avoid straining at stool or coughing, which increases intracranial pressure and can result in intracranial hemorrhage. Obtain prescription for stool softeners, if indicated, to prevent constipation. Teach patient anticonstipation routine as described in **Constipation,** p. 420, in Appendix One, "Caring for Patients on Prolonged Bed Rest."
7. Administer corticosteroids as prescribed to help minimize platelet destruction.
8. Advise patient to use electric razor and soft-bristled toothbrush.
9. Administer platelets as prescribed, and be alert for indicators of transfusion reaction: chills, back pain, dyspnea, hives, wheezing. See Table 7-1.
10. Consult physician about significant findings.

Text continued on page 297.

Table 7-1 Commonly used blood products

Product	Approximate Volume	Indications	Precautions/Comments
Whole blood (WB)	500-510 ml (450 WB; 50-60 anticoagulants)	Acute, severe blood loss; hypovolemic shock; increases both red cell mass and plasma.	Must be ABO and Rh compatible. Do not mix with dextrose solutions; always prime tubing with normal saline. Observe for dyspnea, orthopnea, cyanosis, and anxiety as signs of circulatory overload; monitor VS.
Packed RBCs	250 ml	Increase RBC mass and O_2-carrying capacity of the blood.	Must be ABO and Rh compatible. Leukocyte-depleted RBCs may be used to reduce the risk of antibody formation and nonhemolytic reactions. Irradiated RBCs may be used to prevent graft-versus-host disease in immunocompromised patients. Packed RBCs have less volume than WB, which reduces the risk of fluid overload.

Continued.

Hematologic

Table 7-1 Commonly used blood products—cont'd

Product	Approximate Volume	Indications	Precautions/Comments
Fresh frozen plasma	250 ml	Treatment of choice for combined coagulation factor deficiencies and factor V and XI deficiencies; alternate treatment for factor VII, VIII, IX, and X deficiencies when concentrates are not available.	Must be ABO compatible; supplies clotting factors. Usual dosage is 10-15 ml/kg body weight; transfuse within 24 h of thawing. Do not use if patient needs volume expansion.
Random donor platelet concentrate	50 ml (usual adult dose is 5-6 U)	Treatment of choice for thrombocytopenia; also used for leukemia and hypoplastic anemia.	Usual dosage is 0.1 U/kg body weight to increase platelet count to 25,000/μl; administer as rapidly as tolerated. ABO compatibility is preferable. Effectiveness is reduced by fever, sepsis, and splenomegaly. Febrile reactions are common. Use special platelet tubing and filter. Special filters are available for removing leukocytes and thus reducing the risk of alloimmunization to human leukocyte antigen (HLA). Platelets must be infused within 4 h of initiation.

Platelet concentrate by platelet pheresis (single donor platelets)	200 ml (may vary)	Treatment for thrombocytopenia that is refractory to random donor platelets.	Involves removing donor's venous blood, removing platelets by differential centrifuge, and returning blood to donor. Approximately 3–4 L of whole blood is processed to obtain a therapeutic dose of platelets. May use special donors who are HLA matched to patient.
Cryoprecipitate (factor VIII)	10–25 ml	Routine treatment for hemophilia (factor VIII deficiency) and fibrinogen deficiency (factor XIII deficiency).	Made from fresh frozen plasma; infuse immediately upon thawing.
AHG (factor VIII) concentrates	20 ml	Alternative treatment for hemophilia A.	Allergic and febrile reactions occur frequently. Administer by syringe or component drip set. Can store at refrigerator temperature, making it convenient for hemophiliacs during travel.
Factor II, VII, IX, X concentrate	20 ml	Treatment of choice for hemophilia B and factor IX deficiencies.	Can precipitate clotting. Allergic and febrile reactions occur occasionally. Contraindicated in liver disease.

Continued.

Hematologic

Table 7-1   Commonly used blood products—cont'd

Product	Approximate Volume	Indications	Precautions/Comments
Albumin*	50 or 250 ml	Hypovolemic shock, hypoalbuminemia, protein replacement for burn patients.	Osmotically equal to 5 × its volume of plasma. Used as a volume expander in conjunction with crystalloids. Also used in hypoalbuminemic states. Commercially available.
Plasma protein fraction*	250 ml (83% albumin with some alpha- and beta-globulins)	Volume expansion.	Commercially available; expensive. Certain lots reported to have caused hypotension, possibly related to vasoactive amines used in preparation.
Granulocyte transfusion (collected from a single apheresis donor)	200 ml (may vary)	Leukemia with granulocytopenia related to treatment.	Uncommon treatment; febrile and allergic symptoms are common. Must be ABO compatible.

*No risk of disease transmission. **Note:** When administering blood products, it is important to recognize that delivery of most blood products carries some risk (e.g., transmission of the human immunodeficiency virus [HIV], hepatitis B, hepatitis C, cytomegalovirus, and human T-cell lymphotrophic virus, type I [HTLV-1]).

Note: DNA recombinant technology may reduce complications from factor concentrates.

Altered cerebral, peripheral, and renal tissue perfusion (or risk for same) related to interrupted blood flow secondary to presence of thrombotic component, which results in sensitization and clumping of platelets in blood vessels

Desired outcome: Patient's cerebral, peripheral, and renal perfusion are adequate, as evidenced by orientation to time, place, and person; normoreactive pupillary responses; absence of headaches, dizziness, and visual disturbances; peripheral pulses >2+ on a 0-4+ scale; and urine output ≥30 ml/h.

1. Assess patient for changes in LOC and pupillary responses.
2. Monitor for headaches, dizziness, or visual disturbances.
3. Palpate peripheral pulses. Be alert for pulses ≤2+.
4. Assess urine output. Adequate perfusion is reflected by urine output ≥30 ml/h for 2 consecutive hours.
5. Monitor I&O. Patient should be well hydrated (2-3 L/day) to increase perfusion of small vessels.

Pain related to joint discomfort secondary to hemorrhagic episodes or blood extravasation into tissues.

Desired outcomes: Within 1 h of intervention, patient's subjective perception of discomfort decreases, as documented by a pain scale. Objective indicators, such as grimacing, are absent or diminished.

1. Monitor for fatigue, malaise, and joint pain. Devise a pain scale with patient, rating discomfort on a scale of 0 (no pain) to 10 (worst pain).
2. Maintain a calm, restful environment; provide periods of undisturbed rest.
3. Elevate legs to minimize joint discomfort in lower extremities. Support legs with pillows. Avoid gatching bed at the knees, which could occlude popliteal vessels.
4. Use a bed cradle to reduce pressure on tissues on the lower extremities.
5. Administer analgesics as prescribed. Document relief obtained, using pain scale. **Caution:** Aspirin and other nonsteroidal antiinflammatory drugs are contraindicated because of their antiplatelet action.

Risk for fluid volume deficit related to postsplenectomy bleeding/hemorrhage

Desired outcome: Patient is normovolemic, as evidenced by BP ≥90/60 mm Hg (or within patient's normal range); HR ≤ 100 bpm; RR 12-20 breaths/min with normal depth and pattern (eupnea); soft, nondistended abdomen; and absence of frank bleeding.

1. Monitor postoperative VS for changes that may indicate bleeding (e.g., decreasing BP and increasing HR). Be alert for restlessness as well.
2. Inspect abdomen for distention, and question patient about abdominal pain or tenderness, any of which can signal internal bleeding.
3. Inspect surgical site for frank bleeding.
4. Monitor postoperative platelet count. Approximately 60%-70% of postsplenectomy patients have increased platelet counts. Optimal range for these patients is 200,000-300,000/μl.
5. Consult physician about significant findings.

Hematologic

6. If surgery is performed, see nursing diagnoses and interventions in Appendix One, "Caring for Preoperative and Postoperative Patients," p. 395.

PATIENT-FAMILY TEACHING AND DISCHARGE PLANNING

Give patient and significant others verbal and written information about the following:

1. Importance of preventing trauma, which can cause bleeding.
2. Seeking medical attention for *any* signs of bleeding or infection. Review signs and symptoms of common infections (e.g., upper respiratory infection, urinary tract infection, wound infection). Signs and symptoms of common infections are described in **Risk for infection** in "Care of the Renal Transplant Recipient," p. 85. Also teach patient to assess for hematuria, melena, hematemesis, oozing from mucous membranes, and petechiae.
3. Importance of regular medical follow-up for platelet counts.
4. If patient is discharged on corticosteroids, the potential side effects that require medical attention: acne, moon face, buffalo hump, hypertension, gastric upset, weight gain, thinning of arms and legs, edema, and mood changes. Stress the importance of *not* discontinuing steroids unless directed to by physician.
5. Other medications, including drug name, dosage, purpose, schedule, precautions, drug/drug and food/drug interactions, and potential side effects.

Hemophilia

NURSING DIAGNOSES AND INTERVENTIONS

Altered protection related to increased risk of bleeding secondary to clotting factor deficiency

Desired outcome: Patient is free of bleeding, as evidenced by systolic BP $\geq$90 mm Hg (or within patient's baseline range), HR $\leq$100 bpm, RR 12-20 breaths/min with normal depth and pattern (eupnea), and secretions and excretions negative for blood.

1. Monitor VS for signs of bleeding, including hypotension and increased HR. Also be alert for restlessness.
2. Monitor patient for evidence of bleeding: swollen joints, abdominal pain, hematuria, hematemesis, melena, and epistaxis.
3. If signs of bleeding occur, elevate affected area if possible and apply cold compresses and gentle pressure to the site.
4. When indicated, institute measures to minimize the risk of bleeding from trauma (e.g., keeping side rails up and padded, assisting with ambulation, limiting invasive procedures if possible).
5. Advise patient to use electric razor and soft-bristled toothbrush.
6. Do not administer aspirin; caution patient about its anticoagulant action.
7. Administer clotting factors as prescribed (see Table 7-1).
8. Teach patient the importance of lifetime medical follow-up and

regular factor transfusions. For patient in whom factor VIII prophylaxis is used, teach patient or significant other the procedure for IV administration of factor VIII as appropriate.

Risk for impaired skin integrity and **Impaired tissue integrity** related to altered blood circulation to tissues secondary to bleeding

Desired outcome: Patient's skin and tissue remain intact and show no bruising or swelling.

1. Inspect patient's skin at least q4h, being alert for bruising, pressure areas, and swelling.
2. Apply ice or pressure over sites of intradermal bleeding to promote vasoconstriction.
3. Handle patient gently to minimize risk of tissue trauma.
4. To enhance joint mobility and perfusion to tissues, assist patient with ROM exercises daily. However, avoid exercise for 48 h after bleeding to prevent recurrence.
5. To promote circulation to tissues, assist patient with ambulation when it is tolerated.

Pain related to swollen joints (hemarthrosis)

Desired outcomes: Within 1 h of intervention, patient's subjective perception of discomfort decreases, as documented by a pain scale. Objective indicators, such as grimacing, are absent or diminished.

1. Monitor patient for joint discomfort. Devise a pain scale with patient, rating discomfort on a scale of 0 (no pain) to 10 (worst pain).
2. Apply splints or other supportive devices to joints; immobilize joints in slight flexion.
3. Elevate or position pillows under affected joints to promote comfort.
4. Administer analgesics as prescribed; do not use aspirin because of its anticoagulant action. Document pain relief achieved, using pain scale.
5. Assist patient with ambulation as needed.
6. As needed, use ice for its topical analgesia and ability to constrict vessels, which will reduce swelling. **Caution:** Avoid use of warm thermotherapy for these patients, because it will increase swelling.
7. Discuss with patient the importance of frequent assessment of joint function to allow rapid identification and treatment of hemophilic arthritis.

PATIENT-FAMILY TEACHING
AND DISCHARGE PLANNING

Give patient and significant others verbal and written information about the following:

1. Importance of avoiding trauma, and necessity of seeking medical attention for any bleeding.
2. Phone numbers to call in emergencies.
3. Procedure if bleeding occurs: apply cold compresses and gentle, direct pressure; elevate affected part if possible; seek medical attention promptly.

Hematologic

4. Importance of notifying physician if dental procedures need to be done.
5. Importance of lifetime medical follow-up and regular factor transfusions.
6. Importance of frequent assessment of joint function to allow rapid identification and treatment of hemophilic arthritis.

IN ADDITION

7. In patients for whom factor VIII prophylaxis is used, patient or significant other will require instruction in IV administration of factor VIII.

Disseminated Intravascular Coagulation

NURSING DIAGNOSES AND INTERVENTIONS

Altered cardiopulmonary, peripheral, renal, and cerebral tissue perfusion related to interrupted blood flow secondary to coagulation/fibrinolysis processes

Desired outcome: After treatment, patient has adequate cardiopulmonary, peripheral, renal, and cerebral perfusion, as evidenced by BP ≥90/60 mm Hg and HR ≤100 bpm (or within patient's baseline range); peripheral pulse amplitude >2+ on a 0-4+ scale; urinary output ≥30 ml/h; equal and normoreactive pupils; normal/baseline motor function; and orientation to time, place, and person.

1. Monitor VS. Be alert for and report decreased BP, increased HR, or decreased amplitude of peripheral pulses, which signal that coagulation is occurring.
2. Monitor I&O; report output <30 ml/h despite adequate intake, which is another indicator of the coagulation process.
3. Perform neurologic checks (orientation, pupil function, and motor response) and assess LOC to evaluate cerebral perfusion. If signs of impaired cerebral perfusion occur, protect patient from injury by instituting measures such as keeping bed in lowest position and side rails up.
4. Monitor for hemorrhage from surgical wounds, GI tract, and mucous membranes, which can occur after fibrinolysis.
5. Monitor laboratory studies for values suggestive of disseminated intravascular coagulation (DIC): low fibrinogen (<200 mg/dl), low platelet count (<250,000/μl), increased fibrin split products (>8 g/ml), increased PT (>11-15 sec), and increased PTT (>40-100 sec).
6. Report significant findings to physician; prepare for transfer to ICU if condition worsens.

Altered protection related to increased risk of bleeding secondary to hemorrhagic component of disseminated intravascular coagulation

Desired outcome: Patient is free of signs of bleeding, as evidenced by systolic BP ≥90 mm Hg, HR ≤100 bpm (or within patient's normal range); RR 12-20 breaths/min with normal depth and pattern (eupnea); urinary output ≥30 ml/h; secretions and excretions negative for blood; stable abdominal girth measurements; and orientation to time, place, and person.

1. Monitor VS and LOC at frequent intervals; report significant changes. Be alert for hypotension, tachycardia, dyspnea, and disorientation, which can signal hemorrhage. **Note:** Be careful with pressure used with BP cuffs; frequent BP readings may cause bleeding under the cuff.
2. Monitor coagulation studies; be alert for PTT >40-100 sec.
3. Use a reagent stick to check stool, urine, emesis, and nasogastric drainage for blood.
4. Monitor for internal bleeding by measuring abdominal girth q8h. Also assess for abdominal pain and a boardlike abdomen, other signs of GI bleeding.
5. Assess puncture sites regularly for oozing or bleeding.
6. Be alert for other signs of bleeding: joint pain and headache. Visual changes may signal retinal hemorrhage.
7. Avoid giving IM injections or performing venipunctures for blood drawing.
8. Administer blood products (fresh frozen plasma, packed RBCs, platelets [see Table 7-1]), and IV fluids as prescribed.
9. Advise patient to use electric shavers and soft-bristled toothbrushes.
10. See Table 7-2 for clinical conditions that can activate DIC.

Risk for impaired skin integrity or **Impaired tissue integrity** related to altered circulation secondary to hemorrhage and thrombosis

Desired outcome: Patient's skin and tissue remain intact.

1. Assess patient's skin, noting changes in color, temperature, and sensation, which may signal decreased perfusion and can lead to tissue damage.
2. Eliminate or minimize pressure points by ensuring that patient turns q2h and by using sheepskin on elbows and heels. Do not pull on extremities when turning patient.
3. Keep patient's extremities warm to prevent tissue hypoxia.
4. If patient has areas of breakdown, see "Managing Wound Care," p. 384.

See "Pulmonary Embolus" for **Altered protection** related to increased risk of bleeding or hemorrhage secondary to anticoagulant therapy, p. 7.

PATIENT-FAMILY TEACHING AND DISCHARGE PLANNING

See patient's primary diagnosis.

Table 7-2 Clinical conditions that can activate disseminated intravascular coagulation

Obstetric	GI Disorders	Tissue Damage	Infections	Hemolytic Processes	Vascular Disorders	Miscellaneous
Abruptio placentae	Cirrhosis	Surgery	Viral	Transfusion reaction	Shock	Fat or pulmonary embolism
Toxemia	Hepatic necrosis	Trauma	Bacterial	Acute hemolysis secondary to infection or immunologic disorder	Aneurysm	Snake bite
Amniotic fluid embolism	Pancreatitis	Burns	Rickettsial		Giant hemangioma	Neoplastic disorder
Septic abortion	Peritoneovenous shunts	Prolonged extracorporeal circulation	Protozoal			Acute anoxia
Retained dead fetus	Necrotizing enterocolitis	Transplant rejection				
		Heat stroke				

SECTION TWO: NEOPLASTIC DISORDERS OF THE HEMATOPOIETIC SYSTEM

Lymphomas

NURSING DIAGNOSES AND INTERVENTIONS

Activity intolerance related to imbalance between oxygen supply and demand secondary to decreased oxygen-carrying capacity of the blood due to anemia

Desired outcome: After treatment, patient rates perceived exertion at ≤3 on a 0-10 scale and exhibits tolerance to activity, as evidenced by RR 12-20 breaths/min with normal depth and pattern (eupnea), HR ≤100 bpm, and absence of headache and dizziness.

1. As patient performs ADLs, be alert for indicators of decreased tissue oxygenation: dyspnea on exertion, dizziness, palpitations, headaches, verbalization of increased perceived exertion level (see description, p. 413).
2. Provide frequent rest periods between care activities, allowing time for at least 90 min of undisturbed rest.
3. Reassure patient that symptoms usually are relieved and tolerance for activity increases with therapy.
4. As patient's condition improves, encourage increase in activities to tolerance. Set specific goals with patient (e.g., "Today I would like you to walk from your room to the nurses' station and back three times" [or appropriate number, depending on patient's tolerance]).
5. Administer oxygen as prescribed to increase arterial oxygen content.

Altered nutrition: Less than body requirements related to decreased intake secondary to fatigue, impairment of oral mucosa, or anorexia

Desired outcome: By a minimum of 24 h before hospital discharge, patient exhibits adequate nutrition, as evidenced by maintenance of or return to baseline body weight.

1. Weigh patient daily and document dietary intake.
2. If patient is easily fatigued, encourage small, frequent meals; document intake.
3. Monitor for oral lesions or soreness of gums, tongue, and esophagus. If oral lesions or cracks are present, encourage soft, bland foods.
4. For patient with decreased appetite, encourage significant others to bring in patient's favorite foods and stay with patient during meals to encourage eating.
5. Administer vitamins and minerals as prescribed.

Risk for infection related to inadequate secondary defenses secondary to altered WBC count and patient's decreased resistance to infection due to radiation or chemotherapy

Desired outcome: Patient is free of infection, as evidenced by normothermia, HR ≤100 bpm, RR 12-20 breaths/min with normal depth

Hematologic

and pattern (eupnea), and absence of erythema, warmth, and drainage at any invasive or wound sites.

1. Perform meticulous handwashing before touching patient.
2. Report any signs of systemic infection (e.g., fever); obtain prescription for blood, wound, and urine cultures as indicated. Administer antibiotics as prescribed.
3. Monitor for and report any signs of local infection, such as sore throat or erythematous or draining wounds.
4. Provide oral care at frequent intervals to prevent oral lesions, which may result in bleeding and infection.
5. Provide and encourage adequate perianal hygiene to prevent rectal abscess. Avoid giving medications or taking temperature rectally.
6. Avoid invasive procedures, if possible.
7. Encourage ambulation, deep breathing, turning, and coughing to prevent problems of immobility, which can result in pneumonia and skin breakdown.
8. Teach patient and significant others the signs and symptoms of infection and the importance of notifying staff or physician promptly if they develop.

See "Disseminated Intravascular Coagulation" for **Altered protection** related to increased risk of bleeding, p. 300.

See Appendix One, "Caring for Preoperative and Postoperative Patients," p. 395, and "Caring for Patients with Cancer and Other Life-Disrupting Illnesses," p. 423.

PATIENT-FAMILY TEACHING
AND DISCHARGE PLANNING

Give patient and significant others verbal and written information about the following:

1. For patients in stage I or stage II, resumption of normal life-style with minor adjustments, as prescribed.
2. Continuing radiation or chemotherapy, if prescribed, which is given on an outpatient basis; confirm date and time of next appointment.
3. Signs and symptoms that require medical attention: persistent fever, weight loss, enlarged lymph nodes, malaise, and decreased exercise tolerance.
4. Importance of preventing infection and avoiding exposure to individuals with infection, which is essential because of alterations in WBC count and patient's decreased resistance to infection secondary to therapy. Teach patient the indicators of common infections (e.g., urinary tract, upper respiratory, and wound infection). See **Risk for infection,** p. 85, in "Care of the Renal Transplant Recipient."
5. Importance of maintaining good nutritional habits to increase resistance to infection.
6. Referral to American Cancer Society and local support groups.
7. Avoiding trauma, which can cause bruising, especially with thrombocytopenia, which can occur secondary to chemotherapy.
8. If appropriate, measures for assisting patient with ADLs.

Acute Leukemia

NURSING DIAGNOSES AND INTERVENTIONS

Risk for infection related to inadequate secondary defenses secondary to myelosuppression from disease process or therapy

Desired outcome: Patient is free of infection, as evidenced by normothermia, negative culture results, absence of adventitious breath sounds, HR ≤100 bpm, and well-healing wounds.

1. Monitor patient's temperature frequently. If any infections are suspected, obtain prescription for a culture. Report temperature >38° C (100.4° F) that lasts >24 h and occurs concurrently with chills and/or HR >100 bpm.
2. Be aware that as the neutrophil count decreases, the risk of infection increases. When patient becomes neutropenic, perform reverse (protective) isolation using a gown, mask, and gloves; provide a private room.
3. Perform meticulous handwashing before caring for patient.
4. Avoid all invasive procedures (e.g., catheterization) unless absolutely necessary. When such procedures are performed, use strict asepsis.
5. Assist patient with ambulation when possible. Institute turning, coughing, and deep breathing at frequent intervals to help prevent problems of immobility (e.g., skin breakdown, respiratory dysfunction), which can result in infection.
6. Provide oral hygiene and perianal care at frequent intervals.
7. Monitor I&O, and maintain adequate hydration by encouraging 3 L/day of fluids unless contraindicated.
8. Administer antibiotic therapy if prescribed.
9. Administer transfusion of granulocytes if prescribed.

Altered protection related to increased risk of bleeding secondary to decreased platelet count

Desired outcomes: Patient is free of symptoms of bleeding, as evidenced by BP ≥90/60 mm Hg, HR ≤100 bpm (or within patient's baseline range), and excretions and secretions negative for blood.

1. Monitor platelet counts; with counts <50,000/μl, the risk of bleeding increases dramatically. Monitor Hct and Hgb for values suggestive of bleeding, and consult physician about values outside the normal ranges, which are: *Men:* Hct: 40%-54%; Hgb: 14-18 g/dl; *Women:* Hct: 37%-47%; Hgb: 12-16 g/dl.
2. Request that patient alert staff members to oozing of blood from gums.
3. Inspect patient's skin, mouth, nose, urine, feces, sputum, emesis, and IV sites for signs for bleeding. Test all excretions for occult blood.
4. Monitor VS at frequent intervals, and be alert for signs of bleeding (e.g., hypotension, increased HR).
5. Limit invasive procedures to those that are absolutely necessary.
6. Use small-gauge needle when possible. Maintain gentle pressure on injection site until bleeding stops.

Hematologic

7. If bleeding occurs, elevate affected part, if possible, and apply cold compresses and gentle pressure.
8. Pad side rails to prevent trauma.
9. Administer stool softeners as prescribed to minimize risk of rectal bleeding.
10. Teach patient the signs and symptoms of bleeding and the importance of notifying staff promptly if they occur.
11. Advise patient to use soft-bristled toothbrushes or sponge-tipped applicators and electric shavers.

Activity intolerance related to imbalance between oxygen supply and demand secondary to decreased oxygen-carrying capacity of the blood due to erythrocyte destruction

Desired outcome: After treatment, patient rates his or her perceived exertion at ≤3 on a 0-10 scale and exhibits tolerance to activity, as evidenced by HR ≤100 bpm, RR ≤20 breaths/min, and absence of headache and dizziness.

1. Monitor patient's response to activity, and ask patient to rate his or her perceived exertion. See **Risk for activity intolerance** in Appendix One, p. 413, for a description.
2. If prescribed, administer packed RBCs to restore normal erythrocyte level (see Table 7-1).
3. Assist patient with ADLs as necessary.
4. Provide periods of undisturbed rest.
5. Minimize restlessness, which increases oxygen use, by providing frequent comfort measures, such as back rubs.
6. Administer oxygen if prescribed. Encourage deep-breathing exercises, which may promote oxygenation by enhancing gas exchange.
7. As patient's condition improves, encourage activities to tolerance. Set mutually agreed on goals (e.g., "Can you walk the length of the hall two or three times this morning?" [or appropriate number, depending on tolerance]). Be alert for and document activity intolerance, as evidenced by pallor, weakness, headache, and dizziness. Discontinue activity and help patient get back into bed if these symptoms occur.

Altered renal tissue perfusion related to interrupted blood flow secondary to destruction of RBCs and their precipitation in the kidney tubules

Desired outcome: By a minimum of 24 h before hospital discharge, patient has adequate renal perfusion, as evidenced by balanced I&O, urinary output ≥30 ml/h, and stable weight.

1. Monitor for and report signs of renal insufficiency: positive fluid balance, weight gain, urinary output <30 ml/h despite adequate intake.
2. Maintain adequate hydration of at least 2-3 L/day (unless contraindicated) to enhance urinary flow.
3. Encourage ambulation or in-bed exercises to patient's tolerance to promote renal circulation.
4. Consult physician about significant findings.

See Appendix One for nursing diagnoses and interventions in "Caring for Patients with Cancer and Other Life-Disrupting Illnesses," p. 423.

PATIENT-FAMILY TEACHING AND DISCHARGE PLANNING

Give patient and significant others verbal and written information about the following:

1. Importance of avoiding infections and bleeding and measures to prevent them: avoid exposure to individuals with infection; maintain good hygiene; avoid situations with high risk of trauma or injury; and report any signs of infection to physician (e.g., fever, chills, malaise).

2. Side effects of chemotherapy: constipation, alopecia, nausea, vomiting, anorexia, diarrhea, stomatitis, skin rash, nail changes, hyperpigmentation of the skin, weight gain from steroid use, ecchymosis, and cystitis. For more information, see "Caring for Patients with Cancer and Other Life-Disrupting Illnesses," p. 423.

3. Importance of good nutrition; eating small, frequent meals; consuming 2-3 L/day of fluids (unless contraindicated by cardiac or renal disorder); and using soft-bristled toothbrush and electric razor.

4. Referrals to American Cancer Society, Leukemia Society of America, local support groups, and home care or hospice groups, if appropriate.

Chronic Leukemia

NURSING DIAGNOSES AND INTERVENTIONS

See "Acute Leukemia," p. 305.

Although patients with chronic leukemia survive longer and have less severe symptoms, the same principles and nursing interventions apply as for acute leukemia. If a splenectomy is performed, also see Appendix One, "Caring for Preoperative and Postoperative Patients," p. 395, and "Caring for Patients with Cancer and Other Life-Disrupting Illnesses," p. 423.

PATIENT-FAMILY TEACHING AND DISCHARGE PLANNING

See this section in "Acute Leukemia," above.

Hematologic

Musculoskeletal Disorders

8

SECTION ONE: MUSCULAR AND CONNECTIVE TISSUE DISORDERS

Dislocation/Subluxation

Pain related to joint changes and corrective therapy

Desired outcomes: Within 1-2 h of intervention, patient's subjective perception of pain decreases, as documented by a pain scale. Objective indicators, such as grimacing, are absent or diminished. Patient demonstrates ability to perform ADLs without complaints of discomfort.

1. Devise and help patient use a rating system to evaluate pain and analgesic relief on a scale of 0 (no pain) to 10 (worst pain).
2. Administer analgesics and antiinflammatory agents as prescribed (or 30 min before strenuous activity), and document their effectiveness, using pain scale. As appropriate, teach patient about the function of epidural anesthesia or patient-controlled analgesia (PCA).
3. Teach patient nonpharmacologic methods of pain control: guided imagery; graduated breathing (as in Lamaze); enhanced relaxation; massage; biofeedback; cutaneous stimulation (*via* a counterirritant, such as oil of wintergreen); a transcutaneous electrical nerve stimulation (TENS) device; warm or cool thermotherapy; music therapy; tactile, auditory, visual, or verbal distraction.
4. Use traditional nursing interventions to counteract pain: back rubs, repositioning, encouraging patient to express his or her feelings.
5. Incorporate rest, local warmth or cold, and elevation of affected joints, when possible, to help control discomfort.
6. Advise patient to coordinate the time of peak effectiveness of antiinflammatory agent with periods of exercise or mandatory use of joints.
7. Instruct patient in the use of moist heat and hydrotherapy, which help reduce long-term discomfort.
8. For additional interventions, see this nursing diagnosis in the Appendix One, p. 396.

Impaired physical mobility related to musculoskeletal impairment and adjustment to a new walking gait with an assistive device

Desired outcomes: By hospital discharge, patient demonstrates adequate upper body strength for use of an assistive device. Patient demonstrates appropriate use of assistive device on flat and uneven surfaces.

1. Before ambulation, make sure patient's upper extremities have the necessary strength for an assistive device by incorporating the interventions listed in **Risk for disuse syndrome,** p. 416, in Appendix One. Triceps muscle strength is especially important for ambulation with crutches or a walker. Having patients push down on the bed as they extend their arms to lift their buttocks off the bed strengthens triceps muscles.
2. Use a thorough discussion followed by a demonstration to teach patient how assistive device is used.
3. When fitting crutches, make sure patient is wearing flat-heeled, properly fitting, supportive shoes. With patient standing and with his or her elbows slightly flexed at 10-30 degrees, make sure crutch tops rest 1-1½ in (or the width of two fingers) below the axillae. Be aware that complaints of upper extremity paresthesia may indicate improperly fitted crutches. Ensure that crutches have rubber tips to prevent slipping and rubber axillary pads to reduce pressure at axillae.
4. Once assistive device is in position, repeat instructions and then supervise ambulation. Ambulation should begin in small increments on level ground and eventually progress to all surfaces patient might encounter after hospital discharge.
5. Make sure that before discharge, patient demonstrates independence in ambulation with assistive device on level surfaces, stairs, and getting in and out of a car.

Knowledge deficit: Need for elevation of involved extremity, use of thermotherapy, and prescribed exercises

Desired outcome: Within 8 h of instruction, patient verbalizes understanding of the purpose of treatment and returns a demonstration of the exercise regimen and use of elevation and thermotherapy.

1. Teach patient the pathophysiology of the injury and concomitant inflammatory response.
2. Instruct patient to keep injured extremity elevated until edema is no longer a problem (usually 3-7 days). Explain that the involved extremity should be kept above the level of the heart, with each successively distal joint elevated above the level of the preceding joint.
3. Explain that ice usually is applied for the first 48 h to prevent excessive edema. (**Note:** Ice is contraindicated for patients suspected of having compartment syndrome, as well as for those with peripheral vascular disease, diminished local sensation, coagulation disorders, or similar pathologic conditions that increase the possibility of thermal injury.) Advise patient to apply thermotherapy with at least two thicknesses of terry cloth to protect the skin from injury.
4. Give a detailed explanation of each prescribed exercise and its purpose. The optimum method is to describe the exercise, demonstrate it, and then have the patient return the demonstration. Give the patient written instructions that describe the exercises and that tell how many repetitions of each should be performed and how often the exercises should be done. Include a phone number in case the patient has questions after being discharged from the hospital.

Musculoskeletal

Knowledge deficit: Care and assessment of the casted extremity
Desired outcomes: Within 12 h of instruction, patient verbalizes understanding of the care of the casted extremity and knowledge of self-assessment of neurovascular status. Also, patient returns a demonstration of the use of ambulatory aids, exercise, and general cast care.

1. Explain the function of patient's cast.
2. Instruct patient in the purpose and procedure for neurovascular checks of casted extremity. Explain that they should be performed q2-4h for the first 2 days, and then 4 ×/day until the cast is removed. Advise patient to be alert for and promptly report pallor, cyanosis, coolness, decreased pulse or capillary refill, increasing pain, decreasing sensation, and paralysis of distal portion of casted limb.
3. Make sure patient demonstrates independence in ADLs and ambulation before discharge. If ambulatory aids are used (crutches, walker, cane), be sure patient demonstrates independent use on all surfaces likely to be encountered and that patient understands precautions. Be sure patient will have adequate assistance or is independent in self-care before discharge. If necessary, initiate a referral for home care.
4. Instruct patient to exercise parts of extremity not immobilized by cast (e.g., wiggling toes or fingers and putting the most proximal joints through complete ROM), unless doing so is contraindicated by the injury or the physician. Isometric exercises for muscles beneath the cast will be prescribed for some patients. When prescribed, explain the purpose of these exercises and provide instructions, including written instructions that review the information and give the frequency and number of repetitions of each exercise.
5. Provide patient with a phone number to call if problems or questions arise after he or she is discharged from the hospital.
6. Instruct patient in basic components of cast care:

WITH PLASTER OF PARIS CAST
1. Use plastic bags while showering or in the rain to avoid getting cast wet. Damp cloths can be used to clean soiled cast surfaces, but saturation must be avoided.
2. Use white shoe polish *sparingly* to cover stains.
3. Petal cast edges with tape if they are rough or if cast crumbs are falling into cast. If edges continue to irritate skin, pad them with moleskin, sheepskin, or foam rubber. Notify physician if irritation continues.
4. Avoid putting anything beneath cast because skin there is more susceptible to injury.
5. Report any pain, burning, changes in sensation, drainage on cast, or foul odor because they can signal pressure necrosis.

WITH SYNTHETIC CAST MATERIAL
1. Physician may permit immersion in water, depending on materials used, type of injury, and whether surgery was performed. If immersion is allowed, dry cast thoroughly (using a hair dryer on a cool setting) to prevent skin maceration.

2. If permitted, dirt or sand can be rinsed from the cast.

Knowledge deficit: Potential for joint weakness, and techniques for applying external supports and assessing neurovascular status

Desired outcome: Within 8 h of instruction, patient verbalizes understanding of the potential for joint weakness and returns demonstrations of how to apply external supports and of self-checking neurovascular status.

1. Advise patient about the potential for joint weakness and the need for limiting or omitting activities that aggravate the condition.
2. If physician has prescribed elastic wraps, elastic supports, or orthotic devices to supplement joint strength until exercise has compensated for joint laxity, explain and demonstrate their use and application. Show patient how to apply elastic wraps diagonally from distal to proximal areas with an overlap of two-thirds to one-half the width of the wrap for each successive layer.
3. Teach patient how to self-check neurovascular status 15 min after application and to rewrap joint if a deficit is found. For details, see **Knowledge deficit:** Care and assessment of casted extremity, p. 310.
4. Make sure patient receives two wraps, supports, or orthotic devices to allow for cleaning. These devices typically are washed with mild soap and water and allowed to air dry without stretching (or see manufacturer's recommendations).

Risk for peripheral neurovascular dysfunction related to interrupted arterial flow secondary to compression from circumferential cast or dressing

Desired outcomes: Patient has adequate peripheral neurovascular function in involved extremity, as evidenced by normal color, warmth, brisk capillary refill (<2 sec), distal pulses >2+ on a 0-4+ scale, ability to move the great toe, and absence of numbness or tingling. Patient verbalizes knowledge of signs of impaired neurovascular status and the importance of prompt treatment if they occur.

1. Assess affected extremity for integrity of neurovascular status each time VS are taken (or at least q4h or more frequently as indicated). Impaired neurovascular status requires nursing interventions (e.g., elevation, loosening of restrictive dressings); consult physician promptly if these measures are ineffective.
2. Make sure patient can verbalize the signs and symptoms of impaired neurovascular status and knows that it is important to call the physician if they occur after hospital discharge. These indicators include persistent changes in color (pallor, cyanosis, redness), coolness, delayed capillary refill, paresthesia (numbness, tingling), or inability to move distal areas (great or second toe).
3. For additional interventions, see this nursing diagnosis in "Ischemic Myositis," p. 314.

If surgery was performed, see "Total Knee Arthroplasty," in this chapter, for **Risk for fluid volume deficit** related to postsurgical hemorrhage or hematoma formation, p. 335. Also see Appendix One for nursing diagnoses and interventions in "Caring for Preoperative and Postoperative Patients," p. 395, and "Caring for Patients on Prolonged Bed Rest," p. 413.

Musculoskeletal

PATIENT-FAMILY TEACHING
AND DISCHARGE PLANNING

Give patient and significant others verbal and written information
about the following:

1. At-home therapeutic regimens: thermotherapy, elevation, exercises,
   use of immobilization devices, cast care, drugs.
2. Potential complications: recurrent dislocations, neurovascular deficit, and wound infection (indicated by persistent redness, swelling,
   fever, local warmth, increasing pain, wound discharge, foul odor
   from within cast, burning sensation within cast, drainage from
   cast).
3. Precautions: curtailing activities (as physician directs); checking for
   changes in neurovascular status qid; and following care guidelines
   for cast, splint, or orthotic device.
4. Medications, including drug name, purpose, dosage, schedule, precautions, drug/drug and food/drug interactions, and potential side
   effects.

Meniscal Injuries

NURSING DIAGNOSES AND INTERVENTIONS

See "Dislocation/Subluxation" for **Impaired physical mobility** related
to musculoskeletal impairment and adjustment to new walking gait,
p. 308; **Knowledge deficit:** Need for elevation of involved extremity,
use of thermotherapy, and prescribed exercises, p. 309; and **Risk for
peripheral neurovascular dysfunction** related to interrupted arterial
flow secondary to compression from circumferential cast or dressing,
p. 311.

See "Total Knee Arthroplasty" for **Risk for fluid volume deficit** related to postsurgical hemorrhage or hematoma formation, p. 335. Also
see Appendix One, "Caring for Preoperative and Postoperative Patients," p. 395.

PATIENT-FAMILY TEACHING
AND DISCHARGE PLANNING

Give patient and significant others verbal and written information
about the following:

1. Use of elevation, thermotherapy, and exercises (see "Dislocation/
   Subluxation," p. 309).
2. Use of external support devices (elastic wraps, knee immobilizer,
   brace), including care of the device, care of the skin underneath the
   device, and checking for areas of irritation and neurovascular deficit
   (see "Dislocation/Subluxation," p. 308).
3. Cast care (see p. 310).
4. Medications, including drug name, purpose, dosage, schedule, precautions, drug/drug and food/drug interactions, and potential side
   effects.

5. Indicators of wound infection, which require medical attention: erythema, edema, joint effusion, purulent discharge, local warmth, pain, fever.
6. Ambulation and use of assistive device. Make sure patient can ambulate independently, using assistive device on level surfaces, uneven ground, and stairs, before hospital discharge (see "Dislocation/Subluxation," p. 308).

Torn Anterior Cruciate Ligament

NURSING DIAGNOSES AND INTERVENTIONS

See "Dislocation/Subluxation" for **Pain** related to joint changes and corrective therapy, p. 308; **Impaired physical mobility** related to musculoskeletal impairment and adjustment to new walking gait, p. 308; **Knowledge deficit:** Need for elevation of involved extremity, use of thermotherapy, and prescribed exercises, p. 309; **Knowledge deficit:** Potential for joint weakness, and techniques for applying external supports and assessing neurovascular status, p. 311; and **Risk for peripheral neurovascular dysfunction** related to interrupted arterial flow secondary to compression from circumferential cast or dressing, p. 311.

See Appendix One for nursing diagnoses and interventions in "Caring for Preoperative and Postoperative Patients," p. 395.

PATIENT-FAMILY TEACHING AND DISCHARGE PLANNING

Give patient and significant others verbal and written information about the following:
1. Telephone number of someone to call if patient has questions after being discharged from the hospital.
2. Use of external support devices (elastic wraps, knee immobilizer, orthosis), including care of the device, care of the skin underneath the device, and checking for areas of irritation and neurovascular deficit (see "Dislocation/Subluxation," p. 308).
3. Prescribed exercise regimen: purpose; how exercise is performed; number of repetitions; how often exercise should be done.
4. Medications, including drug name, purpose, dosage, schedule, precautions, drug/drug and food/drug interactions, and potential side effects.
5. Indicators of wound infection, which require medical attention: erythema, edema, joint effusion, purulent discharge, local warmth, pain, fever.
6. Ambulation with assistive device. Make sure patient can ambulate independently, using assistive device on level surfaces, uneven ground, and stairs, before hospital discharge (see "Dislocation/Subluxation," p. 308).

Ischemic Myositis (Compartment Syndrome)

NURSING DIAGNOSES AND INTERVENTIONS

PATIENTS AT RISK FOR ISCHEMIC MYOSITIS

Risk for peripheral neurovascular dysfunction related to interruption of capillary blood flow secondary to increased pressure within the anatomic compartment

Desired outcomes: Patient has adequate peripheral neurovascular function in involved limb, as evidenced by brisk capillary refill (<2 sec); peripheral pulse amplitude >2+ on a 0-4+ scale; normal tissue pressures (<15 mm Hg); and absence of edema, tautness, and the six P's (pain, especially on passive digital movement and with pressure over compartment; paresthesia; paralysis; polar; pallor; and pulselessness) over compartment. Patient verbalizes understanding of the importance of reporting symptoms indicating impaired neurovascular status.

1. Monitor neurovascular status of injured extremity with each VS check (at least q2h). Monitor for sluggish capillary refill, increasing limb edema, and tautness over individual compartments. Also assess for the six P's.
2. Report deficits in neurovascular status promptly. Loosen all circumferential dressings, as indicated, and, when appropriate, apply ice (i.e., if patient *does not* have compartment syndrome). **Caution:** If patient has or is suspected of having compartment syndrome, ice and elevation are contraindicated because they may further compromise vascular supply.)
3. Teach patient the symptoms that must be reported promptly to his or her physician: increasing pain, paresthesia (diminished sensation, hyperesthesia, anesthesia), paralysis, coolness.
4. Continually monitor tissue pressures if an intracompartmental pressure device is present; consult physician about above-normal pressures. Remember that pressures >30 mm Hg may be significantly higher than normal.
5. Ensure that fluid resuscitation is accomplished as necessary to ensure adequate circulation to the involved compartments.
6. In patients with lowered systemic BP, monitor delta pressure (mean arterial pressure minus compartment tissue pressure). Report delta pressure ≤30 mm Hg for 6 h or ≤40 mm Hg for 8 h.

PATIENTS WITH ISCHEMIC MYOSITIS

Pain related to tissue ischemia secondary to compartment syndrome

Desired outcomes: Within 8 h of treatment, patient's subjective perception of discomfort decreases as documented by a pain scale. Nonverbal indicators of discomfort, such as grimacing, are absent or diminished. Patient verbalizes understanding of the need to report uncontrolled or increasing pain.

1. Assess the patient's complaints of pain for onset, duration, progression, and intensity. Devise a pain scale with patient, rating discomfort from 0 (no pain) to 10 (worst pain).

2. Determine if passive stretching of digits and pressure over limb compartments increase the pain because both are likely to occur with compartment syndrome.
3. Adjust the medication regimen to the patient's needs; document medication effectiveness.
4. Prevent pressure on involved compartment and neurovascular structures. When not contraindicated by evidence of impaired circulation, apply ice if it has been prescribed.
5. If patient has had a fasciotomy, be aware that if the pain does not subside after this procedure, it could signal an incomplete fasciotomy. Pain that increases several days after a fasciotomy may signal compartmental infection.
6. Continue to monitor neurovascular function with each VS check to assess recurring compartment syndrome or infection.

Risk for infection related to inadequate primary defenses secondary to necrotic tissue, wide compartmental fasciotomy, and open wound

Desired outcome: Patient is free of infection, as evidenced by normothermia; WBC count $\leq11,000/\mu l$; erythrocyte sedimentation rate (ESR) ≤15 mm/h for men or ≤20 mm/h for women; and absence of wound erythema and other clinical indicators of infection.

1. Monitor for fever, increasing pain, and laboratory values indicating infection (e.g., increased WBC count and ESR).
2. Assess exposed wounds and dressings for erythema, increasing or purulent drainage, increasing wound circumference, edema, and localized tenderness.
3. Monitor distal neurovascular status for deficit (see "Dislocation/Subluxation" for **Risk for peripheral neurovascular dysfunction,** p. 311), which may indicate infection of or pressure on these structures caused by nearby deep infection.
4. After primary closure or grafting of wound, continue to assess wound for signs of infection (see above).
5. Be aware of and assess for chronic infection and osteomyelitis as potential complications after compartment syndrome. Explain the increased potential for infection with this type of wound and that chronic infection and osteomyelitis are late complications after compartment syndrome.
6. Use aseptic technique when changing dressings and providing wound care. As indicated, teach patient aseptic technique before hospital discharge.
7. Consult physician promptly about significant findings.

Body image disturbance related to physical changes secondary to large, irregular fasciotomy wound and skin-grafted scar; loss of function and cosmesis of an extremity; or amputation

Desired outcomes: By the 24 h before hospital discharge, patient acknowledges body changes and demonstrates movement toward incorporating changes into self-concept. Patient does not exhibit maladaptive response to wound or functional loss (e.g., severe depression).

1. Encourage questions about compartment syndrome, therapeutic interventions, and long-term effects.

2. Provide time for patient to express his or her feelings about the change in appearance and function. Encourage discussion of these feelings with patient's significant other.
3. Identify and emphasize patient's strengths to facilitate adaptation to cosmetic and functional loss. Help patient set realistic goals for recovery.
4. Facilitate patient's progression through the grieving process, as appropriate.
5. Recognize individuality in adjustment; let patient determine when to view or discuss the injury.
6. If extremity will be amputated, collaborate with physician about a visit by an amputee who has successfully adapted and who can serve as patient's role model.
7. Encourage maximum self-care. Provide necessary adjunctive aids (e.g., built-up utensils, button hooks, orthotics) to facilitate independence.
8. For additional interventions, see this nursing diagnosis in Appendix One, p. 459.

See "Dislocation/Subluxation," for **Pain** related to joint changes and corrective therapy, p. 308; **Knowledge deficit:** Need for elevation of involved extremity, use of thermotherapy, and prescribed exercises, p. 309; and **Risk for peripheral neurovascular dysfunction** related to interrupted arterial flow secondary to compression from circumferential cast or dressing, p. 311.

If surgery was performed, see Appendix One for nursing diagnoses and interventions in "Caring for Preoperative and Postoperative Patients," p. 395.

PATIENT-FAMILY TEACHING AND DISCHARGE PLANNING

Give patient and significant others verbal and written information about the following:
1. Phone number of appropriate person to call for questions after hospital discharge.
2. Information about the process of ischemic myositis and instructions for use of elevation and ice, and loosening of restrictive dressings.
3. Discharge instructions for patients with fractures (see "Fractures," p. 320).
4. Importance of seeking medical attention promptly if signs and symptoms of wound infection occur.
5. Importance of monitoring for vascular changes in patients who have undergone vascular surgery (exploration or resection). Teach patient to be alert for color changes (pallor, cyanosis, duskiness), coolness, pulselessness, or decreased or absent capillary refill. Stress the importance of promptly reporting these findings to the physician.

SECTION TWO: SKELETAL DISORDERS

Osteomyelitis

NURSING DIAGNOSES AND INTERVENTIONS

Risk for infection *(for others)* related to potential for cross-contamination; *(for patient)* related to disease chronicity
Desired outcomes: Upon hospital discharge, patient, other patients, and staff members are free of symptoms of infection, as evidenced by normothermia and WBC count ≤11,000/μl. Within 24 h of instruction, patient verbalizes knowledge of potential chronicity of disease and the importance of strict adherence to prescribed antibiotic therapy.

1. When appropriate for infecting organism, isolate patient from other patients, especially those with orthopedic disorders.
2. Handle patient's drainage system properly, using infection control technique, and make sure all staff members wash their hands carefully between patients to prevent cross-contamination.
3. Teach patient about the disease and the potential for chronic infection. Stress the importance of complying with the prescribed antibiotic therapy.
4. Use proper infection management (i.e., use gloves) when performing irrigation, changing dressings, or handling contaminated dressings (see Appendix Two, p. 479). Wash hands carefully between patients.

Knowledge deficit: Side effects of prolonged use of potent antibiotics
Desired outcome: Within 24 h of instruction, patient verbalizes knowledge of potential side effects of antibiotic therapy and necessary precautions.

AMINOGLYCOSIDE ANTIBACTERIALS

Gentamicin sulfate, kanamycin sulfate, neomycin, streptomycin, and tobramycin are used to combat gram-negative organisms. Potential toxic reactions include ototoxicity (exhibited by dizziness, vertigo, tinnitus, and decreased auditory acuity); nephrotoxicity (evidenced by rising blood urea nitrogen [BUN] and serum creatinine levels, from progressive renal tubular necrosis, which can progress to renal failure if untreated); and superimposed infections, which occur because of loss of normal body flora protection against bacterial overgrowth.

- Teach patient about potential complications and the need to report symptoms as early as possible.
- Advise patient that with long-term therapy, a baseline audiogram with weekly audiograms should be performed to identify potential hearing deficit; serum creatinine and BUN should be drawn weekly while patient is taking aminoglycosides; and weight should be checked daily to help assess for fluid retention (patients should report weight gain of ≥2 lb/day). Monitor I&O during patient's hospitalization to help assess renal function.

- Advise patient to monitor for superimposed infections, especially fungal infections, by being alert for fever, black or furry tongue, nausea, diarrhea, and oral or vaginal monilial growth. If a venous access device is used for antibiotic administration, the infusion site should be closely monitored for indicators of irritation that do not respond to usual treatments with topical antibiotics. During hospitalization, consult physician about culturing suspicious areas of inflammation.

PENICILLINS

Ampicillin, carbenicillin, cyclacillin, methacillin, mezlocillin, oxacillin, and piperacillin are used to combat organisms that demonstrate sensitivity to them. Potential toxic reactions include anemia, hypersensitivity reactions, and overgrowth of nonsusceptible organisms.

- Teach patient about potential complications and the need to report symptoms promptly.
- Use penicillin cautiously in patients with allergies or allergic pathologic conditions such as asthma, hay fever, or dermatitis. Erythematous, maculopapular rash; urticaria; and anaphylaxis can occur. Caution patient about these potential reactions.
- Instruct patient to seek medical attention if rash, fever, chills, or signs of infection or inflammation develop.

CEPHALOSPORINS

Cefadroxil, cefamandole, cefazolin, cefoperazone, cefotetan, cefoxitin, ceftazidine, ceftriaxone, cefuroxime, cephalothin, cephapirin, and cephradine are used in the treatment of susceptible organisms. Potential toxic reactions include overgrowth of nonsusceptible organisms, photosensitivity, increased BUN, hepatotoxicity, and pseudomembranous colitis.

- Advise patient about potential complications, which require prompt medical attention.
- Explain that patients with suspected renal or hepatic disease should have baseline and serial (weekly) serum liver enzymes (lactate hydrogenase [LDH], serum glutamic-oxaloacetic transminase [SGOT], serum glutamic-pyruvic transminase [SGPT]), BUN, and serum creatinine evaluations. I&O should be monitored, along with daily weight to determine hydration status. Scleral and skin icterus, as well as darkening of the urine (from increased urobilinogen), should be noted. Persistent diarrhea (>3 liquid stools or liquid stools for >2 days) should be reported promptly to the health care provider.
- Advise patient to avoid direct sunlight or sources of ultraviolet light. Suggest that patient use sunscreens to help prevent photosensitivity reactions.
- When oral medications are used, instruct patient to avoid taking them with dairy or iron products, which can inhibit absorption from the gut.

SULFONAMIDES

Sulfadiazine, sulfamethoxazole, sulfapyridine, and sulfisoxazole can cause toxic reactions, including disruption of intestinal flora, which results in diminished production of metabolically active vitamin K and hemorrhagic tendencies, agranulocytosis, nephrotoxicity, and crystalluria.

- Teach patient about potential complications and the importance of seeking prompt medical attention if they occur.
- Advise patients undergoing long-term therapy of the need to have baseline BUN and serum creatinine levels determined, along with weekly levels, to rule out nephrotoxicity. Baseline and serial (weekly) granulocyte determinations also should be performed. Agranulocytosis can manifest as lesions of the throat, mucous membranes, GI tract, and skin. Daily weight and I&O should be evaluated to help assess hydration status.
- Teach patient how to monitor for bleeding, especially epistaxis, bleeding gums, hemoptysis, hematemesis, melena, hematuria, prolonged bleeding from wounds, and ecchymosis. During patient's hospitalization, hematest suspicious secretions, or send them to the laboratory, if prescribed, to determine if blood is present. Teach patient to control bleeding with ice, pressure, or elevation and to seek medical assistance promptly if he or she is unable to control hemorrhage.
- Advise patient to consume at least 2-3 L/day of fluids (unless contraindicated by cardiac or renal disease) to prevent crystalluria. Teach the indicators of urinary calculi and the importance of getting medical attention should they occur: hematuria, pyuria, retention, frequency, urgency, and pain in the flank, lower back, perineum, thighs, groin, labia, or scrotum.

Knowledge deficit: Potential for infection and air embolus related to use of Hickman catheter or other venous access device for long-term intermittent antibiotic therapy

Desired outcome: By a minimum of the 24 h before hospital discharge, patient demonstrates care of the catheter and verbalizes knowledge of the indicators of infection and air embolus.

1. If therapy is to be continued at home, teach patient how to care for the catheter and monitor the entry site for indicators of infection or inflammation. Use sterile technique for dressing changes, following hospital protocol for the procedure, which usually includes defatting the skin with acetone or alcohol, applying povidone-iodine, and covering the site with an air-occlusive dressing. Have patient or significant other return the demonstration before hospital discharge. If appropriate, arrange for a visit by a home health care nurse.

2. Caution patient about the importance of keeping the tubing clamped unless he or she is aspirating or injecting solutions into the catheter. Teach patient and significant others to be alert for indicators of air embolism: labored breathing, cyanosis, cough, chest pain, and syncope. Explain that if air embolism is suspected, patient should be rolled immediately to the left side and placed in Trendelenburg's position, the catheter reclamped, and medical assistance obtained as quickly as possible.

3. Teach patient the importance of preventing inadvertent puncture or breakage of the tubing and of checking for kinks or cracks daily.

Explain the necessity of taping all tube junctions to prevent accidental separation and of positioning the clamp over tape tabs to minimize stress on the tubing.

See "Dislocation/Subluxation" for **Pain,** p. 308; see "Fractures" for **Self-care deficit,** p. 321. See Appendix One for nursing diagnoses and interventions in "Caring for Preoperative and Postoperative Patients," p. 395; "Caring for Patients on Prolonged Bed Rest," p. 413; and "Caring for Patients with Cancer and Other Life-Disrupting Illnesses," p. 450.

PATIENT-FAMILY TEACHING
AND DISCHARGE PLANNING

Give patient and significant others verbal and written information about the following:

1. Necessary patient care after hospital discharge (e.g., dressing changes, warm soaks, ROM exercises). Involve significant others in patient's care during hospitalization to familiarize them with care activities after discharge.
2. When parenteral antibiotic therapy is to be given at home (usually *via* a Hickman catheter, Portacath, or similar long-term vascular access device), the method of administering medications and care of the device.
3. Medications, including drug name, purpose, dosage, schedule, precautions, drug/drug and food/drug interactions, and potential side effects.
4. Involving a public health nurse, visiting nurse, or similar home health care provider to ensure adequate follow-up at home.
5. Indicators of potential complications: recurring infection, pathologic fracture, joint contracture, pressure necrosis, medication reactions, or toxic effects.

Fractures

NURSING DIAGNOSES AND INTERVENTIONS

Fatigue related to state of discomfort, psychoemotional demands, and effects of prolonged immobility
Desired outcome: Within 24 h of admission, patient verbalizes a reduction in fatigue.

1. Assess time fatigue occurs, its relationship to required activities, and activities that relieve or aggravate symptoms.
2. Investigate patient's sleep pattern, and intervene as appropriate to ensure adequate rest (see **Sleep pattern disturbance** in Appendix One, p. 454).
3. Assess for dietary and physiologic sources of fatigue, and correct as needed.
4. Determine whether patient's pain is adequately controlled, and intervene with pharmacologic and nonpharmacologic treatments as indicated.
5. Assess patient for stress or psychoemotional distress; intervene as

necessary or seek assistance from an appropriate clinical specialist in psychiatric nursing.

6. Discuss the reason for a graded exercise regimen to increase endurance and strength (see Appendix One for **Risk for activity intolerance,** p. 413, and **Risk for disuse syndrome,** p. 416). Encourage patient to set realistic goals and post these goals to facilitate participation of associated health care providers.

7. Pace activities and intersperse rest periods of at least 90 min.

8. Teach patient how to use adjunctive and assistive devices.

See "Amputation" for **Knowledge deficit:** Postsurgical exercise regimen, p. 329 (for any patient beginning exercise therapy).

See "Total Hip Arthroplasty" for **Knowledge deficit:** Potential for and mechanism of total hip arthroplasty (THA) dislocation, p. 332 (for patients undergoing hemiarthroplasty for replacement of the femoral head); **Knowledge deficit:** Potential for infection caused by foreign body reaction to an endoprosthesis, p. 333 (useful for any patient with an internal fixation device, especially large devices); and **Risk for peripheral neurovascular dysfunction,** p. 334 (can be adapted for any patient in traction).

See "Total Knee Arthroplasty" for **Risk for fluid volume deficit** related to postsurgical hemorrhage or hematoma formation, p. 335 (for patients with ORIF).

See Appendix One for nursing diagnoses and interventions in "Caring for Preoperative and Postoperative Patients," p. 395, and "Caring for Patients on Prolonged Bed Rest," p. 413.

SPECIFIC NURSING DIAGNOSES FOR PATIENTS WITH CASTS, TRACTION, OPEN REDUCTION WITH INTERNAL FIXATION (ORIF), AND EXTERNAL FIXATORS

Self-care deficit related to physical limitations secondary to cast or surgical procedure (applies to patients with casts, ORIF, and external fixators)

Desired outcome: Within 48 h of surgical procedure or cast application, patient demonstrates independence with ADLs.

1. For patients with insufficient strength to manipulate casted extremities to allow independence in self-care, incorporate a structured exercise regimen that will increase strength and endurance. Direct regimen toward developing muscle groups necessary for patient's activity deficit. See guidelines described for **Knowledge deficit:** Postsurgical exercise regimen, p. 329, in "Amputation," and **Risk for disuse syndrome** related to inactivity secondary to prolonged bed rest, p. 416, in Appendix One.

2. Use assistive devices liberally (e.g., stocking helpers, Velcro fasteners, enlarged handles on eating utensils, pickup sticks, raised toilet seats).

3. As appropriate, ask hospital's social services department for assistance with funding for buying assistive equipment or for home help.

4. Because pain control is essential to resumption of self-care, make sure patient is as comfortable as possible (see "Dislocation/Subluxation" for **Pain,** p. 308).

Musculoskeletal

5. Teach significant others how to help patient with self-care when needed.
6. As appropriate, use adaptive clothing (e.g., with Velcro fasteners) designed to accommodate cast.

Risk for impaired skin integrity and/or **Impaired tissue integrity** related to irritation and pressure secondary to presence of a cast (applies to patients with casts, ORIF, or continuous passive movement [CPM] device)

Desired outcomes: Patient has no discomfort under cast, and skin is intact when cast is removed. Within 8 h of application of cast, patient verbalizes knowledge of indicators of pressure necrosis.

1. When assisting with cast application, ensure that adequate padding is put on affected extremity before cast is applied.
2. While cast is curing (drying), handle it only with the palms of the hands to avoid pressure points caused by finger indentations. Make sure cast surface is exposed to facilitate drying.
3. Petal edges of plaster casts with tape or moleskin to prevent cast crumbs from falling into cast and causing pressure necrosis.
4. Instruct patient never to insert anything between cast and skin. If patient has severe itching, advise him or her to notify physician, who may prescribe a medication to relieve itching.
5. Teach patient the indicators of pressure necrosis within cast: pain, burning sensation, foul odor from cast opening, drainage on cast.

Knowledge deficit: Potential for disuse osteoporosis (appropriate for patient with cast or traction)

Desired outcome: Within 24 h of instruction, patient verbalizes knowledge of the process of and measures to prevent disuse osteoporosis.

1. Teach patient the process of disuse osteoporosis, gearing explanation to patient's level of understanding: The immobilized limb has insufficient stress to stimulate osteoblastic (bone-building) activity.
2. Instruct patient to report any indicators of pain in immobilized limb or findings of spontaneous fracture: bony deformity, pain, lost function, edema, ecchymosis.
3. Consult physician about appropriate alternative methods of bone stress, and teach them to patient: use of a tilt table, sandbags applied intermittently against bone, or having patient push against a foot board or perform isometric exercise of immobilized limb.

Altered cerebral or cardiopulmonary tissue perfusion (or risk for same) related to interrupted arterial flow secondary to fat embolization (applies to patients with multiple trauma, multiple fractures, or surgical repair of fractures)

Desired outcome: Patient has adequate cerebral and cardiopulmonary perfusion, as evidenced by Pao_2 $\geq$80 mm Hg, HR $\leq$100 bpm, RR $\leq$20 breaths/min, normothermia, normal skin color, absence of adventitious breath sounds over tracheobronchial tree, absence of petechial rash, and orientation to time, place, and person.

1. Ensure strict maintenance of fracture immobilization to help prevent embolization.
2. Carefully monitor patient for initial 72 h after injury or surgery for indicators of fat embolism: tachycardia, tachypnea, profuse tracheo-

bronchial secretions, chest pain, cyanosis, fever, petechial rash (involving conjunctiva, trunk, neck, proximal arms, and axilla), anxiety, apprehension, progressive mental dysfunction (confusion, disorientation), fat globules in the retina. Hct may drop, serum lipase will rise, and fat may be noted on urinalysis. Frequent specimens for ABG levels should be drawn on patients at risk for fat embolus for the first 48 h after injury, because the early hypoxemia that signals fat embolism is apparent only in laboratory values. In addition, a platelet count indicating thrombocytopenia ($<150,000/\mu$l) is diagnostic of fat embolism.

3. Because fat embolism is a life-threatening emergency, notify physician immediately if any of the preceding signs occur. Inform patient and significant others of these potential indicators so that they can notify staff if they occur.

4. As prescribed, perform respiratory support measures with oxygen and rigorous pulmonary hygiene. Intubation with ventilation using positive end-expiratory pressure (PEEP) may be necessary. As a general rule, all patients with significant trauma and fractures should receive oxygen at 40% concentration *via* mask or nasal prongs until the threat of fat embolism has been ruled out.

5. Administer IV steroids, diuretics, and dextran as prescribed.

Knowledge deficit: Potential for infection because of orthopedic procedure or presence of the internal or external device (appropriate for patients with ORIF or external fixators)

Desired outcome: Within 24 h of instruction, patient verbalizes knowledge of potential for infection, lists indicators that may occur, and understands the significance of reporting them promptly.

1. Advise patient of potential for infection, which can occur as a result of surgical procedure.

2. Teach patient the following indicators of infection and the importance of reporting them promptly to a health care provider: persistent redness, swelling, increasing pain, wound drainage, local warmth, foul odor from within cast, sensation of burning within cast, drainage from cast, fever.

3. Alert patients with internal fixation devices to the potential for infection for as long as the implant is present. Instruct them to report any of the preceding indicators promptly.

Knowledge deficit: Potential for refracture owing to vulnerability because of the presence of an internal fixator (applies to patients with ORIF)

Desired outcome: By a minimum of the 24 h before hospital discharge, patient verbalizes knowledge about potential for refracture and complies with prescribed regimen for prevention.

1. Advise patient that although the internal fixation device supplements bone strength at the fracture site in the early stages of healing, the implant will compromise the bone's strength later. Larger internal fixation devices alter the vectors of stress placed on the bone, changing the normal physiologic balance between osteoblasts and osteoclasts, which results in a bone that is weakened in the long run by the implant.

2. Be sure patient verbalizes understanding of this process and complies with prescribed regimen of limb use and ambulation.
3. Make sure patient knows that intramedullary nails or rods and large plates probably will be removed within a year.

Knowledge deficit: Function of external fixation, pin care, and signs and symptoms of pin site infection

Desired outcomes: By a minimum of the 24 h before hospital discharge, patient verbalizes knowledge of the rationale for external fixator and demonstrates ways to adapt life-style to fixator. Patient demonstrates knowledge of pin care and verbalizes knowledge of indicators of infection at pin sites.

1. Explain the reason for use of fixator with the type of fracture or injury patient has, emphasizing benefits for patient.
2. Discuss ways patient can adapt his or her life-style to accommodate fixator (e.g., by wearing adaptive clothing that fits the device).
3. Instruct patient and significant others in pin care as prescribed by physician. Some physicians prescribe daily pin site care with hydrogen peroxide or skin prep solutions such as pHisoHex, alcohol, or povidone-iodine. Some physicians request that buildup of crusts from serous drainage be removed when cleaning pin sites, whereas others want crust left intact to minimize risk of infection. If prescribed, teach patient how to apply antibacterial ointments and small dressings to pin site. External fixator pins should be cleansed with alcohol daily. **Note:** Literature supplied with some external fixators cautions against use of iodine-based mixtures, which may cause corrosion of the device.
4. Instruct patient and significant others not to use external fixator as a handle or support for extremity. Teach them to support extremity with pillows, two hands, slings, and other devices as necessary to prevent excessive stress on skeletal pins.
5. Teach patient how to monitor pin sites for indicators of infection (persistent redness, swelling, drainage, increasing pain, temperature >38.3° C [101° F], and local warmth), and to be alert for pin migration or "tenting" of skin on the pin, which can signal movement of pin or infection. Instruct patient to report significant findings promptly to physician.
6. Advise patient of the need for follow-up care to ensure that device is functioning properly and maintaining adequate immobilization of fractures.

PATIENT-FAMILY TEACHING
AND DISCHARGE PLANNING

Give patient and significant others verbal and written information about the following:

1. Medications, including drug name, purpose, dosage, schedule, precautions, drug/drug and food/drug interactions, and potential side effects.
2. Importance of rest, elevation, and use of thermotherapy (see "Dislocation/Subluxation," p. 309).

3. Reason for therapy after discharge, and an explanation of how therapy will be accomplished (e.g., casting, external or internal fixation).

4. Precautions of therapy:
   - *Casts:* Cast care; checking neurovascular status of distal extremity; being alert for signs of pressure necrosis beneath cast; performing prescribed exercises; preventing skin maceration; and preventing disuse osteoporosis (also see "Dislocation/Subluxation" for **Knowledge deficit:** Care and assessment of the casted extremity, p. 310).
   - *External fixation devices:* Wound care; noting signs of wound infection; preventing refracturing of the limb; performing prescribed exercises; and monitoring for delayed infection.
   - *External fixator:* Pin care; knowing when to notify physician of problems with fixator; performing prescribed exercises; checking neurovascular status of the limb; and monitoring pin sites for signs of infection.

5. Ways in which patient can control discomfort (see **Pain,** p. 308).

6. Use of assistive devices and ambulatory aids. Make sure patient returns demonstration and is independent with devices and aids before hospital discharge (see "Dislocation/Subluxation," p. 308). If needed, initiate referral for a home visit early after discharge to ensure patient's safety.

7. Materials necessary for care at home and agencies that supply them.

8. If a patient will require home help, hospital nurses and community care agencies should collaborate to ensure continuity of care. Appropriate agency should see patient before he or she is discharged from the hospital.

Malignant Neoplasms

NURSING DIAGNOSES AND INTERVENTIONS

See "Dislocation/Subluxation" for **Pain,** p. 308, and **Impaired physical mobility** related to musculoskeletal impairment and adjustment to new walking gait, p. 308.

See "Total Knee Arthroplasty" for **Risk for fluid volume deficit** related to postsurgical hemorrhage or hematoma formation, p. 335.

When postoperative casts, use of orthotics, exercises, or similar therapies are prescribed, refer to appropriate nursing diagnoses throughout this chapter. If patient undergoes amputation, see "Amputation," p. 328.

Also see Appendix One for nursing diagnoses and interventions in "Caring for Preoperative and Postoperative Patients," p. 395; "Caring for Patients on Prolonged Bed Rest," p. 413; and "Caring for Patients with Cancer and Other Life-Disrupting Illnesses," p. 423.

PATIENT-FAMILY TEACHING AND DISCHARGE PLANNING

Give patient and significant others verbal and written information about the following:

1. Medications, including drug name, purpose, dosage, schedule, precautions, drug/drug and food/drug interactions, and potential side effects.
2. For surgical patients, indicators of wound infection and the importance of reporting them to the physician: persistent redness, swelling, local warmth, fever, discharge from wound, pain. As appropriate, also see "Dislocation/Subluxation" for **Knowledge deficit:** Need for elevation of involved extremity, use of thermotherapy, and prescribed exercises, p. 309.
3. For patients with casts, orthotics, prosthetics, ambulatory aids, assistive devices, or similar therapies, instructions for their use, including a return demonstration by patient and a phone number to call should any questions arise after hospital discharge. See **Impaired physical mobility** related to musculoskeletal impairment and adjustment to a new walking gait, p. 308, and **Knowledge deficit:** Care and assessment of the casted extremity, p. 310.
4. Referral to hospice or agency that provides home help; this should be done before discharge planning begins to ensure continuity of care.

Osteoporosis

NURSING DIAGNOSES AND INTERVENTIONS

Health-seeking behaviors: Prevention of osteoporosis, its treatment, and the importance of choosing and using calcium supplements effectively

Desired outcome: Within 48 h of instruction, patient verbalizes knowledge of disease process and understanding of the most effective calcium supplements and how they are used.

N O T E : It is important to begin instructing all individuals at risk for osteoporosis as early in their lives as possible because of the prolonged period involved in developing (and thus preventing) this process. Individuals at risk for osteoporosis include those with loss of ovarian function (surgical or physiologic menopause, women athletes), family history, nulliparity, preexisting skeletal disease, underweight, inadequate childhood nutrition (lifelong low calcium intake), high caffeine intake, increased protein intake, sedentary life-style, high alcohol intake, cigarette smoking, and Caucasian or Asian ancestry. The risk of osteoporosis increases with age and is higher in women than men. Secondary causes include metastatic disease, drugs (heparin, alcohol, phosphate-binding antacids, corticosteroids, phenytoin, isoniazid), hyperparathyroidism, immobilization, hypercortisolism, hyperthyroidism, hypogonadism, and connective tissue disease.

---

1. Make sure physician has recommended or approves use of calcium supplements for patient. Increased calcium can result in nephrolithiasis in susceptible individuals.
2. Be sure patient is aware of the silent nature of this disorder and re-

alizes that by the time symptoms arise, it is too late for effective treatment.

3. Teach patient that calcium supplements come in many varieties. The most effective form is calcium carbonate, which delivers about 40% calcium. Bonemeal and dolomite should be avoided because they may contain high amounts of lead or other toxic substances.

4. Teach patient to look for the amount of elemental calcium available when evaluating supplement labels, rather than the weight of the total compound, and to avoid supplements with added vitamin D because hypervitaminosis of this vitamin is possible. Remind patients of the need for 15 min/day of sunlight to allow for activation of vitamin D.

5. Teach patient not to take calcium and iron supplements simultaneously because iron absorption will be impaired. Calcium also may reduce absorption of some medications. Similarly, some foods inhibit absorption of calcium (e.g., red meats, spinach, colas, bran, bread, and whole grain cereals). Therefore, calcium should be taken 2 h before or after other medications or meals. Calcium is best absorbed at night and should be taken at hs.

6. Caution patient to avoid taking more than 500-600 mg of calcium at one time and to spread doses over the entire day. Remind patient to drink a full glass of water with each supplement to minimize the risk of developing renal calculi.

Altered nutrition: Less than body requirements for calcium and vitamin D

Desired outcome: Patient demonstrates intake of adequate amounts of calcium and vitamin D and, within the 24 h before hospital discharge, plans a 3-day menu that provides sufficient intake of both.

1. Ensure that patient demonstrates knowledge of foods high in calcium: cheese; milk; dark green, leafy vegetables; eggs; peanuts; sesame seeds; oysters. Provide patient with a list of these foods, including the relative amounts of calcium in each.

2. Teach patient how to plan menus that provide sufficient daily intake of calcium and vitamin D–fortified foods: eggs, halibut, herring, fortified dairy products, liver, mackerel, oysters, salmon, sardines.

3. Provide patient with sample menus that include adequate daily amounts of calcium and vitamin D. Have patient plan a 3-day menu that incorporates these foods.

4. Provide patient with phone numbers to call if questions arise after hospital discharge.

See "Amputation" for **Knowledge deficit:** Postsurgical exercise regimen, p. 329. Moderate weight-bearing exercise is necessary to stress the bones and activate osteoblastic bone formation.

PATIENT-FAMILY TEACHING
AND DISCHARGE PLANNING

Give patient and significant others verbal and written information about the following:

1. Medications, including drug name, purpose, dosage, schedule, precautions, drug/drug and food/drug interactions, and potential side effects.
2. Instructions for prescribed dietary regimen, including the reason for the diet and foods to include and avoid, if appropriate.
3. Prescribed exercise regimen, including how to perform the exercise, the number of repetitions of each, and the frequency of exercise periods (see **Knowledge deficit:** Postsurgical exercise regimen, p. 329).
4. Importance of establishing measures for preventing falls in the home (e.g., placing a handrail in the bathtub, installing nightlights, avoiding use of throw rugs). Arrange for a home visit for fall prevention as necessary.
5. Importance of reporting to health care provider indicators of pathologic fracture: deformity, pain, edema, ecchymosis, limb shortening, false motion, decreased ROM, crepitus. Stress the importance of promptly reporting indicators of vertebral fractures resulting in spinal cord or nerve compression: paresthesia, weakness, paralysis, loss of bowel or bladder function.

SECTION THREE: MUSCULOSKELETAL SURGICAL PROCEDURES

Amputation

NURSING DIAGNOSES AND INTERVENTIONS

Risk for disuse syndrome related to severe pain and immobility secondary to amputation

Desired outcomes: Within 24 h of instruction, patient verbalizes understanding of exercise regimen and performs exercises independently. Patient is free of symptoms of contracture formation, as evidenced by complete ROM of joints and maintenance of muscle mass.

1. Control patient's pain to ensure appropriate movement.
2. For the first 2 postoperative days, intersperse elevation with periods of ROM to remaining joints. **Caution:** Both elevation and ROM are performed only if prescribed by physician. A stump with marginal vascular supply must not be elevated.
3. Prevent flexion contractures of the knee and hip by assisting patient with lying prone for 1 h 3 ×/day.
4. Another method of preventing flexion contractures is to teach patient to perform exercises that increase the strength of muscle extensors. Consult physician about prescriptions for the following exercises:
   - *Above-the-knee amputation (AKA):* Have patient attempt to straighten hip from a flexed position against resistance or perform gluteal-setting exercises.
   - *Below-the-knee amputation:* Have patient attempt to straighten knee against resistance or perform quadriceps-setting exercises.

These patients also should perform the exercises described above for AKA.

5. For other interventions, see **Risk for disuse syndrome,** p. 416, in Appendix One.

Impaired physical mobility related to altered stance secondary to amputation of lower limb

Desired outcome: Within 2 days of beginning ambulation, patient demonstrates use of muscle-tightening technique to enhance mobilization.

1. Inform patients with lower extremity amputation that difficulty in adjusting to altered stance may occur as a result of amputation. Suggest that to prevent an altered stance, patient should tighten gluteal and abdominal muscles while standing.

2. For other interventions, see "Dislocation/Subluxation" for **Impaired physical mobility** related to musculoskeletal impairment and adjustment to a new walking gait with an assistive device, p. 308.

Knowledge deficit: Postsurgical exercise regimen

Desired outcome: Within 8 h of instruction, patient verbalizes knowledge of exercise regimen and returns demonstration independently.

1. To increase adherence to prescribed exercise regimen, explain the reason for the exercises and how to perform them, and suggest ways to adapt the exercises to home use. Most therapeutic programs include ROM and muscle-strengthening exercises.

2. Demonstrate each exercise until patient can return the demonstration independently. Provide patient with written instructions that describe each exercise and the number of repetitions and number of times a day it should be performed. Also provide a phone number to call if any questions arise after patient is discharged. If necessary, arrange for a postdischarge home visit.

3. If additional equipment is required, provide patient with information about where it can be purchased and, if necessary, seek financial assistance from social services.

Knowledge deficit: Care of the stump and prosthesis; signs and symptoms of skin irritation or pressure necrosis

Desired outcomes: Within the 24 h before hospital discharge, patient verbalizes knowledge of care of stump and prosthesis and independently returns demonstration of wrapping stump. Patient also verbalizes knowledge of indicators of pressure necrosis and irritation from wrapping device or prosthesis.

N O T E : A stump that is inappropriately treated will become edematous and more prone to injury, which will delay proper fitting of the permanent prosthesis.

1. If molding of the stump for eventual prosthetic fitting is prescribed, instruct patient in technique for applying an elastic sleeve or wrap: Application of the elastic wrap is begun with a recurrent turn over the distal end of the stump, and then diagonal circumferential turns are made, overlapping one-half to two-thirds the width of the wrap. Traction applied to the wrap should ensure more pressure on the

distal portion of the stump. The elastic device should be snug but not excessively so, because a tight wrap can impede circulation and healing. Rewrapping should be performed q4h, combined with careful inspection of the stump. Areas prone to pressure, such as bony prominences or prominent tendons, should be assessed for evidence of excess pressure. Ensure that all tissue is contained by the elastic device. If any tissue is allowed to bulge, proper fitting of the prosthesis will be difficult.

2. Teach patient to monitor stump for indicators of skin irritation or pressure necrosis caused by elastic device or prosthesis (e.g., blebs, abrasions, erythemic or tender areas). Explain that if massage fails to alleviate the problem, patient should seek the help of the public health nurse or visiting nurse or notify physician.

3. For areas prone to pressure, provide extra padding with sheet wadding, moleskin, or lamb's wool to prevent irritation.

4. The day after sutures have been removed (and assuming incision is dry and intact), instruct patient to cleanse stump daily with mild soap and water. Caution against use of emollients, which can create skin maceration beneath the prosthesis.

5. Advise patient that when molding is no longer necessary (after 1-6 mo), he or she will be fitted with a stump sock that will allow air to circulate around stump.

6. Make sure patient receives complete instructions in care of prosthesis by certified prosthetist-orthotist or knowledgeable nurse.

Risk for fluid volume deficit related to postsurgical hemorrhage

Desired outcomes: Patient is normovolemic, as evidenced by BP ≥90/60 (or within patient's usual range), HR ≤100 bpm, urinary output ≥30 ml/h, peripheral pulses >2+ on a 0-4+ scale, brisk capillary refill (<2 sec), and drainage ≤50 ml/h in a drainage device. Patient verbalizes knowledge of the importance of reporting bleeding promptly to staff.

1. Inspect cast (or postoperative dressing) for increasing drainage. If stump is elevated, inspect dependent areas for evidence of bleeding. Inform patient of the need to report increasing bleeding to staff. Also monitor VS for systemic evidence of bleeding (hypotension, tachycardia, pallor), as well as decreased amplitude of peripheral pulses and delayed capillary refill in involved limb.

2. If a drain or drainage device is used, document amount of drainage. Report drainage >50 ml/h.

Pain related to phantom limb sensation

Desired outcomes: Within 24 h of intervention, patient has fewer phantom limb sensations, as documented by a pain scale. Objective indicators, such as facial grimacing, are absent or diminished.

1. Explain to patient that continued sensations often arise from amputated part, and they can be painful, irritating, or simply disconcerting. As appropriate, devise a pain scale with patient, rating discomfort from 0 (no pain) to 10 (worst pain).

2. Instruct patient in the basis for pharmacologic interventions. Beta-blockers may be used to control dull, constant aching by increasing central and peripheral nervous system serotonin level. Anticonvul-

sant agents may be used to treat severe lancinating (sharply cutting or tearing) pain by reducing neuronal excitability. Tricyclic antidepressants may be used to elevate amputee's mood. Local anesthetics may be used in trigger zones on contralateral limb.

3. Manage these painful sensations with interventions discussed in **Pain,** p. 308, in "Dislocation/Subluxation." Counterirritation is especially useful for this type of pain. Other phantom limb sensations may respond to similar tactics: distraction, relaxation, biofeedback, psychotherapy, behavior modification, hypnosis, whirlpool, ultrasound, reciprocal motion (cycling), or use of cutaneous stimulation *via* oil of wintergreen, heat, or massage. Transcutaneous electrical nerve stimulation (TENS) has been found to be especially effective in managing phantom limb sensation.

4. Some physicians advocate vigorous stimulation of the end of the stump to alter the feedback loop of the resected nerve. Advise patient that this can be accomplished by hitting the end of a *well-healed* stump with a rolled towel.

5. Chronic phantom limb sensation may require exploration of stump to resect a neuroma at the site of nerve resection. Inform patient that this may be a possibility if phantom limb sensation continues for more than 6 mo. Use of epidural anesthesia in the perioperative period shows promise in reducing phantom limb pain.

6. For additional interventions, see this nursing diagnosis in Appendix One, p. 396.

Body image disturbance and/or **Altered role performance** related to loss of limb

Desired outcome: Within 72 h of surgery, patient begins to show adaptation toward loss of limb and demonstrates role-related responsibilities.

1. Be aware that use of a prosthesis immediately after surgery allows patients to continue to perceive themselves as ambulatory (and thus "whole") individuals.

2. Gently encourage patient to look at and touch stump and express his or her feelings about the amputation. The nurse and other care givers must show an accepting attitude, as well as encourage significant others to accept patient as he or she now appears. Provide privacy for patient and significant others to express their grief.

3. Assist patient with adapting to loss of limb while maintaining a sense of what is perceived as the normal self. This may be accomplished by introducing patient to others who have successfully adapted to a similar amputation. In addition, teaching aids (e.g., audiovisuals, books, pamphlets, and videotapes) can be used to demonstrate how others have adapted to amputation.

4. For patients who continue to have difficulty adapting to amputation, provide a referral to an appropriate resource person, such as a psychologist or psychiatric nurse.

5. For additional interventions, see **Body image disturbance** in Appendix One, p. 459.

See "Fractures" for **Knowledge deficit:** Potential for infection, p. 323.

See Appendix One for nursing diagnoses and interventions in "Car-

Musculoskeletal

ing for Preoperative and Postoperative Patients," p. 395, and "Caring for Patients with Cancer and Other Life-Disrupting Illnesses," p. 423.

PATIENT-FAMILY TEACHING AND DISCHARGE PLANNING

Give patient and significant others verbal and written information about the following:

1. How and where to purchase necessary supplies and equipment for self-care.
2. Care of stump and prosthesis.
3. Indicators of wound infection, which necessitate medical attention: swelling, persistent redness, discharge, local warmth, systemic fever, pain. Suggest that patient use a small hand mirror, if necessary, to examine incision and stump.
4. Medications, including drug name, purpose, dosage, schedule, precautions, drug/drug and food/drug interactions, and potential side effects.
5. Phone number to call should questions arise after hospital discharge.
6. Prescribed exercises; patient should be able to perform them independently before discharge.
7. Referral to appropriate resource person, should maladaptive behaviors associated with grieving or body image disturbance continue.
8. Ambulation with assistive device and prosthesis on level and uneven surfaces and stairs. Patient should demonstrate independence before hospital discharge. For patients with an upper extremity amputation, independence with ADLs should be demonstrated before discharge. If necessary, arrange for a home visit.

Bone Grafting

NURSING DIAGNOSES AND INTERVENTIONS

See "Dislocation/Subluxation" for **Pain,** p. 308; **Impaired physical mobility** related to musculoskeletal impairment and adjustment to new walking gait, p. 308; **Knowledge deficit:** Care and assessment of the casted extremity, p. 309; **Risk for peripheral neurovascular dysfunction** related to interrupted arterial flow secondary to compression from circumferential cast or dressing, p. 311.

See "Total Knee Arthroplasty" for **Risk for fluid volume deficit** related to postsurgical hemorrhage or hematoma formation, p. 335.

See Appendix One for nursing diagnoses and interventions in "Caring for Preoperative and Postoperative Patients," p. 395; "Caring for Patients on Prolonged Bed Rest," p. 413; and "Caring for Patients with Cancer and Other Life-Disrupting Illnesses," p. 450.

Total Hip Arthroplasty

NURSING DIAGNOSES AND INTERVENTIONS

Knowledge deficit: Potential for and mechanism of total hip arthroplasty (THA) dislocation, preventive measures, positional restrictions, prescribed ambulation regimen, potential for loosening, and use of assistive devices

Desired outcome: At a minimum of the 24 h before hospital discharge, patient verbalizes knowledge of potential for THA dislocation and measures to prevent it, as well as the mechanism of dislocation and indicators of implant loosening. Patient demonstrates prescribed regimen for ambulation and performance of ADLs without experiencing dislocation.

N O T E :   The risk of dislocation is high until the periarticular tissues scar down around the endoprosthesis. Once dislocation occurs, the potential for recurrence is greater because of stretching of the periarticular tissues. Dislocation is treated with reduction under anesthesia and immobilization in balanced suspension for 3-6 wk. Recurrent dislocation may require surgical intervention to tighten periarticular tissues or revise the THA. After 6 wk, a properly placed THA has significantly less potential for dislocation. The following discussion relates to the *posterolateral approach* for THA surgery. Other approaches require different positional restrictions.

---

1. Before surgery, advise patient about the potential for dislocation.
2. Show patient what endoprosthesis looks like (using a model or similar implant) and how easily it can be dislocated if positional restrictions are not observed (e.g., flexion of the hip to 90 degrees; internal rotation or adduction of the affected leg).
3. Before surgery, teach patient how to use ambulatory aids and ADL-assistive devices that allow independence without violation of positional restrictions. Explain the use of devices to maintain positional restrictions.
4. After surgery, discuss positional restrictions and activities that involve these restrictions: pivoting on affected leg, sitting on a regular-height toilet seat, bending over to tie shoelaces, crossing the legs.
5. Advise patient about the need for long-handled shoe horn, pickup sticks, stocking helpers, and a raised toilet seat for use after discharge. Provide addresses of stores that sell these items.
6. Be sure patient verbalizes and demonstrates understanding of positional restrictions and is able to ambulate and perform ADLs independently, using assistive devices.
7. Instruct patient to report hip, buttock, or thigh pain or prolonged limp as indicators of implant loosening.

Knowledge deficit: Potential for infection caused by foreign body reaction to endoprosthesis

Desired outcome: Within 24 h of instruction, patient verbalizes knowledge of potential for infection, its indicators, and the importance of seeking prompt medical care if they occur.

1. Advise patient that potential for infection is permanent. Because of foreign body reaction and increased blood supply resulting from associated inflammatory response, these patients are at increased risk for hematogenic (bloodborne) infection. Introduce this as a potential complication during the informed consent process, and review it during preoperative teaching.

2. Before hospital discharge, make sure patient can describe the indicators of wound, UTI, URI, and dental infections (see **Risk for infection** in "Care of the Renal Transplant Recipient," p. 85, and Table 2-5, p. 39).
3. Advise patient to wear a Medic-Alert bracelet and always to request prophylactic antibiotics for procedures that can result in bacterial seeding of the bloodstream (e.g., minor or major surgery or dental extractions).
4. Advise patient to call physician promptly to report indicators of infection from THA: drainage, pain, fever, local warmth, swelling, restricted ROM of joint, feeling of pressure in the hip.

Risk for peripheral neurovascular dysfunction related to interrupted arterial flow secondary to compression from traction or abduction device

Desired outcomes: Patient has adequate peripheral neurovascular function in distal tissues, as evidenced by warmth, normal color, and ability to dorsiflex involved foot and feel sensations on testing of peroneal nerve dermatome. After instruction, patient verbalizes knowledge of potential neurovascular complications and the importance of reporting indicators of impairment promptly.

1. Because traction sling or abduction device can press on neurovascular structures, it is imperative that neurovascular status of the leg in traction, especially peroneal nerve function, be assessed along with VS. The peroneal nerve runs superficially by the neck of the fibula and can be assessed by testing the dermatome of the first web space between the great and second toes and by having patient dorsiflex the foot. Loss of sensation or movement signals impaired peroneal nerve function. Promptly report significant findings to physician.
2. Be sure patient is aware of the potential for neurovascular impairment and the importance of reporting alterations in sensation, movement, temperature, and color of the immobilized extremity.
3. Encourage patient to reposition the leg within the restrictions of the sling and positional limitations.
4. Encourage patient to perform prescribed exercises as a means of stimulating circulation in the area.

See "Dislocation/Subluxation" for **Pain,** p. 308; **Impaired physical mobility** related to musculoskeletal impairment and adjustment to new walking gait, p. 308.

See "Fractures" for **Self-care deficit,** p. 321, and **Knowledge deficit:** Potential for infection, p. 323.

See "Amputation" for **Knowledge deficit:** Postsurgical exercise regimen, p. 329.

See "Total Knee Arthroplasty" for **Risk for fluid volume deficit** related to postsurgical hemorrhage or hematoma formation, p. 335.

Also see Appendix One for nursing diagnoses and interventions in "Caring for Preoperative and Postoperative Patients," p. 395; "Caring for Patients on Prolonged Bed Rest" (particularly **Altered peripheral tissue perfusion,** p. 418, for interventions concerning deep vein thrombosis); and "Caring for Patients with Cancer and Other Life-Disrupting Illnesses," p. 450.

PATIENT-FAMILY TEACHING AND DISCHARGE PLANNING

Give patient and significant others verbal and written information about the following:

1. Prescribed exercise regimen: reason for each exercise, number of repetitions for each, and frequency of exercise periods. Be sure patient independently demonstrates understanding of exercises and gives a return demonstration before hospital discharge.
2. Indicators of types of infections: wound (persistent redness, swelling, discharge, local warmth, restricted hip ROM, feeling of hip pressure, fever, pain); UTI (dysuria; pyuria; fever; malodorous urine; cloudy urine; urgency; frequency; pain in suprapubic, flank, groin, scrotal, or labial area); URI (change in color or amount of sputum, fever, cough, sore throat, malaise, fever); and dental (pain, swelling of the jaw, difficulty with mastication, fever). Advise patient to notify health care provider promptly if any of these indicators occur and to seek prophylactic antibiotics for minor surgical procedures.
3. Use of assistive devices: pickup sticks, stocking helpers, long-handled shoe horns, raised toilet seat. Make sure patient demonstrates independence in their use before hospital discharge.
4. Independent ambulation with crutches on level and uneven surfaces.
5. Getting into a car safely without risking dislocation. Patient should be able to demonstrate this procedure before hospital discharge.
6. Medications, including drug name, purpose, dosage, schedule, precautions, drug/drug and food/drug interactions, and potential side effects.
7. Indications of implant loosening, such as continuing hip, buttock, or thigh pain or prolonged limp.
8. Phone number of a resource person should questions arise after hospital discharge.

Total Knee Arthroplasty

NURSING DIAGNOSES AND INTERVENTIONS

Risk for fluid volume deficit related to postsurgical hemorrhage or hematoma formation
Desired outcome: Within 36 h after surgery, patient is free of symptoms of excessive bleeding or hematoma formation, as evidenced by BP ≥90/60 mm Hg (or within patient's normal range); HR ≤100 bpm; RR ≤20 breaths/min; balanced I&O; output from drainage device ≤50 ml/h; and brisk capillary refill (<2 sec), peripheral pulses >2+ on a 0-4+ scale, warmth, and normal color in involved extremity distal to surgical site.

NOTE: A hematoma is a collection of extravasated blood within tissues after surgery or trauma. During most orthopedic surgeries, a tourniquet is used to restrict blood flow from the operative field. Sometimes the tourniquet is left inflated until after the dressing or cast has been applied; therefore, major bleeding might not be noted during surgery. Even when the tourniquet is deflated, a significant bleeding vessel may be overlooked, or bleeding may begin later during the patient's recovery.

1. When taking VS, monitor drainage from drainage system as well as that on dressings or cast. Report output from drainage system that exceeds 50 ml/h.
2. Because noting amount of drainage on cast does not always provide an accurate assessment of drainage within cast, carefully evaluate patient's VS, subjective complaints, and neurovascular status.
3. Be alert for and report patient's complaints of warmth within cast or beneath dressing, things "crawling" under cast, aching, increasing pressure or pain, or coolness distal to area of surgery, which can occur with hemorrhage or hematoma formation.
4. Monitor for and report VS indicating shock or hemorrhage, including hypotension and increasing pulse rate.
5. Monitor for pallor, decreased posterior tibial or dorsalis pedis pulses, slowed capillary refill, or coolness of distal extremity, which can occur with hemorrhage or hematoma formation.
6. If hemorrhage or hematoma formation is suspected, consult physician promptly. If limb is casted, elevate it above the level of the heart to slow bleeding. If limb is not casted, apply an elastic wrap for direct pressure on the site of bleeding.
7. If hemorrhage or hematoma formation is suspected and patient's VS indicate shock but a physician is unavailable, the surgical area should be exposed by windowing the cast or loosening the dressing to allow direct inspection of the area. Direct pressure usually will control hemorrhage; if not, apply a thigh blood pressure cuff over sheet wadding to serve as a tourniquet until physician arrives for definitive therapy.

Risk for impaired skin integrity related to irritation and/or
Impaired tissue integrity (or risk for same) related to altered circulation secondary to presence of continuous passive movement (CPM) device
Desired outcomes: Skin and tissue of affected leg remain intact and nonerythematous. After instruction, patient verbalizes knowledge of the importance of reporting indicators of skin irritation promptly while undergoing CPM.

1. Preoperatively, assess skin on operant extremity, being alert for areas of irritation or redness.
2. Preoperatively, introduce patient to use of CPM, demonstrating how it will be used postoperatively. Point out areas prone to pressure or irritation from the device. Teach patient to report alterations in sensation or discomfort.
3. Postoperatively, ensure correct positioning of extremity within CPM device (i.e., neutral position of the leg, with the knee resting over the area flexed by the device).
4. Encourage patient to perform quadriceps sets, gluteal sets, and ankle circles to promote extremity circulation.

5. During VS, or more often if erythema is noted, examine medial, lateral, and posterior aspects of extremity in the CPM device for areas of erythema. Also question patient about alterations in sensation or areas of discomfort.
6. Pad areas of excessive pressure, as noted by presence of erythema. Reposition leg within the CPM device. Report areas of erythema that do not resolve.

See all nursing diagnoses (except **Knowledge deficit:** Potential for and mechanism of THA dislocation) in "Total Hip Arthroplasty," p. 332.

PATIENT-FAMILY TEACHING
AND DISCHARGE PLANNING
See "Total Hip Arthroplasty," p. 335.

Musculoskeletal

Reproductive Disorders

9

SECTION ONE: DISORDERS AND SURGICAL PROCEDURES OF THE BREAST

Breast Reduction

NURSING DIAGNOSES AND INTERVENTIONS

Body image disturbance related to breast size
Desired outcome: Before surgery, patient expresses positive, realistic reasons for having breast surgery.

1. Discuss with patient the meaning of her breasts, including likes and dislikes (both ideal and real).
2. Review patient's expectations for outcome of surgery. Patient should not have unrealistic expectations, as evidenced by statements such as, "Surgery will change my life or marriage."
3. Review informed consent form for potential risks of breast reduction (e.g., impaired breast feeding, nipple or skin necrosis, asymmetry).
4. Support patient in her decision to have surgery by spending time with her and encouraging her to discuss her fears and concerns.

Pain related to surgical procedure
Desired outcomes: Within 1 h of intervention, patient's subjective perception of pain decreases, as documented by a pain scale. Objective indicators, such as grimacing, are absent or diminished. Patient is pain free 5-7 days after surgery.

1. Assess and document location, quality, and duration of pain, using a pain scale from 0 (no pain) to 10 (worst pain).
2. Medicate patient with analgesics as prescribed; evaluate and document response, based on pain scale.
3. Make sure patient has a comfortable bra that adequately supports her breasts without binding or constricting.
4. Teach patient relaxation techniques (e.g., slow, diaphragmatic breathing; guided imagery).
5. Provide distractions (television, soothing music).

6. Encourage activity as tolerated.
7. For additional interventions, see this nursing diagnosis in Appendix One, p. 396.

Knowledge deficit: Care of incisional site and need for monthly breast self-examination (BSE)

Desired outcomes: Before hospital discharge, patient verbalizes knowledge of and demonstrates incisional site care and states signs of infection at incisional site. Patient also understands the importance of BSE after incisions have healed.

1. Instruct patient to clean incisional site after sutures have been re- moved, using basic hygiene, such as soap and water. Explain that heavy lotions, medications, or creams should not be used around in- cisional sites (except for transplanted nipples) unless specified by physician.
2. As prescribed, teach patient how to apply lotions or creams to trans- planted nipples.
3. In preparation for hospital discharge, instruct patient in BSE, using models of the breast; emphasize the importance of monthly BSE when incisions have healed.
4. Teach patient the signs of infection to report to a health care pro- vider: redness, foul odor, pain, swelling, discharge, fever.

Ineffective breast-feeding related to breast surgical procedure

Desired outcome: Before surgery, patient verbalizes understanding that this type of surgery may impair her ability to breast-feed.

1. Before surgery, explain that breast reduction surgery may impair breast-feeding in future pregnancies.
2. Arrange for session with lactation consultant if patient requests more information.

See "Breast Reconstruction" for **Risk for fluid volume deficit** re- lated to postsurgical hemorrhage or hematoma formation, p. 341, and Appendix One for "Caring for Preoperative and Postoperative Pa- tients," p. 395.

PATIENT-FAMILY TEACHING
AND DISCHARGE PLANNING

Give patient and significant others verbal and written information about the following:

1. Medications for pain relief, including drug name, purpose, dosage, schedule, precautions, drug/drug and food/drug interactions, and po- tential side effects.
2. Indicators of wound infection, which require follow-up care by health care provider: persistent redness, pain, swelling, drainage at incisional areas.
3. Care of incision site, including cleansing and dressing, if indicated.
4. Changes in the nipple, which may include decreased sensation and loss of color. Nipple sensation gradually may return within 2 yr.
5. Importance of monthly BSE. Teach or review technique as appropri- ate.

Reproductive

6. Activity restrictions, which may include limited use of arms for 2 wk postoperatively and resumption of full activity after 3 wk.

Breast Reconstruction

NURSING DIAGNOSES AND INTERVENTIONS

Knowledge deficit: Surgical procedure, preoperative care, and postoperative regimen
Desired outcome: Before surgery, patient verbalizes knowledge of surgical procedure and expected results, preoperative care, and postoperative regimen.

1. Consult physician to arrange a visit by a woman who has had breast reconstruction surgery to share feelings and demonstrate the cosmetic results. Support patient's decision for the type of procedure and/or implant to be used. Answer any questions that may arise.
2. Before surgery, explain that after surgery a suction apparatus that removes blood will be present to minimize the potential for hematoma formation. Usually this apparatus is removed after 48 h or when drainage is less than 10-20 ml over a 24-h period.
3. Explain that movement and activity may be restricted after surgery, depending on the procedure used. When an implant is placed under ample tissue, recovery is more rapid and hospitalization usually lasts 1-3 days; flap reconstruction is more involved, and movement and activity may be more restricted. Patients with latissimus flap reconstruction usually are discharged after 2-5 days when the drains are removed. A rectus abdominis procedure is more extensive, requiring up to a week of hospitalization and bed rest the day of surgery. The contralateral breast flap procedure usually requires only a few days of hospitalization.
4. Be aware that women who elect immediate reconstruction are more likely to need a follow-up procedure to obtain satisfactory cosmetic results.
5. Teach patient to monitor reconstructed nipple and report delayed capillary refill (≥ 2 sec) and duskiness. Patients who undergo nipple reconstruction usually are more satisfied with the results than those who don't; however, they may have more anxiety during the postrecovery period and thus may require more reassurance.
6. Questions often arise after hospital discharge; give patient the following information/instructions:
   - Incision care: A gauze dressing usually covers the incision until the sutures are removed, on about day 7. After removal of the sutures, micropore tape strips usually are placed over the incision until it heals; these strips are replaced when they loosen. Patient should notify physician of any signs of infection (persistent redness, pain, swelling, drainage) at incision site.
   - Showers: Showers usually are permitted if the suction catheter and sutures have been removed. If a dressing is present, it should be removed before showering and replaced afterward.
   - Activity restrictions: As directed (usually for the first 4-6 wk),

strenuous exercise, contact sports, excessive stretching, and heavy lifting (>10 lb) are prohibited. Activity that involves movement below the waist usually can be resumed after 1 wk but may be delayed, depending on the type of flap created.

Also:

- Avoid putting pressure on the chest wall for 4-6 wk (e.g., patient should use superior position during coitus).
- Wear a comfortable bra after the drains are removed; do not wear underwire bras. It will take 3-6 mo for the reconstructed breast to develop a natural contour.
- Apply the prescribed lotion to the nipple daily if nipple transplantation was performed.
- Perform monthly BSE of both breasts (review procedure with patient).
- Keep follow-up appointments if a tissue expander was used for gradual enlargement of the implant site.
- Depending on the type and placement of the implant, massage the breast with a gentle squeezing and flattening motion to prevent fibrocapsular formation. This usually is done 3 ×/day after the incision has healed.

Risk for fluid volume deficit related to postsurgical hemorrhage or hematoma formation

Desired outcomes: Patient is normovolemic, as evidenced by BP ≥90/60 mm Hg (or within patient's normal range); HR 60-100 bpm; RR ≤20 breaths/min; warm, dry skin; and urinary output ≥30 ml/h. Drainage in suction apparatus is ≤50 ml/h initially and <20 ml/h within 24 h after surgery. If patient develops a hematoma, it is detected and reported promptly.

1. Monitor patient for clinical indicators of hemorrhage (e.g., drop of systolic BP 10-20 mm Hg below trend; rapid HR; cool, clammy skin; pallor; confusion; diaphoresis). Report significant findings.
2. Assess for a hematoma, as evidenced by swelling, pain, and possibly bluish discoloration of the skin. Consult physician about significant findings.
3. Assess suction apparatus for patency, and document amount and character of drainage. Report drainage >50 ml/h for 2 h. Reestablish suction as necessary. Suction apparatus usually is removed after 48 h or if total drainage is <10-20 ml in 24 h.

Body image disturbance related to body changes before and after breast reconstruction surgery

Desired outcome: Patient has realistic expectations before surgery (e.g., that breast will look normal under clothing) and demonstrates movement toward acceptance of body changes after surgery.

1. Review with patient her expectations for the outcome of surgery.
2. Discuss emotional responses women often have after breast reconstruction, such as elation during the early postoperative period followed by depression or confusion.
3. Explain that some of the depression and confusion may be a result of the memory of the mastectomy and fear of cancer. Reassure pa-

tient that these feelings are normal and usually disappear after a short time.

4. Provide emotional support by being with patient when dressing is first removed. Explain that reconstructed breast will not look like the other breast at first, but that the molding process will begin during the recovery period and continue for 3-6 mo.

IF A SILICONE BREAST IMPLANT HAS BEEN USED (EITHER IN THE PAST OR CURRENTLY)

Anxiety related to use of silicone breast implant (silicone leakage, autoimmune disease, mammographic difficulties)

Desired outcome: Within the 24 h before hospital discharge, patient discusses concerns related to silicone implant and identifies potential systemic and local reactions.

1. Advise patient that removal of the silicone breast implant generally is not considered unless problems develop.
2. Inform patient that surgical substitution can be made with saline implants if necessary.
3. Teach patient to report symptoms of body's reaction to silicone: joint swelling and pain; skin erythema and swelling; glandular swelling; unusual fatigue; swelling of the feet or hands.
4. Teach patient to report symptoms of fibrocapsular formation (e.g., breast hardness), which may be painful and result in a displaced breast.
5. Make sure patient is given the name of the type of implant used and the manufacturer's applicable identification number.

See Appendix One for nursing diagnoses and interventions in "Caring for Preoperative and Postoperative Patients," p. 395, and "Caring for Patients with Cancer and Other Life-Disrupting Illnesses," p. 423.

PATIENT-FAMILY TEACHING AND DISCHARGE PLANNING

Give patient and significant others verbal and written information about the following:

1. Care of incision, including applying a gauze dressing until sutures are removed, about day 7. After sutures are removed, micropore tape strips usually are placed over incision until healing has taken place, and are replaced when they loosen. Instruct patient to notify physician if signs of infection (persistent redness, pain, swelling, drainage) appear at incision site.
2. Taking showers, which usually are permitted after suction catheter and sutures are removed. If present, the dressing should be removed from the surgical site before showering and replaced afterward.
3. Activity restriction for the first 4-6 wk or as directed, including strenuous exercise, contact sports, excessive stretching, and heavy lifting (>10 lb).
4. Importance of not putting pressure on the chest wall for 4-6 wk (e.g., patient should use superior position during coitus).

5. Importance of breast massage 3 ×/day for at least the first year after surgery. Explain that it takes 3-6 mo for the reconstructed breast to appear natural in contour.
6. Potential recommendation not to wear a bra for 3 mo to allow for unrestricted movement of implant.
7. Necessity of applying prescribed lotion to nipple daily if nipple transplantation was performed.
8. Importance of monthly BSE of both breasts. Teach or review procedure as appropriate. In addition, stress the importance of follow up care. Successful reconstruction may give a false sense of security.
9. Medications, including drug name, purpose, dosage, schedule, precautions, drug/drug and food/drug interactions, and potential side effects.

Malignant Breast Disorders

NURSING DIAGNOSES AND INTERVENTIONS

Anxiety related to the possibility of cancer and its treatment
Desired outcome: Within 12 h of hospital admission, patient expresses concerns and exhibits increasing psychologic comfort, as evidenced by participation in decisions regarding her care and reporting that she can rest and sleep adequately.
1. Assess patient's understanding of the possible diagnosis and the treatment plan; clarify and explain as appropriate. Also determine what patient has learned about breast cancer from books, TV, or friends and relatives, and correct any misconceptions.
2. Give patient the opportunity to express her feelings and fears about the diagnosis.
3. Evaluate patient's emotional status. The breast may represent nurturance, sexuality, femininity, and desirability to her.
4. Assess your own feelings about the diagnosis of cancer and the psychologic meaning of the breast. Your attitudes may be reflected in patient's care; therefore, a positive attitude is essential for optimal patient support.
5. Provide a nonthreatening, relaxed atmosphere for patient and significant others by using therapeutic communication techniques, such as open-ended questions and reflection.
6. For additional interventions, see this nursing diagnosis in Appendix One, p. 451.

Ineffective individual coping related to situational crisis (diagnosis of breast cancer)
Desired outcomes: Within the 24 h before hospital discharge, patient expresses her feelings, identifies positive coping patterns (e.g., using support systems, planning daily activities), and accepts the support of others.
1. Assist patient in identifying and developing a support system.
2. Provide support to patient's significant other. Refer significant other to a support group that addresses his or her specific concerns.

Reproductive

3. If a mastectomy was performed, recognize the signs of grief: denial, anger, withdrawal, inappropriate affect. Provide emotional support, and describe the stages of grief to patient and significant others. Also explain to significant others, who may misunderstand patient's behavior or actions.

4. Consult with surgeon about a visit from a woman who has had a diagnosis similar to patient's. Reach to Recovery volunteers from the American Cancer Society are trained to share their experiences with breast cancer patients.

5. See "Caring for Patients with Cancer and Other Life-Disrupting Illnesses," p. 450, in Appendix One for this and other psychosocial nursing diagnoses and interventions.

Risk for disuse syndrome related to upper extremity immobilization secondary to discomfort, lymphedema, or infection after mastectomy

Desired outcomes: Before surgery, patient verbalizes knowledge of the importance of and rationale for upper extremity movements and exercises. Upon recovery, patient has full ROM of upper extremity.

1. Consult surgeon before mastectomy to determine the type of surgery expected. With surgeon's help, develop an exercise plan specific to patient's needs and surgical procedure; implement this plan as soon as patient returns from the recovery room.

2. As soon as patient returns to her room, encourage finger, wrist, and elbow movement to help minimize edema.

3. Elevate extremity as tolerated.

4. Encourage progressive exercise by having patient use affected arm for personal hygiene and ADLs the morning after surgery, if indicated. Other exercises (e.g., clasping the hands behind the head and "walking" the fingers up the wall) should be added as soon as patient is ready. After the sutures have been removed (usually 7-10 days after surgery), patient should begin exercises to enhance external rotation and abduction of the shoulder. She should be able to achieve maximum shoulder flexion by touching her fingertips together behind her back. A Reach for Recovery volunteer can visit and provide patient with verbal and written instructions for these exercises.

5. Assist patient with ambulation until her gait is normal. Encourage her to maintain correct posture, keeping back straight and shoulders back.

6. To minimize the risk of lymphedema and infection, do not give injections, check BP, or take blood samples from affected arm. Remind patient of her lowered resistance to infection and the importance of treating any breaks in the skin promptly. To help prevent infection after hospital discharge, advise patient to clean minor cuts and abrasions with soap and water and to notify her health care provider if signs of infection occur: swelling, erythema, warmth in affected arm.

7. Advise patient to wear a Medic-Alert bracelet that cautions against using involved arm for injections and tests.

8. To protect the hand and arm from injury, advise patient to wear a

protective glove when gardening or doing chores that require exposure to harsh chemicals such as cleaning fluids. Instruct her not to cut her cuticles and to use lotion to keep the skin soft.

Pain related to the surgical procedure

Desired outcomes: Within 1 h of intervention, patient's subjective perception of pain decreases, as documented by a pain scale; objective indicators, such as grimacing, are absent or diminished. Patient reports that pain is relieved with IV or IM narcotics for the first 48 h after surgery and with oral medications for the following 2 wk, with pain decreasing daily.

1. Assess and document location, quality, and duration of pain, rating it with patient on a scale of 0 (no pain) to 10 (worst pain).
2. Medicate patient with prescribed analgesics before pain becomes too severe, or provide instructions for individuals using patient-controlled analgesia (PCA). Evaluate and document response, using pain scale.
3. Reassure patient that phantom breast sensations and hyperesthesia and dysesthesia of chest wall are normal.
4. Provide a comfortable in-bed position, and support affected arm with pillows.
5. Encourage movement of fingers on affected arm to increase circulation. Inform patient that although progressive exercise will cause some discomfort, it will help build up mobility of affected arm and enhance recovery.
6. Reassure patient that exercise movements will be adapted to her level of tolerance.
7. If appropriate, instruct patient in relaxation techniques and use of guided imagery.
8. Provide distraction, such as television, radio, or books.
9. Use touch to help relieve tension (e.g., by giving a gentle massage).
10. For additional interventions, see this nursing diagnosis in Appendix One, p. 396.

Body image disturbance related to loss of a breast

Desired outcome: Within the 24 h before hospital discharge, patient verbalizes knowledge of possible emotional reactions and body image implications related to loss of her breast.

1. Recognize that loss of a breast is perceived in different ways by different women.
2. Provide emotional support by being with patient when surgical dressing is removed.
3. As appropriate, explain that sexual relations can be resumed as soon as surgical pain has diminished. Reassure patient that relations that were positive before surgery usually remain positive. However, be aware that sexual relationships that were weak before surgery may not tolerate the added stress. Refer patient to counseling when indicated.
4. Recognize the need for a supportive person, such as a Reach for Recovery volunteer who underwent the same procedure. Consult physician about a visit from such a person, if indicated. Support systems also should be made available to significant others.

Reproductive

5. If reconstruction is to be delayed, or if it is contraindicated or not desired, provide patient with a breast prosthesis after surgery to help her feel "normal." A temporary prosthesis made of nylon and filled with Dacron fluff (usually provided by the Reach for Recovery volunteer) can be worn until the incision heals. Provide patient with information about where to get a breast prosthesis. The American Cancer Society has lists of distributors and types of prostheses available.

6. Be aware that use of touch often enhances patient's self-image.

7. Provide information and answer questions about breast reconstruction (see p. 340).

8. For additional interventions, see this nursing diagnosis in Appendix One, p. 459.

Altered family processes related to breast malignancy and treatment with radiation therapy and/or chemotherapy.

Desired outcome: Within the 24 h before hospital discharge, patient of childbearing age verbalizes accurate information about pregnancy and parenthood after breast cancer and its treatment.

N O T E :   Reproductive counseling should take into account the patient's age, stage of disease, type of cancer treatment, and pretreatment fertility status.

---

1. Explain that childbearing should be delayed for about 2 yr after cancer diagnosis and treatment, or for as long as physician advises. This interval varies, depending on the stage of the disease, use of adjuvant therapies, and other factors.

2. Explain to patient that she can breast-feed with either breast after chemotherapy, but that after radiation therapy she should use only the nonirradiated breast.

3. Explore adoption as an alternative for an infertile couple.

4. As indicated, discuss issues of parental death and single parenthood with patient and significant other. See psychosocial nursing diagnoses and interventions in Appendix One, "Caring for Patients with Cancer and Other Life-Disrupting Illnesses," p. 450.

See Appendix One for nursing diagnoses and interventions in "Caring for Preoperative and Postoperative Patients," p. 395, and "Caring for Patients with Cancer and Other Life-Disrupting Illnesses," p. 423.

PATIENT-FAMILY TEACHING
AND DISCHARGE PLANNING

Give patient and significant others verbal and written information about the following:

1. Medications, including drug name, purpose, dosage, schedule, precautions, drug/drug and food/drug interactions, and potential side effects.

2. Dates and types of follow-up treatments.

3. Resumption of sexual activity, which usually can occur as soon as pain abates.

4. Care of the incision site, including cleansing. Explain the components of good hygiene.
5. Progressive exercise regimen, which should be continued at home. Advise patient to stop the exercise movement if a pulling sensation or pain is felt.
6. Informing health care provider not to measure BP or give injections in affected arm.
7. Indicators of infection (fever, erythema, local warmth, skin discoloration) and the importance of reporting them to health care provider.
8. Permanent breast prosthesis if indicated, including distributors and types available.
9. Name and telephone number of a support person who can be called during the first postoperative year. An ideal individual would be a Reach for Recovery volunteer.
10. Importance of performing monthly breast self-examination (BSE). In addition, as a part of BSE, teach patient to palpate scar, sweep down chest wall, and palpate axillary, supraclavicular, and subclavian lymph nodes to assess for lumps. In addition, teach patient that skin changes (e.g., rashes, erythema) suggest recurrence and that they should be reported promptly.
11. Importance of follow-up care.

SECTION TWO: NEOPLASMS OF THE FEMALE PELVIS

Cancer of the Cervix

NURSING DIAGNOSES AND INTERVENTIONS

Pain related to surgery or radiation implant
Desired outcomes: Within 1 h of intervention, patient's subjective perception of pain decreases, as documented by a pain scale. Objective indicators, such as grimacing, are absent or diminished.
1. Provide back rubs, which are especially helpful for patients who were in the lithotomy position during surgery. Massage shoulders and upper back for patients with radium implants, who are not allowed position changes.
2. For other interventions, see this nursing diagnosis in Appendix One, p. 396.

Risk for fluid volume deficit related to operative, postoperative, or postimplant bleeding
Desired outcomes: Patient is normovolemic, as evidenced by BP $\geq$90/60 mm Hg (or within patient's usual range); HR 60-100 bpm; urinary output $\geq$30 ml/h; RR $\leq$20 breaths/min with normal depth and pattern (eupnea); skin dry and of normal color; and soft, nondistended

abdomen. Patient and significant others verbalize knowledge of the signs and symptoms of excessive bleeding and are aware of need to alert staff promptly if they occur.

1. Monitor VS q2-4h during the first 24 h. Be alert for indicators of hemorrhage and impending shock: hypotension, increased pulse and respirations, pallor, diaphoresis.
2. Assess postoperative bleeding q2-4h by noting amount and quality of drainage on dressings and perineal pads if abdominal approach was used, or on perineal pads alone if vaginal approach was used. Normally postoperative bleeding is minimal. It should be dark (or serosanguineous if an abdominal hysterectomy was performed). If an implant is in place, check for vaginal bleeding.
3. Inspect abdomen for distention, and assess patient for severe abdominal pain; both are indicators of internal bleeding.
4. Review CBC values for evidence of bleeding: decreases in Hgb and Hct. Consult physician about significant findings. Optimal values are Hgb $\geq$12 g/dl and Hct $\geq$37%.
5. Teach patient and significant others the signs of excessive bleeding and the importance of alerting staff immediately if they occur.

Altered urinary elimination (oliguria or anuria) related to inadequate intake, obstruction of indwelling catheter, or ureteral ligation

Desired outcome: Within 24 h of surgery, patient demonstrates a balanced I&O, with urinary output $\geq$30 ml/h immediately after surgery.

1. Monitor I&O and document each shift. Consult physician about urinary output <30 ml/h for 2 consecutive hours despite adequate intake.
2. Ensure patency of indwelling catheter.
3. Administer oral or parenteral fluids as prescribed. Make sure nonrestricted patients get 2-3 L/day.
4. Assess for bladder distention by inspecting suprapubic area and percussing or palpating bladder. **Caution:** For patients with radiation implants, bladder distention can result in radiation burns to the bladder.

Grieving related to actual or perceived loss or changes in body image, body function, or role performance secondary to diagnosis of cancer

Desired outcome: Before hospital discharge, patient and significant others express grief, explain the meaning of the loss, and communicate concerns with each other. Patient completes self-care activities as her condition improves.

1. Anticipate patient's concern about loss of uterus, presence of cancer, potential for recurrence, and "loss of womanhood." Provide emotional support and unhurried atmosphere for patient and significant others to ask questions and express concerns, frustrations, and fears.
2. Recognize covert signs of grief that can accompany self-concept disturbances: anger, withdrawal, demanding behavior, inappropriate affect. Give support to significant others who might misinterpret patient's coping mechanisms.

3. To enhance patient's sense of control over her situation, encourage her to perform ADLs and begin self-care as soon as her condition warrants.
4. Provide materials by organizations such as the American Cancer Society and arrange for a contact person from such an organization, if appropriate.
5. For additional interventions, see this nursing diagnosis in Appendix One, p. 456.

See Appendix One for nursing diagnoses and interventions in "Caring for Preoperative and Postoperative Patients," p. 395, and "Caring for Patients with Cancer and Other Life-Disrupting Illnesses," p. 423.

PATIENT-FAMILY TEACHING
AND DISCHARGE PLANNING

Give patient and significant others verbal and written information about the following:

PATIENTS WITH RADIUM IMPLANTS

1. Necessity of notifying physician if the following problems occur: vaginal bleeding, rectal bleeding, foul-smelling vaginal discharge, abdominal pain or distention, dysuria, urinary frequency, hematuria.
2. Resumption of sexual intercourse, typically 6 wk after surgery or as directed by physician. Describe, as indicated, use of a vaginal dilator to prevent stenosis. It usually is inserted once a day for 5 min.
3. Medications, including drug name, purpose, dosage, schedule, precautions, drug/drug and food/drug interactions, and potential side effects.
4. Need for follow-up care; confirm date and time of next appointment.
5. Patient is *not* radioactive once implant has been removed.
6. Side effects of radium implants: vaginal dryness, burning sensation, vaginal discharge.

PATIENTS WHO HAD A HYSTERECTOMY

1. Necessity of notifying physician if the following indicators of infection occur: incisional swelling, redness, purulent drainage, vaginal bleeding, abdominal pain.
2. Care of incision.
3. Restriction of activities as directed, such as heavy lifting (>10 lb) and sexual intercourse. Advise patient to get maximum amounts of rest and avoid fatigue.
4. Medications, including drug name, purpose, dosage, schedule, precautions, drug/drug and food/drug interactions, and potential side effects.
5. Need for follow-up care; confirm date and time of next appointment.

Reproductive

Ovarian Tumors

NURSING DIAGNOSES AND INTERVENTIONS

See "Cancer of the Cervix" for **Pain,** p. 347; **Risk for fluid volume deficit** (bleeding), p. 347; **Altered urinary elimination,** p. 348; and **Grieving,** p. 348.

Also see Appendix One for nursing diagnoses and interventions in "Caring for Preoperative and Postoperative Patients," p. 395, and "Caring for Patients with Cancer and Other Life-Disrupting Illnesses," p. 423.

PATIENT-FAMILY TEACHING AND DISCHARGE PLANNING

Give patient and significant others verbal and written information about the following:

1. Medications, including drug name, purpose, dosage, schedule, precautions, drug/drug and food/drug interactions, and potential side effects.
2. Importance of reporting indicators of infection (depending on surgery) to physician: fever, vaginal bleeding and discharge, abdominal pain and distention, and incisional redness, purulent drainage, local warmth, and swelling.
3. Activity restrictions related to heavy lifting (>10 lb), exercise, sexual intercourse, or housework, as directed by physician.
4. Necessity of follow-up appointments; confirm date and time of next appointments with physician or for radiation therapy or chemotherapy as appropriate.

Endometrial Cancer

NURSING DIAGNOSES AND INTERVENTIONS

See "Cancer of the Cervix," p. 347.

PATIENT-FAMILY TEACHING AND DISCHARGE PLANNING

See "Cancer of the Cervix," p. 349.

Vulvar Cancer

NURSING DIAGNOSES AND INTERVENTIONS

Sexual dysfunction related to fear after surgical procedure, excision of reproductive tract, and/or pain
Desired outcome: Within the 24 h before hospital discharge, patient communicates concerns with partner and verbalizes a plan for satisfying sexual activity.

1. Determine patient's need to communicate fears and concerns regarding sexual functioning after treatment of vulvar cancer.

2. As indicated, teach patient that vulvectomy usually does not diminish sexual responsiveness; however, sexual functioning may be changed, depending on procedure used and patient's psychosocial adjustments.

3. Advise patient to use medications or relaxation techniques (e.g., hot shower) before sexual activity to help prevent discomfort.

4. If vaginal lubrication is reduced, suggest that patient use a water-soluble lubricant.

5. Suggest the female superior position during coitus to control depth of penetration.

6. Suggest alternative sexual practices, depending on couple's values. Options include vibrators, touching, and massage.

7. As indicated, advise patient that sexual intercourse usually can be resumed after healing has occurred.

For other nursing diagnoses and interventions, see "Cancer of the Cervix," p. 347.

PATIENT-FAMILY TEACHING AND DISCHARGE PLANNING

See "Cancer of the Cervix," p. 349.

SECTION THREE: DISORDERS OF THE FEMALE PELVIS

Endometriosis

NURSING DIAGNOSES AND INTERVENTIONS

Anticipatory grieving related to potential for reproductive infertility
Desired outcome: Within the 24 h before hospital discharge, patient and significant other express grief, participate in decisions about the future, and communicate their concerns to health care team and each other.

1. Assess for and accept patient's stage in the grieving process and behavioral response. Expect reactions such as disbelief, denial, grief, ambivalence, and depression. Recognize that patient and significant other may move from one stage to another, depending on the circumstance (i.e., desire for a child, type of treatment recommended, or stage of endometriosis and subsequent likelihood of infertility).

2. Assess religious and sociocultural expectations related to loss (e.g., Is childbearing of primary importance in the relationship? What are the desires of the family for offspring? Has there been a lifelong desire to have children?).

3. Encourage patient and significant other to explore and communicate feelings about anticipated loss of fertility. Recognize that the

Reproductive

woman often feels a greater sense of loss than the man. Infertility can place a strain on the relationship; treatment options may be expensive and time consuming and may raise ethical issues.

4. Assess couple's coping strategies. Suggest other ways of handling grief if their strategies are ineffective. Common strategies include increasing the space between themselves and reminders of their infertility (i.e., keeping busy), regaining control (seeking information, keeping a positive attitude), giving in to feelings (crying, indulging), and sharing their burden with each other and others.

5. Demonstrate empathy. Provide an open, supportive atmosphere. Patient often is exposed to those who have children and do not value the experience. Recognize that patient may feel hostility toward those who are fertile.

6. Assess for support systems, and describe and provide addresses of groups that share a common interest (e.g., RESOLVE). It also may be helpful to arrange for referrals to specialists with knowledge of infertility (e.g., psychiatric nurse clinician, psychologist).

7. For additional interventions, see this nursing diagnosis in Appendix One, p. 456.

See "Cancer of the Cervix" for **Pain,** p. 347, and **Risk for fluid volume deficit** (bleeding), p. 347. See Appendix One for nursing diagnoses and interventions in "Caring for Preoperative and Postoperative Patients," p. 395.

PATIENT-FAMILY TEACHING AND DISCHARGE PLANNING

See "Ovarian Tumors," p. 350.

Cystocele

NURSING DIAGNOSES AND INTERVENTIONS

See "Urinary Incontinence," p. 94, for related nursing diagnoses. See "Cancer of the Cervix" for **Risk for fluid volume deficit** (bleeding), p. 347.

See "Vulvar Cancer" for **Sexual dysfunction,** p. 350.

See Appendix One for nursing diagnoses and interventions in "Caring for Preoperative and Postoperative Patients," p. 395.

PATIENT-FAMILY TEACHING AND DISCHARGE PLANNING

Give patient and significant others verbal and written information about the following:

1. Medications, including drug name, purpose, dosage, schedule, precautions, drug/drug and food/drug interactions, and potential side effects.

2. Activity limitations during first 6 wk or as physician directs, including no heavy lifting (>10 lb) or strenuous exercise.
3. Forgoing sexual intercourse for 6 wk or as prescribed if vaginal surgery was performed. Discuss alternative methods of sexual expression.
4. Notifying physician if indicators of infection appear: fever; persistent pain; purulent, foul-smelling drainage; foul-smelling, bloody, or cloudy urine.
5. Importance of follow-up appointments; confirm date and time of next appointment.

Rectocele

NURSING DIAGNOSES AND INTERVENTIONS

Constipation related to restriction against straining, low-residue diet, or pain with defecation secondary to surgical procedure
Desired outcomes: After early postoperative period, patient has bowel movements within her normal pattern and with minimal discomfort. Patient verbalizes knowledge of rationale for alerting staff before and after bowel movements and for not straining during defecation.
1. Assess patient for constipation; administer stool softeners or mild laxatives as prescribed.
2. Patient will be on a low-residue diet during the early postoperative period to minimize the potential for disruption of the surgical site. As indicated after early postoperative period, consult physician about introducing high-residue foods to promote bowel movements.
3. Instruct patient not to strain when having a bowel movement, because this can disrupt the surgical repair.
4. Advise patient that defecation may be painful, and tell her to alert staff as soon as the urge to defecate is felt so that she can be medicated before bowel movement.
5. Do not use enemas or rectal tubes, which can disrupt the surgical repair.
6. Provide sitz baths as a comfort measure after bowel movements.
7. Ask patient to notify staff after each bowel movement; document accordingly.

See "Cancer of the Cervix" for **Risk for fluid volume deficit** (bleeding), p. 347. See "Vulvar Cancer" for **Sexual dysfunction,** p. 350. See Appendix One for nursing diagnoses and interventions in "Caring for Preoperative and Postoperative Patients," p. 395.

PATIENT-FAMILY TEACHING AND DISCHARGE PLANNING

Give patient and significant others verbal and written information about the following:
1. Medications, including drug name, purpose, dosage, schedule, pre-

Reproductive

cautions, drug/drug and food/drug interactions, and potential side effects.
2. Limitation of activities during the first 6 wk as directed by physician, including heavy lifting (>10 lb) and exercising. Abstinence from sexual intercourse usually is recommended for 6 wk. Discuss alternative forms of sexual expression with patient. Advise patient that initially coitus may be painful.
3. Indicators of infection: abdominal or rectal pain, foul-smelling vaginal discharge, fever.
4. Dietary recommendations and the importance of an adequate fluid intake.
5. Importance of a regular bowel elimination pattern to prevent constipation and straining.
6. Importance of follow-up care; confirm date and time of next appointment.

Uterine Prolapse

NURSING DIAGNOSES AND INTERVENTIONS

See "Cancer of the Cervix" for **Risk for fluid volume deficit** (bleeding), p. 347, and, if a hysterectomy was performed, **Grieving,** p. 348.

See "Vulvar Cancer" for **Sexual dysfunction,** p. 350, and "Rectocele" for **Constipation,** p. 353.

See Appendix One for nursing diagnoses and interventions in "Caring for Preoperative and Postoperative Patients," p. 395.

PATIENT-FAMILY TEACHING AND DISCHARGE PLANNING

See "Rectocele," p. 353.

SECTION FOUR: INTERRUPTION OF PREGNANCY

Spontaneous Abortion

NURSING DIAGNOSES AND INTERVENTIONS

Risk for fluid volume deficit related to abortive or postsurgical bleeding
Desired outcome: Patient is normovolemic, as evidenced by BP ≥90/60 mm Hg; HR 60-100 bpm; urinary output ≥30 ml/h; RR ≤20 breaths/min with normal pattern and depth (eupnea); warm, dry skin; and orientation to time, place, and person.
1. Assess and document BP, HR, and RR at frequent intervals (typi-

cally q15min × 4; q30min × 2; q1-2h until stable; and then q4h). Consult physician about significant changes. Be alert for hypotension; changes in LOC; cool, clammy skin; and increasing HR and RR.

2. Monitor I&O at least q4h. Be alert for decreasing urinary output, which can signal the onset of shock.

3. Administer parenteral fluids, blood, and blood products as prescribed.

4. If prescribed, administer oxytocin to assist with contraction of uterus and expulsion of products of conception (POC).

5. Inspect perineal pads, and note and document amount and quality of bleeding. If vaginal bleeding increases or expulsion of POC occurs, notify physician at once. Save any tissue or clots expelled. **Note:** Bleeding is considered excessive if 1 or more perineal pads are saturated in 1 h and symptoms of orthostasis are present (i.e., fainting or dizziness upon standing, diaphoresis, pallor).

6. After expulsion of POC, palpate uterine fundus to assess its tone. If it feels soft and boggy, provide light massage, using a circular motion. **Caution:** Do not massage a uterus that is well contracted because this can result in muscle fatigue and uterine relaxation.

Pain related to uterine contractions

Desired outcomes: Within 30 min of intervention, patient's subjective perception of pain decreases, as documented by a pain scale. Objective indicators, such as grimacing, are absent or diminished.

1. Monitor and document frequency and duration of contractions. Assess and document patient's level of pain and response to management, using a scale of 0 (no pain) to 10 (worst pain).

2. Administer analgesics as prescribed. Provide back rubs, which are especially relaxing.

3. Instruct patient in alternative methods of pain relief: deep breathing, relaxation techniques, guided imagery.

4. For additional interventions see this nursing diagnosis in Appendix One, p. 396.

Risk for infection related to retention of part or all of POC

Desired outcome: Patient is free of infection, as evidenced by normothermia and absence of foul-smelling vaginal discharge and abdominal tenderness.

1. Assess temperature q4h; consult physician if it becomes elevated.

2. Be alert for foul-smelling vaginal discharge, a signal of infection.

3. Administer antibiotics as prescribed.

4. Ensure that proper perineal care is performed after voiding and bowel movements.

Altered role performance related to fetal loss

Desired outcome: Before hospital discharge, patient verbalizes realistic acceptance of change in her role as wife or childbearer or verbalizes plans for adaptation.

1. Provide emotional support for patient and significant others. Provide time and a supportive atmosphere that allows patient to feel comfortable expressing feelings and concerns. Do not minimize pa-

tient's feelings of loss. Conversely, if pregnancy was not desired, she may experience feelings of relief or guilt about the loss.

2. Assist patient in identifying concerns, if present, with role performance as wife or childbearer. Assist patient in developing plans for adaptation. Provide referral for genetic counseling if genetics was a factor in pregnancy loss.

3. Involve social services if needed.

Grieving related to anticipated or actual fetal loss

Desired outcome: Before hospital discharge, patient expresses feelings about loss (actual or potential) and shares her grief with significant others.

1. Assess stage of grieving patient is experiencing. Be aware that feelings may be complicated by emotions that preceded the actual or impending fetal loss (e.g., if the woman experienced joy about her pregnancy, her grief may be more than anticipated; conversely, if the pregnancy was viewed negatively, she may experience feelings of guilt and self-blame).

2. Do not minimize patient's feelings of loss. Recognize that an early pregnancy loss may take longer to resolve, because the grieving process is complicated by the absence of a recognizable body.

3. Assist patient and significant others with acknowledging the loss by taking the time to sit and talk with them.

4. Offer emotional support and encourage patient and significant others to discuss the loss among themselves, as well.

5. Ensure privacy for patient and significant others.

6. Refer patient to community-based parent support group.

7. Provide for pastoral or other supportive care if indicated.

8. See psychosocial nursing diagnoses for patients and families in Appendix One, p. 450.

PATIENT-FAMILY TEACHING
AND DISCHARGE PLANNING

Give patient and significant others verbal and written information about the following:

1. Medications, including drug name, purpose, dosage, schedule, precautions, drug/drug and food/drug interactions, and potential side effects.

2. Vaginal bleeding, which should taper gradually during the first 10 days. Advise patient that an increase in bleeding is abnormal and requires medical attention.

3. Indicators of infection, which necessitate medical attention: temperature $\geq 37.78°$ C (100° F), foul-smelling vaginal discharge, and/or abdominal tenderness or pain.

4. Activity limitations as directed by physician, including strenuous exercise and sexual relations.

5. Importance of follow-up care; confirm date and time of next appointment.

6. Names and addresses of community resources.

Ectopic Pregnancy

NURSING DIAGNOSES AND INTERVENTIONS

Risk for fluid volume deficit related to bleeding or hemorrhage with ectopic rupture

Desired outcome: Patient is normovolemic, as evidenced by urinary output ≥30 ml/h; BP ≥90/60 mm Hg; RR ≤20 breaths/min with normal depth and pattern (eupnea); HR ≤100 bpm; warm, dry skin; absent or scant vaginal bleeding.

1. Assess VS at frequent intervals, noting changes in BP, HR, and RR. Be alert for hypotension, increases in HR and RR, and cool, clammy skin as indicators of impending shock.
2. Assess amount and quality of vaginal bleeding. Bright red, frank bleeding, along with abnormal VS, should be reported to physician at once.
3. Review results of CBC, noting values of Hgb and Hct, which decline with blood loss. Optimal values are Hgb ≥12 g/dl and Hct ≥37%.
4. Infuse parenteral and blood products as prescribed.

See "Spontaneous Abortion" for **Grieving,** p. 356, and **Altered role performance,** p. 355. See "Endometriosis" for **Anticipatory grieving,** p. 351. See Appendix One for nursing diagnoses and interventions in "Caring for Preoperative and Postoperative Patients," p. 395. See psychosocial nursing diagnoses and interventions for patient and significant others in "Caring for Patients with Cancer and Other Life-Disrupting Illnesses," p. 450.

PATIENT-FAMILY TEACHING AND DISCHARGE PLANNING

Give patient and significant others verbal and written information about the following, depending on the type of surgery performed:

1. Medications, including drug name, purpose, dosage, schedule, precautions, drug/drug and food/drug interactions, and potential side effects.
2. Importance of monitoring vaginal drainage, including amount, color, consistency, and odor, and of reporting significant changes to physician.
3. Activity limitations as directed by physician, including strenuous exercise, housework, and sexual relations.
4. Indicators of incisional infection: persistent redness, swelling, warmth, fever, purulent discharge, incisional/abdominal pain.
5. Importance of follow-up care and purpose of serial human chorionic gonadotropin (HCG) levels (with the more conservative treatment) or methotrexate management; confirm time and date of next appointment.

Reproductive

SECTION FIVE: DISORDERS AND SURGICAL PROCEDURES OF THE MALE PELVIS

Benign Prostatic Hypertrophy

NURSING DIAGNOSES AND INTERVENTIONS

Risk for fluid volume deficit related to postsurgical bleeding/hemorrhage

Desired outcomes: Patient is normovolemic, as evidenced by balanced I&O, HR ≤100 bpm (or within patient's normal range), BP ≥90/60 mm Hg (or within patient's normal range), RR ≤20 breaths/min, and skin that is warm, dry, and of normal color. After instruction, patient relates actions that might result in hemorrhage of the prostatic capsule and participates in interventions to prevent them.

1. Upon patient's return from the recovery room, monitor VS q15min for the first 30 min; if stable, check q30min for 1 h; and then q4h for 24 h or per agency policy. Be alert for increasing pulse, decreasing BP, diaphoresis, pallor, and increasing respirations, which can occur with hemorrhage and impending shock.
2. Monitor and document I&O q8h. Subtract amount of fluid used with bladder irrigations from total output.
3. Monitor catheter drainage closely for the first 24 h. Watch for dark red drainage that does not lighten to reddish-pink or drainage that remains thick after irrigation, which can signal venous bleeding within the operative site. Drainage should lighten to pink or blood-tinged within 24 h after surgery.
4. Be alert for bright red, thick drainage at any time, which can occur with arterial bleeding within the operative site.
5. Do not take temperature rectally or insert tubes or enemas into rectum. Instruct patient not to strain with bowel movements or sit for long periods. Any of these actions can put pressure on the prostatic capsule and may lead to hemorrhage. Obtain prescription for and provide stool softeners or cathartics as necessary.
6. Surgeon may establish traction on the indwelling urethral catheter in the operating room to help prevent bleeding. Maintain traction for 4-8 h after surgery or as directed.
7. Also monitor patient for signs of disseminated intravascular coagulation, which can occur as a result of the release of large amounts of tissue thromboplastins, which can occur during a transurethral resection of the prostate (TURP). Watch for active bleeding (dark red) without clots and unusual oozing from all puncture sites. Report significant findings promptly if they occur. For more information, see "Disseminated Intravascular Coagulation," p. 300.

Risk for infection (septic shock) related to invasive procedure (cystoscopy or TURP), resulting in risk of introduction of gram-negative bacteria

Desired outcome: Patient is free of gram-negative infection, as evidenced by normothermia; urinary output ≥30 ml/h; RR 12-20 breaths/min; HR and BP within patient's normal range; and orientation to time, place, and person (within patient's normal range).

N O T E :   Accurate assessment of the patient in the early (warm) stage of septic shock greatly improves the prognosis.

1. Monitor patient's VS and mentation status at frequent intervals for indicators of the early (warm) stage of septic shock. During the first 24 h after surgery, be alert for temperatures of 38.3°-40° C (101°-104° F), which occur with infection due to increased metabolic activity and release of pyrogens. Also assess for moderately increased RR and HR and decreased BP. Classic circulatory signs of collapse occur in the late (cold) stage of septic shock: profoundly decreased BP (due to decreased stroke volume); greatly increased and weakened HR (compensatory mechanism to maintain cardiac output), and decreased RR (owing to respiratory center depression). Mental status changes of inappropriate behavior, personality changes, restlessness, increasing lethargy, and disorientation may signal hypoxia due to decreased cerebral perfusion.
2. Monitor patient's skin for flushing and warmth, which are early signs of septic shock due to vasodilatation. In the cold stage of septic shock, skin becomes cool and pale because of sustained vasoconstriction.
3. Monitor patient's urinary output for decrease and for increased concentration (normal specific gravity is 1.010-1.020).
4. Notify physician promptly if septic shock is suspected. Prepare for the following if septic shock is confirmed: IV infusion (e.g., lactated Ringer's or normal saline); oxygen administration; specimens for WBC, ABG, and electrolyte values; and administration of antibiotics.
5. Teach the indicators of infection and early septic shock to patient, and stress the importance of notifying staff promptly if they occur.

Fluid volume excess (or risk for same) related to absorption of irrigating fluid during surgery (TURP syndrome)

Desired outcomes: After surgery, patient is normovolemic, as evidenced by balanced I&O (after subtraction of irrigant total from output); orientation to time, place, and person; BP and HR within patient's normal range; absence of dysrhythmias; and electrolyte values within normal range. Urinary output is ≥30 ml/h, and drainage from Jackson-Pratt drain is >40 ml/h.

1. Monitor and record VS. Watch for sudden increases in BP with corresponding decrease in HR. Monitor pulse for dysrhythmias, including irregular rate and skipped beats.
2. Monitor and record I&O. To determine true amount of urinary output, subtract amount of irrigant from total output. Report discrepancies, which can signal fluid retention or loss.

Reproductive

3. Monitor patient's mental and motor status. Assess for muscle twitching, seizures, and changes in mentation; these are signs of water intoxication and electrolyte imbalance, which can occur within 24 h after surgery because of the high volumes of fluid used in irrigation.
4. Monitor electrolyte values, in particular sodium (Na^+), for evidence of hyponatremia. Normal range for Na^+ is 137-147 mEq/L.
5. Promptly consult physician about indications of fluid overload and electrolyte imbalance.

Pain related to bladder spasms

Desired outcomes: Within 1 h of intervention, patient's subjective perception of pain decreases, as documented by a pain scale. Objective indicators, such as grimacing, are absent or diminished.

1. Assess and document quality, location, and duration of pain. Devise a pain scale with patient, rating pain from 0 (no pain) to 10 (worst pain).
2. Medicate patient with prescribed analgesics, narcotics, and antispasmodics as appropriate; evaluate and document patient's response, using pain scale. If retropubic approach was used, suppositories are contraindicated; oral anticholinergics (e.g., oxybutynin) are used instead.
3. Use warm blankets or heating pad on affected area or warm baths to increase regional circulation and relax tense muscles.
4. Teach technique for slow, diaphragmatic breathing to relax patient and help ease pain.
5. Provide back rubs and encourage use of other nonpharmacologic methods of pain relief: guided imagery, distraction, relaxation tapes, soothing music. Also see p. 27 for **Health-seeking behaviors:** Relaxation technique effective for stress reduction.
6. Monitor for leakage around catheter, which can indicate bladder spasms.
7. If patient has spasms, reassure him they are normal and can be caused by irritation of the bladder mucosa by the catheter balloon or a clot that results in backup of urine into the bladder, with concomitant irritation of the mucosa. Encourage fluid intake to help prevent spasms. If physician has prescribed catheter irrigation for removal of clots, follow instructions carefully to prevent discomfort and injury.
8. Monitor for clots in tubing. If clots are present for patient with continuous bladder irrigation, adjust rate of bladder irrigation to maintain light red urine (with clots). Total output should exceed amount of irrigant instilled. If output equals amount of irrigant or patient complains that his bladder is full, catheter may be clogged with clots. If clots inhibit the flow of urine, irrigate catheter by hand according to agency or physician's directive.

Risk for impaired skin integrity related to wound drainage from suprapubic or retropubic prostatectomy

Desired outcome: Patient's skin remains clear and intact.

1. Monitor incisional dressings frequently during the first 24 h, and change or reinforce as needed. If incision has been made into the

bladder, irritation can result from prolonged contact of urine with skin.
2. Use Montgomery straps rather than tape to secure dressing.
3. If drainage is copious after drain removal, apply wound drainage or ostomy pouch with a skin barrier over incision. Use a pouch with an antireflux valve to prevent contamination from reflux.

Sexual dysfunction related to fear of impotence due to lack of knowledge about postsurgical sexual function
Desired outcome: After instruction, patient discusses concerns about sexuality and has accurate information about sexual function.
1. Assess patient's level of readiness to discuss sexual function; provide opportunities for patient to discuss fears and anxieties.
2. Reassure patient who has had a simple prostatectomy that his ability to obtain and maintain an erection is unaltered. Retrograde ejaculation (backward flow of seminal fluid into the bladder, which is eliminated with the next urination), or "dry" ejaculation, will occur in most patients, but this probably will end after a few months. However, it does not affect the ability to achieve orgasm.
3. Encourage communication between patient and his significant other.
4. Be aware of your own feelings about sexuality. If you are uncomfortable discussing it, request that another staff member take responsibility for discussing feelings and concerns with patient.
5. As indicated, encourage continuation of counseling after hospital discharge. Confer with physician and social services to identify appropriate referral.

Constipation related to postsurgical discomfort or fear of exerting excess pressure on prostatic capsule
Desired outcome: By postoperative day 3 or 4, patient has a bowel movement pattern that is normal for him with minimal pain or straining.

NOTE: A patient who states that he needs to have a bowel movement during the first 24 h after surgery probably has clots in the bladder that are creating pressure on the rectum. Assess for clots (see **Pain,** earlier) and irrigate the catheter as indicated.

1. Document presence and quality of bowel sounds, or absence of sounds, in all four abdominal quadrants.
2. Gather baseline information on patient's normal bowel pattern, and document findings.
3. Unless contraindicated, encourage patient to consume 2-3 L of fluid a day after surgery.
4. Consult physician and dietitian about need for increased fiber in patient's diet.
5. Teach patient to avoid straining when defecating to prevent excess pressure on prostatic capsule.
6. Consult physician about use of stool softeners during postoperative period.
7. See **Constipation,** p. 420, in Appendix One for more information.

Reproductive

Urge incontinence related to urethral irritation after removal of urethral catheter

Desired outcome: Patient reports increasing intervals between
voidings by postoperative day 2 and regains normal pattern of micturi-
tion within 4-6 wk after surgery.

1. Before removing urethral catheter, explain to patient that he may
   void in small amounts for the first 12 h after catheter is removed
   because of irritation from catheter.
2. Instruct patient to save urine in a urinal for the first 24 h after surgery. Inspect each voiding for color and consistency. First urine
   specimens can be dark red from passage of old blood; each successive specimen should be lighter in color.
3. Note and document time and amount of each voiding. Initially patient may void q15-30min, but intervals between voidings should
   increase toward a more normal pattern.
4. Before hospital discharge, inform patient that dribbling may occur
   for 4-6 wk after surgery because of disturbance of the bladder neck
   and urethra during prostate removal. As muscles strengthen and
   healing occurs (urethra reaches normal size and function), dribbling
   stops.
5. Teach patient Kegel exercises (see p. 97) to improve sphincter control.

Acute confusion (or risk for same) related to fluid volume deficit
secondary to postsurgical bleeding/hemorrhage; fluid volume excess
secondary to absorption of irrigating fluid during surgery; or cerebral
hypoxia secondary to infectious process or sepsis.

Desired outcomes: Patient's mental status returns to normal for
patient within 3 days of treatment. Patient has no injury resulting from
his altered mental status.

1. Assess patient's baseline LOC and mental status on admission.
   Ask patient to perform a three-step task (e.g., "Raise your right
   hand, place it on your left shoulder, and then place the right hand
   by your side."). Test short-term memory by showing patient how
   to use call light, having him return the demonstration, and then
   waiting 5 min before having him demonstrate use of call light
   again. Inability to remember beyond 5 min indicates poor short-
   term memory. Document patient's response.
2. Document patient's actions in behavioral terms. Describe "confused" behavior.
3. Obtain description of prehospital functional and mental status from
   sources familiar with patient (e.g., family, friends, personnel at
   nursing home or residential care facility).
4. Identify cause of acute confusion. For example, request oximetry
   or ABG values to determine oxygenation levels; serum glucose or
   finger-stick glucose to determine glucose levels; and electrolytes
   and CBC to ascertain imbalances and/or elevated WBC count as a
   determinant of infection. Assess hydration status by reviewing
   I&O records after surgery. Note any imbalances either way. Output
   should match input. Assess legs for dependent edema, which can
   signal overhydration with poor venous return. Assess cardiac and

lung status for abnormal heart sounds or rhythms and crackles in lung bases, which can indicate fluid excess. Assess mouth for furrowed tongue or dry mucous membranes, signals of fluid deficit.

5. As appropriate, anticipate initiation of oxygen therapy to increase oxygenation; initiation of antibiotics if sepsis occurs; diuretics to increase diuresis; increased fluid intake by mouth or IV to rehydrate patient.

6. As appropriate, have patient wear glasses and hearing aid, or keep them close to bedside and within easy reach.

7. Keep patient's urinal and other frequently used items within easy reach. If patient has a short-term memory problem, do not expect him to use call light.

8. Check on patient at least q30min and whenever passing room.

9. Place patient close to nurse's station if possible. Provide nonstimulating, safe environment. Provide music, but avoid use of TV (individuals who are acutely confused regarding place and time often think the action on the TV is happening in the room).

10. Attempt to reorient patient to surroundings as needed. Keep a clock and calendar at bedside, and remind patient verbally of date and place.

11. Encourage family to bring items familiar to patient to provide a foundation for orientation. These can include blankets, bedspreads, or pictures of family or pets.

12. If patient becomes belligerent, angry, or argumentative during attempt to reorient him, *stop this approach.* Do not argue with patient or his interpretation of environment. Say, "I can understand why you may (hear, think, see) that."

13. If patient displays hostile behavior or misperceives your role (nurse becomes thief, jailer, etc.), leave the room. Return in 15 min. Introduce yourself to patient as though you have never met. Begin dialogue anew. Patients who are acutely confused have poor short-term memory and may not remember the previous encounter or that you were involved in it.

14. If patient attempts to leave the hospital, walk with him and attempt distraction. Ask patient to tell you about destination (e.g., "That sounds like a wonderful place! Tell me about it."). Keep tone pleasant and conversational. Continue walking with patient around unit, away from exits and doors. After a few minutes, attempt to guide him back to his room.

15. If the patient has permanent or severe cognitive impairment, check on him frequently and reorient to baseline mental status as indicated; however, do not argue with patient about his perception of reality. This can make a cognitively impaired person aggressive and combative. **Note:** Patients with severe cognitive impairments (e.g., Alzheimer's disease or dementia) also can experience acute confusional states (i.e., delirium) and can be returned to their baseline mental state.

See "Cancer of the Bladder" for **Altered urinary elimination** related to obstruction of suprapubic catheter, p. 93. See "Prostatic Neoplasm" for **Stress incontinence,** p. 365. See Appendix One for nursing diagnoses and interventions in "Caring for Preoperative and Postoperative Patients," p. 395.

PATIENT-FAMILY TEACHING
AND DISCHARGE PLANNING

Give patient and significant others verbal and written information about the following:
1. Medications, including drug name, purpose, dosage, schedule, precautions, drug/drug and food/drug interactions, and potential side effects.
2. Indicators of UTI, which require medical attention: cloudy or foul-smelling urine, fever, pain, dysuria.
3. Care of incision, if appropriate, including cleansing, dressing changes, and bathing. Advise patient to be aware of indicators of infection: persistent redness, increased warmth along incision, purulent drainage.
4. Care of catheters or drains if patient is discharged with them.
5. Fluid requirement of at least 2-3 L/day in nonrestricted patients.
6. Importance of increasing dietary fiber or taking stool softeners to soften stools. This minimizes risk of damage to prostatic capsule by preventing straining with bowel movements. Caution patient not to use suppositories or enemas to treat constipation.
7. Use of a sofa, reclining chair, or footstool to promote venous drainage from legs and to distribute weight on perineum, not rectum.
8. Avoiding the following activities for period prescribed by physician: sitting for long periods, heavy lifting (>10 lb), sexual intercourse.
9. Kegel exercises (p. 97) to help regain urinary sphincter control for postoperative dribbling.

Prostatic Neoplasms

NURSING DIAGNOSES AND INTERVENTIONS

Sexual dysfunction related to erectile dysfunction (85%-90% risk) after radical prostatectomy
Desired outcome: Patient verbalizes feelings about sexuality within 3 days after surgery.
1. Assess the patient's readiness to discuss sexual concerns. Encourage verbalization and, as indicated, use facilitative communication techniques: open-ended questions, reflective statements, rephrasing of patient's statements for clarification.
2. Be alert for signs of grief (hostility, depression, demanding behavior) and signs of denial (inappropriate affect or acceptance of diagnosis too easily).
3. As appropriate, arrange for care givers who have established rapport with patient to spend time with him and encourage verbalization of his concerns.

4. Be alert for patient and significant other's need for more information about sexual functioning.
5. As indicated, inform physician about patient's need for more information so that counseling can be reinforced.
6. Confer with physician and social services to identify appropriate referrals for counseling after hospital discharge.

Knowledge deficit: Side effects of antiandrogen therapy or bilateral orchiectomy

Desired outcome: Within the 24 h before hospital discharge, patient verbalizes knowledge of the extent and duration of body changes.

1. Inform patient of side effects of estrogen therapy and orchiectomy: breast enlargement and tenderness, loss of sexual desire, impotence. As indicated, teach him about the side effects of alpha-adrenergics (e.g., terazosin, prazosin, and phenoxybenzamine), which include first-dose syncope and mild hypotension.
2. For patients undergoing estrogen therapy, provide reassurance that side effects disappear when therapy is discontinued.
3. If appropriate, explain to patient that before initiating estrogen therapy, physician may prescribe radiation therapy to areolae of breasts to minimize painful gynecomastia. However, this procedure will not diminish other side effects.
4. Reassure patient undergoing orchiectomy that procedure will not affect his ability to have an erection and orgasm, but that he will not ejaculate.

Stress incontinence related to temporary loss of muscle tone in the urethral sphincter after radical prostatectomy

Desired outcome: Within the 24 h before hospital discharge, patient expresses understanding of cause of temporary incontinence and regimen that must be followed to promote bladder control.

1. Explain to patient that urinary incontinence is possible after prostatectomy, but that it should resolve within 6 mo. Describe the reason for the incontinence, using aids such as anatomic illustrations.
2. Encourage patient to maintain an adequate fluid intake of at least 2-3 L/day (unless contraindicated by an underlying cardiac dysfunction or other disorder). Explain that dilute urine is less irritating to prostatic fossa.
3. Instruct patient to avoid fluids that irritate the bladder, such as beverages containing caffeine. Explain that caffeine has a mild diuretic effect, which would make bladder control even more difficult.
4. Establish a bladder routine with patient before hospital discharge (see "Urinary Incontinence," p. 94).
5. Teach patient Kegel exercises to enhance sphincter control (see "Urinary Incontinence," p. 97).
6. Remind patient to discuss any incontinence problems with physician during follow-up examinations.

See "Benign Prostatic Hypertrophy" for **Risk for fluid volume deficit** (bleeding/hemorrhage), p. 358, **Pain,** p. 360, **Risk for infection,** p. 358, **Risk for impaired skin integrity,** p. 360, **Constipation,** p. 361, and **Acute confusion,** p. 362.

Reproductive

See Appendix One for nursing diagnoses and interventions in "Caring for Preoperative and Postoperative Patients," p. 395, and "Caring for Patients with Cancer and Other Life-Disrupting Illnesses," p. 423.

PATIENT-FAMILY TEACHING AND DISCHARGE PLANNING

Give patient and significant others verbal and written information about the following:
1. For patients with radical prostatectomy, referral to a counselor or counseling agency as necessary, and discussion about incontinence after removal of indwelling catheter.
2. See this section in "Benign Prostatic Hypertrophy," p. 364, for more information.

Testicular Neoplasms

NURSING DIAGNOSES AND INTERVENTIONS

Sexual dysfunction related to body changes that occur with orchiectomy
Desired outcome: Before hospital discharge, patient verbalizes feelings and frustrations about orchiectomy and has realistic knowledge of changes that will occur.
1. Provide a calm, unhurried atmosphere for patient and significant others. Use facilitative communication techniques: open-ended questions, reflective statements, rephrasing of patient's statements for clarification.
2. Encourage communication between patient and significant other.
3. Encourage patient to verbalize feelings, fears, and frustrations about sexual attractiveness, impotence, and infertility. Explain that the *surgery* will not impair fertility or potency; however, fertility may be compromised by radiation therapy or chemotherapy, and the impairment can last for 2 yr.
4. For patient undergoing lymphadenectomy, explain that ejaculatory failure may occur if the sympathetic nerve is damaged, but that erection and orgasm will be possible. Explain that if ejaculatory failure does occur, artificial insemination is possible because the semen flows back into the urine, from which it can be extracted, allowing the ovum to become fertilized artificially.
5. If appropriate, explain that a silicone prosthesis may be placed in the scrotum to achieve a normal appearance. Consult physician about potential for this procedure.
6. For patient undergoing radiation therapy or chemotherapy, explain that he can store sperm in a sperm bank. However, the rate of pregnancy is only 50% with this method because some sperm do not survive the freezing process.
Pain related to scrotal swelling secondary to orchiectomy or lymphadenectomy

Desired outcomes: Within 1-2 h of intervention, patient's subjective perception of pain decreases, as documented by a pain scale. Objective indicators, such as grimacing, are absent or diminished.

1. Assess and document quality, duration, and location of pain. Ask patient to rate pain on a scale of 0 (no pain) to 10 (worst pain).
2. Administer prescribed analgesics as indicated. Note and document patient's response, using pain scale to evaluate improvement.
3. Adjust scrotal support as needed to enhance patient's comfort. Scrotal support elevates and supports scrotum to minimize edema.
4. Apply ice gloves or packs to scrotum to reduce swelling.
5. Encourage patient to ambulate as soon as possible. Explain that exercise reduces swelling and pain by improving circulation.

Risk for fluid volume deficit related to postsurgical bleeding/hemorrhage

Desired outcome: Patient remains normovolemic, as evidenced by BP ≥90/60 mm Hg (or within patient's normal range); HR ≤100 bpm (or within patient's normal range); balanced I&O; urinary output ≥30 ml/h; RR ≤20 breaths/min; and warm, dry skin.

1. Monitor patient's VS q15min for 30 min after return from recovery room. Once stable, check q30min for 1 h, then q4h for 24 h (or according to hospital protocol).
2. Be alert for increasing HR, decreasing BP, diaphoresis, pallor, decreasing urinary output, and increasing RR, which signal hemorrhage and impending shock.
3. Monitor I&O. In nonrestricted patients, ensure a fluid intake of at least 2-3 L/day. Immediately after surgery, administer fluids IV and then advance to oral.
4. Measure and document urine, gastric tube, and drainage output; record output amounts separately. Optimally, drainage amounts will decrease gradually and then cease.
5. Check dressing at frequent intervals after surgery, changing it when it becomes damp. Document color and amount of drainage. Consult physician if drainage is heavy (saturates dressings within 1 h after changing), becomes bright red, or forms clots on dressings, any of which can occur with arterial or venous bleeding.

See Appendix One for nursing diagnoses and interventions in "Caring for Preoperative and Postoperative Patients," p. 395, and "Caring for Patients with Cancer and Other Life-Disrupting Illnesses," p. 423.

PATIENT-FAMILY TEACHING
AND DISCHARGE PLANNING

Give patient and significant others verbal and written information about the following:

1. Medications, including drug name, purpose, dosage, schedule, precautions, drug/drug and food/drug interactions, and potential side effects.

2. Care of incision, including cleansing and dressing changes. Advise patient to be alert for signs of infection: fever, persistent redness, swelling, pain, warmth or puffiness along incision, purulent drainage.
3. Care of drains or catheters if patient is discharged with them.
4. Review of postoperative activity restrictions as directed by physician: no heavy lifting (>10 lb), driving, or sexual intercourse for 4-6 wk.
5. Necessity of continued care (radiation therapy, chemotherapy, serial laboratory tests); confirm date and time of next appointment.
6. Importance of self-examination of remaining testicle, since unrelated cancer could develop in remaining testis.

Caring for Patients with Special Needs 10

SECTION ONE: CARING FOR PATIENTS WITH HUMAN IMMUNODEFICIENCY VIRUS (HIV) DISEASE

NURSING DIAGNOSES AND INTERVENTIONS

Risk for infection related to inadequate secondary defenses of the immune system, malnutrition, or side effects of chemotherapy

Desired outcome: Patient is free of additional infections during hospitalization, as evidenced by appropriate cultures or biopsies.

1. Assess for indicators of opportunistic infection: persistent fever, dry cough, diarrhea, night sweats, fatigue, involuntary weight loss. See Table 10-1 for the common opportunistic infections and organisms that infect individuals with HIV disease.

2. Monitor laboratory data, especially CBC, differential, ESR, and cultures, to evaluate course of infection. Consult physician about significant findings.

3. Maintain strict asepsis for all invasive procedures to prevent introduction of new pathogens.

4. Assist patient in maintaining meticulous body hygiene to prevent spread of organisms from body secretions into skin breaks, especially if patient has diarrhea.

5. Monitor temperature and VS at frequent intervals for evidence of fever or sepsis. In addition to increase in temperature, be alert for diaphoresis, confusion, decrease in LOC, increased HR, and decreased BP secondary to vasodilatory effect of increased body temperature. Perform a complete physical assessment at least q8h to identify changes from baseline assessment. Assess for changes in breath sounds, which may indicate an increasing level of infiltrates.

6. Promote pulmonary toilet by encouraging patient to engage in frequent breathing or incentive spirometry exercises. Use caution when

Table 10-1   Opportunistic infections and organisms affecting individuals with HIV disease

Viral	Fungal	Protozoal	Bacterial
Herpes (types 1 and 2)	*Candida*	*Pneumocystis carinii*	*Treponema pallidum* (syphilis)
Cytomegalovirus	*Histoplasma capsulatum*	*Toxoplasma gondii*	*Neisseria gonorrhoeae*
Varicella	*Cryptococcus*	*Entamoeba histolytica*	*Shigella*
Epstein-Barr	*Coccidioides*	*Giardia lamblia*	*Salmonella*
Hepatitis A, B, and C		*Cryptosporidium enteritidis*	*Mycobacterium avium-intracellulare* (MAI)
			Mycobacterium tuberculosis

performing postural drainage and chest physiotherapy, if prescribed, because patient may be too ill to tolerate these activities.

7. Monitor sites of invasive procedures for signs of infection: erythema, swelling, tenderness, purulent exudate.

8. Ensure good handwashing technique before contact with patient to minimize risk of infectious organisms being transmitted from staff and other patients.

9. Teach patient methods to use at home to prevent infection after hospital discharge (see "Patient-Family Teaching and Discharge Planning," p. 377.

Impaired gas exchange related to altered oxygen supply secondary to presence of pulmonary infiltrates, hyperventilation, and sepsis

Desired outcomes: After treatment or intervention, patient has adequate gas exchange, as evidenced by RR 12-20 breaths/min with normal depth and pattern (eupnea) and absence of adventitious sounds, nasal flaring, and other clinical indicators of respiratory dysfunction. By hospital discharge, patient's ABG results are: Pao_2 ≥80 mm Hg; $Paco_2$ 35-45 mm Hg; pH 7.35-7.45.

1. Assess respiratory status q2h during patient's awake period, noting rate, rhythm, depth, and regularity of respirations. Observe for use of accessory muscles, flaring of nares, adventitious sounds, cough, or cyanosis, which occur with respiratory dysfunction.

2. Monitor ABG results closely for decreased $Paco_2$ (<35 mm Hg) and increased pH (>7.4), which can occur with hyperventilation.

3. Adjust oxygen therapy to attain optimal oxygenation, as determined by ABG values.

4. Instruct patient to report changes in cough and dyspnea that increases with exertion.

5. To maintain adequate tidal volume, provide chest physiotherapy as prescribed; encourage use of incentive spirometry at frequent intervals.

6. Reposition patient q2h to help prevent stasis of lung fluids.
7. Obtain sputum for culture and sensitivity as indicated.
8. Group nursing activities to provide patient with uninterrupted periods of rest, optimally 90-120 min at a time.
9. When administering sulfa for *Pneumocystis carinii* pneumonia (PCP), monitor closely for side effects such as rash or bone marrow suppression (leukopenia, neutropenia). If administering pentamidine, be alert for side effects such as hypotension or hypoglycemia, which require frequent BP checks and finger sticks for blood sugar levels.
10. Administer humidified oxygen to relieve mucous membrane irritation, which can predispose patient to coughing spells.
11. Administer sedatives and analgesics judiciously to help prevent or minimize respiratory depression.

C A U T I O N :   Wear a high-efficiency (particulate respirator) mask and protect mucous membranes when caring for patients diagnosed as having active tuberculosis. See p. 12 for more information.

Altered nutrition: Less than body requirements related to diarrhea and nausea associated with side effects of medications, malabsorption, anorexia, dysphagia, and fatigue

Desired outcome: By hospital discharge, patient has adequate nutrition, as evidenced by stable weight, serum albumin 3.5-5.5 g/dl, transferrin 180-260 mg/dl, thyroxine-binding prealbumin 20-30 mg/dl, retinol-binding protein 4-5 mg/dl, and a state of nitrogen balance or a positive nitrogen state.

1. Assess nutritional status daily, noting weight, caloric intake, and protein and albumin values. Be alert for progressive weight loss, wasting of muscle tissue, loss of skin tone, and decreases in both total protein and albumin, which can adversely affect wound healing and impair patient's ability to withstand infection.
2. Provide small, frequent, high-calorie, high-protein meals, allowing patient sufficient time to eat. Offer supplements between feedings. As a rule, these patients are kept in a slightly positive nitrogen state (after resolution of the critical phases of this illness) by ensuring a daily calorie intake of 50 kcal/kg ideal body weight, with an additional 1.5 g of protein/kg (e.g., a man weighing 70 kg should receive 3,500 kcal plus 105 g of protein per day).
3. Provide supplemental vitamins and minerals as prescribed to replace deficiencies.
4. To minimize anorexia and help treat stomatitis, which can occur as a side effect of chemotherapy, provide oral hygiene before and after meals.
5. If patient feels socially isolated, encourage significant others to visit at mealtimes and bring in patient's favorite high-calorie, high-protein foods from home.
6. If patient is nauseated, provide instructions for deep breathing and voluntary swallowing, which help diminish stimulation of vomiting center. Administer antiemetics as prescribed.

Special Needs

7. Encourage dysphagic patient to drink high-calorie, high-protein fluids; provide different flavors and textures for variation.

8. As prescribed, provide isotonic tube feeding for patient unable to eat. Isotonic fluids help prevent diarrhea associated with hypertonic or hypotonic fluids. Check placement of gastric tube before each feeding; assess absorption by evaluating amount of residual feeding q4h. Do not deliver feeding if residual is >50-100 ml. Keep HOB elevated 30 degrees while feeding, and place patient in right side-lying position to facilitate gastric emptying.

9. If patient's caloric intake is insufficient, discuss potential need for TPN with physician.

Diarrhea related to gastrointestinal (GI) infection, chemotherapy, or tube feeding intolerance
Desired outcome: By hospital discharge, patient has formed stools and a bowel elimination pattern normal for him or her.

1. Ensure minimal use of antidiarrheal medications, which promote intestinal concentration of infectious organisms.

2. Teach patient to avoid consuming large amounts of caffeine (>300 mg/day), which increases peristalsis and can promote diarrhea.

3. Maintain accurate I&O records to monitor for changes in fluid volume status. Be alert for signs of hypovolemia: cool, clammy skin; increased HR (>100 bpm); increased RR (>20 breaths/min); decreased urinary output (<30 ml/h).

4. Assess stool for blood, fat, and undigested material.

5. Monitor stool cultures for evidence of new infectious organisms.

6. Monitor patient for indicators of electrolyte imbalance: anxiety, confusion, muscle weakness, cramps, dysrhythmias, weak pulse, decreased BP.

7. If patient is receiving tube feedings, dilute strength or reduce rate of infusion to prevent "solute drag," which may be the cause of the diarrhea.

8. Encourage patient to eat foods high in sodium (Table 1-4, p. 18) and potassium (Table 3-2, p. 72) to replace any decrements of these ions.

9. Protect anorectal area by keeping it clean and applying compounds, such as zinc oxide, that prevent or retard skin excoriation.

Impaired tissue integrity (or risk for same) related to cachexia and malnourishment, diarrhea, side effects of chemotherapy, Kaposi's sarcoma (KS) lesions, negative nitrogen state, and reduced mobility due to arthralgia and fatigue
Desired outcome: Upon hospital discharge, patient's tissue is intact.

1. Assess and document skin integrity, noting temperature, moisture, color, vascularity, texture, lesions, and areas of excoriation or poor wound healing. Evaluate KS lesions for location, dissemination, weeping, or significant changes. Note and record presence of herpes lesions, especially perirectal ones.

2. Prevent prolonged pressure on dependent body parts by turning and positioning patient q2h; encourage patient to change position at frequent intervals.

3. Provide patient with a pressure-relief mattress, as indicated.
4. Teach patient to use mild, hypoallergenic, nondrying soaps or lano-lin-based products for bathing and to pat rather than rub skin to dry it. When appropriate, use lotions and emollients to soften and re-lieve itching of dry, flaky skin.
5. Use soft sheets on bed, avoiding wrinkles. If patient is incontinent, use some type of rectal device (e.g., fecal incontinence bag, rectal tube) to protect skin and prevent perirectal excoriation and skin breakdown.
6. To enhance healing of skin and tissue, assist patient toward a state of nitrogen balance by promoting adequate amounts of protein and carbohydrates (see **Altered nutrition,** p. 371).
7. Make sure patient receives minimum daily requirements of vitamins and minerals; supplement them as necessary.
8. Encourage ROM and weight-bearing mobility, when possible, to in-crease circulation to skin and tissue.

Pain related to physical and chemical factors associated with pro-longed immobility, side effects of chemotherapy, infections, peripheral neuropathy, and frequent venipunctures

Desired outcomes: Within 1 h of intervention, patient's subjective perception of pain decreases, as documented by a pain scale. Nonver-bal indicators of discomfort, such as grimacing, are absent or dimin-ished.

1. Assess and record location, onset, and duration of pain, and factors that precipitate or alleviate it. With patient, establish a pain scale, rating pain from 0 (no pain) to 10 (worst pain). Use scale to evalu-ate degree of pain and to document degree of relief obtained.
2. Administer analgesia as prescribed.
3. Provide heat or cold applications to affected areas (e.g., apply heat to painful joints, and cold packs to reduce swelling associated with infections or multiple venipunctures).
4. Encourage patient to engage in diversional activities as a means of increasing pain tolerance and decreasing its intensity (e.g., soothing music, quiet conversation, reading, and slow, rhythmic breathing).
5. To reduce intensity of pain, teach patient techniques that reduce skeletal muscle tension: deep breathing, biofeedback, relaxation ex-ercises (see **Health-seeking behaviors:** Relaxation technique effec-tive for stress reduction, p. 27).
6. If frequent venipunctures are the cause of patient's discomfort, dis-cuss with physician the desirability of a capped venous catheter for long-term blood withdrawal.
7. Administer anticonvulsant agents as prescribed to relieve peripheral neuropathy.
8. Promote relaxation and comfort with back rubs and massage.
9. For other interventions, see this diagnosis in Appendix One, p. 396.

Activity intolerance related to generalized weakness secondary to fluid and electrolyte imbalance, arthralgia, myalgia, dyspnea, fever, pain, hypoxia, and effects of chemotherapy

Desired outcome: Before hospital discharge, patient rates per-ceived exertion at ≤3 on a 0-10 scale and exhibits tolerance to activity,

Special Needs

as evidenced by HR ≤20 bpm over resting HR, RR ≤20 breaths/min, and systolic BP ≤20 mm Hg over or under resting systolic BP.

1. Assess patient's tolerance to activity by assessing HR, RR, and BP before and immediately after activity, and ask patient to rate his or her perceived exertion. See this nursing diagnosis in Appendix One, p. 413, for details.
2. Plan adequate rest periods (90-120 min) between patient's scheduled activities. Adjust activities as appropriate to reduce energy expenditure.
3. As much as possible, encourage regular periods of exercise to help prevent cardiac intolerance to activities, which can occur quickly after periods of prolonged inactivity.
4. Monitor electrolyte levels to ensure that patient's muscle weakness is not caused by hypokalemia.
5. Monitor ABG values to ensure that patient is oxygenated adequately; adjust oxygen delivery accordingly.
6. Advise patient to keep anecdotal notes (perhaps in journal format) on exacerbation and remission of signs and symptoms.
7. For more information, see this nursing diagnosis in Appendix One, "Caring for Patients on Prolonged Bed Rest," p. 413.

Anxiety related to threat of death and social isolation

Desired outcome: After intervention, patient expresses feelings and is free of harmful anxiety, as evidenced by HR ≤100 bpm, RR ≤20 breaths/min with normal depth and pattern (eupnea), and BP within patient's normal range.

1. Monitor patient for verbal or nonverbal expressions of the following: inability to cope, apprehension, guilt for past actions, uncertainty, concerns about rejection and isolation, and suicide ideation.
2. Spend time with patient and encourage him or her to express feelings and concerns.
3. Support effective coping patterns (e.g., by allowing patient to cry or talk rather than denying legitimate fears and concerns).
4. Provide accurate information about HIV disease and related diagnostic procedures.
5. If patient hyperventilates, teach him or her to mimic your normal respiratory pattern (eupnea).

Body image disturbance related to biophysical changes secondary to KS lesions, chemotherapy, and emaciation

Desired outcome: Before hospital discharge, patient expresses positive feelings about self to family, significant others, and primary nurse.

1. Encourage patient to express feelings, especially the way he or she views or feels about self.
2. Provide patient with positive feedback; help patient focus on facts rather than myths or exaggerations about self.
3. Provide patient with access to clergy, psychiatric nurse, social worker, psychologist, or HIV counselor as appropriate.
4. Encourage patient to join and share feelings with HIV support group.

5. For additional information, see this nursing diagnosis in Appendix One, p. 459.

Knowledge deficit: Disease process, prognosis, life-style changes, and treatment plan

Desired outcome: Before hospital discharge, patient verbalizes accurate information about the disease process, prognosis, behaviors that increase the risk of transmitting the virus to others, and treatment plan.

1. Assess patient's knowledge about HIV disease, including pathophysiologic changes that will occur, ways the disease is transmitted, necessary behavioral changes, and side effects of treatment. Correct misinformation and misconceptions as necessary.
2. Inform patient of private and community agencies available to help with such tasks as handling legal affairs, cooking, housecleaning, and nursing care. Provide telephone numbers and addresses for HIV support groups and self-help groups.
3. Provide literature that explores the myths and realities of HIV disease process.
4. Teach patient the importance of informing sexual partners of HIV condition and of modifying high-risk behavior known to transmit the virus (see Table 10-2).
5. Involve significant others in the teaching and learning process.
6. Provide patient and significant others with names and addresses or phone numbers of HIV resources (see "Patient-Family Teaching and Discharge Planning" below).

Social isolation related to altered state of wellness, societal rejection, loss of support system, feelings of guilt and punishment, fatigue, and changed patterns of sexual expression

Desired outcome: Before hospital discharge, patient communicates and interacts with others.

1. Keep patient and significant others well informed about patient's status and treatment plan.
2. Provide private time for patient to communicate and interact with significant others.
3. Encourage significant others to share in patient's care.
4. Encourage physical closeness between patient and significant others. Provide privacy as much as possible.
5. Involve patient in unit or group activities as appropriate.
6. Explain significance of isolation precautions to patient.

Table 10-2   High-risk sexual behaviors

Unprotected anonymous sex
Unprotected oral sex with transfer of body fluids
Unprotected receptive anal/vaginal sex
Unprotected oral-anal contact (rimming)
Manual anal/vaginal penetration (fisting)
Sharing sexual aids or needles
Unprotected sex with multiple partners

Special Needs

Impaired environmental interpretation syndrome related to physiologic changes and impaired judgment secondary to infection, space-occupying lesion in the CNS, or HIV dementia

Desired outcomes: After intervention, patient verbalizes orientation to time, place, and person. Optimally, by hospital discharge, patient correctly completes exercises in logical reasoning, memory, perception, concentration, attention, and sequencing of activities.

1. Assess patient for minor alterations in personality traits that cannot be attributed to other causes such as stress or medication.
2. Assess patient for signs of dementia: slowing of all cognitive functioning, with problems in attention, concentration, memory, perception, logical reasoning, and sequencing of activities.
3. Encourage patient to report persistent headaches, dizziness, or seizures, which may signal CNS involvement.
4. Note any cranial nerve involvement that differs from patient's past medical history. Most commonly cranial nerves V (trigeminal), VII (facial), and VIII (acoustic) are involved in infectious processes of the CNS.
5. Assess patient for signs of mental aberration, blindness, aphasia, hemiparesis, or ataxia, which may signal a demyelinating disease.
6. Divide activities into small, easily accomplished tasks.
7. Maintain a stable environment so patient can familiarize himself or herself with the immediate surroundings (e.g., do not change location of furniture in room).
8. Write notes as reminders; maintain a calendar of appointments.
9. Provide some mechanism (e.g., pill boxes) to ensure that patient takes medications as prescribed.
10. Teach patient the importance of reporting changes in neurologic status (e.g., increasing severity of headaches, blurred vision, gait disturbances, or blackouts). Consult physician about all significant findings.

For other nursing diagnoses and interventions, see "Providing Nutritional Support," p. 378; "Managing Wound Care," p. 384; "Caring for Patients on Prolonged Bed Rest," p. 413; and "Caring for Patients with Cancer and Other Life-Disrupting Illnesses," p. 450.

PATIENT-FAMILY TEACHING
AND DISCHARGE PLANNING

Give patient and significant others verbal and written instructions about the following:

1. Importance of avoiding use of recreational drugs, which are believed to potentiate the immunosuppressive process and lower resistance to infection.
2. Significance and importance of refraining from donating blood.
3. Necessity of modifying high-risk sexual behavior. See Tables 10-2 and 10-3 for specific information.
4. Principles and importance of maintaining a balanced diet, and ways to supplement diet with multivitamins and other food sources

Table 10-3   Safer sex guidelines

Safer Sexual Practices
Social (dry) kissing
French (wet) kissing
Hugging
Massage
Mutual masturbation
Body-to-body contact (except mucous membrane areas)
Activities not involving direct body contact

Sexual Practices of Questionable Safety
Anal-oral contact (rimming) using a latex barrier
Anal or vaginal intercourse using latex condoms*
Fellatio (mouth to penis) without ejaculation
Cunnilingus (mouth to vaginal area)
Watersports (enemas, urination)

Unsafe Sexual Practices
Anal or vaginal intercourse without latex condom
Oral contact with bodily fluids (semen, urine, feces, vaginal secretions)
Contact with blood
Oral-anal contact (rimming)
Manual anal/vaginal penetration (fisting)
Sharing of sexual aids or needles

*Petroleum-based lubricants have been shown to increase the risk of condom rupture. Water-based products, such as K-Y Jelly and similar products, are preferred. Use of viricidal spermicides, such as nonoxynol-9, is strongly urged as added protection.

such as high-calorie substances (e.g., Isocal and Ensure). Because of increased susceptibility to foodborne opportunistic organisms, fruit and vegetables should be washed thoroughly; meats should be cooked thoroughly at appropriate temperatures; raw eggs, raw fish (sushi), and unpasteurized milk should be avoided.
5. Because of reduced resistance to infection, the importance of limiting contact with individuals known to have active infections. In addition, pets may harbor various fungal, protozoal, and bacterial organisms in their excrement. Therefore, contact with bird cages, cat litter, and tropical fish tanks should be avoided.
6. Necessity for meticulous hygiene to prevent spread of any current or new infectious organisms. To avoid exposure to fungi, damp areas in bathrooms (e.g., shower) should be cleaned with bleach solution; refrigerators should be cleaned thoroughly with soap and water; and leftover food should be disposed of within 2-3 days.
7. Techniques for self-assessment of early signs of infection (e.g., erythema, tenderness, swelling, purulent exudate) in all cuts, abrasions, lesions, or open wounds.

8. Care of venous access device, including technique for self-administration of TPN or medications (see Appendix One, "Caring for Patients with Cancer and Life-Disrupting Illnesses," p. 427); care of gastric tube and administration of enteral tube feedings, if appropriate.

9. Importance of avoiding fatigue by limiting participation in social activities, getting maximum amounts of rest, and minimizing physical exertion.

10. Prescribed medications, including drug name, purpose, dosage, schedule, precautions, drug/drug and food/drug interactions, and potential side effects.

11. Importance of maintaining follow-up appointments.

12. Advisability of keeping anecdotal notes (perhaps in journal format) on exacerbation and remission of signs and symptoms.

13. Importance of reporting changes in neurologic status (e.g., increasing severity of headaches, blurred vision, gait disturbances, or blackouts).

14. Advisability of sharing feelings with significant others or within a support group.

15. In addition, provide the following information about HIV resources:
    - Public Health Service AIDS Hotline: (800) 342-AIDS, (800) 342-2437.
    - AZT Information Hotline: (800) 843-9388.
    - Local Red Cross, or American Red Cross AIDS Education Office, 1730 D Street NW, Washington, DC 20006; (202) 737-8300.
    - Centers for Disease Control AIDS Activity, Building 6, Room 292, 1600 Clifton Road, Atlanta, GA 30333; (404) 329-3479.
    - National Gay Task Force AIDS Information Hotline: (800) 221-7044.
    - National Sexually Transmitted Diseases Hotline/American Social Health Association: (800) 227-8922.
    - National AIDS Network, 729 Eighth Street SE, Suite 300, Washington, DC 20003; (202) 546-2424.

SECTION TWO: PROVIDING NUTRITIONAL SUPPORT

Altered nutrition: Intake less than body requirements related to inability to ingest, digest, or absorb nutrients

Desired outcome: Patient has adequate nutrition, as evidenced by stabilization of weight at desired level or steady weight gain of approximately ¼-½ lb/day; improved or normal protein stores (serum albumin 3.5 g/dl, transferrin 180-260 mg/dl, thyroxine-binding prealbumin 20-30 mg/dl, retinol-binding protein 4-5 mg/dl); state of nitrogen balance, as measured by nitrogen balance studies; wound granulation (pinkish white tissue around wound edges that grows to fill in wound); and absence of infection (see **Risk for infection,** p. 383).

GENERAL INTERVENTIONS

1. Ensure nutritional screening and assessment of patient within 72 h of admission; document and reassess weekly. Standard criteria used to identify patient's potential for nutritional risk include:
   - Age (pregnancy, advanced adulthood).
   - Drug or alcohol use.
   - History of inadequate nutrient intake.
   - Underweight condition (<80% of ideal body weight).
   - Overweight status (>20% above ideal body weight).
   - Recent, unplanned weight loss (>10%).
   - Serum albumin <3.5 g/dl.
   - IV support with dextrose and/or saline alone for >5 days.
   - Medications that affect nutritional status (e.g., chemotherapy).
   - Chronic illness (e.g., COPD, renal disease, diabetes mellitus, pancreatitis, arthritis).
   - Trauma (e.g., fractured mandible), surgery (e.g., radical head and neck dissection), disease of the GI tract (e.g., malabsorption syndrome).

2. Take a dietary history to determine adequacy of usual and recent food intake. Note excesses or deficiencies. Dietary history should include:
   - Comprehensive review of usual dietary intake, including food sensitivities, food and drug allergies, food aversions, and use of nutritional supplements.
   - Assessment of special eating patterns (various types of vegetarian or prescribed diets).
   - Use of fad diets (especially for weight loss).
   - Use of vitamin and mineral supplementation.
   - Identification of anything that impairs adequate selection, preparation, ingestion, digestion, absorption, and excretion of nutrients.
   - Assessment of intake *via* calorie counts.

3. Perform a physical assessment, noting loss of muscle or adipose tissue and changes in hair, skin, or neuromuscular function.

4. Gather anthropometric data: height, weight, triceps skinfold thickness, midarm circumference.

5. Assess biochemical data: serum albumin, transferrin, thyroxine-binding prealbumin, retinol-binding protein, creatinine-height index, nitrogen balance studies.

6. Monitor electrolyte, BUN, and blood sugar levels daily until they stabilize. Make sure serum albumin and transferrin or prealbumin and trace elements are monitored weekly; document.

7. Reassess status weekly using assessment guidelines discussed above.

ADDITIONAL INTERVENTIONS FOR ORAL NUTRITION

1. Follow General Interventions above.

2. Provide small, frequent feedings of diet compatible with disease state and patient's ability to ingest foods.

Special Needs

3. Respect patient's food aversions, and try to maximize food preferences. Have significant others bring in patient's favorite foods.
4. Position patient appropriately for eating. Assist with feeding as necessary. Involve significant others in meal rituals for patient's com-
   panionship.
5. Provide liquid nutritional supplements as prescribed. Serve cold or
   over ice to enhance palatability.

ADDITIONAL INTERVENTIONS FOR ENTERAL/PARENTERAL NUTRITION
1. Follow General Interventions.
2. Administer formula within 10%-20% of rate as prescribed using an
   infusion pump. Check rate and volume infused qh.
3. Record I&O carefully, tracking fluid balance trends.
4. Weigh patient daily and document.
5. Make sure patient receives prescribed calories.

Risk for aspiration related to GI feeding, delayed gastric emptying,
and site of feeding tube

Desired outcome: Patient is free of aspiration problems, as evidenced by auscultation of clear lung sounds, VS within patient's baseline limits, and absence of signs of respiratory distress.

1. Determine placement of feeding tube before each feeding. Check
   x-ray for position of feeding tube before each feeding. Insuffla-
   tion with air and aspiration of stomach contents do *not* confirm
   placement of feeding tubes. Mark and secure tubing for future reference.
2. Assess respiratory status q4h for unexplained pulmonary infiltrates,
   noting respiratory rate and effort and adventitious breath sounds.
3. Monitor for fever of unexplained origin q4h.
4. Auscultate bowel sounds, percuss abdomen, and assess abdominal
   contour and girth q8h. Consult physician if bowel sounds are absent
   or high pitched, abdomen becomes distended, or nausea and vomiting occur.
5. Elevate HOB ≥30 degrees during and 1 h after feeding. If this is
   not possible or comfortable for patient, turn patient into slightly elevated right side-lying position to enhance gravity flow from greater
   stomach curve to pylorus.
6. Consult physician if residual feeding is >50% of hourly feed. Hold
   feeding for 1 h and recheck residual.
7. Stop tube feeding 30 min to 1 h before chest physical therapy, suctioning, or placing patient supine.
8. Discuss with physician the possibility of placing feeding tube well
   beyond the pylorus.
9. As prescribed, administer metoclopramide HCl to promote gastric
   motility.

Diarrhea (or risk for same) related to bolus feeding, lactose intolerance, bacterial contamination, osmolality intolerance, medications,
and low fiber content

Desired outcome: Patient has formed stools within 24-48 h of intervention.

N O T E :   Diarrhea is defined as more than 3 liquid stools a day.

1. Assess abdomen and GI status: bowel sounds, distention, consistency and frequency of bowel movements, cramping, skin turgor, other indicators of hydration.
2. Monitor I&O status carefully.
3. Bolus feeding: Switch to intermittent or continuous feeding method.
4. Lactose intolerance: As prescribed, switch to lactose-free products.
5. Bacterial contamination:
   ■ Obtain stool sample for culture and sensitivity.
   ■ Use clean technique in handling feeding tube, enteral products, and feeding sets.
   ■ Change all equipment q24h.
   ■ Refrigerate all opened products, but discard after 24 h.
   ■ Discard feedings hanging >8 h.
6. Osmolality intolerance:
   ■ Determine osmolality of feeding formula. Most are isotonic (plasma osmolality 300 mOsm). If hypertonic, reduce rate. If problem continues, dilute to ½ formula and ½ water, but maintain rate.
7. Medications:
   ■ Monitor use of antibiotics, antacids, antidysrhythmics, aminophylline, cimetidine, and potassium chloride, and use of sorbitol in liquid medications.
   ■ As prescribed, administer *Lactobacillus acidophilus* to restore GI flora, or use antidiarrheal agents to reduce GI motility.
8. Low fiber content: Add bulk-forming agents (psyllium husks or fiber preparations).

Constipation (or risk for same) related to inadequate fluid and fiber in diet
Desired outcome: Patient has a bowel movement within 2-3 days of this diagnosis.
1. Assess intake of free water. Optimally, it should be 1 ml/calorie intake, or 30-50 ml/kg body weight.
2. Give free water q2h as prescribed.
3. Recommend changing formula to one that has fiber added.

Impaired tissue integrity (or risk for same) related to mechanical irritant (presence of enteral tube)
Desired outcome: At hospital discharge, patient's tissue is intact and shows no erosion around orifices, excoriation, skin rash, or breakdown of mucous membranes.

Gastric/Enteral Tube
1. Assess skin for irritation or tenderness q8h.
2. Use tube with smallest bore possible.
3. If long-term support is needed, discuss potential for using gastrostomy or jejunostomy tube with physician.
4. Give ice chips, chewing gun, or hard candies prn if permitted.
5. Apply petrolatum ointment to lips q2h.
6. Brush teeth and tongue q4h.
7. Apply water-soluble lubricant to naris prn.
8. Alter position of tube daily to prevent pressure on underlying tissue.

GASTROSTOMY TUBE
1. Assess site for erythema, drainage, tenderness, and odor q4h.
2. Monitor placement of tube q4h.
3. Secure tube to prevent tension on tissue and skin.
4. Wash skin with soap and water daily; pat dry.

JEJUNOSTOMY TUBE
1. Assess site for erythema, drainage, tenderness, and odor q4h.
2. Secure tube to prevent tension. Coil tube on top of dressing if necessary.
3. Cleanse skin with half-strength solution of hydrogen peroxide and water; rinse hydrogen peroxide from skin and dry. Apply povidone-iodine ointment around insertion site daily and prn.
4. Dress site with split 4×4s and tape with paper or hypoallergenic tape.

Impaired swallowing (or risk for same) related to decreased or absent gag reflex, facial paralysis, mechanical obstruction, fatigue, and decreased strength or excursion of muscles involved in mastication

Desired outcome: Before foods or fluids are initiated, patient demonstrates adequate cough and gag reflexes and ability to ingest food *via* phases of swallowing, as instructed.

1. Assess oral motor function within 72 h of patient's admission or upon progression to oral diet.
2. Assess cough and gag reflexes before first feeding. Initially, liquids and solids may be difficult for patient to manage. Offer semi-solid foods and progress to thicker texture as tolerated. Assist patient through phases of ingesting food: opening mouth, inserting food, closing lips, chewing, transferring food from side to side in mouth and then to back of oral cavity, elevating tongue to roof of mouth, and swallowing between breaths.
3. Order extra sauces, gravies, or liquids if dryness of oral cavity impairs patient's ability to swallow. Suggest that patient use these to moisten each bite of food.
4. If tolerated, keep patient in high Fowler's position for 30 min to minimize risk of aspiration.
5. Provide mouth care before and after meals and dietary supplements.
6. Provide small, frequent meals.
7. Provide foods at temperatures acceptable to patient.
8. Respect food aversions, and provide food preferences whenever possible.
9. Provide oral supplements or tube feeding supplements as prescribed. Advise patient of transition status; praise his or her progress.
10. In conjunction with PT or OT, assist in retraining or facilitating patient's swallowing.
11. Monitor and record patient's intake (*via* calorie count, daily weight) and output.

Risk for infection related to invasive procedures
Desired outcome: Patient is free of infection, as evidenced by temperature and VS within normal limits, total lymphocytes 25%-40% (1,500-4,500/μl), WBC count $\leq$11,000/μl, and absence of clinical signs of sepsis: erythema and swelling at insertion site, chills, fever, glucose intolerance, leukocytosis.

1. Ensure adequate nutritional support based on individual needs. For guidelines see **Altered nutrition,** p. 378. Reassess weekly.
2. Twice weekly and prn, monitor total lymphocyte count, WBC count, and differential for values outside normal range.
3. Check blood glucose q6h for values outside normal range.
4. Examine catheter insertion sites q8h for erythema, swelling, or purulent drainage.
5. Use meticulous sterile technique when changing central line dressing, containers, or lines. Cleanse insertion sites with tincture of iodine (1%-2%), followed by 70% alcohol or povidone-iodine solution.
6. Do not use central line used for nutritional support to draw blood, monitor pressure, or administer medications or other fluids.
7. Change all administration sets within the time frame established by agency.
8. Culture specimens from catheter tip and exit site prn.
9. Take blood specimens for culture, if sepsis is suspected, and administer antibiotics as prescribed.
10. Hang fat emulsion for time frame established by agency.

Altered cardiopulmonary tissue perfusion (or risk for same) related to interruption of venous flow (air embolus)
Desired outcome: Patient has adequate cardiopulmonary tissue perfusion, as evidenced by VS, ABG values, and arterial oximetry within normal limits and absence of dyspnea, tachypnea, cyanosis, chest pain, tachycardia, and hypotension.

1. Administer D_5W solution until chest x-ray shows proper catheter position.
2. Position patient in Trendelenburg's position when changing tubing or when neck vein catheters are inserted or removed.
3. If possible, teach patient Valsalva's maneuver for use during tubing changes, or apply abdominal pressure.
4. Use Luer-Lok connectors on all connections.
5. Tape all tubing connections longitudinally to prevent disconnection.
6. Monitor patient for chest pain, tachycardia, tachypnea, cyanosis, and hypotension.
7. If air embolus is suspected, clamp catheter and turn patient to left side-lying Trendelenburg position to trap air in right ventricle. Ensure adequate oxygenation. Consult physician immediately.
8. Use occlusive dressing over insertion site for 24 h after catheter is removed to prevent air entry *via* catheter sinus tract.

Risk for fluid volume deficit related to failure of regulatory mechanisms, hyperglycemia, and hyperglycemic hyperosmotic nonketotic syndrome   (HHNK)

Desired outcome: Patient's hydration status is adequate, as evidenced by baseline VS, glucose <300 mg/dl, balanced I&O, urine specific gravity 1.010-1.025, and electrolytes within normal limits.

1. Assess rate and volume of nutritional support hourly. Reset to prescribed rate as indicated. To minimize risk of HHNK, increase rate by no more than 10%-20%.
2. Weigh patient daily; monitor I&O hourly.
3. Consult physician for urine output <1 ml/kg/h.
4. Check urine specific gravity; consult physician for value >1.035.
5. Monitor serum osmolality and electrolytes daily and prn; consult physician for abnormalities. See Table 10-4 for assessment of metabolic disorders.
6. Monitor for circulatory overload during fluid replacement.
7. Monitor for indicators of hyperglycemia. Perform finger stick q6h prn until blood glucose is stable. Administer insulin (usually a sliding scale) as prescribed to keep blood glucose levels <220 mg/dl.
8. Provide 1 ml of free water for each calorie of enteral formula provided (or 30-50 ml/kg body weight).

SECTION THREE: MANAGING WOUND CARE

Wounds Closed by Primary Intention

NURSING DIAGNOSES AND INTERVENTIONS

Impaired tissue integrity: Wound, related to altered circulation, metabolic disorders (e.g., diabetes mellitus [DM]), alterations in fluid volume and nutrition, and medical therapy (chemotherapy, radiation therapy, and steroid administration)

Desired outcome: Patient shows signs of wound healing: well-approximated wound edges; good initial postinjury inflammatory response (erythema, warmth, induration, pain); no inflammatory response after day 5 postinjury; no drainage (without drain present) 48 h after closure; healing ridge present by postoperative day 7-9. See Table 10-5.

1. Assess wound for indications of impaired healing: absence of healing ridge; drainage or purulent exudate; delayed or prolonged inflammatory response. Monitor VS for signs of infection, including elevated temperature and HR. Document findings.
2. Use aseptic technique when changing dressings. If a drain is present, keep it sterile, maintain patency, and handle it gently to prevent dislodgment. If wound care will be necessary after hospital discharge, teach patient and significant others the procedure for dressing changes (see Appendix Two, "Infection Prevention and Control," p. 479.)

Table 10-4 Possible electrolyte imbalances in enteral and parenteral nutrition

Sodium: Daily requirement is 60-150 mEq. Sodium is the primary extracellular cation in maintaining concentration and volume of extracellular fluid.

Complication	Pathophysiology/Strategy
Hypernatremia	In protein-calorie malnutrition (PCM), patients have increased sodium owing to extravascular volume expansion and intravascular volume depletion. Monitor sodium levels as depletion resolves, edema decreases, and diuresis occurs. Hypernatremia also occurs in patients receiving hypertonic tube feedings without adequate water supplements. **Sources:** Amino acid solutions contain varying amounts of sodium (up to 70 mEq/L; some antibiotics (e.g., sodium penicillin) also have a high sodium content (31-200 mEq/dl). Corticosteroids may cause sodium retention, and blood products can contain increased levels (130-160 mEq/L).
Hyponatremia	Can be a problem in patients with gastric suctioning and in those receiving diuretic agents or those with syndrome of inappropriate antidiuretic hormone (SIADH). **Replacement:** TPN solutions can replace sodium by using acetate, phosphate, or chloride salt form, depending on underlying disease state. Phosphate form should not be used in patients with renal failure. In acidemia, the acetate form is preferred to correct the imbalance.

Potassium: Daily requirement is 50-100 mEq. Potassium is the major intracellular cation required for neurotransmission, protein synthesis, cardiac and renal function, and carbohydrate metabolism.

Complication	Pathophysiology/Strategy
Hyperkalemia	May be caused by excessive parenteral or enteral potassium supplementation or increased tissue catabolism, especially in renal insufficiency. Elevated potassium levels occur in patients receiving angiotensin-converting enzyme (ACE) inhibitors, heparin, cyclosporin, and potassium-sparing diuretics.

Continued

Table 10-4 Possible electrolyte imbalances in enteral and parenteral nutrition—cont'd

Complication	Pathophysiology/Strategy
Hypokalemia	May occur during anabolism (tissue synthesis) in patients being refed. Potassium shifts into intracellular space, and patients require supplementation. It also may occur in patients with high GI losses or increased loss from diuretics. Potassium levels in patients with acid-base disorders may be misleading: potassium decreases by 0.4-1.5 mEq/L for every 0.1 increase in pH. **Replacement:** In daily TPN solutions, 80-120 mEq may be given to patients without renal problems. Potassium can be replaced using acetate, phosphate, and chloride forms, depending on underlying disease state, but it should be titrated separately to avoid wasting of TPN solutions. Infusion rates >0.5 mEq/kg/h are associated with cardiac irregularities.

Phosphorus: Daily requirement is 2.5-4.5 mg/dl. Phosphorus is required for release of oxygen from hemoglobin in the form of 2,3-diphosphoglycerate and for bone deposition, calcium regulation, and synthesis of carbohydrates, fats, and protein.

Complication	Pathophysiology/Strategy
Hyperphosphatemia	Occurs in catabolic stress, renal failure, and hypocalcemia. Treatment involves ingestion of aluminum antacids, which bind phosphate in the intestine. **Sources:** Phosphorus-rich solutions, antacids, diuretic agents, and steroids.
Hypophosphatemia	A complication with a high mortality rate, often found in malnourished patients upon refeeding. As patient receives fluids containing dextrose, phosphorus shifts rapidly into intracellular space, causing hypophosphatemia. **Replacement:** Phosphate-rich TPN solutions.

Magnesium: Daily requirement is 18-30 mEq. Magnesium is required for carbohydrate and protein metabolism and enzymatic reactions.

Complication	Pathophysiology/Strategy
Hypermagnesemia	Transient elevations can occur with use of diuretics or extracellular volume depletion. **Source:** Magnesium-containing antacids.
Hypomagnesemia	Low levels commonly occur in patients with severe malnutrition or lower GI losses and in those given insulin for hyperglycemia. For anabolism to occur, the body requires 2 mEq of magnesium per gram of nitrogen. **Replacement:** Parenteral magnesium.

Calcium: Daily requirement is 1,000-1,500 mg. Calcium is a necessary ingredient of the cells that play a major role in neurotransmission.

Complication	Pathophysiology/Strategy
Hypercalcemia	Occurs in thiazide diuretic use, prolonged immobilization, and decreased excretion. **Source:** Side effect of diuretic use.
Hypocalcemia	May occur from reduced total body calcium or reduced ionized calcium. It also occurs with hyperphosphatemia. A deficit can be misleading, inasmuch as serum calcium is bound to protein and varies with changing albumin levels. Also, in acidosis, a lower pH results in release of more calcium from protein, which elevates serum calcium levels. The opposite is true as pH rises. **Replacement:** Calcium-rich parenteral solutions.

Table 10-5   Assessment of healing by primary intention

Normal Findings	Abnormal Findings
Edges well approximated	Edges not well approximated
Good initial inflammatory response: redness, warmth, induration, pain	Diminished or no inflammatory response, or response persists or occurs after day 5
No drainage 48 h after closure (if drain is present)	Drainage continues >48 h after closure
Healing ridge present by postoperative day 7-9	No healing ridge by postoperative day 9; hypertrophic scar or keloid developing

3. Maintain blood glucose within normal range for persons with DM by performing serial monitoring of blood glucose and administering insulin to keep glucose level <200 mg/dl.
4. Explain to patient that deep breathing promotes oxygenation, which enhances wound healing. If indicated, provide incentive spirometry at least 4 ×/day. Stress the importance of position changes and activity as tolerated to promote ventilation. Splint incision as needed.
5. Monitor perfusion status by checking BP, HR, capillary refill time in the tissue adjacent to incision, moisture of mucous membranes, skin turgor, volume and specific gravity of urine, and I&O.
6. For nonrestricted patients, ensure a fluid intake of at least 2-3 L/day.
7. Encourage ambulation or ROM exercises as allowed to enhance circulation to wound.
8. To promote positive nitrogen state, which enhances wound healing, provide a diet with adequate protein, vitamin C, and calories. Encourage between-meal supplements. If patient complains of feeling full with three meals a day, give more frequent, small feedings instead.

PATIENT-FAMILY TEACHING AND DISCHARGE PLANNING

Give patient and significant others verbal and written information about the following:
1. Local wound care: type of equipment necessary, wound care procedure, therapeutic and negative side effects of topical agents used. Have patient or significant other demonstrate dressing change procedure before hospital discharge.
2. Signs and symptoms of improvement in wound status (see Table 10-5).
3. Signs and symptoms of deterioration in wound status, including those that should be reported to a health care provider (see Table 10-5).

4. Diet that promotes wound healing. Discuss the importance of adequate protein and calorie intake. See "Providing Nutritional Support," p. 378. Involve dietitian, patient, and significant others as necessary.

5. Activities that maximize ventilatory status: a planned regimen for ambulatory patients, and deep breathing and turning (at least q2h) for those on bed rest.

6. Importance of taking multivitamins, antibiotics, and iron and zinc supplements as prescribed. For all medications to be taken at home, provide drug name, purpose, dosage, schedule, precautions, drug/drug and food/drug interactions, and potential side effects.

7. Importance of follow-up care with physician; confirm date and time of next appointment.

IN ADDITION

8. If needed, arrange for a visit by a home health nurse before hospital discharge.

Surgical or Traumatic Wounds Healing by Secondary Intention

NURSING DIAGNOSES AND INTERVENTIONS

Impaired tissue integrity: Wound, related to presence of contaminants, metabolic disorders (e.g., DM), medical therapy (e.g., chemotherapy or radiation therapy), altered perfusion, or malnutrition
Desired outcomes: Patient's wound shows signs of healing: initially postinjury, wound edges are inflamed, indurated, and tender; with epithelialization, edges become pink within 1 wk of injury; granulation tissue develops (identified by pink tissue that becomes beefy red) within 1 wk of injury; absence of odor, exudate, and necrotic tissue. Patient or significant other successfully demonstrates wound care procedure before hospital discharge, if appropriate. See Table 10-6.

1. Monitor for signs of impaired healing: initially postinjury, decreased inflammatory response or inflammatory response that lasts >5 days; epithelialization slowed or mechanically disrupted and noncontinuous around wound; granulation tissue remaining pale or excessively dry or moist; presence of odor, exudate, and/or necrotic tissue.

2. Apply prescribed dressings (see Table 10-7). Insert dressing into all tracts to promote gradual closure of those areas. Wash hands wellbefore and after dressing changes, and dispose of contaminated dressings appropriately.

3. When a drain is used, maintain patency, prevent kinking of tubing, and secure tubing to prevent drain from becoming dislodged. Use aseptic technique when caring for drains.

4. To help prevent contamination, cleanse skin surrounding wound with a mild disinfectant (e.g., soap and water). Do not use friction with cleansing if tissue is friable.

5. If irrigation is prescribed to reduce contaminants, administer high-pressure irrigation using a 35-ml syringe with an 18-gauge needle, and follow proper infection control technique (see p. 479). If tissue is

Special Needs

Table 10-6   Assessment of healing by secondary intention

Normal Findings	Abnormal Findings
Initially postinjury, wound edges inflamed, indurated, and tender; with epithelialization, edges become pink	Initially postinjury, decreased inflammatory response or inflammation around wound continues after day 5 postinjury; epithelialization slowed or mechanically disrupted and not continuous around wound
Granulation tissue initially avascular and moist and then turns pink; becomes beefy red over time	Granulation tissue remains pale or is excessively dry or moist
No odor	Odor
No exudate or necrotic tissue	Exudate or necrotic tissue

friable or wound is located over a major organ or blood vessel, use extreme caution with irrigation pressure. To remove contaminants effectively, use a large amount of irrigant (100-150 ml).

6. Topically applied antiinfective agents (e.g., neomycin and iodophors) are absorbed by the wound and can produce systemic side effects. When these agents are used, be alert for side effects such as toxicity to cells in the wound, nephrotoxicity, and acidosis.

7. When a hydrophilic agent such as Debrisan or Bard Absorption Dressing is prescribed, remove it with high-pressure irrigation. If these agents were removed with a 4 × 4 or surgical sponge, the friction would disrupt capillary budding and delay healing.

8. When topical enzymes are prescribed, use them on necrotic tissue only and follow package directions carefully. Be aware that some agents (e.g., povidone-iodine) deactivate enzymes. Protect surrounding undamaged skin with zinc oxide or aluminum hydroxide paste.

9. Teach patient or significant other the prescribed wound care procedure, if indicated.

PATIENT-FAMILY TEACHING AND DISCHARGE PLANNING

See teaching and discharge planning interventions in "Wounds Closed by Primary Intention," p. 388.

Pressure Ulcers

NURSING DIAGNOSES AND INTERVENTIONS

Impaired tissue integrity (or risk for same) related to excessive tissue pressure, shearing forces, or altered circulation

Table 10-7   Dressings used for wound care

Dressing	Advantages	Limitations
Dry to dry* (insert dry and remove dry)	Highly absorbent; debridement	Excessively drying to tissue; disrupts new tissues; removal is painful
Wet to dry* (insert wet and remove dry)	Good absorption but not as good as dry to dry; good debridement	Drying of tissues but not as much as dry to dry; disrupts new tissue; removal is painful
Moist to moist* (insert and remove moist)	Provides topical antiinfective agent; no wound desiccation; good debridement; removal painless; inexpensive	Less effective at removing exudate; if too wet, can cause tissue maceration; if dries out, must be moistened before removal
Xeroform gauze	Provides topical antiseptic; keeps tissue hydrated; minimal pain with removal	If too moist, can cause tissue maceration
Porcine skin dressing	Can provide topical antibiotic; keeps tissue hydrated; removal painless; often used before closure of wound with tissue grafts	Expensive; usually stored in refrigerator until use

Continued

Table 10-7 Dressings used for wound care—cont'd

Dressing	Advantages	Limitations
Transparent dressing (e.g., Op-Site, Tegaderm, Biooclusive)	Prevents loss of wound fluid; protects wound from external contamination; protects from friction and fluid loss; minimal pain with removal	Excess drainage must be removed and dressing resealed; appearance of drainage erroneously suggests infection
Hydrocolloid dressing (e.g., Duoderm, Restore, Intact)	Maintains moist wound surface while minimizing pooling; easy to apply; minimal pain with removal	Wound cannot be directly assessed without removing dressing; "melts" when used under radiant heat; limited absorption
Hydrophilic gel (e.g., Vigilon, Intrasite Gel)	Maintains moist wound surface; nonadherent; absorbs some exudate; compatible with topical medications; easy to apply; minimal pain with removal	Maceration with direct contact with normal tissue; expensive; may require frequent changing; minimal absorption of exudate
Alginates (e.g., Sorbsan)	Physiologic; maintains moisture; removal painless	Not good for dry wounds
Foams (e.g., Lyofoam, Allevin)	Maintains moist wound surface; insulates wound; nonadherent	Poor barrier; opaque; not good for wounds with copious viscous drainage

*All dressings are sterile, coarse mesh gauze without cotton fiber fill and are covered with a dry, sterile outer layer to prevent ingress of organisms. When moisture is prescribed, it is provided with an antiinfective agent or physiologic solution.

Desired outcomes: Patient's tissue remains intact. Patient participates in preventive measures and verbalizes understanding of the rationale for these interventions.

1. Identify individuals at risk, and systematically assess skin over bony prominences daily; document.
2. Establish and post a position-changing schedule.
3. Assist patient with position changes. There is an inverse relationship between pressure and time in ulcer formation; therefore, heavier patients need to change position more frequently. Position changes include turning bed-bound patient q1-2h and having wheelchair-bound patient (who is able) perform pushups in chair q15min to ensure periodic relief from pressure on buttocks. Use pillows or foam wedges to protect bony prominences from direct pressure. In addition, patients with history of previous tissue injury require pressure-relief measures more frequently. Because high Fowler's position results in increased shearing, use low Fowler's position and alternate supine position with prone and 30-degree elevated side-lying positions.
4. For immobile patients, totally relieve pressure on heels by raising them off bed surface *via* pillows inserted under length of lower leg.
5. Minimize friction on tissue during activity. Friction causes shearing of vessels, which leads to tissue disruption. Lift rather than drag patient during position changes and transferring; use draw sheet to facilitate patient movement. Do not massage over bony prominences, since this can result in tissue damage.
6. Minimize exposure of skin to moisture. Cleanse at time of soiling and at routine intervals. Use moisture barriers and disposable briefs as needed.
7. Use mattress that reduces pressure (e.g., foam, alternating air, gel, water).

Table 10-8   Grading of pressure ulcers

Grade	Description
I	Nonblanchable erythema of intact skin; in people with dark skin, heat may be the only indication of a grade I pressure ulcer
II	Partial-thickness skin loss that involves the epidermis or dermis, or both; seen as an abrasion, blister, or shallow crater
III	Full-thickness skin loss that involves subcutaneous tissue but does not extend through the fascia
IV	Full-thickness injury that involves muscle, bone, or supporting structures

Special Needs

8. To enhance circulation, encourage patient to maintain current level of activity.

Impaired tissue integrity: Presence of pressure ulcer, with increased risk for further breakdown related to altered circulation and presence of contaminants or irritants (chemical, thermal, or mechanical)

Desired outcomes: Grade I and grade II ulcers heal within 7-10 days; grade III and grade IV ulcers may require months to heal. After intervention and instruction, patient verbalizes causes and preventive measures for pressure ulcers and successfully participates in plan of care to promote healing and prevent further breakdown.

1. Evaluate grade of pressure ulcer (see Table 10-8).
2. Maintain a moist physiologic environment to promote tissue repair and minimize contaminants. Change dressings as prescribed.
3. Be sure patient's skin is kept clean with regular bathing, and be especially conscientious about washing urine and feces from skin. Soap should be used and then thoroughly rinsed from skin.
4. If patient has excessive perspiration, ensure frequent bathing and change bedding as needed.
5. To absorb moisture and prevent shearing when patient is moved, apply heel and elbow covers as needed.
6. Use lamb's wool to keep areas between toes dry. Change wool periodically, depending on amount of moisture present.
7. Do not use a heat lamp because it increases the metabolic rate of tissues, resulting in increased demand for blood flow in an area with impaired perfusion. As a result, ulcer diameter and depth can increase.
8. Teach patient and significant others the importance of and measures for preventing excess pressure as a means of preventing pressure ulcers.
9. Provide wound care as needed (see "Surgical or Traumatic Wounds Healing by Secondary Intention").

See "Surgical or Traumatic Wounds Healing by Secondary Intention" for **Impaired tissue integrity:** Wound, related to presence of contaminants, metabolic disorders, or medical therapy, p. 389.

PATIENT-FAMILY TEACHING AND DISCHARGE PLANNING

Give patient and significant others verbal and written information about the following:

1. Location of local medical supply stores that have pressure-reducing mattresses and wound care supplies.
2. Planning a schedule for changing patient's position.

For other teaching and discharge planning interventions, see "Wounds Closed by Primary Intention," p. 388.

Patient Care

SECTION ONE: CARING FOR PREOPERATIVE AND POSTOPERATIVE PATIENTS

Knowledge deficit: Surgical procedure, preoperative routine, and postoperative care

Desired outcome: Patient verbalizes knowledge of the surgical procedure, including preoperative preparations and sensations and postoperative care and sensations, and demonstrates postoperative exercises and use of devices before surgical procedure or, with emergency surgery, during immediate postoperative period.

1. Assess patient's understanding of the diagnosis, surgical procedure, preoperative routine, and postoperative regimen. Evaluate patient's desire for information about diagnosis and procedure (some individuals find detailed information helpful; others prefer very brief, simple explanations). Assess for factors that would affect patient's ability to learn. Determine past surgical experiences and their positive or negative effect on patient. Assess nature of any concerns or fears related to surgery. Document this assessment and share it with others involved in patient's care.

2. Clarify and explain diagnosis and surgical procedure as needed. When possible, emphasize sensations (e.g., dry mouth, thirst, muscle weakness), since information often is helpful in reducing stress and anxiety. Allow ample time for instruction and clarification, and reinforce physician's explanation of procedure. Use anatomic models, diagrams, and other audiovisual aids when possible. Provide simply written information to reinforce learning. Provide written and verbal information in patient's native language for non-English-speaking patients. **Note:** Evaluate patient's reading comprehension before providing written materials.

3. Explain preoperative events. Review the following with patient and significant others:

   ■ Where patient will be before, during, and immediately after surgery (i.e., postanesthesia care unit, ICU, other specialty unit). Clarify sounds and other sensations (e.g., dry mouth, sore throat, cool temperature, hard stretcher) patient may experience during

immediate postoperative period. If possible, take patient to the new unit and introduce him or her to the nursing staff.
- Preoperative medications and timing of surgery (scheduled time, expected duration).
- Pain management, including sensations to expect and methods of relief. If patient-controlled analgesia (PCA) will be prescribed, have patient return demonstration of use of delivery device.
- Placement of tubes, catheters, drains, and oxygen-delivery devices. Show patient these devices when possible.
- Use of pneumatic compression stockings.
- Dietary alterations, including NPO status followed by clear liquids until full gastrointestinal (GI) function returns.
- Restrictions of activity and positions.
- Need to refrain from smoking during perioperative period.
- Visiting hours and location of waiting room.

4. Explain postoperative activities, exercises, and precautions. Have patient return demonstration of the following devices and exercises as appropriate:
   - Deep-breathing and coughing exercises (see **Ineffective airway clearance**, p. 401). **Caution:** If increased intracranial, intrathoracic, or intraabdominal pressure is contraindicated, patient should not cough.
   - Use of incentive spirometry and other respiratory devices.
   - Calf-pumping, ankle-circling, and footboard-pressing exercises to enhance circulation and prevent thrombophlebitis in the lower extremities (see "Venous Thrombosis/Thrombophlebitis," p. 61, for more information).
   - Use of PCA infusion device.
   - Movement in and out of bed.

5. Before patient is discharged, teach him or her prescribed activity precautions: getting maximum amounts of rest, increasing activities gradually to tolerance, avoiding heavy lifting ($>$10 pounds), refraining from driving a car (often for as long as 4-6 wk).

6. Provide time for patient to ask questions and express feelings of anxiety; be reassuring and supportive. Be certain to address his or her main concerns.

Pain or **Chronic pain** related to disease process, injury, or surgical procedure

Desired outcomes: Within 1 h of intervention, patient's subjective perception of discomfort decreases, as documented by a pain scale. Patient does not exhibit nonverbal indicators of pain (Table A-1). Autonomic indicators (Table A-2) are diminished or absent. Verbal responses, such as crying or moaning, are absent.

1. Develop a systematic approach to pain management for each patient. To achieve the best results, the primary nurse should collaborate with the pain control team, surgeon, anesthesiologist, and patient.

2. Monitor patient at frequent intervals for discomfort. Use a formal method of assessing pain. One method is to have patient rate discomfort on a scale of 0 (no discomfort) to 10 (worst pain). Other

Table A-1   Nonverbal indicators of pain

Masklike, grimacing, tense facial expression
Guarding or protective behavior
Restlessness or increase in motor activity
Withdrawal or decrease in motor activity
Skeletal muscle tension
Short attention span
Irritability
Anxiety
Sleep disturbances

Table A-2   Autonomic indicators of pain

Diaphoresis
Vasoconstriction
Increased systolic and diastolic BP
Increased pulse rate (>100 bpm)
Pupillary dilatation
Change in respiratory rate (usually increased, >20 breaths/min)
Muscle tension or spasm
Decreased intestinal motility, evidenced by nausea, vomiting, abdominal distention, and possibly ileus
Endocrine imbalance, evidenced by sodium and water retention and mild hyperglycemia

    methods may be used, but the method selected should be used consistently.
3. Evaluate patients with acute and chronic pain for nonverbal indicators of discomfort (see Table A-1).
4. Evaluate patient with acute pain for autonomic indicators of discomfort (see Table A-2). Be aware that patients with chronic pain (>6 mo) may not exhibit an autonomic response.
5. Evaluate patient's health history for use of alcohol or drugs (prescribed or OTC). A positive history of addiction to alcohol or drugs affects effective doses of analgesics (i.e., more or less may be required). Consult pain control team if available. All care providers must be consistent in setting limits while providing effective pain control through pharmacologic and nonpharmacologic methods. Psychiatric consultation may be necessary.
6. Administer opioid analgesics (e.g., morphine) and related mixed agonist-antagonist analgesics (e.g., butorphanol) as prescribed (Table A-3). When possible, morphine or related "mu" receptor agonists are preferred to meperidine (Demerol) for moderate to severe postoperative pain. Monitor for side effects: respiratory depression, excessive sedation, nausea, vomiting, constipation. Be aware that meperidine may produce excitation, muscle twitching,

Table A-3 Use of opioid and agonist-antagonist analgesia

Route	Commonly Prescribed Medications	Advantages	Disadvantages
Continuous infusion	morphine, fentanyl (Sublimaze)	Useful for severe, predictable pain or as a basal dose with bolus supplements for fluctuating pain Relieves pain with lower doses than IV bolus Avoids peaks and valleys of pain found with IV bolus and IM injections	Requires frequent observation to monitor flow rate VS must be monitored often
IV bolus	morphine, meperidine (Demerol), fentanyl	Useful for severe, intermittent pain (i.e., for procedures, treatments) Rapid onset of action; may be controlled by patient using specialized pump	Relatively short duration of pain relief Fluctuating levels Possibility of excessive sedation as drug levels peak
Epidural	morphine, fentanyl, hydromorphone, meperidine	Very effective relief of moderate to severe pain Delivery close to opiate receptors provides pain control with small doses May be delivered with local anesthetic (e.g., bupivacaine) for increased effectiveness	Catheter must be inserted by anesthetist or anesthesiologist Specialized delivery system must be used Side effects include urinary incontinence, hypotension, respiratory depression, pruritus, nausea, and vomiting

Patient-controlled analgesic	morphine, meperidine, fentanyl, buprenorphine (Buprenex)	Useful for moderate to severe pain Enables titration by patient for effective analgesia without excessive sedation Relief of pain with lower dosages of medication Immediate delivery of medication Patient's sense of self-control lowers anxiety Less nursing time spent preparing medications	Pumps necessary to deliver drug are expensive Patient must have clear mental status Health care provider resistance to self-administration by patient
IM injection	meperidine, morphine, pentazocine (Talwin), nalbuphine (Nubain), butorphanol (Stadol), buprenorphine	Useful for moderate to severe pain Longer duration of action than with IV route Used for postoperative pain	Variable absorption and fluctuating levels, especially in hypotensive and critically ill patients Possibility of excessive sedation as drug levels peak Potential delay in administration
Oral	codeine, oxycodone (Percodan), meperidine, pentazocine, propoxyphene (Darvon), hydromorphone (Dilaudid), morphine (MS Contin)	Useful for mild to moderate acute pain or chronic severe pain (large doses necessary)	Variable absorption Cannot be used until GI function returns; lengthy interval before onset of action
Transdermal	fentanyl (Duragesic)	Long duration of action (3 days) Useful when pain is moderate to severe and constant	Delayed onset of action (up to 36 h) Prolonged effects after removal Must be used with rapid-action supplement for variable pain

Appendix One

and seizures, especially in conjunction with phenothiazines. **Note:** Do not administer mixed agonist-antagonist analgesic concurrently with morphine or other pure agonist, because analgesic effects may be obviated.

7. With patients receiving opioid analgesics, assess at frequent intervals for evidence of excessive sedation when awake or respiratory depression (i.e., RR <10 breaths/min or Sao_2 <85%). If respiratory depression develops, reduce amount or frequency of dose as prescribed. Have naloxone (Narcan) readily available to reverse severe respiratory depression.

C A U T I O N :   Reduce doses and titrate carefully if patient has limited pulmonary reserve (i.e., chronic obstructive pulmonary disease, asthma) or hepatic or renal insufficiency, or is an older adult.

---

8. Administer nonnarcotic (acetaminophen [Tylenol, Tempra]) and nonsteroidal antiinflammatory drugs (acetylsalicylic acid [aspirin], ibuprofen [Motrin, Advil, Nuprin], indomethacin [Indocin], naproxen [Naprosyn, Anaprox], and ketorolac [Toradol]) as prescribed to relieve mild to moderate pain during postoperative recovery (see Table A-4). Nonsteroidal antiinflammatory drugs (NSAIDs) are especially effective when pain is associated with inflammation and soft tissue injury. Make sure GI function has returned before administering oral agents. Ketorolac may be given IM for patients unable to tolerate oral agents. Monitor for side effects: epigastric pain, nausea, dyspepsia, gastric bleeding. **Note:** Because NSAIDs have peripheral effects and a different mechanism of action, they are very effective when combined or used with centrally acting opioid analgesics.

9. Check patient's analgesia record for the last dose and amount of medication given during surgery and in postanesthesia recovery room. Coordinate timing and dose of postoperative analgesics with previously administered medication. **Note:** Combined fentanyl and droperidol (Innovar) anesthesia potentiates the effects of opioids for up to 10 h after administration; patient should be monitored carefully when opioid analgesia is used.

10. Administer prn analgesics before pain becomes severe. Consider converting to scheduled dosing with supplemental prn analgesia.

Table A-4   Common nonnarcotic and nonsteroidal antiinflammatory analgesics

Nonsteroidal Antiinflammatory Drugs	Nonnarcotic Drugs
acetylsalicylic acid (aspirin) ibuprofen (Motrin, Advil, Nuprin) indomethacin (Indocin) ketorolac (Toradol) naproxen (Naprosyn, Anaprox)	acetaminophen (Tylenol, Tempra)

Prolonged stimulation of pain receptors increases sensitivity to painful stimuli, necessitating a larger dose of medication to relieve pain. Remember that becoming addicted to narcotics is uncommon in hospitalized patients.

11. Plan to administer intermittently scheduled analgesics before painful procedures and ambulation and at bedtime. Schedule them so that peak effect is achieved at the start of the activity or procedure.

12. Augment analgesic therapy with sedatives and tranquilizers to prolong and enhance analgesia. Do not substitute sedatives or tranquilizers for analgesics.

13. Wean patient from opioid analgesics by reducing the dose or frequency of administration. Convert to oral therapy as soon as possible. When changing the drug or route of administration, be sure to use equianalgesic doses of new drug (Table A-5).

14. Augment action of drug with nonpharmacologic methods of pain control (Table A-6). Many of these techniques can be taught to and implemented by patient and significant others.

15. Maintain a quiet environment to promote rest. Plan nursing activities to allow long periods of uninterrupted rest at night.

16. Evaluate for and correct nonsurgical sources of discomfort (e.g., position, full bladder, infiltrated IV site).

17. Position patient comfortably, and reposition often to relieve discomfort due to pressure and improve circulation.

18. Sudden or unexpected changes in pain intensity can signal complications such as internal bleeding or leakage of visceral contents. Carefully evaluate patient and notify surgeon immediately.

19. Document efficacy of analgesics and other pain control interventions, using pain scale or other formalized method.

Ineffective airway clearance related to increased tracheobronchial secretions secondary to effects of anesthesia; ineffective coughing secondary to central CNS depression or pain and muscle splinting; and possible laryngospasm secondary to endotracheal tube or allergic reaction to anesthetics

Desired outcome: Patient's airway is clear, as evidenced by normal breath sounds on auscultation, RR 12-20 breaths/min with normal depth and pattern (eupnea), normothermia, and normal skin color.

1. Assess respiratory status, including breath sounds, q1-2h during immediate postoperative period and q8h during recovery. Note and report rhonchi that do not clear with coughing, labored breathing, tachypnea (RR >20 breaths/min), restlessness, cyanosis, and fever (≥38.3° C [101° F]).

2. Encourage deep breathing and coughing q2h or more often for the first 72 h postoperatively. If fine crackles are present (and if not contraindicated), have patient cough to expectorate secretions. Facilitate deep breathing and coughing by demonstrating how to splint abdominal and thoracic incisions with the hands or a pillow. If indicated, medicate patient ½ h before deep breathing, coughing, or ambulation to enhance compliance.

Table A-5   Equianalgesic doses of narcotic analgesics

Class/Name	Route	Equianalgesic Dose (mg)*	Average Duration (h)
Morphinelike Agonists			
codeine	IM, SC	130†	3
	PO	180†	3
hydromorphone (Dilaudid)	IM, SC	1.5-2	4
	PO	6-7.5	4
levorphanol (Levo-Dromoran)	IM, SC	2	6
	PO	4	6
morphine	IM, SC	10	4
oxycodone (Percodan)	PO	30†	4
oxymorphone (Numorphan)	IM, SC	1-1.5	4
	Rectal	10	4
Meperidine-like Agonists			
fentanyl (Sublimaze)	IV, IM, SC	0.1-0.2	1‡
meperidine (Demerol)	IM, SC	100	3
	PO	300†	3
Methadone-like Agonists			
methadone (Dolophine)	IM, SC	10	6
	PO	10-20	6
propoxyphene (Darvon)	PO	130-250†	4
Mixed Agonist-Antagonists§			
buprenorphine (Buprenex)	IM	0.3-0.6	4
butorphanol (Stadol)	IM, SC	2-3	3
nalbuphine (Nubain)	IM, SC	10-20	4
pentazocine (Talwin)	IM	30-60	3
	PO	10-200†	3

Adapted from Baumann T, Lehman M: In DiPrio J et al: *Pharmacotherapy: a pathophysiologic approach,* New York, 1988, Elsevier; and Koda-Kimble MA et al: *Applied therapeutics: the clinical use of drugs,* ed 5, Vancouver, Wash, 1992, Applied Therapeutics.

*Recommended starting dose; actual dose must be titrated to patient's response.
†Starting doses lower (codeine 30 mg, oxycodone 5 mg, meperidine 50 mg, propoxyphene 65-130 mg, pentazocine 50 mg).
‡Respiratory depressant effects persist longer than analgesic effects.
§Mixed agonist-antagonist analgesics may precipitate withdrawal in narcotic-dependent patients.

Table A-6   Common nonpharmacologic methods of pain control*

Sensory Interventions

Massage: To relax muscular tension and increase local circulation; back and foot massage are especially relaxing

ROM exercises (passive, assisted, or active): To relax muscles, improve circulation, and prevent pain related to stiffness and immobility

Applications of heat or cold: Cold used initially to diminish tissue injury response and alter pain threshold; heat used to facilitate clearance of tissue toxins and mobilize fluids

Transcutaneous electrical nerve stimulation (TENS): A battery-operated device used to send weak electrical impulses *via* electrodes placed on the body; reduces sensation of pain during and sometimes after treatment

Emotional Interventions

Prevention and control of anxiety: Limiting anxiety reduces muscle tension and increases patient's pain tolerance; anxiety and fear contribute to autonomic stimulation and pain responses; progressive relaxation exercises and slow, controlled breathing may be helpful

Promoting self-control: Feelings of helplessness and lack of control contribute to anxiety and pain; techniques such as PCA and promoting self-helping behavior contribute to feelings of self-control

Cognitive Interventions

Cognitive preparations: Preparing patient by explaining what can be expected, thereby reducing stress and anxiety (e.g., preoperative teaching)

Patient education: Teaching methods for preventing or reducing pain (e.g., suggesting comfortable postoperative positions, methods of ambulation, and splinting of incisions when coughing)

Distraction: Encouraging patient to focus on something unrelated to pain (e.g., conversing, reading, watching TV or videos, listening to music, employing relaxation techniques [see **Health-seeking behaviors:** Relaxation technique effective for stress reduction, p. 27])

Humor: Can be an excellent distraction and may help patient cope with stress

Guided imagery: Patient uses a mental process that uses images to alter a physical or emotional state; a technique that promotes relaxation and reduces pain sensations

*Many of these techniques can be taught to and implemented by the patient and significant others.

C A U T I O N : Vigorous coughing may be contraindicated for some individuals (e.g., those undergoing intracranial surgery, spinal fusion, eye or ear surgery, or similar procedures). Coughing after a herniorrhaphy and some thoracic procedures should be done in a controlled manner, with the incision supported carefully.

---

3. Make sure emergency airway equipment (i.e., intubation tray, endotracheal tubes, suctioning equipment, tracheostomy tray) is readily available in case of sudden airway obstruction or ventilatory failure.
4. Administer humidified oxygen as prescribed to prevent further drying of respiratory passageways and secretions.

Risk for aspiration related to entry of secretions, food, or fluids into tracheobronchial passages secondary to CNS depression, depressed cough and gag reflexes, decreased GI motility, abdominal distention, recumbent position, presence of gastric tube, and possible impaired swallowing in individuals with oral, facial, or neck surgery

Desired outcome: Patient's upper airway remains unobstructed, as evidenced by clear breath sounds, RR 12-20 breaths/min with normal depth and pattern (eupnea), and normal skin color.

1. See interventions 1-3 under **Ineffective airway clearance,** above.
2. If sedated patient has nausea or vomiting, turn immediately into side-lying position. Fully alert patients may remain upright. As necessary, suction oropharynx with Yankauer or similar suction device to remove vomitus.
3. Check placement and patency of gastric tubes q8h and before instillation of feedings and medication.

N O T E : Use caution when irrigating and otherwise manipulating GI tubes of patients who recently have had esophageal, gastric, or duodenal surgery, because the tubes may be displaced or the surgical incision disrupted by such activity. Consult surgeon before irrigating tubes for these individuals.

---

4. Assess patient's abdomen for distention (increasing size, firmness, increased tympany, decreased bowel sounds) q4-8h using inspection, auscultation, palpation, and percussion. Consult physician if distention has rapid onset or is associated with pain.
5. Encourage early and frequent ambulation to improve GI motility and reduce abdominal distention caused by accumulated gases.
6. Introduce oral fluids cautiously, especially in patients who had oral, facial, and neck surgery.
7. Administer antiemetics and metoclopramide (Reglan) as prescribed.
8. For additional information, see this nursing diagnosis in "Providing Nutritional Support," p. 380.

Ineffective breathing pattern (or risk for same) related to deceased lung expansion secondary to CNS depression, pain, muscle splinting, recumbent position, and effects of anesthesia

Desired outcome: Patient exhibits effective ventilation, as evidenced by relaxed breathing, RR 12-20 breaths/min with normal depth and pattern (eupnea), clear breath sounds, normal color, Pao_2 ≥80 mm Hg, pH 7.35-7.45, $Paco_2$ 35-45 mm Hg, and HCO_3^- 22-26 mEq/L.

1. See interventions under **Ineffective airway clearance**, above.
2. Perform preoperative baseline assessment of patient's respiratory system, noting rate, rhythm, degree of chest expansion, quality of breath sounds, cough, and sputum production. Note preoperative ABG values as available.
3. If appropriate, encourage patient to refrain from smoking for at least 1 wk after surgery. Explain the effects of smoking on the body.
4. Monitor Sao_2 continuously in high-risk patients (e.g., older adults, patients who are heavily sedated or have preexisting lung disease) and periodically in other patients as indicated. Consult physician about Sao_2 <85%-90%.
5. Evaluate ABG values and consult physician about low or decreasing Pao_2 and high or increasing $Paco_2$.
6. Assist patient with turning and deep-breathing exercises q2h for the first 72 h after surgery to promote lung expansion. Be aware that opioid analgesics depress the respiratory system.
7. If patient has an incentive spirometer, provide instructions and ensure compliance with its use q2h or as prescribed.
8. Unless contraindicated, assist patient with ambulation by postoperative day 2 to enhance ventilation.
9. For other interventions, see this nursing diagnosis in "Atelectasis," p. 1.

Risk for fluid volume deficit related to postoperative bleeding/hemorrhage

Desired outcomes: Patient is normovolemic, as evidenced by BP ≥90/60 mm Hg (or within patient's preoperative baseline), HR 60-100 bpm, RR 12-20 breaths/min with normal depth and pattern (eupnea), brisk capillary refill (<2 sec), warm extremities, distal pulses >2+ on a 0-4+ scale, and urinary output ≥30 ml/h. Patient verbalizes orientation to time, place, and person.

1. Monitor VS at frequent intervals during the first 24 h of postoperative period. Be alert for indicators of internal hemorrhage and impending shock: decreasing pulse pressure (difference between systolic and diastolic BP), decreasing BP, increasing HR, increasing RR.
2. Assess patient at frequent intervals during the first 24 h of postoperative period for indicators of internal hemorrhage and impending shock: pallor, diaphoresis, cool extremities, delayed capillary refill, diminished intensity of distal pulses, restlessness, agitation, disorientation. Also note subjective complaints of thirst, anxiety, or a sense of impending doom.
3. Monitor and measure urinary output q4-8h during initial postoperative period. Report average hourly output <30 ml/h. Be alert for progressive urine concentration.
4. Inspect surgical dressing for evidence of frank bleeding (i.e., rapid saturation of dressing with bright red blood). Record saturated dressings, and report significant findings to surgeon. If initial postoperative dressing becomes saturated, reinforce and consult sur-

geon because he or she may wish to perform initial dressing change.

5. Note amount and character of drainage from gastric and other tubes at least q8h. If drainage appears to contain blood (e.g., bright red, burgundy, or dark coffee-ground appearance), perform an occult blood test. If test is newly or unexpectedly positive, consult surgeon. **Note:** After gastric and some other GI surgeries, patient will have small amounts of bloody or blood-tinged drainage for the first 12-24 h. Be alert for large or increasing amounts of bloody drainage.

6. Review CBC values for evidence of bleeding: decreases in hemoglobin (Hgb) from normal (men, 14-18 g/dl; women, 12-16 g/dl); and decreases in hematocrit (Hct) from normal (men, 40%-54%; women, 37%-47%).

7. Maintain a patent 18-gauge or larger IV catheter for use should hemorrhagic shock develop. See "Cardiac and Noncardiac Shock," p. 44, for management.

Risk for fluid volume deficit related to *active loss* secondary to presence of indwelling drainage tubes, wound drainage, or vomiting; *inadequate intake of fluids* secondary to nausea, NPO status, CNS depression, or lack of access to fluids; or *failure of regulatory mechanisms* with third spacing of bodily fluids secondary to effects of anesthesia, endogenous catecholamines, blood loss during surgery, and prolonged recumbency

Desired outcomes: Patient is normovolemic, as evidenced by BP ≥90/60 mm Hg (or within patient's preoperative baseline), HR 60-100 bpm, distal pulses >2+ on a 0-4+ scale, urinary output ≥30 ml/h, stable or increasing weight, good skin turgor, warm skin, moist mucous membranes, and normothermia. Patient verbalizes orientation to time, place, and person.

1. Monitor VS q4-8 h during recovery phase. Be alert for indicators of dehydration: decreasing BP, increasing HR, slightly increased body temperature.

2. Assess patient's physical status q4-8h. Be alert for indicators of dehydration: dry skin, dry mucous membranes, excessive thirst, diminished intensity of peripheral pulses, alteration in mental status. Assess skin turgor by lifting a section of skin along the forearm, abdomen, or calf. Release the skin and watch its return to original position. With good hydration, it will return quickly; with dehydration, the skin will remain in the lifted position (tenting) or return slowly. **Note:** This test may be less reliable in older adults who have less skin elasticity and subcutaneous fat.

3. Monitor urinary output q4-8h. Be alert for a concentrated urine and low or decreasing output (average normal output is 60 ml/h or 1,400-1,500 ml/day).

4. Measure, describe, and document any emesis. Be alert for and document excessive perspiration. Include assessment of both with documentation of urinary, fecal, and other drainage for a total estimation of patient's fluid balance.

5. Measure and record output from drains, ostomies, wounds, and other

sources. Ensure patency of gastric and other drainage tubes. Record quality and quantity of output. Report and replace excessive losses.

6. Monitor patient's weight daily, using results as an indicator of patient's hydration and nutritional status. Always weigh patient at the same time every day, using the same scale and same type and amount of bed clothing. Be aware that this method is not useful in detecting intravascular fluid loss due to third spacing.

7. If nausea and vomiting are present, assess potential causes: administration of opioid analgesics, loss of patency of gastric tube, environmental factors (e.g., unpleasant odors or sights). Administer antiemetics or metoclopramide (Reglan) as prescribed.

8. Monitor serum electrolytes. Be alert for low potassium levels (K^+ <3.5 mEq/L) and signs and symptoms of hypokalemia: lethargy; irritability; anorexia; vomiting; muscle weakness and cramping; paresthesia; weak, irregular pulse; respiratory dysfunction. Also assess for low calcium levels (Ca^{2+} <8.5 mg/dl) and signs and symptoms of hypocalcemia, including Trousseau's or Chvostek's sign. Chvostek's sign is elicited by tapping the face just below the temple where the facial nerve emerges. The sign is positive if twitching occurs along the nose, lip, or side of the face. Trousseau's sign is tested by applying a BP cuff to the arm, inflating it to slightly higher than the systolic BP, and leaving it inflated for 1-4 min. Carpopedal spasms are indicative of hypocalcemia. Report significant findings to physician. Other signs and symptoms of hypocalcemia include tetany, muscle cramps, fatigue, irritability, and personality changes.

9. Administer and regulate IV fluids and electrolytes as prescribed until patient can resume oral intake. When IV fluids are discontinued, encourage intake of oral fluids, at least 2-3 L/day in nonrestricted patients. Respect patient's preference in oral fluids, and keep them readily available in patient's room.

Fluid volume excess related to compromised regulatory mechanisms after major surgery

Desired outcome: After intervention/treatment, patient becomes normovolemic, as evidenced by BP within normal range of patient's preoperative baseline, distal pulses ≤3 on a 0-4+ scale, eupnea, clear breath sounds, absence of or barely detectable edema (≤1+ on a 0-4+ scale), and body weight near or at preoperative baseline.

1. Assess for and report any indicators of fluid overload: elevated BP, bounding pulses, dyspnea, crackles, pretibial or sacral edema.

2. Maintain record of 8-h and 24-h I&O. Note and report significant imbalance. Remember that normal 24-h output is 1,400-1,500 ml, and normal 1-h output is 60 ml/h.

3. Weigh patient daily, using the same scale and same type and amount of bed clothing. Note significant weight gain. Remember that 1 L of fluid equals approximately 1 kg (2.2 lb).

4. Expect postoperative diuresis approximately 48-72 h after surgery because of mobilization of third-space (interstitial) fluid.

5. Administer furosemide (Lasix) as prescribed to mobilize interstitial fluid.

N O T E : Diuretic therapy may cause dangerous potassium (K^+) depletion. See **Risk for fluid volume deficit,** above, for signs and symptoms of hypokalemia.

---

6. Be aware that older adults and individuals with cardiovascular disease are at high risk for developing postoperative fluid volume excess.

Risk for infection related to inadequate primary defenses (broken skin, traumatized tissue, decrease in ciliary action, stasis of body fluids), invasive procedures, or chronic disease

Desired outcome: Patient is free of infection, as evidenced by normothermia; HR ≤100 bpm; RR ≤20 breaths/min with normal depth and pattern (eupnea); negative cultures; clear, normal-smelling urine; clear, thin sputum; orientation to time, place, and person; and absence of unusual erythema, warmth, or drainage at surgical incision.

1. Monitor VS for evidence of infection: elevated HR and RR, increased body temperature. Consult surgeon if these are new findings.
2. Evaluate orientation and LOC q8h. Consider infection if altered LOC is unexplained by other factors such as medication or disease process.
3. Evaluate IV sites for evidence of infection: erythema, warmth, swelling, unusual drainage. Change IV line and site if evidence of infection is present and according to agency protocol (q48-72h).
4. Evaluate patency of all surgically placed tubes or drains. Irrigate or attach to low-pressure suction as prescribed. Promptly report unrelieved loss of patency.
5. Note color, character, and odor of all drainage. Report foul-smelling or abnormal drainage.
6. Evaluate incisions and wound sites for evidence of infection: unusual erythema, warmth, delayed healing, purulent drainage.
7. Change dressings as prescribed, using sterile technique. Prevent cross-contamination of wounds in the same patient by changing one dressing at a time and washing hands between dressing changes.
8. If patient develops evisceration, do not reinsert tissue or organs. Place a sterile, saline-soaked gauze over evisceration and cover with a sterile towel until surgeon can evaluate wound.
9. Prevent reflux of urine into bladder by keeping drainage collection container below level of patient's bladder. Help prevent urinary stasis by avoiding kinks or obstructions in drainage tubing.
10. Do not open closed urinary drainage system unless absolutely necessary; irrigate catheter only with physician prescription and when obstruction is known cause.
11. Assess for indicators of urinary tract infection (UTI), including chills, fever (>37° C [100° F]), flank or labial pain, cloudy or foul-smelling urine.
12. Encourage fluid intake of 2-3 L/day in nonrestricted patients to minimize potential for UTI by diluting urine and maximizing urinary flow.

13. Make sure patient's perineum and meatus are cleansed during daily bath and that perianal area is cleansed after bowel movements. Do not hesitate to remind patient of these hygiene measures. Be alert for indicators of meatal infection: swelling, purulent drainage, persistent meatal redness. Intervene if patient is unable to perform self-care.

14. Change catheter according to established protocol, or sooner if sandy particles can be felt in distal end of catheter or if patient develops UTI. Change drainage collection container according to established protocol, or sooner if it becomes foul smelling or leaks.

15. Obtain cultures of suspicious drainage or secretions (e.g., sputum, urine, wound) as prescribed. For urine specimens, be sure to use sampling port at proximal end of drainage tube. Cleanse area with an antimicrobial wipe, and use a sterile syringe with a 25-gauge needle to aspirate urine.

16. Prevent transmission of infectious agents by washing hands well before and after caring for patient and by wearing gloves when contact with blood, drainage, or other body substance is likely.

Constipation related to immobility, opioid analgesics and other medications, effects of anesthesia, lack of privacy, disruption of abdominal musculature, or manipulation of abdominal viscera during surgery

Desired outcome: Patient returns to presurgical bowel elimination pattern, as evidenced by return of active bowel sounds within 48-72 h after most surgeries, absence of abdominal distention or sensation of fullness, and elimination of soft, formed stools.

1. Monitor for and document elimination of flatus or stool, which signals returning intestinal motility.

2. Assess for evidence of decreased GI motility: abdominal distention, tenderness, absent or hypoactive bowel sounds, sensation of fullness. Consult surgeon about gross distention, extreme tenderness, and prolonged absence of bowel sounds.

3. To stimulate peristalsis, encourage in-bed position changes, exercises, and ambulation to patient's tolerance unless contraindicated.

4. If a nasogastric (NG) tube is in place, perform the following:
   - Check placement of tube after insertion, before any instillation, and q8h. For a larger-bore tube, either insert air into proximal end of tube to elicit a *whoosh* sound, which can be heard while ausculating over epigastric area, or aspirate gastric contents. If tube is in the trachea, patient will exhibit signs of respiratory distress and tube should be repositioned immediately. For smaller-bore tubes, check a recent x-ray to confirm position before instilling anything into tube.
   - Prevent migration of tube by keeping it securely taped to patient's nose and reinforcing placement by attaching tube to patient's gown with a safety pin or tape.
   - Measure and record quantity and quality of output. Typically the color will be green. For patients who have undergone gastric surgery, it may be brownish initially because of small amounts of bloody drainage but should change to green after about 12 h. Test

reddish or brown output for blood, which can signal the development of a stress ulcer or indicate that a tube opening is compressed against the stomach lining. Reposition tube as necessary. **Note:** If patient had gastric, esophageal, or duodenal surgery, consult surgeon before manipulating tube.

- Maintain patency of NG tube with gentle instillation of normal saline as prescribed. Ensure low intermittent suction of gastric sump tubes by maintaining patency of sump port (usually blue). If sump port becomes occluded by gastric contents, flush sump port with air until a *whoosh* sound is heard over epigastric area. **Caution:** Never clamp or otherwise occlude sump port, because excessive pressure may accumulate and damage gastric mucosa. If patient had gastric, esophageal, or duodenal surgery, consult surgeon before irrigating tube.
- When tube is removed, monitor patient for abdominal distention, nausea, and vomiting.

5. Monitor and document patient's response to diet advancement from clear liquids to regular or other prescribed diet.
6. Encourage oral fluid intake, especially of prune juice.
7. Administer stool softeners, mild laxatives, and enemas as prescribed. Monitor and record results.
8. Arrange for privacy during patient's attempts at bowel elimination.

Sleep pattern disturbance related to preoperative anxiety, stress, postoperative pain, noise, and altered environment

Desired outcome: After intervention/treatment, patient has minimal or no difficulty falling asleep and reports feeling well rested.

1. Administer sedative/hypnotic as prescribed. Be aware that these agents may cause CNS depression and contribute to respiratory depressant effects of opioid analgesics. Also be aware that active metabolites of many of the benzodiazepines may accumulate and result in greater physiologic effects or toxicity. **Note:** Use caution when administering sedative/hypnotic to patients with COPD due to its respiratory depressant effects. Monitor respiratory function at frequent intervals in these individuals.
2. After administering sedative/hypnotic, be sure to raise side rails and caution patient not to smoke in bed.
3. Administer analgesics at bedtime to reduce pain and augment effects of hypnotic.
4. Make sure consent for surgery is signed before administering sedative/hypnotic.
5. Use nonpharmacologic measures to promote sleep (Table A-7).

Impaired physical mobility related to postoperative pain, decreased strength and endurance secondary to CNS effects of anesthesia or blood loss, musculoskeletal or neuromuscular impairment secondary to disease process or surgical procedure, perceptual impairment secondary to disease process or surgical procedure (e.g., ocular surgery, neurosurgery), or cognitive deficit secondary to disease process or effects of opioid analgesics and anesthetics

Desired outcome: Optimally, by hospital discharge (depending on type of surgery), patient returns to preoperative baseline physical mo-

Table A-7 Nonpharmacologic measures to promote sleep

Activity	Examples
Mask or eliminate environmental stimuli	Use eyeshields or ear plugs; play soothing music; dim lights at bedtime; mask odors from dressings/drainage; change dressing or drainage container as indicated
Promote muscle relaxation	Encourage ambulation as tolerated throughout the day; teach and encourage in-bed exercises and position changes; perform back massage at bedtime; if not contraindicated, use heating pad
Reduce anxiety	Ensure adequate pain control; keep patient informed of progress and treatment measures; avoid overstimulation by visitors or other activities immediately before bedtime; avoid stimulant drugs (e.g., caffeine)
Promote comfort	Encourage patient to use own pillows and bedclothes if not contraindicated; adjust bed; rearrange linens; regulate room temperature
Promote usual presleep routine	Offer oral hygiene at bedtime; provide warm beverage at bedtime; encourage reading or other quiet activity
Minimize sleep disruption	Maintain quiet environment throughout the night; plan nursing activities to allow long periods (at least 90 min) of undisturbed sleep; use dim lights when checking on patient during the night

bility, as evidenced by ability to move in bed, transfer, and ambulate independently or with minimal assistance.

1. Assess patient's preoperative physical mobility by evaluating coordination and muscle strength, control, and mass. Be aware of medically imposed restrictions on movement, especially with orthopedic, neurosurgical, or ocular conditions or surgical procedures.

2. Evaluate and correct factors limiting physical mobility: oversedation with opioid analgesics, failure to achieve adequate pain control, poorly arranged physical environment.

3. Initiate movement from bed to chair and ambulation as soon as possible after surgery, depending on postoperative prescriptions, type of surgery, and patient's recovery from anesthetics (usually 12-24 h after surgery). Assist patient with moving slowly to a sitting position in bed and then standing at bedside before attempting ambulation.

For more information, see **Altered cerebral tissue perfusion,** p. 419.

N O T E : Many anesthetics depress normal vasoconstrictor mechanisms and can result in sudden hypotension with quick changes in position.

---

4. Encourage frequent movement and ambulation after surgery. Provide assistance as indicated.
5. Explain the importance of movement in bed and ambulation in reducing postoperative complications, including atelectasis, pneumonia, thrombophlebitis, and depressed GI motility.
6. For additional information, see "Caring for Patients on Prolonged Bed Rest" for **Risk for activity intolerance,** p. 413, and **Risk for disuse syndrome,** p. 416.

Risk for trauma related to weakness, balancing difficulties, and reduced muscle coordination secondary to anesthetics and postoperative opioid analgesics
Desired outcome: Patient does not fall and remains free of trauma, as evidenced by absence of bruises, wounds, or fractures.

1. Orient and reorient patient to time, place, and person during initial postoperative period. Inform patient that surgery is over. Repeat information until patient is fully awake and oriented (usually several hours but may be days with heavily sedated or otherwise obtunded individuals).
2. Maintain side rails on stretchers and beds in upright and locked positions. Be aware that some individuals experience agitation and thrash about as they emerge from anesthesia.
3. Secure all IV lines, drains, and tubing to prevent dislodgment.
4. Put bed in lowest position before leaving patient's room.
5. Make sure call mechanism is within patient's reach; instruct patient in its use.
6. Caution patient and visitors to avoid smoking in rooms when oxygen is in use.
7. Identify patients at high risk for falling by assessing the following (correct or compensate for risk factors):
   ■ *Time of day:* Night shift, peak activity periods (e.g., meals, bedtime).
   ■ *Medications:* Opioid analgesics, sedatives, hypnotics, and anesthetics.
   ■ *Impaired mobility:* Individuals requiring assistance with transfer and ambulation.
   ■ *Sensory deficits:* Diminished visual acuity due to disease process or environmental factors; changes in kinesthetic sense due to disease or trauma.
8. Use restrains and protective devices only if necessary and prescribed.

Risk for impaired skin integrity related to presence of secretions/excretions around percutaneous drains and tubes.

Desired outcome: Patient's skin around percutaneous drains and tubes remains clear and intact.
1. Change dressings as soon as they become wet. Surgeon may prefer to perform first dressing changes at surgical incision. Use sterile technique for all dressing changes.
2. Keep area around drain or T-tube as clean as possible (e.g., the presence of bile can quickly lead to skin excoriation). Sterile normal saline or a solution of saline and hydrogen peroxide or other prescribed solution may be used to clean around drain site.
3. If some external drainage is present, position a pectin-wafer skin barrier around drain or tube. Ointments also may be used (e.g., zinc oxide, petrolatum, aluminum paste). Consult with enterostomal therapy (ET) nurse if drainage is excessive or skin excoriation develops. For additional information, see "Managing Wound Care," p. 384.

Altered oral mucous membrane related to NPO status and/or presence of NG or endotracheal tube
Desired outcome: Upon hospital discharge, patient's oral mucosa is intact, without pain or evidence of bleeding.
1. Provide oral care and oral hygiene q4h and prn. Arrange for patient to gargle, brush teeth, and cleanse mouth with sponge-tipped applicators as necessary to prevent excoriation and excessive dryness.
2. Use a moistened, cotton-tipped applicator to remove encrustations. Carefully lubricate lips and nares with antimicrobial ointment, petroleum jelly, or emollient cream.
3. If patient's throat is irritated from presence of NG tube, obtain a prescription for a lidocaine gargling solution.

For more information about preventing surgical complications, see "Atelectasis," p. 1; "Pneumonia," p. 2; "Venous Thrombosis/Thrombophlebitis," p. 61; "Urinary Retention," p. 99; "Providing Nutritional Support," p. 378; "Managing Wound Care,"; p. 384; and "Caring for Patients on Prolonged Bed Rest," p. 413.

For psychosocial nursing diagnoses and interventions, see "Caring for Patients with Cancer and Other Life-Disrupting Illnesses," p. 450.

SECTION TWO: CARING FOR PATIENTS ON PROLONGED BED REST

Risk for activity intolerance related to deconditioned status (see Table A-8)
Desired outcomes: Patient exhibits cardiac tolerance to activity or exercise, as evidenced by HR $\leq$20 bpm over resting HR; systolic BP

Appendix One

Table A-8   Physiologic effects of prolonged bed rest (deconditioning)

Increased HR and BP for submaximal work load
Decrease in functional capacity
Decrease in circulating volume
Orthostatic hypotension
Reflex tachycardia
Modest decrease in pulmonary function
Increase in thromboemboli
Loss of muscle mass
Loss of muscle contractile strength
Negative protein state
Negative nitrogen state

≤20 mm Hg over or under resting systolic BP; RR ≤20 breaths/min with normal depth and pattern (eupnea); normal sinus rhythm; warm, dry skin; and absence of crackles, new murmurs, new dysrhythmias, gallop, or chest pain. Patient rates perceived exertion (RPE) at ≤3 on a scale of 0 (none) to 10 (maximal).

1. Perform ROM exercises 2-4 ×/day on each extremity. Individualize exercise plan based on the following guidelines:

   ■ *Mode or type of exercise:* Begin with passive exercises, moving joints through motions of abduction, adduction, flexion, and extension. Progress to active-assisted exercises in which you support the joints while patient initiates muscle contraction. When patient is able, supervise him or her in active isotonic exercises, during which patient contracts a selected muscle group, moves extremity at a slow pace, and then relaxes the muscle group. Have patient repeat each exercise 3-10 times.

C A U T I O N :   Stop any exercise that produces muscular or skeletal pain. Consult physical therapist (PT) about necessary modifications. Do not use isometric exercises with cardiac patients.

   ■ *Intensity:* Begin with 3-5 repetitions as tolerated by patient. Assess exercise tolerance by measuring HR and BP at rest, peak exercise, and 5 min after exercise. If HR or systolic BP increased >20 bpm (or 20 mm Hg) over resting level, reduce the number of repetitions. A decrease in HR or systolic BP >10 bpm (or 10 mm Hg) at peak exercise could be a sign of left ventricular failure, denoting that the heart cannot meet this work load. For other adverse signs and symptoms, see "Assessment of exercise tolerance," below.
   ■ *Duration:* Begin with 5 min or less of exercise. Gradually increase exercise to 15 min as tolerated.
   ■ *Frequency:* Begin with exercises 2-4 ×/day. As duration increases, frequency can be reduced.

■ *Assessment of exercise tolerance:* Be alert for signs and symptoms that the cardiovascular and respiratory systems are unable to meet demands of low-level ROM exercises. Excessive SOB may occur if (1) transient pulmonary congestion occurs secondary to ischemia or left ventricular dysfunction; (2) lung volumes are decreased; (3) oxygen-carrying capacity of the blood is reduced; or (4) there is shunting of blood from the right to the left side of the heart without adequate oxygenation. If cardiac output does not increase to meet the body's needs during modest levels of exercise, systolic BP may fall; the skin may become cool, cyanotic, and diaphoretic; dysrhythmias may be noted; crackles may be auscultated; or a systolic murmur of mitral regurgitation may occur. If patient tolerates exercise, increase intensity or number of repetitions each day.

2. Ask patient to rate perceived exertion during exercise, using the following scale developed by Borg (1982):

    0 nothing at all
    1 very weak effort
    2 weak (light) effort
    3 moderate
    4 somewhat stronger effort
    5 strong effort
    7 very strong effort
    9 very, very strong effort
    10 maximal effort

Patient should not have RPE >3 while performing ROM exercises. Reduce intensity of exercise and increase frequency until RPE of ≤3 is attained.

3. As patient's condition improves, increase activity as soon as possible to include sitting in a chair. Assess for orthostatic hypotension, which can occur as a result of decreased plasma volume and difficulty in adjusting immediately to postural change. Prepare patient for this change by increasing time spent in high Fowler's position and moving patient slowly and in stages. The following describes activity progression in hospitalized patients.

Level I: Bed rest	Flexion and extension of extremities 4 ×/day, 15 × each extremity; deep breathing 4 ×/day, 15 breaths; position change from side to side q2h
Level II: Out of bed to chair	As tolerated, 3 ×/day for 20-30 min; may perform ROM exercises 2 ×/day while sitting in chair
Level III: Ambulate in room	As tolerated, 3 ×/day for 3-5 min
Level IV: Ambulate in hall	Initially, 50-200 ft 2 ×/day; progressing to 600 ft 4 ×/day; may incorporate slow stair climbing in preparation for hospital discharge

Appendix One

Signs of activity intoler-ance:	Decrease in BP >20 mm Hg; increase in HR to >120 bpm (or >20 bpm above resting HR in patients under-going beta-blocker therapy)

4. Increase activity level by having patient perform self-care activities such as eating, mouth care, and bathing as tolerated.
5. Teach significant others the purpose and interventions for prevent-ing deconditioning. Involve them in patient's plan of care.
6. To help allay fears of failure, pain, or medical setbacks, provide emotional support to patient and significant others as patient's activ-ity level is increased.

Risk for disuse syndrome related to paralysis, mechanical immobi-lization, prescribed immobilization, severe pain, or altered LOC

Desired outcome: Patient exhibits complete ROM of all joints without pain and limb girth measurements congruent with or increased over baseline measurements.

N O T E : ROM exercises should be performed every day for all im-mobilized patients with *normal* joints. Modification may be required for patients with flaccidity (i.e., immediately after cerebrovascular ac-cident [CVA] or spinal cord injury [SCI]) to prevent subluxation; or for patient with spasticity (i.e., during the recovery period for patients with CVA or SCI) to prevent an increase in spasticity. Consult with PT or occupational therapist (OT) for assistance in modifying exercise plan for these patients. Also, be aware that ROM exercises are restricted or contraindicated for patients with rheumatologic disease during the in-flammatory phase and for dislocated or fractured joints.

---

1. Be alert for the following areas that are especially prone to joint contracture; *shoulder,* which can become "frozen," limiting abduc-tion and extension; *wrist,* which can "drop," prohibiting extension; *fingers,* which can develop flexion contractures that limit exten-sion; *hips,* which can develop flexion contractures that affect the gait by shortening the limb or develop external rotation or adduc-tion deformities that affect the gait; *knees,* which can develop flex-ion contractures that limit extension and affect the gait; and *feet,* which can "drop" as a result of plantarflexion, which limits dorsi-flexion and alters the gait.
2. Make sure patient changes position at least q2h. Post a turning schedule at patient's bedside. Position changes not only maintain correct body alignment, thereby reducing strain on joints, but also prevent contractures, minimize pressure on bony prominences, and promote maximal chest expansion.
   ■ Try to place patient in a position that achieves proper standing alignment: head neutral or slightly flexed on the neck, hips ex-tended, knees extended or minimally flexed, and feet at right angles to the legs. Maintain this position with pillows, towels, or other positioning aids.
   ■ To prevent hip flexion contractures, make sure patient is prone

or side-lying, with the hips extended, for the same amount of
time patient spends in the supine position.

- When HOB must be elevated 30 degrees, extend patient's shoulders and arms, using pillows to support the position, and allow fingertips to extend over the edge of the pillows to maintain normal arching of the hands. **Caution:** Because elevating HOB promotes hip flexion, make sure patient spends equal time with hips in extension (see intervention earlier).
- When patient is in side-lying position, extend lower leg from hip to help prevent hip flexion contracture.
- When patient can be placed in prone position, move him or her to the end of the bed and allow the feet to rest between the mattress and footboard. This prevents not only plantarflexion and hip rotation, but also injury to heels and toes. Place thin pads under angles of axillae and lateral aspects of clavicles to prevent internal rotation of shoulders and to maintain anatomic position of the shoulder girdle.

3. To maintain joints in neutral position, use pillows, rolled towels, blankets, sandbags, antirotation boots, splints, and orthotics as indicated. When using adjunctive devices, monitor involved skin at frequent intervals for alterations in integrity, and implement measures to prevent skin breakdown.

4. Assess for footdrop by inspecting feet for plantarflexion and evaluating patient's ability to pull toes upward toward nose. Since the feet naturally lie in plantarflexion, be particularly alert for inability to pull toes up. Document this assessment daily.

5. Teach patient the purpose and procedure for ROM exercises, and have patient return demonstrations. Review **Risk for activity intolerance,** earlier, to make sure patient does not exceed his or her tolerance. Provide passive exercises for patients unable to perform active or active-assistive exercises. In addition, incorporate movement patterns into care activities, such as position changes, bed baths, getting patient on and off the bedpan, or changing patient's gown. Make sure joints especially prone to contracture are exercised more stringently. Provide patient with a handout that reviews the exercises and lists the repetitions for each.

6. Perform and document limb girth measurements, dynamography, and ROM, and establish exercise baseline limits to assess patient's existing muscle mass and strength and joint motion.

7. Explain to patient that muscle atrophy often occurs because of disuse or failure to use joint due to immediate or anticipated pain. Eventually disuse may result in a decrease in muscle mass and blood supply and a loss of periarticular tissue elasticity, which in turn can lead to increased muscle fatigue and joint pain with use.

8. Emphasize the importance of maintaining or increasing muscle strength and periarticular tissue elasticity through exercise. If unsure about patient's complicating condition, consult physician about appropriate form of exercise.

9. Explain the need to participate maximally in self-care as tolerated

to help maintain muscle strength and enhance a sense of participation and control.

10. For noncardiac patients needing greater help with muscle strength, assist with resistive exercises (e.g., moderate weightlifting to increase size, endurance, and strength of muscles). For patients in beds with Balkan frames, provide means for resistive exercise by implementing a system of weights and pulleys. First determine patient's baseline level of performance on a given set of exercises, then set realistic goals with patient for repetitions (e.g., if patient can do 5 repetitions of lifting a 5-lb weight with the biceps muscle, the goal may be to increase the repetitions to 10 within a week, to an ultimate goal of 20 within 3 wk, and then advance to 7½-lb weights).

11. If joints require rest, isometric exercises can be used. With these exercises, teach patient to contract a muscle group and hold the contraction for a count of 5 or 10. The sequence is repeated for increasing numbers or repetitions until an adequate level of endurance has been achieved. Thereafter, maintenance levels are performed.

12. Provide a chart to show patient's progress, and combine this with large amounts of positive reinforcement. Post exercise regimen at bedside to ensure consistency by all health care providers.

13. As appropriate, teach transfer or crutch-walking techniques and use of a walker, wheelchair, or cane so that patient can maintain the highest possible level of mobility. Include significant others in demonstrations, and stress the importance of good body mechanics.

14. Provide periods of uninterrupted rest between exercises and activities to allow patient to replenish energy stores.

15. Seek a referral to a PT or OT as appropriate.

Altered peripheral tissue perfusion related to interrupted venous flow secondary to prolonged immobility

Desired outcomes: At a minimum of 24 h before hospital discharge, patient has adequate peripheral perfusion, as evidenced by normal skin color and temperature and adequate distal pulses (>2+ on a 0-4+ scale) in peripheral extremities. Patient performs exercises independently, adheres to prophylactic regimen, and maintains a fluid intake of 2-3 L/day unless contraindicated.

1. Teach patient that pain, redness, swelling, and warmth in involved area and coolness, unnatural color or pallor, and superficial venous dilatation distal to involved area are all indicators of deep vein thrombosis (DVT) and should be reported to staff member promptly if they occur.

2. Monitor for the indicators listed above, along with routine VS checks. If patient is asymptomatic for DVT, assess for positive Homans' sign: flex knee 30 degrees and dorsiflex foot. Pain elicited with dorsiflexion may be a sign of DVT, and patient should be referred to physician for further evaluation. Additional signs of DVT may include fever, tachycardia, and elevated erythrocyte sedimentation rate (ESR). Normal ESR (Westergren method) in men <50 yr

is 0-15 mm/h, >50 yr 0-20 mm/h; in women <50 yr 0-20 mm/h, and >50 yr 0-30 mm/h.

3. Teach patient calf-pumping (ankle dorsiflexion-plantarflexion) and ankle-circling exercises. Instruct patient to repeat each movement 10 times, performing each exercise qh during extended periods of immobility, provided that patient is free of symptoms of DVT. Help promote circulation by performing passive ROM or encouraging active ROM exercises.

4. Encourage deep breathing, which increases negative pressure in the lungs and thorax to promote emptying of large veins.

5. When not contraindicated by peripheral vascular disease (PVD), make sure patient wears antiembolic hose or pneumatic sequential compression stockings. Remove them for 10-20 min q8h and inspect underlying skin for evidence of irritation or breakdown. Put hose back on after elevating patient's legs at least 10 degrees for 10 min.

6. Instruct patient not to cross feet at ankles or knees while in bed, because doing so may cause venous stasis. If patient is at risk for DVT, elevate foot of bed 10 degrees to increase venous return.

7. In nonrestricted patient, increase fluid intake to at least 2-3 L/day to reduce hemoconcentration, which can contribute to the development of DVT. Educate patient about need to drink large amounts of fluid. Monitor I&O to ensure compliance.

8. Patients at risk for DVT, including those with chronic infection and a history of PVD and smoking, as well as older adults and obese or anemic individuals, may require pharmacologic interventions (aspirin, sodium warfarin, phenindione derivatives, or heparin). Administer medication as prescribed, and monitor appropriate laboratory values (e.g., prothrombin time [PT], partial thromboplastin time [PTT]). Teach patient to self-monitor for and report bleeding (epistaxis, bleeding gums, hematemesis, hemoptysis, melena, hematuria, ecchymoses).

9. In patients prone to DVT, acquire bilateral baseline measurements of midcalf, knee, and midthigh and record them on patient's Kardex. Monitor measurements daily and compare them to baseline values to rule out extremity enlargement caused by DVT.

Altered cerebral tissue perfusion (orthostatic hypotension) related to interrupted arterial flow to the brain secondary to prolonged bed rest
Desired outcome: When getting out of bed, patient has adequate cerebral perfusion, as evidenced by HR <120 bpm and BP ≥90/60 mm Hg (or within 20 mm Hg of patient's normal range) immediately after position change, dry skin, normal skin color, and absence of vertigo and syncope, with return of HR and BP to resting levels within 3 min of position change.

1. Assess patient for factors that increase the risk of orthostatic hypotension because of fluid volume changes (recent diuresis, diaphoresis, or change in vasodilator therapy), altered autonomic control (diabetic cardiac neuropathy, denervation postheart transplant, or advanced age), or severe left ventricular dysfunction.

2. Explain the cause of orthostatic hypotension and measures for preventing it.

3. Antiembolic hose, which are used to prevent DVT, may be useful in preventing orthostatic hypotension once patient is mobilized. If patient continues to have difficulty with orthostatic hypotension, it may be necessary to supplement hose with elastic wraps to groin when patient is out of bed. Make sure wraps encompass entire surface of the legs.
4. When patient is in bed, provide instructions for leg exercises as described under **Risk for activity intolerance,** p. 413.
5. Prepare patient for getting out of bed by encouraging position changes within necessary confines. It is sometimes possible and advisable to use a tilt table to reacclimate patient to upright positions.
6. Follow these guidelines for mobilization:
   - Check BP in any high-risk patient for whom this will be the first time out of bed.
   - Have patient dangle legs at bedside. Be alert for indicators of orthostatic hypotension: diaphoresis, pallor, tachycardia, hypotension, syncope. Question patient about lightheadedness or dizziness.
   - If indicators of orthostatic hypotension occur, check VS. A drop in systolic BP of 20 mm Hg and an increased pulse rate, combined with symptoms of vertigo and impending syncope, signal the need to return to a supine position.
   - If leg dangling is tolerated, have patient stand at bedside with two staff members in attendance. If no adverse signs or symptoms occur, have patient progress to ambulation as tolerated.

Constipation related to less than adequate fluid or dietary intake and bulk, immobility, lack of privacy, positional restrictions, and use of narcotic analgesics
Desired outcomes: Within 24 h of this diagnosis, patient verbalizes knowledge of measures that promote bowel elimination. Within 3-5 days of this diagnosis, patient reports return of his or her normal pattern and character of bowel elimination.
1. Assess patient's bowel history to determine normal bowel habits and interventions used successfully at home.
2. Monitor and document patient's bowel movements, diet, and I&O. Be alert for indications of constipation: fewer than patient's usual number of bowel movements, abdominal discomfort or distention, straining at stool, feeling of rectal pressure or fullness. Fecal impaction may be manifested by oozing of liquid stool and confirmed *via* digital examination.
3. Auscultate each abdominal quadrant for at least 1 min to determine if bowel sounds are present. Normal sounds are clicks or gurgles occurring at a rate of 5-34/min. **Note:** Bowel sounds are decreased or absent with paralytic ileus. High-pitched, rushing sounds may be heard during abdominal cramping, indicating an intestinal obstruction.
4. If a rectal impaction is suspected, use a gloved, lubricated finger to remove stool from rectum. This stimulation may be adequate to stimulate bowel movement. Oil-retention enemas may soften impacted stool.

5. Teach patient the importance of a high-roughage diet and a fluid intake of at least 2-3 L/day (unless this is contraindicated by a renal, hepatic, or cardiac disorder). High-roughage foods include bran, whole grains, nuts, raw and coarse vegetables, and fruits with skins.
6. Maintain patient's normal bowel habits whenever possible by offering bedpan, ensuring privacy, and timing medications, enemas, or suppositories so that they take effect at the time of day patient normally has a bowel movement. Provide warm fluids before breakfast and encourage toileting to gain advantage of gastrocolic or duodenocolic reflexes.
7. To promote peristalsis, maximize patient's activity level within limitations of endurance, therapy, and pain.
8. Request pharmacologic intervention from physician when necessary. To help prevent rebound constipation, make a priority list of interventions to ensure minimal disruption of patient's normal bowel habits. The following is a suggested hierarchy of interventions:
   (1) Bulk-building additives (psyllium), bran
   (2) Mild laxatives (apple or prune juice, milk of magnesia)
   (3) Stool softeners (docusate sodium or docusate calcium)
   (4) Potent laxatives and cathartics (bisacodyl, cascara sagrada)
   (5) Medicated suppositories
   (6) Enemas
9. Discuss the role that narcotic agents and other medications have in constipation. Teach alternative methods of pain control (see Table A-6, p. 403).

Diversional activity deficit related to prolonged illness and hospitalization

Desired outcome: Within 24 h of intervention, patient engages in diversional activities and relates the absence of boredom.

1. Be alert for patient indicators of boredom: wishing for something to read or do, daytime napping, expressed inability to perform usual hobbies because of hospitalization.
2. Assess patient's activity tolerance as described on p. 413.
3. Collect a database by assessing patient's normal support systems and relationship patterns with significant others. Question patient about his or her interests, and explore diversional activities that may be suitable for hospital setting and patient's level of activity tolerance.
4. Personalize patient's environment with favorite objects and photographs of significant others.
5. Provide low-level activities commensurate with patient's tolerance (e.g., books or magazines pertaining to patient's recreational or other interests, television, or writing for short intervals).
6. Initiate activities that require little concentration and proceed to more complicated tasks as patient's condition allows (e.g., if reading requires more energy or concentration than patient is capable of, suggest that significant others read to patient or bring in audiotapes and books, such as those marketed for the visually impaired).
7. Encourage discussion of past activities or reminiscence as a substitute for performing favorite activities during convalescence.

8. As patient's endurance improves, obtain appropriate diversional activities such as puzzles, model kits, handicrafts, and computerized games and activities, and encourage patient to use them.

9. Encourage significant others to visit within limits of patient's endurance and to involve patient in activities that are of interest to him or her, such as playing cards or backgammon. Encourage significant others to stagger their visits throughout the day.

10. Spend extra time with patient.

11. Suggest that significant others bring in a radio or, if appropriate, rent a TV or radio from the hospital, if not part of the standard room charge.

12. If appropriate for patient, arrange for hospital volunteers to visit, play cards, read books, or play board games.

13. As appropriate for patient who desires social interaction, consider relocation to a room in an area of high traffic.

14. As patient's condition improves, help him or her to a chair near a window to watch outside activities. When patients are able, provide opportunities to sit in a solarium so that they can visit with other patients. If physical condition and weather permit, take patient outside for brief periods.

15. Request consultation from social services, OT, pastoral services, and psychiatric nurse for interventions as appropriate.

16. Increase patient's involvement in self-care to provide a sense of purpose, accomplishment, and control. Performing in-bed exercises (e.g., deep breathing, ankle circling, calf pumping), keeping track of I&O, and similar activities can and should be accomplished routinely by these patients.

Altered sexuality pattern related to actual or perceived physiologic limitations on sexual performance secondary to disease, therapy, or prolonged hospitalization

Desired outcome: Within 72 h of this diagnosis, patient reports satisfaction with sexuality and/or understanding of ability to resume sexual activity.

1. Assess patient's normal sexual function: importance placed on sex in the relationship, frequency of interaction, normal positions used, and couple's ability to adapt to change to meet requirements of patient's limitations.

2. Identify patient's problem diplomatically, and clarify it with patient. Indicators of sexual dysfunction can include regression, acting-out with inappropriate behavior (grabbing, pinching), sexual overtures toward hospital staff, and self-enforced isolation.

3. Encourage patient and significant other to verbalize feelings and anxieties about sexual abstinence, having sexual relations in hospital, hurting the patient, or having to use new or alternative methods for sexual gratification. Develop strategies with patient and significant other.

4. Encourage acceptable expressions of sexuality (e.g., for women, wearing makeup and jewelry).

5. Inform patient and significant other that it is possible to have time alone together for intimacy. Provide that time by putting a "Do Not

Disturb" sign on the door, enforcing privacy by restricting staff and visitors from the room, or arranging for temporary private quarters.

6. Encourage patient and significant other to seek alternate methods of sexual expression when necessary. This may include mutual masturbation, altered positions, vibrators, and identification of other erotic areas for the partner.

7. Refer patient and significant other to professional sexual counseling as necessary.

Altered role performance: Dependence versus independence

Desired outcome: Within 48 h of this diagnosis, patient collaborates with care givers in planning realistic goals for independence, participates in own care, and takes responsibility for self-care.

1. Encourage patient to be as independent as possible within limits of endurance, therapy, and pain. However, be aware that temporary periods of dependence are appropriate because they enable the individual to restore energy reserves needed for recovery.

2. Ensure that all health care providers are consistent in conveying their expectations of eventual independence.

3. Alert patient to areas of overdependence, and involve him or her in goal-setting to achieve independence.

4. Do not minimize patient's feelings of depression. Allow patient to express emotions, but provide support, understanding, and realistic hope for a positive role change.

5. If indicated, provide self-help devices to increase patient's independence with self-care.

6. Provide positive reinforcement when patient meets or advances toward goals.

For interventions related to preventing atelectasis and pneumonia, see those sections in "Respiratory Disorders."

See "Pressure Ulcers" for **Impaired tissue integrity** (for patients without pressure ulcers who are at risk because of immobility)," p. 390.

For psychosocial nursing diagnoses and interventions, see "Caring for Patients with Cancer and Other Life-Disrupting Illnesses," p. 450.

SECTION THREE: CARING FOR PATIENTS WITH CANCER AND OTHER LIFE-DISRUPTING ILLNESSES

Chemotherapy and Immunotherapy

Risk of injury (to staff and environment) related to preparation, handling, administration, and disposal of chemotherapeutic agents

Desired outcome: Chemotherapy exposure of staff and environment is minimized by proper preparation, handling, administration, and disposal by individuals familiar with these agents.

1. Make sure chemotherapy is prepared by pharmacists and administered by nurses familiar with these agents. Keep institutional guidelines readily available for safe preparation, handling, and potential complications, such as spills or individual contact with these drugs. **Note:** A chemotherapy approval course is highly recommended for nurses who will be administering these drugs.
2. Make sure pregnant nurses exercise extreme caution when handling these drugs. Check with individual agencies for policies about administration of these drugs by women who are pregnant or are considering becoming pregnant.
3. Implement measures to minimize aerosolization and direct contact with these drugs during preparation: using a biological safety cabinet, placing an absorbent pad on the work area, and wearing latex gloves, full-length gown with cuffed sleeves, and goggles. Gloves and gowns should always be worn during handling and disposal of these agents.
4. Prime IV tubing with a 50-ml bag of diluent, or prime tubing into a sterile bag, using gauze to absorb excess liquid.
5. When removing IV administration set, wear latex gloves and wrap sterile gauze around needle to prevent direct contact with drug. Place all needles, drugs, drug containers, and related material in a puncture-proof container clearly marked *Biohazardous Waste.* **Note:** Follow this procedure in disposing of immunotherapy waste as well.
6. Wear latex gloves when handling all body excretions for 48 h after chemotherapy, because drug is excreted through urine and feces.
7. To clean up a chemotherapy spill, double-glove and wear eye protection and a full-length gown. Use absorbent pads to absorb liquid. Then, cleanse 3 times with a detergent solution. Dispose of all waste in a biohazardous waste container.
8. To prevent oral contamination with drug, avoid any activity in which the hand goes to the mouth (e.g., eating, drinking, smoking) in any area where the chemical is given or prepared.
9. In the event of skin contact with drug, wash affected area with soap and water. Consult physician about follow-up care.
10. If eye contact occurs, irrigate eye with water for 15 min and consult physician about follow-up care.

Impaired tissue integrity (or risk for same) related to extravasation of vesicant or irritating chemotherapy agents

Desired outcome: Patient's tissue remains intact, without evidence of inflammation or pain along injection site.

N O T E : Vesicant drugs that can cause tissue damage include dactinomycin, daunomycin, doxorubicin, mitomycin-C, epirubicin, estramustine, idarubicin, mechlorethamine, vinblastine, vincristine, and vindesine. Drugs that can cause pain along the injection site with or without inflammation include amsacrine, carmustine, dacarbazine, etoposide, plicamycin, streptozocin, and teniposide.

---

1. Make sure vesicant chemotherapy is administered by a nurse experienced in venipuncture and knowledgeable about chemotherapy.
2. Select IV site carefully, using a new site if possible. Avoid sites such as the antecubital fossa, wrist, or dorsal side of the hand, where the risk of damage to underlying tendons or nerves is greater.
3. Check patency of IV before and during administration of the drug. Instruct patient to report burning or pain immediately.
4. Give infusions of vesicant drugs through a central venous catheter to minimize risk of extravasation. Assess entry site frequently. Pain, burning, and stinging are common with extravasation, as are erythema and swelling around needle site. Do not use blood return as an indicator that extravasation has not occurred because blood return is possible with extravasation. Instruct patient to report discomfort at site promptly.
5. Keep an extravasation kit readily available, along with institutional guidelines for extravasation management.
6. If extravasation occurs, follow these general guidelines:
   - Stop infusion immediately, and aspirate any remaining drug from needle. To do this, first put on latex gloves, then attach syringe to tubing and aspirate drug.
   - Consult physician.
   - Leave needle in place if an antidote is to be used with extravasated drug.
   - Attach a syringe containing recommended antidote, and instill antidote. Remove IV needle from site.
   - If recommended, inject extravasated site with antidote, using a TB syringe and a 25- to 27-gauge needle.
   - Do not apply pressure to site. Apply a sterile occlusive dressing, elevate site, and apply heat or cold as recommended.
   - Document incident, noting date, time, insertion site of needle, drug, approximate amount of drug that extravasated, management of extravasation, and appearance of site. Check institutional guideliness regarding need for photodocumentation. Monitor site frequently.
   - Provide patient with information about site care and follow-up appointments for evaluating severity of extravasation.

Knowledge deficit: Chemotherapy and the purpose, expected side effects, and potential toxicities associated with chemotherapeutic drugs, appropriate self-care measures for minimizing side effects, and available community and educational resources

Desired outcome: Before specific chemotherapeutic drugs are administered, patient and significant others verbalize knowledge of their potential side effects and toxicities, appropriate self-care measures for minimizing side effects, and available community and educational resources.

1. Establish patient's and significant others' current level of knowledge about patient's health status and prescribed therapies.
2. Assess patient's and significant others' cognitive and emotional readiness to learn.

Appendix One

3. Recognize barriers to learning: ineffective communication, neurologic deficit, sensory alterations, fear, anxiety, lack of motivation. In particular, clarify misunderstandings about side effects and toxicities of chemotherapy. Define all terminology as needed, and correct any misconceptions.

4. Assess patient's and significant others' learning needs and establish short- and long-term goals with these individuals. Identify their preferred methods of learning and the amount of information they would like to receive. Develop a teaching plan based on this information.

5. Use individualized verbal and audiovisual strategies to promote learning and enhance understanding. Give simple, direct instructions; reinforce this information often.

6. Provide an environment free of distractions and conducive to teaching and learning.

7. Discuss drugs patient will receive, including route of administration, duration of treatment, schedule, most common side effects and toxicities, and appropriate self-care. Provide both written and verbal information.

8. Provide emergency phone numbers for use should patient develop a fever or other side effects.

9. Provide material from educational resources such as the American Cancer Society, National Cancer Institute, and drug companies. Make sure materials are at the reading level appropriate for patient.

10. Identify appropriate community resources that assist with transportation, costs of care, and skilled care as needed.

Knowledge deficit: Immunotherapy and its purpose, potential side effects and toxicities, appropriate self-care measures to minimize side effects, and available community and education resources

Desired outcome: Before immunotherapy is administered, patient and significant others verbalize understanding of its purpose, potential side effects and toxicities, appropriate self-care measures to minimize side effects, and available community and education resources.

1. First see interventions 1-6 under **Knowledge deficit,** above.

2. Provide information about route of administration, expected action, and potential side effects. Because these patients often given their own injections of interferon, instruct them in the proper technique and site rotation schedule. Teach patient to record site and time of administration, side effects, self-management of side effects, and any medications taken. Teach them proper disposal of needles.

3. Arrange for pharmacy delivery of medication because it must be refrigerated. As appropriate, arrange for community nursing follow-up for additional supervision and instruction.

4. Teach patient and significant others to be alert for side effects of interferon: fever, chills, flulike symptoms. Suggest that patient take acetaminophen, with physician's approval, to manage these symptoms; warn patient not to take aspirin or NSAIDs because they may interfere with the action of interferon.

5. Teach patient to monitor and record temperature 2 ×/day and drink

extra fluids. Anorexia and weight loss, which are dose related, are other common side effects of interferon. Provide information about nutritional supplementation.

6. Provide educational materials available through drug companies.

Venous Access Devices

Knowledge deficit: Purpose and management of venous access device (VAD)

Desired outcome: Within the 24 h before hospital discharge, patient and significant others verbalize understanding of VAD, including its purpose, appropriate management measures, and potential complications.

1. Determine patient's and significant others' level of understanding of purpose of a VAD. As appropriate, explain that device can be used for administration of drugs, fluids, and blood products and drawing of blood samples and that it eliminates the need for frequent venipunctures.

2. Show patient a model of the device and explain insertion procedure. Silicone elastic atrial catheters and implanted venous ports are inserted in the operating room using local anesthetic. Patient may feel mild discomfort, similar to a toothache, for 48 h after procedure. Reassure patient that discomfort responds readily to mild pain medication.

3. If possible, introduce patient and significant others to another individual who has the device so that they can see first-hand what the VAD looks like and discuss their concerns.

4. Teach patient about VAD care. Provide both verbal and written instructions, including educational materials provided by the VAD manufacturer. Have patient or significant other demonstrate dressing care, flushing technique, and cap-changing routine before hospital discharge. Make sure patient has 24-h emergency number to call in case of problems.

5. For silicone elastic atrial catheter:
    - *Hickman:* Maintenance involves flushing 3 ×/week with 2.5 ml heparin solution (100 U/ml). Care after blood drawing involves flushing with 5 ml of normal saline solution followed by 2.5 ml of heparin solution (100 U/ml).
    - *Groshong:* Maintenance involves flushing with 5 ml of normal saline solution weekly. Care after blood drawing involves flushing with 20 ml of normal saline solution.

6. For subcutaneous implanted port:
    - *Port-a-Cath:* Maintenance involves flushing monthly and after each use with 5 ml of heparin (100 U/ml). Care after blood drawing involves flushing with 20 ml of normal saline followed by 5 ml of heparin solution (100 U/ml).

7. Discuss potential complications associated with VAD, along with appropriate self-management measures.
    - *Infection:* Teach patient to assess exit site for erythema, swelling, discomfort, purulent drainage, and temperature >38° C (100.5° F).

- *Bleeding:* Teach patient to apply pressure to site. Instruct patient to notify health team member if bleeding does not stop in 5 min.
- *Clot in catheter:* Teach patient to flush catheter without using excessive pressure, which could damage or dislodge catheter (particularly an implanted port). If flushing does not dislodge clot, instruct patient to notify health team member. **Note:** It is not unusual for small blood clots or fibrin sheaths to develop on the end of the catheter. The most common manifestation of a fibrin sheath is ability to infuse fluids and inability to aspirate blood. Both fibrin sheaths and small blood clots respond readily to urokinase therapy. The usual dose of urokinase is 5,000-10,000 U. The suggested dwell time in the catheter is ≥30-60 min.
- *Disconnected cap:* Instruct patients to tape all connections and to carry hemostats with them at all times.
- *Extravasation:* Although a relatively rare complication, it can cause severe damage if a sclerosing agent such as adriamycin is involved. Therefore, it is important to instruct patients to report pain, burning, and stinging in the chest, clavicle, or port pocket, or along subcutaneous tunnel during drug administration.

Radiation Therapy

Risk for injury to staff, other patients, and visitors related to potential for exposure to sealed sources of radiation, such as cesium-137 (^{137}Cs), gold-198 (^{198}Au), iridium-192 (^{192}Ir), iodine-125 (^{125}I), or unsealed sources of radiation, such as iodine-131 (^{131}I) or phosphorus-32 (^{32}P).

Desired outcome: Staff and visitors verbalize understanding of potential dangers of radiation therapy and measures that must be taken to ensure safety.

N O T E : Most institutions have a radiation safety committee that assists in providing and enforcing guidelines that minimize radiation risk to employees and the environment (committee guidelines should be kept readily available). The committee approves certain rooms that can be used for patients undergoing radioactive treatment to minimize exposure of employees and other patients.

1. Assign patient a private room, and place an appropriate radiation precaution sign on patient's chart, door, and ID bracelet.
2. Follow radiologist's or agency's protocol for visitor restrictions. Visitors usually are restricted to 1 h/day and should stand 6 ft from the bed.
3. Make sure pregnant women and children <18 yr of age do not enter the room.
4. To ensure optimal care planning, recognize type and amount of radiation source. The two major principles are time and distance.
   - *Time:* Plan care to minimize amount of time spent in patient's room. Staff members should not spend more than 30 min/shift with patient and should not care for more than two patients with

implants at the same time. Staff should perform nondirect care activities in the hall (e.g., opening food container, preparing food tray, opening medications). Linen should be changed only when soiled, rather than routinely, and complete bed baths should be avoided.

  ■ *Distance:* Maximize distance from implant (e.g., if implant is in patient's prostate, stand at HOB).

5. Wear gloves when in contact with secretions/excretions of all patients treated with unsealed radiation sources, which are radioactive. Flush toilet several times after depositing urine or feces from commode.

N O T E :   Urine from individuals with sealed radiation is *not* radioactive and can be discarded in the usual manner. However, patients with implanted ^{125}I seeds should save all urine so that it can be assessed for the presence of seeds.

---

6. Save all linen, dressings, and trash from patients with sealed sources of radiation. They will be analyzed by the safety committee representative before discarding to ensure that seeds have not been misplaced.

7. Keep long, disposable forceps and a sealed box in the room at all times in case displaced seeds are found. Caution all staff members to use forceps, never the hands, to pick up seeds.

8. Use disposable products for all patients with unsealed radiation. These patients will be radioactive for several days. Cover all articles in the room with paper to prevent contamination.

9. Attach a radiation badge (dosimeter) to your clothing before entering the room to monitor amount of radiation exposure. According to federal regulations, radiation should not exceed 400 mrem/mo. Nurses who care for patients with radiation implants rarely receive this much exposure.

Knowledge deficit: Type and purpose of radiation implant (internal radiation) and measures for preventing and managing complications

Desired outcome: Before radiation implant is inserted, patient and significant others verbalize understanding of its type and identify measures for preventing and managing complications.

1. Determine patient's and significant others' level of understanding of radiation implant. Explain the following, as indicated:

  ■ *After loading:* Implant carrier is inserted in the operating room, and radioactive source is inserted later.

  ■ *Preloading:* Radioactive source is implanted with carrier.

2. Explain that implant is used to provide high doses of radiation therapy to one area, thereby sparing normal tissue.

3. Explain that radiation precautions (see **Risk for injury,** earlier) are required to protect health care team, other patients, and visitors.

4. Explain the following assessment guidelines and management interventions for specific types of implants:

Appendix One

Gynecologic Implants

1. Explain that the following can occur: vaginal drainage, bleeding, or tenderness; impaired bowel or urinary elimination; phlebitis. Instruct patient to report any of these signs and symptoms.
2. Teach patient to perform isometric exercises while on bed rest to minimize the risk of contractures or muscle atrophy.
3. Explain the importance and purpose of wearing antiembolic hose while on bed rest.
4. Explain that ambulation will be increased gradually when bed rest no longer is required (see "Caring for Patients on Prolonged Bed Rest," p. 413, for guidelines to use after prolonged immobility).
5. Explain that after radiation source has been removed, patient should dilate vagina *via* either sexual intercourse or vaginal dilator to prevent fibrosis or stenosis.

Head and Neck Implants

1. After a complete nutritional assessment and assessment of oropharyngeal area, discuss measures for nutritional support during implantation (e.g., soft or liquid diet, high-protein diet, optimal hydration).
2. Teach patient the signs and symptoms of infection: fever, pain, erythema, and purulent drainage at site of implantation.
3. Encourage patient to take analgesics routinely for pain rather than wait until pain becomes severe.
4. Identify alternative means of communication if patient's speech deteriorates (e.g., cards, slate). Consult speech therapist as appropriate.

Breast Implants

1. Teach patient the signs of infection that may appear over the breast: erythema, warmth, drainage at insertion site.
2. Teach patient the importance of avoiding trauma at implant site and of keeping skin clean and dry to help maintain skin integrity.

Prostate Implants

1. Explain that urinary output will be measured every shift and that staff member will inspect urine for radiation seeds.
2. Caution patient that linen, dressings, and trash will be saved and examined for radioactive seeds.
3. Explain that care givers will limit amount of time spent at implant site.

Knowledge deficit: Purpose and procedure for external beam radiation therapy, appropriate self-care measures after treatment, and available educational and community resources

Desired outcome: Before external radiation beam therapy is begun, patient and significant others identify its purpose and describe procedure, appropriate self-care measures, and available educational and community resources.

1. See interventions 1-6 under **Knowledge deficit:** Chemotherapy, p. 425.

2. Provide information about treatment schedule, duration of each treatment, and number of treatments planned.
   - Radiation therapy usually is given 5 days/wk, Monday through Friday.
   - The treatment itself lasts only a few minutes; most of the time is spent preparing patient for treatment. Immobilization devices and shields are positioned before treatment to ensure proper delivery of radiation and minimize radiation o surrounding normal tissue.
3. Explain that the skin will be marked to facilitate delivery of radiation to desired area. Usually small skin tattoos (small pinpoint marks) are used. These tattoos are permanent and are used to ensure precise delivery of the radiation. However, if gentian violet is used, explain the importance of not washing the marks (see **Impaired skin/tissue integrity**, p. 446, for more information). Caution patient that it is important not to use skin lotions or soaps unless approved by radiation therapy.
4. Discuss side effects that may occur with radiation treatment and appropriate self-care measures. Systemic side effects include fatigue and anorexia; however, the most common side effects appear locally (e.g., side effects associated with head and neck radiation include mucositis, xerostomia, altered taste sensation, dental caries, sore throat, hoarseness, dysphagia, headache, and nausea and vomiting). See subsequent nursing diagnoses and interventions for more detail about local side effects.
5. Provide patient with a written copy of the side effects for his or her site of radiation therapy. Explain that the National Cancer Institute has a book titled *Radiation and You*, which lists side effects and their management.
6. Provide information about community resources for transportation to and from radiation center and for skilled nursing care as needed.

General Care of Patients with Cancer

Body image disturbance related to alopecia secondary to radiation therapy to the head and neck or administration of chemotherapeutic agents

Desired outcome: Patient discusses effects alopecia may have on self-concept, body image, and social interaction and identifies measures for preventing, minimizing, or adapting to alopecia.

N O T E : Commonly used chemotherapeutic agents that cause alopecia are actinomycin D, amsacrine, bleomycin, cyclophosphamide, daunomycin, doxorubicin, epirubicin, idarubicin, ifosfamide, teniposide, vinblastine, vincristine, and etoposide (VP 16).

---

1. Discuss potential for hair loss with patient before treatment.
   - Radiation therapy of 1,500-3,000 rad to the head and neck will produce either partial or complete hair loss. Explain that this is temporary and that onset usually occurs within 5-7 days; regrowth begins 2-3 mo after the final treatment.

- Radiation therapy >4,500 rad usually results in permanent hair loss.
- Hair loss associated with chemotherapy is temporary and related to the specific agent, dose, and duration of administration. Regrowth usually begins 1-2 mo after the last treatment. However, the hair often grows back a different color or texture.

2. Explore the impact hair loss has on patient's self-concept, body image, and social interaction. Recognize that alopecia is an extremely stressful side effect for most patients.

3. Encourage measures to minimize the impact or severity of alopecia: use a mild shampoo, conditioner, soft-bristled brush or wide-toothed comb; sleep on a silk pillowcase to minimize tangles; wash hair less often; and avoid irritants and mechanical stress (dyes, permanent wave solutions, hair dryers, curling irons, clips, hair sprays).

4. Explain that scalp hypothermia and tourniquet applications during IV infusion may reduce the severity of hair loss. A significant decrease in alopecia has been found in individuals who use a hypothermia cap. These techniques are contraindicated with hematologic malignancy and with solid tumors with scalp metastasis because they may prevent adequate absorption of the drug where it is needed.

5. Suggest measures that may help minimize the psychological impact of hair loss: cut hair short before treatment; select a wig before hair loss occurs (to match color and style of own hair); wear a hairnet or turban during hair loss to collect hair that falls out; use scarves, hats, caps, and turbans to cover head; use makeup and accessories to enhance self-concept. **Note:** Wigs are tax deductible and often are reimbursed by insurance companies with the appropriate prescription.

6. Inform patient that hair loss may occur on body parts other than the head, including the axillae, groin, legs, face, and eyes (eyelashes and eyebrows).

7. Instruct patient to keep head covered during the summer to minimize sunburn and during the winter to prevent heat loss.

8. Provide information about alopecia available through community resources, such as the American Cancer Society.

Ineffective breathing pattern related to decreased lung expansion secondary to fluid accumulation in the lungs (pleural effusion)
Note: For Desired Outcome and interventions, see this nursing diagnosis in "Pleural Effusion," p. 6.

N O T E : Patients with corresponding cancers (lymphoma, leukemia, mesothelioma, lung and breast cancers, metastasis to the lung from other primary cancers) have a greater risk of developing pleural effusion.

Ineffective breathing pattern related to decreased lung expansion secondary to pulmonary fibrosis
Note: For Desired Outcome and interventions, see this nursing diagnosis in "Pulmonary Fibrosis," p. 20.

N O T E : Some chemotherapeutic drugs (bleomycin sulfate, busulfan, carmustine, chlorozotocin, cytarabine, L-asparaginase, semustine) can cause pulmonary toxicity, an inflammatory reaction that causes fibrotic lung changes, damages cells, and reduces lung capacity. Although much rarer, pulmonary toxicity also can occur with cyclophosphamide, chorambucil, melphalan, mitomycin, methotrexate, mercaptopurine, procarbazine hydrochloride, and zinostatin.

Chronic pain related to direct tumor involvement; infiltration of tumor into nerves, bones, or hollow viscus; or postchemotherapy or post-radiotherapy syndromes

Desired outcome: Within 1-2 h of intervention, patient participates in a prescribed pain regimen and reports that pain associated with direct involvement or infiltration of the tumor and side effects associated with the prescribed therapy are reduced or at an acceptable level, based on pain scale.

1. After a complete medical evaluation of the cause of the pain (Tables A-9 and A-10) and after the most effective pain-relief strategies have been determined, review evaluation and strategies with patient and significant others to assess their level of understanding.
2. Continual assessment of pain is essential and should include the following:
   - Characteristics (e.g., "burning" or "shooting" often describes nerve pain).
   - Location and sites of radiation.
   - Onset and duration.

Table A-9   Physiologic causes of acute pain in cancer patients

Tumor compression or infiltration of nerves
Tumor obstruction of hollow viscera or ductal system
Infiltration/obstruction of blood vessels
Exacerbation of alterated body functions unrelated to cancer (e.g., preexisting conditions such as chronic headaches, arthritis)
Pain associated with treatments
Postsurgical pain, stomatitis, or peripheral neuropathies

Table A-10   Physiologic causes of chronic pain in cancer patients

Tumor unresponsive to therapy
Postsurgical pain
Postchemotherapy pain
Postradiation pain
Postherpetic neuralgia
Altered body functions (e.g., chronic arthritis, back pain, or any musculoskeletal disorder)

Appendix One

- Severity: Use a pain scale, and have patient rate pain from 0 (none) to 10 (worst).
- Aggravating and relieving factors.
- Previous strategies that have relieved pain.

3. Assess patient's and significant others' attitudes and knowledge about pain medication regimen. Many patients and their families have fears related to patient's ultimate addiction to narcotics. Dispel any misperceptions about narcotic-induced addiction when chronic pain therapy is necessary.

4. Pharmacologic management often is the mainstay of treatment of chronic cancer pain. Incorporate the following principles:
   - *Administer nonnarcotic and narcotic analgesics in the correct dose, at the correct frequency, and via the correct route.* Chronic cancer analgesia often is administered orally, and if pain is present most of the day, it should be given around the clock rather than as needed.
   - *Recognize and treat side effects of narcotic analgesia early.* Side effects include nausea and vomiting, constipation, sedation, itching, and respiratory depression. The development of these side effects does not necessarily preclude continued use of the drug.
   - *Use prescribed adjuvant medications to help increase efficacy of narcotics.* These include tricyclic antidepressants, antihistamines, dextroamphetamines, steroids, phenothiazines, and anticonvulsants.
   - *Monitor for signs and symptoms of tolerance, and when it occurs, discuss treatment with physician.* Patients with chronic pain often require increasing doses of narcotics. Respiratory depression rarely occurs in these patients.
   - *Be aware of the potential for physical dependence in patients taking narcotics for a prolonged period.* Narcotics should not be stopped abruptly in these patients because withdrawal may occur.
   - *Evaluate the effectiveness of analgesics at regular and frequent intervals after administration, particularly after the initial dose.*
   - *Use nonpharmacologic approaches when appropriate.* See Table A-6, p. 403, and **Pain,** p. 396.

Constipation related to treatment with vinca alkaloid chemotherapy, narcotic analgesics, tranquilizers, and antidepressants; less than adequate intake because of anorexia; hypercalcemia; spinal cord compression; mental status changes; decreased mobility; or colonic disorders

Note: For Desired Outcomes and interventions, see this nursing diagnosis in "General Care of Patients with Neurologic Disorders," p. 196; "Caring for Preoperative and Postoperative Patients," p. 409; and "Caring for Patients on Prolonged Bed Rest," p. 420.

N O T E :   Cancer patients should not go >2 days without having a bowel movement. Patients receiving vinca alkaloid are at risk for ileus in addition to constipation. Preventive measures, such as use of senna products (e.g., Peri-Colace or Senokot), especially for patients taking narcotics, are highly recommended. In addition, all individuals taking narcotics should receive a prophylactic home regimen.

Risk for infection related to inadequate secondary defenses (neutropenia) secondary to malignancy, chemotherapy, radiation therapy, or immunotherapy

Desired outcomes: Patient is free of infection, as evidenced by normothermia, BP $\geq$90/60 mm Hg, and HR $\leq$100 bpm. Patient identifies risk factors for infection, verbalizes early signs and symptoms of infection and reports them promptly to health care provider if they occur, and demonstrates appropriate self-care measures to minimize the risk of infection.

1. Identify patients at risk for infection by obtaining the absolute neutrophil count (ANC). Calculate ANC by using the following formula:

   ANC = (% of segmented neutrophils + % bands)
   $\times$ total WBC count

   - 1,500-2,000/mm^3 ANC = no significant risk.
   - 1,000-1,500/mm^3 ANC = minimal risk.
   - 500-1,000/mm^3 ANC = moderate risk; initiate neutropenic precautions.
   - <500/mm^3 ANC = severe risk; initiate neutropenic precautions.
2. Assess each body system thoroughly to determine potential and actual sources of infection.
3. Monitor VS and temperature q4h. Be alert for temperature $\geq$38° C (100.4° F) $\times$ 2, temperature <35.6° C (96° F) $\times$ 1, temperature >38.3° C (101° F) $\times$ 1, increased HR, decreased BP, and the following clinical signs of infection: tenderness, erythema, warmth, swelling, and drainage at invasive sites; chills; malaise. **Note:** Signs of infection may be absent with neutropenia.
4. Place sign on patient's door indicating that neutropenic precautions are in effect for patients with ANC $\leq$1,000/mm^3.
5. Instruct all persons entering patient's room to wash hands thoroughly.
6. Restrict individuals from entering who have contagious diseases, such as colds or flu.
7. Instruct patient to wear a mask when out of the hospital room.
8. Consult physician immediately if patient's temperature is >38° C (100.4° F) $\times$ 2, >38.3° C (101° F) $\times$ 1, or <35.6° C (96° F). Initiate antibiotic therapy as prescribed within 1 h when ANC is $\leq$500/mm^3.
9. Implement oral care routine to minimize the risk of infection due to nonintact mucosa or tongue. Teach patient to use a soft-bristled toothbrush after meals and before bed (bristles may be softened even more by running them under hot water). Inspect oral cavity daily, noting white patches on the tongue or mucous membrane. Mycostatin swish and swallow or swish and spit may be prescribed to prevent the development of oral candidiasis. Individuals with prolonged neutropenia are at high risk for candidiasis and other

bacterial and viral infections. Monitor for vesicles and crusted lesions that may signal herpes simplex. Acyclovir may be initiated, as prescribed, to prevent or minimize herpetic infections in patients with prolonged neutropenia who are at risk for herpes.

10. Do not use rectal suppositories, rectal temperature methods, or enemas, to minimize the risk of traumatizing rectal mucosa and thereby increasing the risk of infection. Be aware that patients with prolonged neutropenia are at increased risk for perirectal infection; monitor for it accordingly. Caution patient to avoid straining at stool. Suggest use of stool softener.

11. Implement measures that maintain skin integrity, and instruct patient accordingly: use electric shaver rather than razor blade; avoid vaginal douche and tampons; use emery board rather than clipper for nail care; check with physician before dental care; avoid all invasive procedures; use antimicrobial skin preparations before injections; change IV sites q48h; use steel-tipped rather than plastic catheters (minimizes the risk of infection); use water-soluble lubricant before sexual intercourse; and avoid oral and anal manipulation during sexual activities.

12. Teach patient to avoid potential sources of infection during periods of neutropenia (e.g., avoid foods with high bacterial count [raw eggs, raw fruits and vegetables, foods prepared in a blender that cannot adequately be cleaned]; bird, cat, and dog excreta; and plants, flowers, and sources of stagnant water).

13. Be alert for signs of impending sepsis, including subtle changes in mental status: restlessness or irritability; warm, flushed skin; chills, fever, or hypothermia; increased urine output; bounding pulse; tachypnea; glycosuria. These symptoms often precede the classic signs of septic shock: cold, clammy skin; thready pulse; decreased BP; oliguria.

14. As prescribed, administer colony-stimulating factors to minimize the risk of myelosuppression with chemotherapy, especially for patients with a history of neutropenia with severe infections in the past.

Altered nutrition: Less than body requirements, related to nausea and vomiting or anorexia occurring with chemotherapy or radiation therapy

Desired outcome: At least 24 h before hospital discharge, patient has adequate nutrition, as evidenced by stable weight and a positive or balanced nitrogen state.

ANOREXIA

1. Monitor for clinical signs of malnutrition. See **Altered nutrition,** p. 378, in "Providing Nutritional Support," Weigh patient daily.

2. Assess patient's food likes and dislikes, as well as cultural and religious preferences related to food choices.

3. Explain that anorexia can be caused by pathophysiology of cancer, surgery, and side effects of chemotherapy and radiation therapy.

4. Teach patient the importance of increasing caloric intake to increase energy and minimize weight loss.

5. Teach patient the importance of increasing protein intake to facilitate repair and regeneration of cells.
6. Suggest that patient eat several small meals at frequent intervals throughout the day.
7. Encourage use of nutritional supplements.
8. Consider use of megestrol acetate or hydralazine sulfate. These agents have proved to have a positive influence on appetite stimulation and weight gain in individuals with cancer. Consult patient's physician accordingly.

NAUSEA AND VOMITING

1. Assess pattern of nausea and vomiting: onset, frequency, duration, intensity, amount and character of emesis.
2. Explain to patient that nausea and vomiting are side effects of chemotherapy and radiation therapy (they also can occur with advanced cancer). See Table A-11 for a list of antineoplastic agents known to have an emetic effect.
3. Administer antiemetics (Table A-12) as prescribed. Instruct patient to take prescribed antiemetic 1-12 h before chemotherapy, and to take the drug q4-6h for at least 12-24 h after chemotherapy for as long as nausea persists.
4. Teach patient to eat cold foods or food served at room temperature because the odor of hot food may aggravate nausea.
5. Suggest intake of clear liquids and bland foods.
6. Teach patient to avoid sweet, fatty, highly salted, and spicy foods, as well as foods with strong odors, any of which may increase nausea.
7. Minimize such stimuli as smells, sounds, or sights, all of which may promote nausea.

Table A-11   Antineoplastic agents with emetic action

Mild Emetic Action	Moderate Emetic Action	Severe Emetic Action
L-asparginase	hexamethylmelamine	nitrosourea
bleomycin	azacitidine	dactinomycin
chlorambucil	daunorubicin	cisplatin
hydroxyurea	doxorubicin	cyclophosphamide
melphalan	etoposide (VP 15)	dacarbazine
mercaptopurine	5-fluorouracil (5 FU)	mitomycin-C
tamoxifen	procarbazine	methotrexate
thioguanine	streptozotocin	mithramycin
thiotepa	carboplatin	mechlorethamine
vinblastine		
vincristine		
steroids		
cytarabine		
L-phenylalanine		

Table A-12 Common antiemetic agents

Agent	Generic Name	Trade Name
phenothiazine	prochlorperazine	Compazine
steroids	dexamethasone	Decadron
antihistamine	diphenhydramine	Benadryl
butyrophenon derivatives	haloperidol	Haldol
benzodiazepines	lorazepam	Ativan
benzamide	metoclopramide*	Reglan
serotonin antagonist	ondansetron	Zofran

*Metoclopramide blocks the neurotransmitter sites to reduce stimulation of an area in the medulla known as the chemoreceptor trigger zone.

8. Encourage patient to eat sour or mint candy during chemotherapy to diminish the unpleasant, metallic taste.
9. Encourage patient to experiment with various dietary patterns:
   ■ Avoid eating or drinking for 1-2 h before and after chemotherapy.
   ■ Follow a clear liquid diet for 1-2 h before and 1-24 h after chemotherapy.
   ■ Avoid contact with food while it is being cooked; avoid being around people who are eating.
   ■ Eat light meals at frequent intervals (5-6 ×/day).
10. Suggest that patient sit near an open window to breathe fresh air when feeling nauseated.
11. Help patient find appropriate distraction technique (e.g., music, television, reading).
12. Teach patient to use relaxation techniques. See **Health-seeking behaviors:** Relaxation technique effective for stress reduction, p. 27. This technique also may help prevent anticipatory nausea and vomiting.
13. Teach patient to stay NPO for 4-8 h if frequent episodes of vomiting occur.
14. Instruct patient to sip liquids (broth, ginger ale, cola, tea) or eat Jello slowly; to suck on ice chips; and not to drink large amounts of water.

Altered oral mucous membrane related to treatment with chemotherapy agents (especially antibiotics), antimetabolites, and vinca alkaloids; radiation therapy to head and neck; and ineffective oral hygiene.
Desired outcomes: Patient complies with therapeutic regimen within 12-24 h of instruction. Patient's oral mucosal condition improves as evidenced by intact mucous membrane, moist and intact tongue and lips, and absence of pain and lesions.
1. With myelosuppression, caution patient not to floss the teeth.

2. Patients with moderate to severe stomatitis may require parenteral analgesics (e.g., morphine).

3. Patients with xerostomia (dryness of the mouth from a lack of normal salivary secretion) caused by radiation may benefit from chewing sugarless gum, sucking sugarless candy, or taking frequent sips of water. Saliva substitutes are another option, although they are expensive and do not last long.

4. Close dental follow-up is essential because the lack of or reduction in salivary fluid predisposes the patient to caries. Fluoride treatment is recommended.

Pain related to cancer or its treatment

Note: For Desired Outcome and interventions, see this nursing diagnosis in "Caring for Preoperative and Postoperative Patients," p. 396. Also:

■ Explain that acute pain is short term and is relieved when the underlying cause is treated.

Impaired physical mobility related to musculoskeletal or neuromuscular impairment secondary to bone metastasis or spinal cord compression; pain and discomfort, intolerance to activity, or perceptual or cognitive impairment

Note: For Desired Outcome and interventions, see this nursing diagnosis in "Dislocation/Subluxation," p. 308.

Also see diagnoses and interventions in "Spinal Cord Injury," p. 142; "General Care of Patients with Neurologic Disorders," p. 187; "Fractures," p. 320; "Malignant Neoplasms," p. 325; "Pressure Ulcers," p. 390; and "Caring for Patients on Prolonged Bed Rest," p. 413.

Altered protection related to risk of bleeding/hemorrhage secondary to thrombocytopenia (for all patients receiving chemotherapy and radiation therapy, as well as those with cancer, particularly involving the bone marrow)

Desired outcome: Patient is free of signs and symptoms of bleeding, as evidenced by negative occult blood tests; HR ≤100 bpm; and systolic BP ≥90 mm Hg.

1. Identify platelet counts that place individuals at increased risk for bleeding:
   ■ Platelets 150,000-300,000/μl = normal risk for bleeding.
   ■ Platelets <50,000/μl = moderate risk for bleeding; initiate thrombocytopenic precautions.
   ■ Platelets <20,000/μl = severe risk of bleeding; may develop spontaneous bleeding; initiate thrombocytopenic precautions.

2. Perform a baseline physical assessment for evidence of bleeding: petechiae, ecchymoses, hematuria, coffee-ground emesis, tarry stools, hemoptysis, heavy menses, headaches, blurred vision. Also monitor VS every shift, being alert for hypotension and tachycardia. Do not use rectal thermometer, which can cause rectal bleeding.

3. Test all secretions and excretions for occult blood.

4. Perform a psychosocial assessment, including patient's past expe-

rience with thrombocytopenia; the effect of thrombocytopenia on patient's life-style; and changes in patient's work pattern, family relationships, and social activities. Identify learning needs and need for skilled care after hospital discharge.

5. Hang sign on patient's door indicating that thrombocytopenic precautions are in effect (for patients with platelet count <50,000/μl).

6. With bleeding, begin pad count for heavy menses; measure amount of vomitus and stool; apply direct pressure to site of bleeding (VAD, venipuncture); and deliver platelet transfusion as prescribed.

7. Initiate oral care at frequent intervals to promote integrity of gingiva and mucosa. Advise patient to brush with soft-bristled toothbrush after meals and before bed (hot water run over bristles may soften them further). With gum bleeding, teach patient to use sponge-tipped applicator rather than toothbrush, avoid use of dental floss, and avoid mouthwash with alcohol content >6%. Suggest use of normal saline solution mouthwashes 4 ×/day and water-based ointment for lubricating the lips.

8. Implement bowel program and check with patient daily for bowel movement. Assess need for stool softeners to prevent constipation; encourage adequate hydration (at least 2 L/day) and high-fiber foods to promote bowel function; avoid use of rectal suppositories, enemas, or harsh laxatives to minimize the risk of bleeding.

9. Implement measures that prevent bleeding. Avoid bladder catheterization if possible. Teach patient to use electric shaver; apply direct pressure for 3-5 min after injections and venipuncture; avoid vaginal douche and tampons, constrictive clothing, aspirin or aspirin-containing products because of aspirin's antiplatelet action, alcohol ingestion, anticoagulants, and indomethacin (Indocin), which is a GI irritant. Caution patient to blow nose gently, use emery board rather than clippers for nail care, and check with physician before seeking dental care.

10. Caution patient to avoid activities that may predispose him or her to trauma or injury; remove hazardous objects or furniture from patient's environment. Assist with ambulating if patient's physical mobility is impaired. When patient's platelet count is <20,000/μl, teach patient to avoid activities involving Valsalva's maneuver, which increases intracranial pressure. These activities include moving up in bed, straining at stool, bending at the waist, and lifting heavy objects (>10 lb). Suggest bed rest if patient's platelet count is <10,000/μl.

11. See "Thrombocytopenia," p. 292, for more information.

Sensory/perceptual alterations: Auditory and kinesthetic impairment related to use of cisplatinum or vinca alkaloids

Desired outcome: Patient reports early signs and symptoms of ototoxicity and peripheral neuropathy; measures are implemented promptly to minimize these side effects.

1. Explain that tinnitus or decreased hearing can occur with use of cisplatinum. It usually is dose related and a result of cumulative side effects. Most commonly, high-frequency hearing loss occurs, al-

though with cumulative doses, speech frequency hearing range also may be affected. Affected individuals may have difficulty hearing speech if there is background noise. Suggest that patient face the speaker during conversation. A hearing aid also may be helpful. In instances of hearing loss from cisplatinum, which usually is irreversible, refer patient to community resources for the hearing impaired.

2. Monitor patient for the development of peripheral neuropathy, which can occur with cisplatinum and vincristine use. The first symptom usually is numbness and tingling of fingers and toes, which can progress to difficulty with fine motor skills, such as buttoning shirts or picking up objects. The most severely affected individuals may lose sensation at hip level and have difficulty with balance and ambulation. Instruct patient to report early signs and symptoms. Suggest consultation with PT or OT to assist with maintaining function.

3. Put individuals at risk for paralytic ileus associated with the neuropathy (i.e., those taking vincristine, vinblastine) on daily bowel checks. Administer stool softeners and laxatives daily if patient has not had a bowel movement within 48 h, or as prescribed.

Sexual dysfunction (impaired sexual self-concept and infertility) related to radiation therapy to the lower abdomen, pelvis, and gonads; or chemotherapeutic agents, especially actinomycin D, alkylating agents, amsacrine, bleomycin, cytarabine, daunorubicin, epirubicin, methotrexate, mitomycin, procarbazine, and vinblastine

Desired outcome: After instruction, patient identifies potential treatment side effects on sexual and reproductive function and identifies acceptable methods of contraception during treatment.

1. Initiate discussion about effects of treatment on sexuality and reproduction. The PLISSIT model provides an excellent framework for discussion. This four-step model includes: (1) Permission—give patient permission to discuss issues of concern; (2) Limited Information—provide patient with information about expected treatment effects on sexual and reproductive function, without going into complete detail; (3) Specific Suggestions—provide suggestions for managing common problems that occur during treatment; and (4) Intensive Therapy—although most individuals can be managed by nurses using the first three steps in this model, some patients may require referral to an expert counselor.

2. Assess the impact of the diagnosis and treatment on patient's sexual functioning and self-concept.

3. Determine the possibility of pregnancy before treatment is initiated. Pregnancy will delay treatment. If treatment cannot be delayed, a therapeutic abortion may be recommended.

4. Discuss the possibility of reduced sexual response or desire, which may result from side effects of chemotherapy. Encourage patients to maintain open communication with their partners about needs and concerns. Explore alternate methods of sexual fulfillment: hugging, kissing, talking quietly together, massage. If symptoms are related to therapy, such interventions as taking a nap before sexual activity

or using pain or antiemetic medication may help reduce symptoms. Other suggestions include using a water-based lubricant if dyspareunia or fatigue is a problem, changing the usual time of day for intimacy, or using supine or side-lying positions, which require the least expenditure of energy.

5. Discuss the possibility of temporary or permanent sterility resulting from treatment. Explore the possibility of sperm banking for men before chemotherapy treatment or oophoropexy (surgical displacement of the ovaries outside the radiation field) for women undergoing abdominal radiation therapy.

6. Teach patients the importance of contraception during treatment and for 2 yr after completion of therapy to ensure adequate time for renewal of sperm and to determine individual's response to treatment.

7. Inform patients that healthy children have been born to parents who have received radiation therapy or chemotherapy, but long-term effects have not been clearly identified. Suggest that patients seek genetic counseling before becoming parents, as indicated.

Impaired skin integrity related to pigmentation changes (malignant skin lesions)

Desired outcome: After instruction, patient verbalizes measures that promote comfort and skin integrity.

1. Identify populations at risk for malignant lesions: individuals with primary tumors of the breast, lung, colon/rectum, ovary, or oral cavity; patients with malignant melanoma, lymphoma, or leukemia.

2. Identify common sites of cutaneous metastases: anterior chest, abdomen, head (scalp), neck.

3. Inspect skin lesions, and note and document general characteristics, location and distribution, configuration, size, morphologic structure (e.g., nodule, erosion, fissure), drainage (color, amount, character), and odor.

4. Monitor for indicators of infection: local warmth, erythema, tenderness, purulent drainage.

5. Perform the following skin care for nonulcerating lesions, and teach these interventions to patient and significant others as indicated:
   - Wash affected area with tepid water and pat dry.
   - Avoid pressure on area.
   - Apply dry dressing to protect area against exposure to irritants and mechanical trauma (e.g., scratching).
   - To enhance penetration of topical medications, apply occlusive dressings, such as Telfa, using paper tape.
   - Teach patient not to wear irritating fabrics, such as wool and corduroy.

6. Perform the following skin care for ulcerating lesions, and teach these interventions to patient and significant others as indicated:

CLEANSING AND DEBRIDING
   1. May use half-strength hydrogen peroxide and normal saline solution for irrigation, followed by a normal saline rinse.

2. May use cotton swabs or sponges to apply gentle pressure, thereby debriding ulcerated area.
3. If ulcerated area is prone to bleeding, irrigate only, using a syringe.
4. May use soaks (wet dressings) of saline, water, Burow's solution (aluminum acetate), or hydrogen peroxide for debridement. **Note:** Failure to rinse hydrogen peroxide or aluminum acetate off skin may cause further skin breakdown.
5. May use wet-to-dry dressings for gentle debridement.

PREVENTION AND MANAGEMENT OF LOCAL INFECTION
1. Irrigate and scrub with antibacterial agents, such as acetic acid solution or povidone-iodine.
2. Perform wound cultures as prescribed.
3. Apply topical antibacterial agents as prescribed.
4. Administer systemic antibiotics as prescribed.

TO MAINTAIN HEMOSTASIS
1. For capillary oozing, use silver nitrate sticks.
2. For larger surface-area bleeding, use oxidized cellulose or pack wound with Gelfoam or similar product.

TO CONTROL ODOR
1. Clean wound and change dressings as frequently as necessary.
2. Perform cultures and sensitivities of the wound, as prescribed.
3. Use antiodor agents (e.g., open a bottle of oil of peppermint or place a tray of activated charcoal) in patient's room.

Impaired skin integrity and **Impaired tissue integrity (or risk for same)** related to treatment with chemical irritants (chemotherapy)
Desired outcome: Before chemotherapy, patient identifies potential side effects of chemotherapy on the skin and tissue and measures that promote comfort and integrity.

N O T E : Alterations of the skin or nails that occur in conjunction with chemotherapy are a result of the destruction of the basal cells of the epidermis (general) or of cellular alterations at the site of chemotherapy administration (local). The reactions are specific to the agent used and vary in onset, severity, and duration. Skin reactions include transient erythema/urticaria, hyperpigmentation, telangiectasis, photosensitivity, hyperkeratosis, acnelike reaction, ulceration, and radiation recall.

TRANSIENT ERYTHEMA/URTICARIA
Transient erythema/urticaria may be generalized or localized at the site of chemotherapy administration. Usually it occurs within several hours after chemotherapy and disappears in several hours. It is caused by doxorubicin hydrochloride (Adriamycin), bleomycin, L-asparaginase, mithramycin, and mechlorethamine.
1. Perform and document a pretreatment assessment of patient's skin for posttreatment comparison.
2. Assess onset, pattern, severity, and duration of reaction after treatment.

3. Compare posttreatment and pretreatment findings to determine if the cause of the erythema/urticaria is related to the chemotherapy or to herpes zoster, bacterial or fungal embolic lesions, skin metastasis, allergic reaction, or parasitic infestation.

HYPERPIGMENTATION

This reaction is believed to be caused by increased levels of melanin-stimulating hormone. It can occur on the nail beds, on oral mucosa, and along the veins used for chemotherapy administration, or it can be generalized. It is caused by doxorubicin hydrochloride (Adriamycin), carmustine, bleomycin, cyclophosphamide, daunorubicin, fluorouracil, and melphalan. This reaction also can occur with tumors of the pituitary gland.

1. Inform patient before treatment that this reaction is to be expected and that it will disappear gradually when the course of treatment is finished.

TELANGIECTASIS (SPIDER VEINS)

This reaction is believed to be caused by destruction of the capillary bed. It occurs as a result of application of topical carmustine and mechlorethamine.

1. Inform patient that this reaction is permanent, but that the configuration of veins will become less severe over time.

PHOTOSENSITIVITY

This reaction is enhanced when the skin is exposed to ultraviolet light. Acute sunburn and residual tanning can occur with short exposure to the sun. Photosensitivity can occur during the time the agent is administered, or it can reactivate a skin reaction caused by sun exposure when the agent is administered in close proximity to sun exposure. It is caused by dactinomycin, daunorubicin, doxorubicin hydrochloride (Adriamycin), bleomycin, dacarbazine, fluorouracil, methotrexate, and vinblastine.

1. Assess onset, pattern, severity, and duration of reaction.
2. Teach patient to avoid exposing skin to the sun. Advise patient to wear protective clothing and to use an effective sunscreen (SPF 15 or higher).
3. If burn occurs, advise patient to treat it like a sunburn (e.g., tepid bath, moisturizing cream, consultation with physician).

HYPERKERATOSIS

This reaction manifests as a thickening of the skin, especially over the hands, feet, face, and areas of trauma. Hyperkeratosis is disfiguring and causes loss of fine motor function of the hands. It occurs with bleomycin administration and should be considered an indicator of more severe fibrotic changes in the lungs. This condition is reversible when treatment with bleomycin is discontinued.

1. For patients taking bleomycin, assess for skin thickening and loss of fine motor function of the hands.

2. With skin thickening, be aware that fibrotic changes may be present in the lungs. Assess for this condition accordingly (see "Pulmonary Fibrosis," p. 20).

3. Reassure patient that this condition subsides when bleomycin is discontinued.

ACNELIKE REACTION

This reaction manifests as erythema, especially of the face, and progresses to papules and pustules, which are characteristic of acne. It occurs with administration of dactinomycin and disappears when the drug is discontinued.

1. Reassure patient that this reaction disappears when treatment with dactinomycin is discontinued.

2. Suggest that patient use a commercial preparation such as benzoyl peroxide lotion, gel, or cream to conceal blemishes.

3. Teach patient about proper skin care.
   - Avoid hard scrubbing.
   - Avoid use of antibacterial soap because removing nonpathogenic bacteria on the skin results in replacement by pathogens, which are implicated in the genesis of acne. Use a plain soap, such as Ivory or Camay.
   - Avoid use of oil-based cosmetics.

ULCERATION

This reaction appears as a generalized, shallow lesion of the epidermal layer. It is caused by bleomycin, methotrexate, and mitomycin-C.

1. Assess for ulceration.

2. If present, cleanse ulcers with a solution of ¼-strength hydrogen peroxide and ¾-strength normal saline q4-6h; rinse with normal saline solution.

3. Expose ulcer to air, if possible.

4. Be alert for signs of infection at ulcerated site: local warmth, erythema, purulent drainage.

5. Teach patient the treatment and assessment interventions.

RADIATION RECALL REACTION

This occurs when chemotherapy is given at the same time as or after treatment with radiation therapy. It manifests as erythema, followed by dry desquamation. More severe reactions can progress to vesicle formation and wet desquamation. After the skin heals, it is permanently hyperpigmented. This reaction is caused by doxorubicin hydrochloride (Adriamycin), bleomycin, cyclophosphamide, dactinomycin, fluorouracil, hydroxyurea, and methotrexate.

1. Teach patient the following skin care routine:
   - Cleanse skin gently at the site of recall reaction, using mild soap, tepid water, and a soft cloth; pat dry.
   - Use A&D ointment on areas with dry desquamation.
   - If edema and wet desquamation are present, cleanse area with half-strength hydrogen peroxide and normal saline, and rinse with normal saline solution.
   - To promote healing, use hydrocolloid occlusive dressing on uninfected sites to promote healing.

Appendix One

2. Teach patient to protect skin at site of recall reaction in the following ways:
   - Avoid wearing tight-fitting clothes.
   - Avoid harsh fabrics, such as wool or corduroy.
   - Use mild detergents, such as Ivory Snow.
   - Avoid exposing site of recall reaction to heat and cold.
   - Avoid swimming in saltwater or chlorinated pools.
   - Avoid use of all medications (except A&D ointment and topical steroids), deodorants, perfumes, powders, or cosmetics on skin at recall site.
   - Avoid shaving site of recall reaction; if shaving is absolutely necessary, use an electric razor.

Impaired skin integrity and **Impaired tissue integrity** related to radiation therapy

Desired outcome: Within 24 h of instruction, patient identifies potential skin reactions and management interventions that promote comfort and skin integrity.

1. Assess degree and extensiveness of the skin reaction as follows:
   Stage I: Inflammation, mild erythema, slight edema.
   Stage II: Inflammation; dry desquamation; dry, scaly, itchy skin.
   Stage III: Inflammation, edema, wet desquamation, blisters, peeling.
   Stage IV: Skin ulceration and necrosis, permanent loss of hair in treatment field, suppression of sebaceous glands. *Late effects:* Fibrosis and atrophy of the skin, fibrosis of lymph glands.
2. Teach patient the following skin care over the treatment field:
   - Cleanse skin gently and in a patting motion, using a mild soap, tepid water, and a soft cloth. Rinse area and pat dry.
   - Apply A&D ointment to skin with stage II reaction.
3. For patients with stage III skin reaction, teach the following regimen:
   - Cleanse area with half-strength hydrogen peroxide and normal saline, using an irrigation syringe. Rinse with saline or water and pat dry gently.
   - Use nonadhesive absorbent dressings, such as Telfa or Adaptic and ABD, for draining areas. Be alert for indicators of infection.
   - To promote healing, use hydrocolloid occlusive dressings on noninfected areas.
4. Teach the following interventions for protecting patient's skin:
   - Avoid tight-fitting clothing.
   - Avoid wearing harsh fabrics, such as wool and corduroy.
   - Avoid sun exposure.
   - Use gentle detergents (e.g., Ivory Snow).
   - Avoid exposure to heat and cold.
   - Avoid swimming in chlorinated pools or saltwater.

- Avoid using medications, deodorants, perfumes, powders, or cosmetics on skin in treatment field.
- Avoid shaving hair on skin in treatment field; if shaving is absolutely necessary, use an electric razor.

5. For stage IV reaction, teach the following interventions:
   - Debride wound of eschar (necessary before healing can occur).
   - After removing eschar (results in yellow-colored wound), keep wound clean to prevent infection (wet-to-dry dressings often are used for this purpose).
   - See interventions for alopecia under **Body image disturbance,** p. 431.

Impaired swallowing related to esophagitis secondary to radiation therapy to the neck, chest, and upper back or use of chemotherapy agents, especially antimetabolites; or obstruction (tumors of the esophagus)

Desired outcomes: Before food or fluids are given, patient exhibits gag reflex and is free of symptoms of aspiration, as evidenced by RR 12-20 breaths/min with normal depth and pattern (eupnea), normal skin color, and ability to speak. After instruction, patient verbalizes early signs and symptoms of esophagitis, alerts health care team as soon as they occur, and identifies measures for maintaining nutrition and comfort.

1. Monitor patient for evidence of impaired swallowing with concomitant respiratory difficulties.
2. Teach patient the early signs and symptoms of esophagitis and the importance of reporting them promptly to the staff if they occur: sensation of lump in the throat with swallowing, difficulty with swallowing solid foods, discomfort or pain with swallowing.
3. Monitor patient's dietary intake and provide the following guidelines: maintain a high-protein diet; eat foods that are soft and bland; add milk or milk products to the diet to coat the esophageal lining (for individuals without excessive mucus production); and add sauces and creams to foods, which may facilitate swallowing.
4. Ensure an adequate fluid intake of at least 2 L/day.
5. Implement the following measures, which promote comfort, and discuss them with patient:
   - Use a local anesthetic, as prescribed, to minimize pain with meals. Lidocaine 2% or diclone and diphenhydramine may be taken *via* swish and swallow before eating. **Caution:** These anesthetics may diminish patient's gag reflex.
   - Suggest that patient sit in an upright position during meals and for 15-30 min after eating.
   - Mild analgesics, such as liquid ASA or acetaminophen, can be very helpful. Administer them as prescribed.
   - For severe discomfort, narcotic analgesics may be required. Administer as prescribed. **Note:** If pain is severe or persistent, a barium swallow may be performed to evaluate for infection.

Common causative agents are *Candida* organisms and herpes. Appropriate medical treatment may be initiated (e.g., low-dose amphotericin, ketoconazole, or acyclovir).

■ Encourage frequent oral care with normal saline or sodium bicarbonate solution.

■ Teach patient to avoid irritants such as alcohol, tobacco, and alcohol-based commercial mouthwashs.

6. Keep suction equipment readily available in case patient aspirates. Educate patient in ways to manage oral secretions.

■ Suction mouth as needed, using low continuous suction.

■ Have patient expectorate saliva into tissues and dispose of tissues in nearby waste cans.

Desired outcome: During activity, patient rates perceived exertion at ≤3 on a 0-10 scale and exhibits cardiac tolerance to activity, as evidenced by systolic BP within 20 mm Hg of resting systolic BP, RR ≤20 breaths/min, HR ≤20 bpm above resting HR, and absence of chest pain or new dysrhythmia.

1. Monitor patient for evidence of activity intolerance and ask him or her to rate perceived exertion. For details, see p. 413.

2. Make sure patient maintains bed rest during febrile period and understands the rationale for doing so.

3. Anticipate patient's needs by placing personal articles within easy reach.

4. Advise patient about the importance of frequent rest periods during convalescence.

5. Monitor VS for changes indicating cardiac or pulmonary decompensation: decreasing BP, increasing HR and RR.

Altered peripheral tissue perfusion related to interrupted blood flow secondary to lymphedema

Desired outcome: After intervention/treatment, patient exhibits adequate peripheral perfusion, as evidenced by edema <2+ on a 0-4+ scale, peripheral pulses >2+ on a 0-4+ scale, normal skin color, decreasing or stable circumference of edematous site, bilaterally equal sensation, and ability to perform complete ROM in involved extremity.

N O T E :   Patients at risk for lymphedema include those who have had a radical mastectomy, lymph node dissection (upper and lower extremities), blockage of the lymphatic system from tumor burden, radiation therapy to the lymphatic system, or any combination of these.

---

1. Assess involved extremity for degree of edema, quality of peripheral pulses, color, circumference, sensation, and ROM.

2. Assess for signs of infection: tenderness, erythema, warmth at edematous site.

3. Evaluate and position involved extremity on a pillow in slight abduction.

4. Encourage wearing of loose-fitting clothing.

5. Consult PT and physician about development of exercise plan for ensuring mobility. Suggest use of elastic bandages to promote a decrease in mild, chronic lymphedema, or use of compressive bandages for more severe cases of swelling.

Altered urinary elimination related to hemorrhagic cystitis secondary to cyclophosphamide/ifosfamide treatment; oliguria or renal toxicity secondary to cisplatinum or high-dose methotrexate administration; renal calculi secondary to hyperuricemia; or dysuria secondary to cystitis

Desired outcomes: Patients receiving cyclophosphamide/ifosfamide test negatively for blood in urine, and patients receiving cisplatinum exhibit urine output of $\geq$100 ml/h 1 h before treatment and 4-12 h after treatment. Patients with leukemia and lymphomas and those taking methotrexate exhibit urine pH of 7.5

1. For patients taking cyclophosphamide (Cytoxan), ifosfamide, methotrexate, or cisplatinum, ensure adequate hydration during treatment and for at least 24 h afterward. Teach patient the importance of a fluid intake of at least 2-3 L/day. IV hydration also may be required, especially with high-dose chemotherapy.

2. Administer cyclophosphamide early in the day to minimize retention of antimetabolites in the bladder during the night. Encourage patients to void q2h during the day and before going to bed. Test urine for blood; report positive results to physician. Monitor I&O q8h during high-dose treatment for 48 h after treatment. Be alert for decreasing urinary output.

3. Mesna is administered before ifosfamide and then 4 h and 8 h after the infusion (or *via* a continuous infusion) to minimize the risk of hemorrhagic cystitis. Test all urine for blood. Promote fluid intake to maintain urine output at 100 ml/h. Monitor I&O during infusion and for 24 h after therapy to ensure that this level of urinary output is attained.

4. For patients receiving cisplatinum, prehydrate with $\geq$150-200 ml/h of IV fluid. Cisplatinum can be administered as soon as patient's urine output is $\geq$100-150 ml/h. Monitor I&O qh for 4-12 h after therapy to ensure that urine output is maintained at $\geq$100-150 ml/h. Patients may require diuretics to maintain this output. Promote fluid intake to ensure a positive fluid state for at least 24 h after treatment, especially for patients taking diuretics. Consult physician promptly if urine output drops to <100 ml/h. Urine output should be kept at a relatively high level because nephrotoxicity can occur as a side effect of this treatment.

5. Alkaline urine enhances excretion of methotrexate and of the uric acid that results from tumor lysis, which is associated with leukemia and lymphoma. Monitor I&O q8h, being alert for decreasing output, and test urine pH with each voiding to ensure that it is 7.5. Sodium bicarbonate or acetazolamide (Diamox) is used to alkalinize the urine. Allopurinol prevents formation of uric acid and often is administered before chemotherapy to patients with leukemia or lymphoma.

6. Renal calculi can occur as a result of hyperuricemia due to chemotherapy treatment for leukemia and lymphoma, which causes rapid cell lysis and increased excretion of uric acid. For more information, see "Renal Calculi," p. 67, and "Ureteral Calculi," p. 87.
7. Teach patient the signs of cystitis, which can occur as a result of cyclophosphamide and ifosfamide treatment: fever, pain with urination, malodorous or cloudy urine, urinary frequency and urgency. Instruct patient to notify health care provider if these signs and symptoms occur.

See nursing diagnoses and interventions in the following:

For patients with myelosuppression: see "Atelectasis," p. 1, and "Pneumonia," p. 2.

For patients undergoing bleomycin therapy: see "Pulmonary Fibrosis," p. 20.

For patients with cardiotoxicity who are taking chemotherapeutic agents (e.g., doxorubicin, daunorubicin): see "Heart Failure," p. 34.

For patients taking hepatotoxic drugs (e.g., cyclophosphamide, methotrexate): see "Hepatic and Biliary Disorders," p. 272.

Psychosocial Care of the Patient

Knowledge deficit: Current health status and therapies

Desired outcome: Before invasive procedure, surgical procedure, or hospital discharge (as appropriate), patient verbalizes understanding of his or her current health status and therapies.

1. Assess patient's current level of knowledge about his or her health status.
2. Assess cognitive and emotional readiness to learn.
3. Recognize barriers to learning: ineffective communication, neurologic deficit, sensory alterations, fear, anxiety, lack of motivation.
4. Assess learning needs, and establish short- and long-term goals.
5. Use individualized verbal or written information to promote learning and enhance understanding. Give simple, direct instructions. As indicated, use audiovisual tools as supplemental information.
6. Encourage significant others to reinforce correct information about diagnosis and therapies.
7. As appropriate, facilitate referral of neurologically impaired patient to neurologic clinical nurse specialist, case manager, or neuropsychologist.
8. Encourage patient's interest in health care information by involving him or her in planning of care. Explain the purpose of treatments.
9. Talk with patient often to evaluate comprehension of information given. Ask patient to repeat what he or she has been told. Individuals in crisis often must have explanations repeated several times before they can comprehend the information. Remember that many individuals may not understand seemingly simple medical terms

(e.g., terminal, malignant, constipation). Provide written information to reinforce teaching.

10. As appropriate, stress understanding of informed consent. Help patient use information he or she receives to make informed health care decisions (e.g., about invasive procedures, surgery, resuscitation).

Anxiety related to actual or perceived threat of death, change in health status, threat to self-concept or role, unfamiliar people and environment, or the unknown

Desired outcomes: Within 1-2 h of intervention, patient's anxiety has resolved or declined, as evidenced by patient's verbalization of same, HR ≤100 bpm, RR ≤20 breaths/min, and absence of or decrease in irritability and restlessness.

1. Engage in honest communication with patient; provide empathetic understanding. Listen closely, and establish an atmosphere that allows free expression.

2. Assess patient's level of anxiety. Be alert for verbal and nonverbal cues:
   - *Mild:* Restlessness, irritability, increase in questions, focusing on environment.
   - *Moderate:* Inattentiveness, expressions of concern, narrowed perceptions, insomnia, increased HR.
   - *Severe:* Expression of feelings of doom, rapid speech, tremors, poor eye contact; patient may be preoccupied with the past and unable to understand the present, and may have tachycardia, nausea, and hyperventilation.
   - *Panic:* Inability to concentrate or communicate, distortion of reality, increased motor activity, vomiting, tachypnea.

3. If patient is in severe anxiety or panic state, refer to psychiatric case manager, clinical nurse specialist, or other health team member as appropriate.

4. If patient is hyperventilating, have him or her mimic you in taking slow, deep breaths, and have patient concentrate on a focal point.

5. Validate nursing assessment of anxiety with patient (e.g., "You seem distressed; are you feeling uncomfortable now?").

6. After an episode of anxiety, review and discuss with patient the thoughts and feelings that led to the episode.

7. Identify patient's current coping behaviors: denial, anger, repression, withdrawal, daydreaming, or dependence on narcotics, sedatives, or tranquilizers. Review coping behaviors patient has used in the past. Assist patient with using adaptive coping to manage anxiety (e.g., "I understand that your wife reads to you to help you relax. Would you like to spend a part of each day alone with her?").

8. Encourage patient to express fears, concerns, and questions (e.g., "I know this room looks like a maze of wires and tubes; please let me know when you have any questions.").

9. Reduce sensory overload by providing an organized, quiet environment (see **Sensory/perceptual alterations,** p. 453).

10. Introduce yourself and other health care team members; explain each individual's role as it relates to patient's care.

11. Teach patient relaxation and imagery techniques. See **Health-seeking behaviors:** Relaxation technique effective for stress reduction, p. 27.
12. Allow support persons to be in attendance whenever possible.
13. Engage in and promote awareness of touch to significant others when appropriate. Kinds of touch are described in Table A-13.

Impaired verbal communication related to neurologic or anatomic deficit, psychologic or physical barriers (e.g., tracheostomy, intubation), or cultural or developmental differences

Desired outcome: At the time of intervention, patient communicates needs and feelings, and reports no or less frustration over communication barriers.

1. Assess cause of impaired communication (e.g., tracheostomy, cerebrovascular accident, cerebral tumor, Guillain-Barré syndrome).
2. Involve patient and significant others in assessing patient's ability to read, write, and understand English. If patient speaks another language, work with English-speaking family member or interpreter to establish effective communication.
3. When communicating with patient, face him or her, make direct eye contact, and speak in a clear, normal voice.
4. If patient is unable to speak because of a physical barrier (e.g., tracheostomy, wired mandibles) provide reassurance and acknowledge his or her frustration (e.g., "I know this is frustrating for you, but please do not give up. I want to understand you.").
5. Provide slate, word cards, pencil and paper, alphabet board, pictures, or other device to assist patient with communication. Adapt call system to meet patient's needs. Document meaning of signals patient uses to communicate.
6. Explain source of patient's communication impairment to significant others; teach them effective communication alternatives (see above).

Table A-13   Kinds of touch

Instrumental Touch
Related to task or procedure
May be negatively perceived but accepted as impersonal

Affective Touch
Expressive, personal
Caring
Comforting
May be positively or negatively perceived
Influenced by cultural patterns

Therapeutic Touch
Deliberate intervention to accomplish a therapeutic outcome (e.g., massage, reflexology, acupressure)
Manipulation/mobilization of energy fields

7. Be alert for nonverbal messages: facial expressions, hand movements, nodding of the head. Validate their meaning with patient.
8. Recognize that inability to speak may foster maladaptive behavior. Encourage patient to communicate needs; reinforce independent behavior.
9. Be honest with patient; do not pretend to understand if you are unable to interpret patient's communication.

Sensory/perceptual alterations related to therapeutically or socially restricted environment; psychologic stress; altered sensory reception, transmission, or integration; or chemical alteration

Desired outcome: At the time of intervention, patient verbalizes orientation to time, place, and person; reports ability to concentrate; and expresses satisfaction with degree and type of sensory stimulation being received.

1. Assess factors contributing to patient's sensory-perceptual alteration.
   - *Environmental:* Excessive noise in the environment; constant, monotonous noise; restricted environment (immobility, traction, isolation); social isolation (restricted visitors, impaired communication); therapies.
   - *Physiologic:* Altered organ function, sleep or rest pattern disturbance, medication, previous history of altered sensory perception.
2. Determine sensory stimulation appropriate for patient, and plan care accordingly.
3. Manage factors that contribute to environmental overload (e.g., avoid constant lighting [maintain day/night patterns]; reduce noise whenever possible [decrease alarm volumes, avoid loud talking, keep room door closed, provide earplugs]).
4. Provide meaningful sensory stimulation.
   - Display clocks, large calendars, and meaningful photographs and objects from home.
   - Depending on patient's preference, provide a radio, music, reading materials, or tape recordings of family and significant others. Earphones help block out external stimuli.
   - Position patient to look toward window when possible.
   - Discuss current events, time of day, holidays, and topics of interest during patient care activities (e.g., "Good morning, Mr. Smith. I'm Ms. Stone, your nurse for the afternoon and evening, 3 PM to 11 PM. It's sunny outside. Today is the first day of summer.").
   - As needed, orient patient to surroundings. Direct patient to reality as necessary.
   - Establish personal contact by touch to help promote and maintain patient's contact with environment.
   - Encourage significant others to communicate with patient frequently, using a normal tone of voice.
   - Convey concern and respect for patient. Introduce yourself, and call patient by name.
   - Stimulate patient's vision with mirrors, colored decorations, and pictures.

- Stimulate patient's sense of taste with sweet, salty, and sour substances as allowed.
- Encourage use of eyeglasses and hearing aids.
5. Inform patient before initiating therapies and using equipment.
6. Encourage patient to participate in health care planning and decision making whenever possible. Allow for choice when possible.
7. Assess patient's sleep-rest pattern to evaluate its contribution to sensory-perceptual disorder. Make sure patient has at least 90 min of uninterrupted sleep as often as possible. For more information, see next nursing diagnosis.

Sleep pattern disturbance related to environmental changes, illness, therapeutic regimen, pain, immobility, or psychological stress

Desired outcomes: After discussion, patient identifies factors that promote sleep. Within 8 h of intervention, patient attains 90-min periods of uninterrupted sleep and verbalizes satisfaction with his or her ability to rest.

1. Assess patient's usual sleeping patterns: bedtime routine, hours of sleep per night, sleeping position, use of pillows and blankets, napping during the day.
2. Explore relaxation techniques that promote patient's rest/sleep: imagining relaxing scenes, listening to soothing music or taped stories, using muscle relaxation exercises.
3. Identify causative factors and activities that contribute to patient's insomnia, awaken patient, or adversely affect sleep patterns: pain, anxiety, therapies, depression, hallucinations, medications, underlying illness, sleep apnea, respiratory disorder, caffeine, fear.
4. Organize procedures and activities to allow for 90-min periods of uninterrupted rest/sleep. Limit visiting during these periods.
5. Whenever possible, maintain a quiet environment by providing earplugs or reducing alarm volume. "White noise" (i.e., low-pitched, monotonous sounds such as an electric fan or soft music) may facilitate sleep. Dim lights for a time each day by drawing drapes or providing blindfolds.
6. If appropriate, limit patient's daytime sleeping. Attempt to establish regularly scheduled daytime activity (e.g., ambulation, sitting in chair, active ROM), which may promote nighttime sleep.
7. Investigate and provide nonpharmacologic comfort measures known to promote sleep (see Table A-7, p. 411).

Fear related to diagnosis and treatments, separation from support systems, unfamiliarity with environment or therapeutic regimen, or loss of sense of control

Desired outcome: After intervention, patient expresses fears and concerns and reports feeling greater psychological and physical comfort.

1. Assess patient's perceptions of the environment and health status, and determine factors contributing to patient's feelings of fear. Evaluate patient's verbal and nonverbal responses.
2. Acknowledge patient's fears (e.g., "I understand that this equipment frightens you, but it is necessary to help you breathe.").

3. Provide opportunities for patient to express fears and concerns (e.g., "You seem very concerned about receiving more blood today."). Listen closely to patient. Recognize that anger, denial, occasional withdrawal, and demanding behavior may be coping responses.

4. Encourage patient to ask questions and gather information about the unknown. Provide information about equipment, therapies, and routines according to patient's ability to understand.

5. To promote an increased sense of control, encourage patient to participate in care planning whenever possible. Provide continuity of care by establishing a routine and arranging for consistent care givers whenever possible. Appoint a case manager or primary nurse and associate nurses.

6. Discuss with health care team the appropriateness of medication therapy for patients with disabling fear or anxiety.

7. Explore patient's desire for spiritual or psychological counseling.

8. When there is a question of patient's surviving the illness or surgery, consult physician about a visit by another individual with the same disorder who has survived the surgery or disorder.

Ineffective individual coping related to health crisis, sense of vulnerability, or inadequate support systems

Desired outcome: Within 24 h of this diagnosis, patient verbalizes feelings, identifies strengths and coping behaviors, and does not demonstrate ineffective coping behaviors.

1. Assess patient's perceptions and ability to understand current health status.

2. Establish honest communication with the patient (e.g., "Please tell me what I can do to help you."). Help patient identify strengths, stressors, inappropriate behavior, and personal needs.

3. Support positive coping behaviors (e.g., "I see that reading that book seems to help you relax.").

4. Provide opportunities for patient to express concerns; gather information from nurses and other support systems. Provide patient with explanations about prescribed routine, therapies, and equipment. Acknowledge patient's feelings and assessment of current health status and environment.

5. Identify factors that inhibit patient's ability to cope (e.g., unsatisfactory support system, knowledge deficit, grief, fear).

6. Recognize maladaptive coping behavior: severe depression; dependence on narcotics, sedatives, or tranquilizers; hostility; violence; suicidal ideations. Confront patient about behavior (e.g., "You seem to be needing more pain medication. Are you having more physical pain, or does it help you cope with your situation?"). Refer patient to psychiatric liaison, clinical nurse specialist, case manager, or clergy as appropriate.

7. As patient's condition allows, assist with reducing anxiety. See **Anxiety,** p. 451.

8. Help reduce patient's sensory overload by maintaining an organized, quiet environment. See **Sensory/perceptual alterations,** p. 453.

9. Encourage regular visits by significant others. Encourage them to talk with patient to help minimize patient's emotional and social isolation.

10. Assess significant others' interactions with patient. Attempt to mobilize support systems by involving them in patient care whenever possible.

11. As appropriate, explain to significant others that increased dependency, anger, and denial may be adaptive coping behaviors used by patient in early stages of crisis until effective coping behaviors are learned.

Anticipatory grieving related to perceived potential loss of physiologic well-being (e.g., expected loss of body function or part, changes in self-concept or body image, chronic illness, or death)

Desired outcome: After intervention, patient and significant others express grief, participate in decisions about the future, and discuss their concerns with health care team and each other.

1. Assess factors contributing to anticipated loss.

2. Assess and accept patient's behavioral response. Expect reactions such as disbelief, denial, guilt, anger, and depression. Determine patient's stage of grieving as described in Table A-14.

3. Assess spiritual, religious, and sociocultural expectations related to loss (e.g., "Is religion an important part of your life? How do you and your family deal with serious health problems?"). Refer to clergy or community support groups as appropriate.

4. Encourage patient and significant others to share their concerns (e.g., "Is there anything you'd like to talk about today?"). Also respect their desire not to speak.

Table A-14   Stages of grieving

Protest stage	Denial ("No, not me.")
	Disbelief ("But I just saw her this morning!")
	Anger
	Hostility
	Resentment
	Bargaining to postpone loss
	Appeal for help to recover loss
	Loud complaints
	Altered sleep and appetite
Disorganization	Depression
	Withdrawal
	Social isolation
	Psychomotor retardation
	Silence
Reorganization	Acceptance of loss
	Development of new interests and attachments
	Restructuring of life-style
	Return to preloss level of functioning

5. Demonstrate empathy (e.g., "This must be a very difficult time for you and your family."). Touch when appropriate (see Table A-13).
6. In selected circumstances, explain the grieving process. This approach may help patient and family better understand and acknowledge their feelings.
7. Assess grief reactions of patient and significant others, and identify individuals with potential for dysfunctional grieving reactions (e.g., absence of emotion, hostility, avoidance). If potential for dysfunctional grieving is present, refer individual to psychiatric clinical nurse specialist, case manager, clergy, or other source of counseling as appropriate.
8. Determine patient's wishes about end of life decisions. Document these advance directives as appropriate.
9. When appropriate, determine patient's wishes about tissue donation.

Dysfunctional grieving related to loss of physiologic well-being or chronic fatal illness

Desired outcomes: Within 24 h of this diagnosis, patient and significant others express grief, explain the meaning of the loss, and communicate concerns with each other. Patient completes necessary self-care activities.

1. Assess grief stage (see Table A-14) and previous coping abilities. Discuss with patient and significant others their feelings, the meaning of the loss, and their goals (e.g., "How do you feel about your condition/illness? What do you hope to accomplish in these next few days/weeks?").
2. Acknowledge and permit anger; set limits on expression of anger to discourage destructive behavior (e.g., "I understand that you must feel very angry, but for the safety of others, you may not throw equipment.").
3. Identify suicidal behavior (e.g., severe depression, statements of intent, suicide plan, previous history of suicide attempt). Ensure patient's safety, and refer patient to psychiatric clinical nurse specialist, psychiatrist, clergy, or other support system.
4. Encourage patient and significant others to participate in ADLs and diversional activities. Identify physiologic problems related to loss (e.g., eating or sleeping disorders), and intervene accordingly.
5. If there is a question of patient's surviving the illness, consult physician about a visit by another individual with the same disorder who has survived the surgery or illness.

Powerlessness related to health care environment or illness-related regimen

Desired outcome: Within 24 h of this diagnosis, patient makes decisions about care and therapies and reports an attitude of realistic hope and a sense of self-control.

1. Assess with patient personal preferences, needs, values, and attitudes.
2. Before providing information, assess patient's knowledge and understanding of his or her condition and care.
3. Recognize patient's expressions of fear, lack of response to events,

and lack of interest in information, any of which may signal a sense of powerlessness.

4. Evaluate care giver practices, and adjust them to support patient's sense of control (e.g., if patient always bathes in the evening to promote relaxation before bedtime, modify care plan to include an evening bath rather than follow hospital routine of giving a morning bath).
5. Ask patient to demonstrate activities he or she can perform independently.
6. Whenever possible, offer alternatives to routine hygiene, diet, diversional activities, visiting hours, and treatment times.
7. Ensure patient's privacy and preserve his or her territorial rights whenever possible (e.g., when distant relatives and casual acquaintances request information about patient's status, check with patient and family members before sharing that information).
8. Discourage dependency on staff, and avoid overprotection and parenting behavior. Instead, act as an advocate for patient and significant others.
9. Assess support system; involve significant others in patient care whenever possible.
10. Offer realistic hope for the future. On occasion, encourage patient to direct his or her thoughts beyond the present.
11. Refer to clergy or other support systems as appropriate.
12. Determine patient's wishes about end of life decisions. Document these advance directives as appropriate.

Spiritual distress related to separation from religious ties or cultures or challenged belief and value system

Desired outcome: Within 24 h of this diagnosis, patient verbalizes his or her religious beliefs and expresses hope for the future, attainment of spiritual well-being, and resolution of conflicts.

1. Assess patient's spiritual or religious beliefs, values, and practices (e.g., "Do you have a religious preference? How important is it to you? Are there any religious or spiritual practices you wish to participate in while in the hospital?"). If patient expresses a desire, volunteer to read Scripture or other religious literature.
2. Inform patient and significant others of availability of spiritual resources, such as a chapel or volunteer chaplain.
3. Display a nonjudgmental attitude toward patient's religious or spiritual beliefs and values. Attempt to create an environment conducive to free expression.
4. Identify available support systems that may assist in meeting patient's religious or spiritual needs (e.g., clergy, fellow church members, support groups).
5. Be alert for comments related to spiritual concerns or conflicts (e.g., "I don't know why God is doing this to me." "I'm being punished for my sins.").
6. Listen closely and ask questions to help patient resolve conflicts related to spiritual issues (e.g., "I understand you want to be baptized. We can arrange to do that here.").

7. Provide privacy and opportunities for religious practices, such as prayer and meditation.
8. If spiritual beliefs and therapeutic regimens are in conflict, provide patient with honest, concrete information to encourage informed decision making (e.g., "I understand that your religion discourages receiving blood transfusions. Do you understand that by refusing blood, you make your condition more difficult to treat?").

Social isolation related to altered health status, inability to engage in satisfying personal relationships, altered mental status, altered physical appearance, or body image change

Desired outcome: Within 24 h of this diagnosis, patient demonstrates interaction and communication with others.

1. Assess factors contributing to patient's social isolation:
   - Restricted visiting hours.
   - Absence of or inadequate support system.
   - Inability to communicate (e.g., presence of intubation/tracheostomy).
   - Physical changes that affect self-concept.
   - Denial or withdrawal.
   - Critical care environment.
2. Recognize patients at high risk for social isolation: older adult, disabled, chronically ill, economically disadvantaged.
3. Help patient identify feelings associated with loneliness and isolation (e.g., "You seem very sad when your family leaves the room. Can you tell me more about your feelings?").
4. Determine patient's need for socialization, and identify available and potential support systems. Explore methods for increasing social contact (e.g., TV, radio, tapes of loved ones, intercom system, more frequent visitations, scheduled interaction with nurse or support staff).
5. Provide positive reinforcement for socialization that lessens patient's feelings of isolation and loneliness (e.g., "Please continue to call me when you need to talk to someone. Talking will help both of us to better understand your feelings.").
6. Facilitate patient's ability to communicate with others (see **Impaired verbal communication,** p. 452).

Body image disturbance related to loss or change in body parts or function or physical trauma

Desired outcomes: Within the 24 h before hospital discharge, patient acknowledges body changes and demonstrates movement toward incorporating changes into self-concept. Patient does not demonstrate maladaptive response, such as severe depression.

1. Establish open, honest communication with patient. Promote an environment conducive to free expression (e.g., "Please feel free to talk to me whenever you have any questions."). Assess patient for indicators suggesting body image disturbance, as listed in Table A-15.
2. When planning patient's care, be aware of therapies that may influence patient's body image (e.g., medications or invasive procedures and monitoring).

Appendix One

Table A-15 Indicators suggesting body image disturbance

Nonverbal Indicators

Missing body part, internal or external (e.g., splenectomy or amputated extremity)

Change in structure (e.g., open, draining wound)

Change in function (e.g., colostomy)

Refusal to look at or touch body part

Hiding or exposing body part

Verbal Indicators

Expression of negative feelings about body

Expression of feelings of helplessness, hopelessness, or powerlessness

Personalization or depersonalization of missing or mutilated part

Refusal to acknowledge change in structure or function of body part

3. Assess patient's knowledge of the pathophysiologic process that has occurred and his or her present health status. Clarify any misconceptions.

4. Discuss the loss or change with patient. Recognize that what may seem to be a small change may be of great significance to patient (e.g., arm immobilizer, catheter, hair loss, ecchymoses, facial abrasions).

5. Explore with patient concerns, fears, and feelings of guilt (e.g., "I understand that you are frightened. Your face looks very different now, but you will see changes, and it will improve. Gradually you will begin to look more like yourself.").

6. Encourage patient and significant others to interact with one another. Help family avoid reinforcing loved one's unhappiness over changed body part or function (e.g., "I know your son looks very different to you now, but it would help if you speak to him and touch him as you would normally.").

7. Encourage patient to participate gradually in self-care activities as he or she becomes physically and emotionally able. Allow for some initial withdrawal and denial behavior (e.g., when changing dressings over traumatized part, explain what you are doing but do not expect patient to watch or participate initially).

8. Discuss opportunities for reconstruction of loss or change (e.g., surgery, prosthesis, grafting, cosmetic therapies, organ transplant).

9. Recognize manifestations of severe depression: sleep disturbances, change in affect, change in communication pattern. As appropriate, refer to psychiatric clinical nurse specialist, case manager, clergy, or support group.

10. Help patient attain a sense of autonomy and control by offering choices and alternatives whenever possible. Emphasize patient's strengths, and encourage activities that interest him or her.

11. Offer realistic hope for the future.

Risk for violence related to sensory overload, suicidal behavior, rage reactions, temporal lobe epilepsy, perceived threats, or toxic reaction to medications

Desired outcome: Patient does not harm self or others.

1. Assess factors that may contribute to or precipitate violent behavior: medication reactions, inability to cope, suicidal behavior, confusion, hypoxia, postictal states.

2. Try to prevent or treat causative factors. For example, provide patient teaching, reorient patient, ensure delivery of prescribed oxygen therapy, and reduce or prevent sensory overload (see **Sensory/perceptual alterations,** p. 453).

3. Assess for history of physical aggression or family violence as maladaptive coping behavior.

4. Monitor for early signs of increasing anxiety and agitation: restlessness, verbal aggressiveness, inability to concentrate. Assess for body language indicative of violent behavior: clenched fists, rigid posture, increased motor activity.

5. Approach patient in a positive manner, and encourage verbalization of feelings and concerns (e.g., "I understand that you are frightened. I will be here from 3 PM to 11 PM to care for you.").

6. Offer patient as much personal and environmental control as situation allows (e.g., "Let's discuss the care you will need today. What fluids would you like to drink? Would you prefer a bath in the morning or evening?").

7. Help patient distinguish reality from altered perceptions. Orient patient to time, place, and person. Alter environment to promote reality-based thought processes (e.g., provide clocks, calendars, pictures of loved ones, familiar objects).

8. For patients with acute confusion who become aggressive, do not attempt to reorient them, and avoid arguing with them. Instead, state, "I can understand why you may [hear, think, see] that." Use nonthreatening mannerisms, facial expressions, and tone of voice.

9. Initiate measures that prevent or reduce excessive agitation.
   - Reduce environmental stimuli (e.g., alarms, loud or unnecessary talking).
   - Before touching patient, explain procedures and care, using short, concise statements.
   - Speak quietly (but firmly, as necessary), and project a caring attitude toward patient (e.g., "We are very concerned for your comfort and safety. Can we do anything to help you feel more relaxed?").
   - Avoid crowding (e.g., of equipment, visitors, health care providers) in patient's personal environment.
   - Avoid direct confrontation.

10. Explain and discuss patient's behavior with significant others. Acknowledge frustration, concerns, fears, and questions. Review safety precautions with significant others (see next intervention).

11. In the event of violent behavior, institute safety precautions as discussed in Table A-16.

Hopelessness related to prolonged isolation or activity restriction,

Table A-16 Safety precautions for potentially violent patients

Patient safety	Remove harmful objects from the environment, such as heavy or sharp instruments
	Apply padding to side rails according to agency protocol
	Use restraints as necessary and prescribed; monitor patient's neurovascular status at frequent intervals
	Set limits on patient's behavior, using clear, simple commands
	As prescribed, consider chemical sedation when unable to control patient's behavior by other means
	Explain safety precautions to patient and family
Care giver safety	Alert hospital security department when risk of violence is present
	Do not approach violent patient without adequate assistance from others
	Never turn your back on a violent patient
	Use a calm, matter-of-fact tone of voice
	Monitor security measures often
	Remain alert

failing or deteriorating physiologic condition, long-term stress, or loss of faith in God or belief system

Desired outcome: Within the 24 h before hospital discharge, patient verbalizes hopeful aspects of health status and reports that feelings of despair are absent or lessened.

1. Develop open, honest communication with patient. Listen closely, provide empathetic understanding of fears and doubts, and promote an environment conducive to free expression.
2. Assess patient's and significant others' understanding of patient's health status and prognosis; clarify any misperceptions.
3. Assess for indicators of hopelessness: unwillingness to accept help, pessimism, withdrawal, lack of interest, silence, loss of gratification in roles, previous history of hopeless behavior, hypoactivity, inability to accomplish tasks, expressions of incompetence, closing eyes, and turning away.
4. Provide opportunities for patient to feel cared for, needed, and valued by others (e.g., emphasize importance of relationships "Tell me about your grandchildren." "It seems that your family loves you very much.").
5. Support significant others who seem to spark or maintain patient's feelings of hope (e.g., "Your husband's mood seemed to improve after your visit.").
6. Recognize discussions and factors that promote patient's sense of

hope (e.g., discussions about family members, reminiscing about better times).

7. Explore patient's coping mechanisms; assist patient in expanding positive coping behavior (see **Ineffective individual coping,** p. 455).

8. Assess patient's spiritual needs (see **Spiritual distress,** p. 458).

9. Promote anticipation of positive events (e.g., mealtime, grandchildren's visits, bath time, extubation, discontinuation of traction).

10. Help patient recognize that although there may be no hope for returning to original life-style, there *is* hope for a new, but different life.

11. Avoid insisting that patient assume a positive attitude. Encourage hope for the future, even if it is the hope for a peaceful death.

12. Set realistic, attainable goals, and reward achievement.

Psychosocial Care of the Patient's Family and Significant Others

Altered family processes related to situational crisis (patient's illness)

Desired outcome: After intervention, significant others demonstrate effective adaptation to change/traumatic situation, as evidenced by seeking external support when necessary and sharing concerns within the family unit.

1. Assess family's character: social, environmental, ethnic, and cultural factors; relationships; and role patterns. Identify family developmental stage (e.g., the family may be dealing with other situational or maturational crises, such as an elderly parent or a teenager with a learning disability).

2. Assess previous adaptive behaviors (e.g., "How does your family react in stressful situations?"). Discuss observed conflicts and communication breakdown (e.g., "I noticed that your brother would not visit your mother today. Has there been a problem we should be aware of? Knowing about it may help us better care for your mother.").

3. Acknowledge the family's involvement in patient care, and promote strengths (e.g., "You were able to encourage your wife to turn and cough. That is very important to her recovery."). Encourage family to participate in patient care conferences. Promote frequent, regular patient visits by family members.

4. Provide family with information and guidance related to critically ill patient. Discuss the stresses of hospitalization, and encourage family to discuss feelings of anger, guilt, hostility, depression, fear, or sorrow (e.g., "You seem to be upset since being told that your husband is not leaving the hospital today."). Refer to clergy, clinical nurse specialist, or social services as appropriate.

5. Evaluate patient and family responses to one another. Encourage family to reorganize roles and establish priorities as appropriate (e.g., "I know your husband is concerned about his insurance policy

Appendix One

and seems to expect you to investigate it. I'll ask the financial counselor to talk with you.").

6. Encourage family to schedule periods of rest and activity outside the hospital and to seek support when necessary.

Family coping: Potential for growth, related to use of support systems and referrals and choosing experiences that optimize wellness.

Desired outcomes: At the time of patient's diagnosis, significant others express their intent to use support systems and resources and identify alternative behaviors that promote family communication and strengths. Significant others express realistic expectations and do not demonstrate ineffective coping behaviors.

1. Assess family relationships, interactions, support systems, and individual coping behaviors. Permit movement through stages of adaptation. Encourage further positive coping.

2. Acknowledge family expressions of hope, future plans, and growth among family members.

3. Encourage development of open, honest communication within family. Provide opportunities in a private setting for family interactions, discussions, and questions.

4. Refer family to community or support groups (e.g., ostomy support group, head injury rehabilitation group).

5. Encourage family to explore outlets that foster positive feelings (e.g., periods of time outside hospital area, meaningful communication with patient or support individuals, and relaxing activities such as showering, eating, exercising).

Ineffective family coping: Compromised, related to inadequate or incorrect information or misunderstanding, temporary family disorganization and role change, exhausted support systems, unrealistic expectations, fear, or anxiety

Desired outcome: After intervention, significant others verbalize feelings, identify ineffective coping patterns, identify strengths and positive coping behaviors, and seek information and support from nurse or other support systems outside the family.

1. Establish open, honest communication within the family. Assist family in identifying strengths, stressors, inappropriate behaviors, and personal needs (e.g., "I understand your mother was very ill last year. How did you manage the situation?" "I know your loved one is very ill. How can I help you?").

2. Assess family members for ineffective coping (e.g., depression, chemical dependency, violence, withdrawal), and identify factors that inhibit effective coping (e.g., inadequate support system, grief, fear of disapproval by others, knowledge deficit). For example, "You seem to be unable to talk about your husband's illness. Is there anyone with whom you can talk about it?"

3. Assess family's knowledge of patient's current health status and treatment. Provide information frequently, and allow sufficient time for questions. Reassess the family's understanding at frequent intervals.

4. Provide opportunities in a private setting for family to talk and

share concerns with nurses. If appropriate, refer family to psychiatric clinical nurse specialist for therapy.

5. Offer realistic hope. Help family develop realistic expectations for the future and identify support systems that will assist them with planning for the future.

6. Assist family with reducing anxiety by encouraging diversional activities (e.g., period of time outside of hospital) and interaction with support systems outside the family (e.g., "I know you want to be near your son, but if you would like to go home to rest, I will call you if *any* changes occur.").

Ineffective family coping: Disabling, related to unexpressed feelings, ambivalent family relationships, or disharmonious coping styles among family members

Desired outcome: Within the 24 h before hospital discharge, significant others verbalize feelings, identify sources of support as well as ineffective coping behaviors that create ambivalence and disharmony, and do not demonstrate destructive behaviors.

1. Establish open, honest communication and rapport with family members (e.g., "I am here to care for your mother and to help your family as well.").

2. Identify ineffective coping behavior (e.g., violence, depression, substance abuse, withdrawal). For example, "You seem to be angry. Would you like to talk to me about your feelings?" Refer to psychiatric clinical nurse specialist, clergy, or support group as appropriate.

3. Identify perceived or actual conflicts (e.g., "Are you able to talk freely with your family members?" "Are your brothers and sisters able to help and support you during this time?").

4. Assist family in search for healthy functioning within the family unit (e.g., facilitate open communication among family members and encourage behaviors that support family cohesiveness). For example, "Your mother enjoyed your last visit. Would you like to see her now?"

5. Assess family's knowledge of patient's current health status. Provide opportunities for questions; reassess family's understanding at frequent intervals.

6. Assist family in developing realistic goals, plans, and actions. Refer them to clergy, psychiatric nurse, social services, financial counseling, and family therapy as appropriate.

7. Encourage family members to spend time outside the hospital and to interact with support individuals. Respect family's need for occasional withdrawal.

8. Include family in patient's plan of care. Offer them opportunities to become involved in patient care (e.g., ROM exercises, patient hygiene, and comfort measures, such as a back rub).

Fear related to patient's life-threatening condition or knowledge deficit

Desired outcome: After intervention, significant others report that fear has abated.

1. Assess family's fears and their understanding of patient's clinical situation. Evaluate verbal and nonverbal responses.

2. Acknowledge family's fear (e.g., "I understand these tubes must frighten you, but they are necessary to help nourish your son.").
3. Assess family's history of coping behavior (e.g., "How does your family react to difficult situations?"). Determine resources and significant others available for support (e.g., "Who usually helps your family during stressful times?").
4. Provide opportunities for family members to express fears and concerns. Recognize that anger, denial, withdrawal, and demanding behavior may be adaptive coping responses during initial period of crisis.
5. Provide information at frequent intervals about patient's status and treatments. Demonstrate a caring attitude.
6. Encourage family to use positive coping behaviors by identifying fears, developing goals, identifying supportive resources, facilitating realistic perceptions, and promoting problem solving.
7. Recognize anxiety, and encourage family members to describe their feelings (e.g., "You seem very uncomfortable tonight. Can you describe your feelings?").
8. Be alert for maladaptive responses to fear: potential for violence, withdrawal, severe depression, hostility, and unrealistic expectations for staff or of patient's recovery. Provide referrals to psychiatric clinical nurse specialist or other as appropriate.
9. Offer *realistic* hope, even if it is hope for the patient's peaceful death.
10. Explore family's desire for spiritual or other counseling.
11. Assess your own feelings about patient's life-threatening illness. Acknowledge that your attitude and fear may be reflected to the family.
12. For other interventions, see nursing diagnoses **Altered family processes** and **Ineffective family coping.**

Knowledge deficit: Patient's current health status or therapies

Desired outcome: After intervention, significant others verbalize knowledge and understanding of patient's current health status or treatment

1. At frequent intervals, inform family about patient's current health status, therapies, and prognosis. Use individualized verbal, written, and audiovisual strategies to promote family's understanding.
2. Evaluate family at frequent intervals for understanding of information that has been provided. Assess factors for misunderstanding, and adjust teaching as appropriate. Some individuals in crisis need repeated explanations before comprehension can be assured (e.g., "I have explained many things to you today. Would you mind summarizing what I've told you so that I can be sure you understand your husband's status and what we are doing to care for him?").
3. Encourage family to relay correct information to patient; this reinforces comprehension for family and patient.
4. Ask family members if their needs for information are being met (e.g., "Do you have any questions about the care your mother is receiving or about her condition?").
5. Help family members use information they receive to make health

care decisions about patient (e.g., surgery, resuscitation, organ donation).
6. Promote family's active participation in patient care when appropriate. Encourage family to seek information and express feelings,
concerns, and questions.

SECTION FOUR: CARING
FOR OLDER ADULTS

Risk for aspiration related to delayed gag reflex secondary to age-
related changes
Desired outcomes: Patient swallows independently without choking. Patient's airway is patent and lungs are clear to auscultation before
and after meals.

1. Assess patient's LOC on admission and then routinely during hospital stay.
2. Assess patient's ability to swallow by asking if he or she has any
difficulty swallowing or if any foods or fluids are difficult to swallow or cause gagging. If patient is unable to answer, consult care
giver or significant other. Document findings.
3. Assess for gag reflex by *gently* touching posterior pharynx. Document findings.
4. Place patient in upright position while eating or drinking, and support this position with pillows.
5. Monitor patient when he or she is swallowing. Watch for limited
lip, tongue, or jaw movement, as indicated by drooling of saliva or
food or inability to close lips around a straw. Check for retention
of food in sides of mouth, an indication of poor tongue movement.
6. Monitor patient for coughing or choking before, during, or after
swallowing; this signals aspiration of material into airway.
7. Monitor patient for a wet or gurgly sound when talking after a
swallow; this indicates aspiration into airway and signals a delayed
or absent swallow reflex and a delayed or absent gag reflex.
8. Monitor for double swallowing with each bite, which can indicate
difficulty.
9. If patient has poor swallowing reflex, have patient tilt head forward 45 degrees during swallowing to close off airway and help
prevent inadvertent aspiration. **Note:** If patient has hemiplegia, tilt
head toward unaffected side.
10. Keep patient upright while eating and for 30 min afterward to prevent reflux.
11. As indicated, request evaluation by speech therapist for further assessment of gag and swallow reflex.
12. Anticipate use of swallowing video fluoroscopy to evaluate patient's gag and swallow reflex. Using four consistencies of barium,
the radiologist and speech therapist watch for reduced or ineffec-

tive tongue function, reduced peristalsis in pharynx, delayed or absent swallow reflex, and poor or limited ability to close sphincters that protect airway. This procedure is done to determine if patient is aspirating, the consistency of the materials most likely to be aspirated, and the cause of the aspiration.

13. Provide adequate rest periods before meals. Fatigue increases the risk of aspiration.

14. Monitor intake of food. Document consistencies and amount of food eaten, where patient places food in the mouth, how patient manipulates or chews before swallowing, and length of time before patient swallows the bolus of food.

15. Remind patients with dementia to chew and swallow with each bite.

16. Make sure patient has dentures in place, if appropriate, and that they fit correctly.

17. Make sure someone stays with patient during meals or fluid intake.

18. Provide patient with adequate time to eat and drink. Generally, patients with swallowing deficits require twice as much time for eating and drinking as those whose swallowing is adequate.

19. Monitor patient for signs of aspiration: crackles, SOB, decreasing LOC, increasing temperature.

20. Be aware of location of suction equipment to be used in case of aspiration.

21. If patient aspirates, implement the following:
   - Follow American Heart Association (AHA) Standards if patient displays characteristics of complete airway obstruction (i.e., choking).
   - For partial airway obstruction, encourage patient to cough as needed.
   - For partial airway obstruction in unconscious/nonresponsive individual who is not coughing, suction airway with a large-bore catheter (e.g., Yankauer).
   - For either a complete or partial aspiration, inform physician and obtain order for chest x-ray.
   - Protect patient by implementing NPO until diagnosis is confirmed.
   - Monitor breathing pattern and RR q1-2h after suspected aspiration for alterations (i.e., increased RR) that signal a change in the patient's condition.
   - Anticipate use of antibiotics to prevent infection.
   - Encourage patient to cough and deep breathe q2h while awake and q4h during the night to promote expansion of available lung tissue.

Constipation related to changes in diet, activity, and psychosocial factors secondary to hospitalization

Desired outcomes: Within 3-4 days of this diagnosis, patient states that bowel habits have returned to normal. Stool appears soft, and patient does not strain in passing stools.

1. Upon admission, assess and document patient's normal bowel elimination pattern. Include frequency, time of day, associated hab-

its, and successful methods used to correct constipation in the past. Consult with patient's care giver or significant other if patient is unable to provide this information.

2. Inform patient that changes that occur with hospitalization may increase the potential for constipation. Urge patient to institute successful nonpharmacologic methods used at home as soon as this problem is noticed, or prophylactically as needed.

3. Teach patient the relationship between fluid intake and constipation. Unless otherwise contraindicated, encourage fluid intake of 2-3 L/day. Monitor and record bowel movements.

4. Teach patient the relationship between types of foods consumed and constipation. When possible, encourage patient to include roughage in each meal (e.g., raw fruits and vegetables, whole grains, nuts, and fruits with skins). For a patient unable to tolerate raw foods, encourage intake of bran *via* cereals, muffins, and breads. Titrate amount of roughage to degree of constipation.

5. Teach patient the relationship between constipation and activity level. Encourage optimum activity for all patients. Establish and post an activity program to enhance participation; include devices necessary to permit independence.

6. Advise patient about the need to maintain normal bowel elimination pattern. Provide any materials or support environments the patient normally uses (e.g., cup of coffee first thing upon arising, privacy, short walk).

7. Ask patient if toilet seat height seems the same as at home. If toilet is higher, provide a footstool to raise patient's feet off the floor comfortably. A high-rise toilet seat may be used to increase toilet's height.

8. Schedule interventions to coincide with patient's habit. If patient's habit occurs in the early morning, use gastrocolic or gastroduodenal reflexes to promote colonic emptying. If patient's habit occurs in the evening, ambulate patient just before appropriate time. Digital stimulation of anal sphincter also may facilitate bowel movement.

9. Attempt to use methods patient has used successfully in the past. Follow the maxim "go low, go slow" (i.e., use the lowest amount of nonnatural intervention and advance to more powerful interventions slowly). Older adults tend to focus on the loss of habit as an indicator of constipation, rather than on the number of stools. Do not intervene pharmacologically until patient has not had a stool for 3 days.

10. When requesting pharmacologic intervention, use the more benign, oral methods first. A suggested hierarchy is
    - Bulk-building additives (psyllium, bran)
    - Mild laxatives (apple or prune juice, milk of magnesia)
    - Stool softeners (docusate sodium or docusate calcium)
    - Potent laxatives or cathartics (bisacodyl or cascara sagrada)
    - Medicated suppositories (glycerine or bisacodyl)
    - Enema (tap water, saline, sodium biphosphate/phosphate)

11. After diagnostic imaging of GI tract with barium, make sure pa-

tient receives postexamination laxative to facilitate removal of barium. After any procedure involving a bowel cleanout, rebound constipation may occur because of the severe disruption of bowel habit. Monitor hydration status for signs of dehydration, which can occur from osmotic agents used. Emphasize diet, fluid, activity, and resumption of routines. If no bowel movement occurs in 3 days, begin with mild laxatives to try to regain normal pattern.

12. Also see this diagnosis in "Caring for Patients on Prolonged Bed Rest," p. 420.

Risk for fluid volume deficit related to inability to obtain fluids by self secondary to illness, placement of fluid, or presence of chronic illness; or related to use of osmotic agents during radiologic tests

Desired outcomes: Patient's mental status, VS, and urine specific gravity, color, consistency, and concentration remain within normal limits for patient. Patient's mucous membranes remain moist, and intake equals output.

1. Monitor fluid intake. In nonrestricted individuals, encourage intake of 2-3/L day. Specify amount to be consumed during the day, evening, and night.

2. Assess and document skin turgor. Check hydration status by pinching skin over sternum or forehead. Dehydration is indicated by skin that remains in lifted position (tenting) and returns slowly to original position. A furrowed tongue is a signal of severe dehydration.

3. Assess and document urine specific gravity and color q8h.

4. Assess and document color, amount, and frequency of any fluid output, including emesis, urine, diarrhea, or other drainage.

5. Monitor patient's orientation, ability to follow commands, and behavior. Loss of ability to follow commands, decrease in orientation, and confused behavior can be signals of a dehydrated state.

6. Weigh patient daily at the same time of day (preferably before breakfast) using the same scale and bed clothing. Be alert to wide variations in weight (e.g., $\geq$2.5 kg [5 lb]).

7. In dehydrated patient, expect elevation in serum sodium (Na^+), blood urea nitrogen (BUN), and serum creatinine.

8. If patient is receiving IV therapy, monitor cardiac and respiratory systems for signs of overload, which could precipitate congestive heart failure (CHF) or pulmonary edema. Assess apical pulse and listen to lung fields during every VS assessment. A rising HR and crackles in lungs can be signals of CHF or pulmonary edema.

9. Monitor I&O when patient is receiving dyes for contrast or tube feedings. These agents act osmotically to pull fluid into interstitial tissue. Watch for evidence of third spacing of fluids: increasing peripheral edema, especially sacral; output significantly less than intake (1:2); and urine output <30 ml/h.

10. Offer patient fluid whenever in the room. Older adults have a decreased sense of thirst and need encouragement to drink. Offer a variety of drinks the patient likes, but limit caffeine because it tends to act as a diuretic.

11. Assess patient's ability to obtain and drink fluids by himself or herself. Place fluids within easy reach. Use cups with tops to minimize concern about spilling.

12. Ensure access to toilet, urinal, commode, or bedpan at least q2h when patient is awake and q4h at night. Answer call light quickly. The time between recognition of need to void and urination gets shorter with age.

Impaired gas exchange (or risk for same) related to decreased functional lung tissue secondary to age-related changes

Desired outcomes: Patient's respiratory pattern and mental status remain normal for patient. Patient's ABG or pulse oximetry values are within patient's normal limits.

1. Assess and document the following upon admission and routinely thereafter: respiratory rate, pattern, and depth; breath sounds; cough; sputum; and sensorium.

2. Assess patient for subtle changes in mentation: increased restlessness, anxiety, disorientation, hostility. If available, monitor oxygenation status *via* ABG findings (optimally Pao_2 ≥80%-95%) or pulse oximetry (optimally ≥90%).

3. Assess lungs for adventitious sounds. **Note:** The aging lung has decreased elasticity. The lower part of the lungs is no longer adequately aerated. As a result, crackles commonly are heard in individuals ≥75 yr. This sign alone does not mean that a pathologic condition is present. Crackles that do not clear with coughing in an individual with no other clinical signs (e.g., fever, increasing anxiety, increasing respiratory depth) are considered benign.

4. Encourage patient to cough and breathe deeply to promote alveolar expansion and clear secretions from bronchial tree.

5. Reduce potential for increased oxygen consumption by treating fevers promptly, reducing pain, minimizing pacing activity, and ceasing anxiety.

6. Instruct patient in use of support equipment such as oxygen masks or cannulas.

7. Schedule and pace patient's activities according to tolerance. Document patient's ability to accomplish ADLs.

Hopelessness related to slow recovery from illness or surgery secondary to decreased physiologic reserve

Desired outcome: Within 2-4 days of intervention, patient verbalizes knowledge of his or her strengths, feelings about health, and understanding of a potentially long recovery.

1. Monitor patient for signs of depression: refusal to participate in own care; refusal to answer questions; statements such as "I don't care," "Leave me alone," and "Let me die."

2. Encourage patient to verbalize feelings of despair, frustration, fear, and anger and concerns about hospitalization and health. Reassure patient and significant others that such feelings and concerns are normal.

3. Discuss normal age changes with patient. Inform patient and significant others that recovery periods are longer for older adults because

of decreased physiologic reserve. More energy is spent in maintaining normal status, and thus the body has less capacity to rebuild strength and endurance.

4. Encourage short-term goals and praise small steps, such as participation in own care.

5. Arrange a care conference to discuss discharge requirements specific to patient. Involve patient and significant others in the conference. Set realistic goals with patient based on his or her condition and desires.

Hypothermia related to age-related changes in thermoregulation and/or environmental exposure

Desired outcome: After intervention, patient's temperature and mental status remain within patient's normal limits or return to those limits at a rate of 1° F/h.

1. Monitor patient's temperature, using a low-range thermometer if possible. Be aware that older adults can have a normal temperature of 35.6° C (96° F).

2. Assess patient's temperature orally by placing thermometer far back in the mouth. To ensure proper placement, slide thermometer along buccal membrane and position under back of tongue. **Note:** Do not take axillary temperature in the older adult because they have decreased peripheral circulation and the skin under the arms will be cooler than the core temperature. If unable to take patient's temperature orally, take it *via* rectum or ear, which are measures of the core temperature.

3. Assess and document patient's mental status. Increasing disorientation or atypical behavior can signal hypothermia.

4. Be alert for patients taking sedatives, hypnotics (including anesthetics), and muscle relaxants because these drugs decrease shivering, putting these patients at risk for environmental hypothermia. In addition, all older adults are at risk for environmental hypothermia at ambient temperatures of 22.2°-23.9° C (72°-75° F).

5. Make sure patient is sent to radiology and other departments with enough blankets to keep warm.

6. Initiate slow rewarming using external methods: raising room temperature to at least 23.9° C (75° F), warm blankets, head covers, warm circulating air blankets.

7. If patient's temperature falls below 35° C (95° F), warm patient internally by administering warm oral or IV fluids. Also anticipate use of warmed saline gastric irrigations or introduction of warmed humidified air into airway.

8. Be alert for signs of too-rapid rewarming: irregular HR, dysrhythmias, and very warm extremities caused by vasodilatation in the periphery, which causes heat loss from the core.

9. If patient's temperature fails to rise 1° F qh with these techniques, suspect a cause other than environmental factors. In this event, anticipate laboratory tests, including WBC count for possible sepsis, thyroid test for hypothyroidism, and glucose level for hypoglycemia.

10. As prescribed, administer antibiotics for sepsis, initiate thyroid

therapy, or administer glucose for hypoglycemia. Patient's temperature will not return to normal unless underlying condition is treated.

Risk for infection related to age-related changes in immune and integumentary system; related to suppressed inflammatory response secondary to chronic medication use (e.g., antiinflammatory agents, steroids, analgesics); related to slowed ciliary response; or related to poor nutrition

Desired outcome: Patient remains free of infection, as evidenced by orientation to time, place, and person, and behavior within patient's normal limits; RR and pattern within patient's normal limits; urine that is straw-colored, clear, and of characteristic odor; core temperature and HR within patient's normal limits; sputum that is clear to whitish in color; and skin that is intact and of normal color and temperature for patient.

N O T E : WBC count $\geq 11,000/\mu l$ can be a late sign of infection in older adults because the immune system is slow to respond to insult.

---

1. Assess patient's baseline VS, including LOC and orientation. A change in mentation is a leading sign of infection in older adults. Also be alert for HR >100 bpm and RR >24 breaths/min. Auscultate lung fields for adventitious sounds. Be aware, however, that crackles may be a normal finding when heard in lung bases.
2. Monitor patient's temperature, using a low-range thermometer if possible. Be aware that a temperature of 35.6° C (96° F) may be normal for patient. In that case, a patient with a temperature of 36.7°-37.2° C (98°-99° F) may be considered febrile.
3. To ensure that patient's core temperature is being accurately determined, obtain temperature readings rectally or *via* ear probe if the oral reading does not match the clinical picture (i.e., patient's skin is very warm, patient is restless, mentation is depressed), or if the temperature reads $\geq 36.1°$ C (97° F).
4. Assess patient's skin for tears, breaks, redness, or ulcers. Document condition of skin on admission and as an ongoing assessment (see **Risk for impaired skin integrity,** below).
5. Assess quality and color of the patient's urine. UTI, as manifested by cloudy, foul-smelling urine without painful urination, is the most common infection in older adults. Document changes and consult physician about findings. Also be alert for urinary incontinence, which can signal UTI.
6. Because of increased risk of infection, avoid insertion of urinary catheters when possible.
7. Obtain drug history in reference to use of antiinflammatory or immunosuppressive drugs or chronic use of analgesics or steroids, because these drugs mask fever.
8. If infection is suspected, anticipate initiation of IV fluid therapy to maintain fluid balance; blood cultures, urinalysis, and urine culture to isolate bacteria type; and WBC count to determine immune response. Expect a chest x-ray to rule out pneumonia if patient's chest

sounds are not clear. If infection is present, prepare for initiation of broad-spectrum antibiotic therapy, oxygen therapy to maintain adequate oxygenation to the brain, and use of acetaminophen to reduce temperature and cardiac output, which will decrease cardiac load.

Powerlessness related to hospital environment

Desired outcome: Within 2-4 days after intervention, patient participates in care and verbalizes feelings of control over his or her environment.

1. Encourage patient to verbalize feelings about hospitalization and illness.
2. Assist patient in identifying factors that contribute to feelings of powerlessness.
3. Encourage patient to participate in ADLs as much as possible. Provide adequate time for patient to complete activities.
4. As often as possible, allow patient to participate in scheduling of activities.
5. Discuss with patient and significant others realistic goals of care, and encourage patient's participation in care planning.
6. Explain procedures and routines to patient. Inform patient when changes in plan of care are necessary.
7. Provide flexibility in patient's plan of care when possible (e.g., if patients want to wear their own clothes, enable them to do so).

Risk for impaired skin integrity related to decreased subcutaneous fat and decreased peripheral capillary networks secondary to age-related changes in the integumentary system

Desired outcome: Patient's skin remains clear and intact.

1. Assess patient's skin on admission and routinely thereafter. Note any areas of redness or any breaks in skin surface.
2. Make sure patient turns frequently (at least q2h). Lift or roll patient across sheets when repositioning. Pulling, dragging, or sliding patient across sheets can lead to shear (loss of skin).
3. Monitor skin over bony prominences (i.e., sacrum, heels, spine, hips, knees, costal margins, occiput) for erythema. Apply skin barrier paste to reddened areas for additional protection. Use pillows or pads around bony prominences to protect overlying skin, even when patient is up in a wheelchair or sits for long periods (ischial tuberosities are prone to breakdown when patient is in the seated position).
4. Use lotions on dry skin to promote suppleness.
5. Use alternating pressure mattress, air-fluidized mattress, waterbed, or airbed for older adults who are on bed rest or unable to get out of bed, to protect skin from injury caused by prolonged pressure.
6. Avoid placing tubes under patient's limbs or head. Excess pressure from tubes can create a pressure ulcer. Place pillow or pad between patient and tube for cushioning.
7. Optimize patient mobility; get patient out of bed as often as possible. If patient is unable to get out of bed, assist with position changes q2h.
8. Make sure patient's face, axillae, and genital areas are washed

daily. Complete baths dry out older adults' skin and should be given every other day instead. Use tepid water and super-fatted soaps, which help prevent dry skin. Avoid hot water, which can burn older individuals, who have decreased pain sensitivity and decreased sensation to temperature.

9. Minimize use of protective pads under patient; these pads trap moisture and heat and can lead to skin breakdown.
10. Document percentage of food intake with meals. Encourage significant others to provide patient's favorite foods. Suggest snacks high in protein and vitamin C if patient's diet is not restricted.
11. Obtain nutritional consultation with dietitian as needed.
12. Monitor serum albumin for evidence of protein status (normal value is 3 g/dl for older adults).
13. For more information see "Providing Nutritional Support," p. 378, and "Managing Wound Care," p. 384.

Sleep pattern disturbance related to unfamiliar surroundings and hospital routines

Desired outcomes: Within 24 h of intervention, patient reports getting adequate rest. Patient's mental status remains normal for patient.

1. Assess and document patient's usual sleeping pattern, obtaining information from patient or patient's care giver or significant others. Ask questions about naps and activity levels. Individuals who take naps and have a low level of activity frequently sleep only 4-5 h/night.
2. Try to have patient follow usual nighttime routine.
3. Inform patient of necessary interruptions during hospitalization.
4. Attempt to group activities together (medications, VS, toileting) to reduce the number of interruptions.
5. Provide comfort measures: pain medications, back rub, conversation at bedtime.
6. Provide patient with compatible roommate when possible.
7. Monitor patient's activity level. If patient complains of being tired after activities or displays behavior such as irritability, yelling, or shouting, encourage napping after lunch or early in the afternoon. Otherwise, discourage daytime napping by involving patient in care or activities.
8. Avoid stimulants such as coffee, cola, and tea after 6 PM.
9. Provide a quiet environment by eliminating loud noises and use of overhead lights and minimizing interruptions during sleep hours.

Impaired memory or **Acute confusion** related to decreased cerebral perfusion secondary to age-related decreased physiologic reserve or cardiac dysfunction; related to electrolyte imbalance secondary to age-related decreased renal function; related to altered sensory/perceptual reception secondary to poor vision or hearing; or related to decreased brain oxygenation secondary to illness and decreased functional lung tissue

Desired outcomes: Within 3 days of treatment, patient's mental status returns to normal for patient. Patient suffers no injury as a result of mental status.

1. Assess patient's baseline LOC and mental status on admission. Ask patient to perform a three-step task (e.g., "Raise your right

hand, place it on your left shoulder, and then place the right hand by your right side."). Test short-term memory by showing patient how to use the call light, having patient return the demonstration, and then waiting at least 5 min before having patient demonstrate use of call light again. Inability to remember beyond 5 min indicates poor short-term memory. Document patient's response.

2. Document patient's actions in behavioral terms. Describe "confused" behavior.

3. Determine preconfusion functional and mental status abilities by asking significant others.

4. Identify cause of acute confusion (e.g., check oximetry or ABG values to assess oxygenation levels; serum glucose or finger-stick glucose to determine glucose level; and electrolytes and CBC to ascertain imbalances and/or elevated WBC count as a determinant of infection). Assess hydration status by pinching skin over sternum or forehead for turgor and checking for dry mucous membranes and furrowed tongue.

5. Review cardiac status. Assess apical pulse, and consult physician about any irregular pulse that is new to patient. If patient is on a cardiac monitor, watch for dysrhythmias and notify physician accordingly.

6. Review current medications, including OTC drugs, with pharmacist. Toxic levels of certain medications (e.g., digoxin or theophylline) cause acute confusion. Drugs that are anticholinergic also can cause confusion, as can drug interactions.

7. Monitor I&O at least q8h. Output should match intake. Anticipate/encourage a creatinine clearance test to assess renal function. **Note:** BUN and serum creatinine are affected by hydration status. Serum creatinine is affected by the aging process, because lower mass produces lower creatinine. Normal serum creatinine levels in a well-hydrated older adult can therefore signal renal insufficiency.

8. Have patient wear glasses and hearing aid, or keep them close to bedside and within easy reach.

9. Keep patient's urinal and other routinely used items within easy reach. If patient has short-term memory problems, do not expect him or her to use call light. Toilet or offer patient urinal or bedpan q2h while awake and q4h during the night.

10. Check on patient at least q30min and whenever passing the room.

11. Place patient close to nurses' station if possible. Provide an environment that is nonstimulating and safe. Provide music but not TV (patients who are confused regarding place and time often think the action on the TV is happening in the room).

12. Attempt to reorient patient to surroundings as needed. Keep a clock or calendar at bedside, and verbally remind patient of date and day as needed.

13. Tell patient in simple terms what is occurring (e.g., "It's time to eat breakfast," "This medicine is for your heart," "I'm going to help you get out of bed.").

14. Encourage patient's significant others to bring items familiar to patient, including blanket, bedspread, pictures of family and pets.

15. If patient becomes belligerent, angry, or argumentative during attempt at reorientation, **stop this approach.** Do not argue with patient or patient's interpretation of the environment. State, "I can understand why you may (hear, think, see) that."

16. If patient displays hostile behavior or misperceives your role (nurse becomes thief, jailer, etc.), leave the room. Return in 15 min. Introduce yourself to patient as though you had never met. Begin dialogue anew. Patients who are acutely confused have poor short-term memory and may not remember the previous encounter or that you were involved in it. When you return, allow patient to share feelings about previous encounter as appropriate.

17. If patient attempts to leave the hospital, walk with him or her and attempt distraction. Ask patient to tell you about the destination (e.g., "That sounds like a wonderful place! Tell me about it."). Keep tone pleasant and conversational. Continue walking with patient away from exits and doors around unit. After a few minutes, attempt to guide patient back to room. Offer refreshments and a rest (e.g., "We've been walking for a while and I'm a little tired. Why don't we sit and have some juice while we talk.").

18. If patient has a permanent or severe cognitive impairment, check on him or her at least q30min and reorient to baseline mental status as indicated; however, do not argue with patient about his or her perception of reality, since this can cause a cognitively impaired person to become aggressive and combative. **Note:** Individuals with severe cognitive impairment (e.g., Alzheimer's disease or dementia) also can experience acute confusional states (i.e., delirium) and can be returned to their baseline mental state.

19. If patient tries to climb out of bed, he or she may need to use the toilet; offer urinal or bedpan, or assist to commode. Alternatively, if patient is not on bed rest, place him or her in chair or wheelchair at nurses' station for added supervision.

20. Bargain with patient. Try to establish an agreement to stay for a defined period of time, such as until physician, breakfast or lunch, or significant others arrive.

21. Have patient's significant others talk with patient by phone or come in and sit with patient if patient's behavior requires checking more often than q30min.

22. If patient is attempting to pull out tubes, hide them (e.g., under blankets). Put stockinette mesh dressing over IV lines. Tape feeding tubes to side of face using paper tape, and drape tube behind patient's ear. Remember: out of sight, out of mind.

23. Evaluate continued need for therapy that may have become an irritating stimulus (e.g., if patient is now drinking, discontinue IV; if patient is eating, discontinue feeding tube; if patient has an indwelling urethral catheter, discontinue catheter and begin toileting routine).

24. Use restraints with caution. Patients can become more agitated when wrist and arm restraints are used.

25. Use medications cautiously for controlling behavior. Neuroleptics, such as haloperidol, can be used successfully in calming patients

with dementia or psychiatric illness (contraindicated for individuals with parkinsonism). However, if patient is experiencing acute confusion or delirium, short-acting benzodiazepines (e.g., lorazepam) are more effective in reducing anxiety and fear. Anxiety or fear usually triggers destructive or dangerous behavior in an acutely confused older adult. A short-acting benzodiazepine will reduce feelings of anxiety and calm patient after 1 or 2 doses. **Note:** Neuroleptics can cause akathisia, an adverse drug reaction marked by increased restlessness.

Infection Prevention and Control

For several decades, infection prevention and control have focused on the use of barriers (e.g., gloves, gowns, and masks) to prevent transmission of organisms among patients and health care providers.

Systems for Isolation Precautions

Five different systems of isolation precautions have been used in hospitals (Table B-1). In 1995 the Centers for Disease Control and Prevention (CDC) revised its guidelines for isolation precautions, with the following objectives in mind: (1) to devise epidemiologically sound practices; (2) to recognize the importance of all body fluids, secretions, and excretions in the transmission of nosocomial pathogens; (3) to establish adequate precautions for infections transmitted by the airborne, droplet, and contact routes; (4) to design procedures that were as easy as possible; and (5) to use new terms, so as to avoid confusion with existing infection control and isolation systems.

The 1995 guidelines (Table B-2) have two tiers of precautions: **Standard Precautions,** designed for the care of all hospital patients regardless of their diagnosis or presumed infection status; and **Transmission-based Precautions,** which are divided into Airborne, Droplet, and Contact categories and are used with patients known to be or suspected of being infected or colonized with epidemiologically important pathogens that can be transmitted by the airborne or droplet route or by contact with dry skin or contaminated surfaces.

The 1995 guidelines have replaced the 1983 standards for isolation precautions in hospitals that previously offered three options: a Category-Specific System, a Disease-Specific System, and a Hospital-Designed System. Body Substance Isolation (BSI) is a Hospital-Designed System that many hospitals in the United States and elsewhere have adopted. In 1987-1988, the CDC introduced Universal Precautions to reduce the risk to health care providers of exposure to bloodborne pathogens.

The 1995 Standard Precautions synthesize the major features of Universal Precautions and Body Substance Isolation. Standard Precautions apply to (1) blood, (2) all body fluids, secretions, and excretions, regardless of whether they contain visible blood, (3) skin that is not intact, and (4) mucous membranes. Standard Precautions are designed to reduce the risk of transmission of microorganisms from both recognized and unrecognized sources of infection.

Transmission-based Precautions are designed for patients who have

Text continued on p. 492.

Table A-17   Five systems of infection precautions (as applied to different situations)*

	Category-Specific	Disease-Specific	Body Substance Isolation (BSI)	Universal Precautions†	Standard Precautions and Transmission-based Precautions‡
Patient known to have HBV, HCV, HIV, or other blood-borne disease	Blood and Body Fluid Precautions replaced by Universal Precautions in 1987 (revised 1988); superseded by 1995 Standard Precautions	Use 1995 Standard Precautions	Principles incorporated into 1995 Standard Precautions	Use 1995 Standard Precautions	See Table A-18: 1995 Standard Precautions
Patient not known to have HBV, HCV, HIV, or other blood-borne disease	Use 1995 Standard Precautions	Use 1995 Standard Precautions	Use 1995 Standard Precautions	Use 1995 Standard Precautions	See Table A-18: 1995 Standard Precautions

| Patient diagnosed with enteric disease (e.g., shigellosis) | Enteric Precautions (plus sign on door); superseded by 1995 Standard Precautions | Recommendations for specific disease from 1983 CDC guidelines; sign on door; superseded by 1995 Standard Precautions | Use of barriers depended on interaction with body substances, not diagnosis; principles incorporated into 1995 Standard Precautions | Did not apply to feces except with visible blood, and were not intended for fecal-to-oral diseases; 1995 Standard Precautions apply to feces whether or not fecal-to-oral disease is diagnosed | See Table A-18: 1995 Standard Precautions |
| Patient not known to have enteric disease | No diagnosis, therefore no special precautions; routine care practices; superseded by 1995 Standard Precautions (which apply to diagnosed and undiagnosed patients) | No special precautions because disease-specific precautions were used only for diagnosed patients; superseded by 1995 Standard Precautions (which apply to diagnosed and undiagnosed patients) | Same as above; BSI principles and practices apply to diagnosed and undiagnosed patients | Same as above | See Table A-18: 1995 Standard Precautions |

Continued.

Table A-17   Five systems of infection precautions (as applied to different situations)*—cont'd.

	Category-Specific	Disease-Specific	Body Substance Isolation (BSI)	Universal Precautions†	Standard Precautions and Transmission-based Precautions‡
Patient diagnosed with varicella (chickenpox)	Strict Isolation (plus sign on door); superseded by 1995 Transmission-based Precautions (Airborne, Contact)	Recommendations for specific disease from 1983 CDC guidelines; superseded by 1995 Transmission-based Precautions (Airborne, Contact)	Susceptible individuals prohibited from providing care; immune care givers; BSI precautions only; door closed with sign restricting entry; similar to 1995 Transmission-based Precautions: Airborne	Did not apply to airborne communicable diseases such as chickenpox	See Table A-18: 1995 Transmission-based Precautions: Airborne, and Transmission-based Precautions: Contact; susceptible individuals should not enter room

| Patient diagnosed with or suspected of having pulmonary or laryngeal tuberculosis | AFB Isolation, door closed with sign restricting entry, special room ventilation; superseded by 1995 Transmission-based Precautions: Airborne | Recommendations for specific disease from 1983 CDC guidelines; superseded by 1995 Transmission-based Precautions: Airborne | Airborne Precautions, door closed with sign restricting entry, special room ventilation; similar to 1995 Transmission-based Precautions: Airborne | Did not apply to airborne communicable diseases such as tuberculosis | See Table A-18: 1995 Transmission-based Precautions: Airborne |

*Table based on CDC draft guidelines from: Draft guideline for isolation precautions in hospitals: notice of comment period, *Federal Register* 59(214):55552-55570, Nov 7, 1994. **Note:** Final version may differ.

†Revised by the CDC in 1988; regulated by OSHA's 1991 Bloodborne Pathogens Standard.

‡Proposed in the 1995 CDC draft guidelines to replace all previous systems (these precautions incorporate OSHA's Bloodborne Pathogens Standard).

Appendix Two

Table A-18 Projected recommendations for isolation precautions in hospitals (CDC, 1995)*

| | Standard Precautions | Transmission-based Precautions | | |
		Airborne	Droplet	Contact
Use	Care of all patients	Use in addition to Standard Precautions for patients diagnosed with or suspected of being infected by microorganisms transmitted by airborne nuclei (≤ 5 μm) of evaporated droplets, which can remain suspended in air and can be widely dispersed by air currents	Use in addition to Standard Precautions for patients diagnosed with or suspected of being infected by microorganisms transmitted by airborne nuclei (≥ 5 μm) that can be produced by coughing, sneezing, talking, or performing procedures	Use in addition to Standard Precautions for specified patients diagnosed with or suspected of being colonized by epidemiologically important organisms that can be transmitted by direct contact (e.g., during patient care) or indirect contact (e.g., by touching surfaces or equipment in patient's environment)
Handwashing	Wash hands after touching blood, body fluids, secretions, excretions, or contaminated items, whether or not gloves were worn;			

wash hands immediately after removing gloves and between patient contacts, and to avoid transferring microorganisms to other patients or environments

Gloves

Wear nonsterile gloves when touching blood, body fluids, secretions, excretions, or contaminated items; put on clean gloves just before touching mucous membranes and broken skin; remove gloves promptly after use, and wash hands thoroughly before touching uncontaminated items or environmental surfaces, and before going to another patient

In addition to glove use described under Standard Precautions; wear gloves for direct patient care or when touching potentially contaminated surfaces or items in patient's environment

Continued.

Table A-18   Projected recommendations for isolation precautions in hospitals (CDC, 1995)*—cont'd

| | Standard Precautions | Transmission-based Precautions | | |
		Airborne	Droplet	Contact
Mask, eye protection, face shield	Wear a mask and eye protection or face shield to protect mucous membranes of eyes, nose, and mouth during procedures and patient care activities likely to cause splashing or spraying	Wear respiratory protection when entering the room of a patient diagnosed with or suspected of having TB (particulate-type respirator is recommended) Susceptible individuals should not enter the room of a patient diagnosed with or suspected of having measles (rubeola) or varicella (chickenpox)	Wear a mask when working within 3 ft of patient	
Gown	Wear a clean, nonsterile gown to protect skin and prevent soiling of clothing for procedures or patient care activities likely to soil clothing or cause			Wear a clean, nonsterile gown if substantial contact is likely with patient or with surfaces or items in patient's environment; wear a gown if pa-

	splashing or spraying of blood, body fluids, secretions, or excretions; remove gown promptly when tasks are finished; wash hands thoroughly	tient is incontinent or has diarrhea, an ileostomy, a colostomy, or uncontained wound drainage; remove gown carefully when tasks are finished; wash hands thoroughly
		When possible, dedicate use of noncritical equipment to one patient; if equipment or items must be shared, make sure they are adequately cleaned and disinfected between uses
Patient care equipment	Handle used equipment in a manner that prevents skin and mucous membrane exposure to pathogens, contamination of clothing, and environmental soiling	
Linen	Handle, transport, and process used linen in a manner that prevents skin and mucous membrane exposure to pathogens, contamination of clothing, and environmental soiling	

Continued.

Table A-18   Projected recommendations for isolation precautions in hospitals (CDC, 1995)*—cont'd.

| | Standard Precautions | Transmission-based Precautions | | |
		Airborne	Droplet	Contact
Patient placement	If possible, assign patient to a private room if he or she contaminates the environment, or if patient does not (or cannot) help maintain appropriate hygiene or environmental control; consult infection control professionals for other options	Assign patient to a private room if he or she: (1) has monitored negative air pressure relative to surrounding area; (2) needs a minimum of 6 air changes per hour; or (3) requires either appropriate discharge of air outdoors or monitored, high-efficiency filtration of room air before air is circulated to other parts of the hospital Keep room door closed when patient is in the room	Assign patient to a private room, if possible; if one is not available, maintain a spatial separation of at least 3 ft between infected patient and other patients and visitors; consult infection control professionals for other options	Assign patient to a private room, if possible; if one is not available, consult infection control professionals about selecting suitable roommates or making other arrangement

Patient transport	If a private room is not available, patient can be placed in a room with a patient who has an active infection with the same microorganism; consult infection control professionals for other options		
	Limit movement and transport from room to essential trips only; if transport is necessary, have patient wear a surgical mask, if possible, to minimize dispersal of droplet nuclei	Limit movement and transport from room to essential trips only; if transport is necessary, mask patient, if possible, to minimize dispersal of droplets	Limit movement and transport from room to essential trips only; if transport is necessary, meticulously follow precautions for minimizing contamination of environmental surfaces and equipment
Environmental control			Make sure patient care items, bedside equipment, and frequently touched surfaces are cleaned thoroughly each day

Continued.

Table A-18   Projected recommendations for isolation precautions in hospitals (CDC, 1995)*—cont'd.

| | Standard Precautions | Transmission-based Precautions | | |
		Airborne	Droplet	Contact
OSHA Bloodborne Pathogens Standard (1991)	■ Take care to prevent injuries when (1) using needles, scalpels, or other sharp instruments or devices; (2) handling sharp instruments after procedures; (3) cleaning used instruments; and (4) disposing of used needles ■ Never recap used needles or manipulate them with both hands; do not handle them in any way that involves pointing a needle toward any part of the body ■ If a procedure requires recapping, use			

a one-handed "scoop" technique, or use a mechanical device to hold the needle sheath

■ Do not remove used needles from disposable syringes by hand; do not bend, break, or manipulate used needles by hand

■ Place used sharps in appropriate, puncture-resistant containers kept as close as practical to the site of use

■ Use mouthpieces, resuscitation bags, or other ventilation devices as an alternative to mouth-to-mouth resuscitation in areas where the need is predictable

*Table based on CDC draft guidelines from: Draft guideline for isolation precautions in hospitals: notice of comment period, *Federal Register* 59(214): 55552-55570, Nov 7, 1994. **Note:** Final version may differ.

been documented as being or are suspected of being infected or colonized either by organisms transmitted by the airborne or droplet route, or by epidemiologically important organisms. Transmission-based Precautions have replaced the 1983 Category-Specific and Disease-Specific systems of isolation precautions.

In 1995-1996, the CDC began to encourage all hospitals to review and consider adopting Standard Precautions and Transmission-based Precautions and to discontinue use of the previous forms of isolation precautions. As always, the CDC offers hospitals the option of modifying the recommendations according to their needs and circumstances, and as directed by federal, state, or local regulations. For example, the Bloodborne Pathogens Standard instituted by the Occupational Safety and Health Administration (OSHA) in 1991 still pertains, and all facilities are required to comply with its provisions. The CDC's Standard Precautions incorporate all of the OSHA requirements.

Isolation Precautions for Patients with Pulmonary or Laryngeal Tuberculosis

In 1990, in response to the increasing incidence of pulmonary tuberculosis (TB) in the United States, the CDC established guidelines for preventing transmission of TB in the health care setting. These guidelines were revised in 1994. One component, Airborne Precautions, was designed for individuals diagnosed as having or suspected of having pulmonary or laryngeal TB that can be transmitted to others *via* the airborne route. The revised TB guidelines focus on early identification and treatment of individuals diagnosed as having or suspected of having active TB. In addition, the CDC spelled out requirements for special ventilation and use of masks that provide better filtration and a tighter fit than standard surgical masks. Masks of this type, called particulate respirators (PRs), originally were developed for industrial use to protect workers from dust, fumes, and other hazards that could affect the respiratory tract. The efficacy of PRs in protecting susceptible individuals from infection with TB has not been proven; however, research is under way. In the meantime, OSHA is in the process of developing a Tuberculosis Control Standard for health care settings that will include requirements for risk assessment, special ventilation, PRs, skin testing programs, exposure management, training programs, and other elements similar to the Bloodborne Pathogens Standard.

Management of Devices and Procedures to Reduce the Risk of Nosocomial Infection

Use of barriers is but one of many strategies for reducing the risk of nosocomial infection to patients and health care providers. Studies from the CDC show that a major factor in reducing infection risks is careful management of devices and procedures frequently used in patient care. For example, many patients need intravascular devices for the delivery of therapeutic drugs, but these patients are put at risk for site infections and bacteremias when such devices are used. It is well known that rotating the access site at appropriate intervals reduces the risk to the patient; new catheter materials that are more "vein friendly" also reduce trauma to the vascular system. Also, using a needle to deliver drugs and fluids to patients through these intravascular devices can put the health care provider at risk for puncture injury. Needle-free IV access devices are now available for accessing line ports, so that needles are not necessary once the intravascular catheter is in place. These newer and safer intravascular devices and procedures benefit both patient and health care provider by reducing the risk of infection.

Research studies on ways to reduce the risk of nosocomial infections are published in general and specialty journals and are presented at professional meetings each year. Infection control practitioners (ICPs) and hospital epidemiologists use these studies to recommend changes in nursing and medical practice. The Joint Commission on Accreditation of Healthcare Organizations (JCAHO) requires all accredited facilities to have a person on staff qualified to provide infection surveillance, prevention, and control services. The national associations for these professionals are the Association for Professionals in Infection Control and Epidemiology, Inc. (APIC), which publishes the *American Journal of Infection Control,* and the Society for Healthcare Epidemiology of America (SHEA), which publishes the journal *Infection Control and Hospital Epidemiology.*

Selected Bibliography

Bennett JV, Brachman PS, editors: *Hospital infections,* ed 3, Boston, 1992, Little, Brown.

Centers for Disease Control and Prevention: Guidelines for preventing the transmission of *Mycobacterium tuberculosis* in health care facilities, *MMWR* 43(RR-13):1-133, 1994.

Centers for Disease Control and Prevention: Draft guideline for isolation precautions in hospitals: notice of comment period, *Federal Register* 59(214):55552-55570, 1994.

Centers for Disease Control: Guidelines for preventing the transmission of tuberculosis in health care settings, with special focus on HIV-related issues, *MMWR* 39(RR 1-17), 1990.

Centers for Disease Control: Update: Universal Precautions for prevention of transmission of human immunodeficiency virus and other bloodborne pathogens in health care settings, *MMWR* 37:377-388, 1988.

Centers for Disease Control: Recommendations for prevention of HIV transmission in health care settings, *MMWR* 36(suppl 2):1-18, 1987.

Centers for Disease Control: Guideline for isolation precautions in hospitals, *Infection Control* 4:245-325, 1983.

Department of Labor, Occupational Safety and Health Administration: Occupational exposure to bloodborne pathogens; final rule, 29 CFR part 1910:1030, *Federal Register* 56:64003-64182, 1991.

Jackson MM: Infection prevention and control, *Crit Care Nurs Clin North Am* 4(3):401-409, 1992.

Jackson MM, Lynch P: Development of a numeric health care worker risk-assessment scale to evaluate potential for bloodborne pathogen exposures, *Am J Infect Control* 23:13-17, 1995.

Jackson MM, Lynch P: An attempt to make an issue less murky: a comparison of four systems for infection precautions, *Infect Control Hosp Epidemiol* 12:448-450, 1991.

Jackson MM, Lynch P: In search of a rational approach, *Am J Nurs* 90(10):65-73, 1990.

Jackson MM, Lynch P: Infection control: too much or too little? *Am J Nurs* 84:208-210, 1984.

Jackson MM et al: Why not treat all body substances as infections? *Am J Nurs* 87:1137-1139, 1987.

Lynch P et al: Rethinking the role of isolation practices in the prevention of nosocomial infections, *Ann Intern Med* 107:243-246, 1987.

Lynch P et al: Implementing and evaluating a system of generic infection precautions: body substance isolation, *Am J Infect Control* 18:1-12, 1990.

Martone WJ, Garner JS, editors: Proceedings of the Third Decennial International Conference on Nosocomial Infections, *Am J Med* 91(3B):1-333, 1991.

Pugliese G, Lynch P, Jackson MM, editors: *Universal Precautions: policies, procedures, and resources,* Chicago, 1990, American Hospital Publishing.

Wenzel RP: *Prevention and control of nosocomial infections,* ed 2, Baltimore, 1993, Williams & Wilkins.

Abbreviations Used in This Pocket Guide

ABG: arterial blood gas
ac: before meals
ACBaE: air contrast barium enema
ACTH: adrenocorticotropic hormone
AD: autonomic dysreflexia
ADA: American Diabetes Association
ADH: antidiuretic hormone
ADL: activities of daily living
AFB: acid-fast bacillus
AHA: American Heart Association
AIDS: acquired immunodeficiency syndrome
AKA: above-the-knee amputation
ANC: absolute neutrophil count
ANS: autonomic nervous system
ARDS: adult respiratory distress syndrome
ARF: acute respiratory failure; acute renal failure
ASA: acetylsalicylic acid (aspirin)

BCNU: carmustine
BEE: basal energy expenditure
bid: twice a day
BP: blood pressure
BPH: benign prostatic hypertrophy
bpm: beats per minute
BSE: breast self-examination
BUN: blood urea nitrogen

C: cervical; Centigrade
CABG: coronary artery bypass grafting
Ca/C^{2+}: calcium
CAD: coronary artery disease
CBC: complete blood count
CBI: continuous bladder irrigation
CCU: coronary care unit
CDC: Centers for Disease Control
CEA: carcinoembryonic antigen
CHF: congestive heart failure
Cl: chloride
cm: centimeter

CNS: central nervous system
CO_2: carbon dioxide
COPD: chronic obstructive pulmonary disease
CPM: continuous passive movement
CPP: cerebral perfusion pressure; coronary perfusion pressure
CPR: cardiopulmonary resuscitation
CRF: chronic renal failure
CSF: cerebrospinal fluid
CT: computerized axial tomography
CVA: cerebrovascular accident; costovertebral angle
CVP: central venous pressure

D&C: dilatation and curettage
DDAVP: desmopressin
DI: diabetes insipidus
DIC: disseminated intravascular coagulation
DKA: diabetic ketoacidosis
dl: deciliter
DM: diabetes mellitus
DSA: digital subtractive angiography
DTR: deep tendon reflex
DVT: deep vein thrombosis
D_5NS: 5% dextrose in normal saline
D_5W: 5% dextrose in water
D_{50}: 50% dextrose

ECG: electrocardiogram
EEG: electroencephalogram
e.g.: for example
EMG: electromyography
EP: evoked potentials
ESR: erythrocyte sedimentation rate
ESRD: end-stage renal disease
ET: endotracheal

F: Fahrenheit
FBS: fasting blood sugar
FDA: Food and Drug Administration
FIo_2: fraction of inspired oxygen
Fr: French
ft: foot or feet

g: gram
G-BS: Guillain-Barré syndrome
GH: growth hormone
GI: gastrointestinal
GN: glomerulonephritis

h: hour
HAV: hepatitis A virus

HBV: hepatitis B virus
HCG: human chorionic gonadotropin
HCl: hydrochloric acid
HCO$_3$/HCO$_3$$^-$: bicarbonate
Hct: hematocrit
HCV: hepatitis C virus
HDV: hepatitis D virus
HEV: hepatitis E virus
Hgb: hemoglobin
HHNK: hyperosmolar hyperglycemic nonketotic syndrome
HI: head injury
HIV: human immunodeficiency virus
HOB: head of bed
HR: heart rate
hs: hour of sleep
HTLV-1: human T-cell lymphotrophic virus
H$_2$O: water

ICP: intracranial pressure
ICU: intensive care unit
ID: identification
IDDM: insulin-dependent diabetes mellitus
IICP: increased intracranial pressure
IM: intramuscular
in: inch
I&O: intake and output
IPPB: intermittent positive pressure breathing
IU/iu: international unit
IV: intravenous
IVP: intravenous pyelogram

K/K$^+$: potassium
KCl: potassium chloride
kg: kilogram
KS: Kaposi's sarcoma

L: liter; lumbar
LAD: left arterial descending
lb: pound
LCTs: long-chain triglycerides
LDH: lactate dehydrogenase (also abbreviated LD)
LES: lower esophageal sphincter
LLQ: left lower quadrant
LMN: lower motor neuron
LOC: level of consciousness
LP: lumbar puncture
LUQ: left upper quadrant

Abbreviations

MAO: monoamine oxidase
MCTs: medium-chain triglycerides
mEq: milliequivalent
mg: milligram
Mg/Mg^{2+}: magnesium
MI: myocardial infarction
min: minute
ml: milliliter
mm: millimeter
mm Hg: millimeters of mercury
mmol: millimol
mOsm: milliosmol
MRI: magnetic resonance imaging
MS: multiple sclerosis
μg: microgram
μm: micrometer
μm^3: cubic micrometer

N: nitrogen
Na/Na$^+$: sodium
NaCl: sodium chloride
NaHCO$_3$: sodium bicarbonate
NCV: nerve conduction velocity
ng: nanogram
NG: nasogastric
NIDDM: non-insulin-dependent diabetes mellitus
NPO: nothing by mouth
NSAID: nonsteroidal antiinflammatory drug
NTG: nitroglycerin

O$_2$: oxygen
ORIF: open reduction with internal fixation
OSHA: Occupational Safety and Health Administration
OT: occupational therapist
OTC: over the counter

PaCO_2: partial pressure of dissolved carbon dioxide in arterial blood
PaO_2: partial pressure of dissolved oxygen in arterial blood
PCA: patient-controlled analgesia
PCP: *Pneumocystis carinii* pneumonia
PE: pulmonary embolus
PEEP: positive end-expiratory pressure
PET: positron emission tomography
pg: picogram
pH: hydrogen ion concentration
PO: by mouth
POC: products of conception
PPN: peripheral parenteral nutrition
prn: as needed
PSA: prostate-specific antigen

PT: physical therapist; prothrombin time
PTCA: percutaneous transluminal coronary angioplasty
PTH: parathyroid hormone
PTT: partial thromboplastin time
PTU: propylthiouracil
PVC: premature ventricular complexes; peripheral venous catheter
PVD: peripheral vascular disease

q: every
qid: four times a day

RBC: red blood cell
RDA: Recommended Daily Allowance; Recommended Dietary Allowance
RLQ: right lower quadrant
ROM: range of motion
RPE: rate perceived exertion
RR: respiratory rate
RUQ: right upper quadrant

S: sacral
Sao$_2$: oxygen saturation of hemoglobin
SC: subcutaneous (also abbreviated SQ)
SCI: spinal cord injury
sec: second
SGOT: serum glutamic-oxaloacetic transaminase
SGPT: serum glutamic-pyruvic transaminase
SIADH: syndrome of inappropriate antidiuretic hormone
SNS: sympathetic nervous system
SOB: shortness of breath
stat: immediately

T: thoracic
TB: tuberculosis
Tbsp: tablespoon
TENS: transcutaneous electrical nerve stimulation
THA: total hip arthroplasty
tid: three times a day
TKA: total knee arthroplasty
TPN: total parenteral nutrition
TPR: temperature, pulse, respirations
TSH: thyroid-stimulating hormone
TURBT: transurethral resection of the bladder and tumor
TURP: transurethral resection of the prostate

u/U: unit
UMN: upper motor neuron
URI: upper respiratory infection
UTI: urinary tract infection

Abbreviations

VAD: venous access device; ventricular assist device
VS: vital signs

WBC: white blood cell
wk: week
WOB: work of breathing

×: times

Index

Disuse syndrome, risk for—cont'd
  in malignant breast disorders,
      344-345
  in patients on prolonged bed
      rest, 416-418
  in spinal cord injury, 145-146
Diuretics, 35, 72
Diversional activity deficit in
      patients on prolonged
      bed rest, 421-422
Diverticulitis, 251-252
Diverticulosis, 251-252
DKA; see Diabetic ketoacidosis
DM; see Diabetes mellitus
Dolophine; see Methadone
Dopamine agonists, 129
Dressings for wound care,
      391-392
Dry to dry dressing in wound
      care, 391
DSA; see Digital subtraction
      angiography
Duoderm dressing in wound
      care, 392
Dymelor; see Acetohexamide
Dysfunctional grieving in cancer,
      457
Dysreflexia
  autonomic, 102-103, 142
  risk for
    in neurogenic bladder,
        102-103
    in spinal cord injury, 142-143
Dysrhythmias and conduction
      disturbances, 45-48

E

Ectopic pregnancy, 357
Edema
  cranial nerve, brain tumors and,
      163
  pulmonary, 49-51
Education, patient, pain control
      and, 403
EEG; see Electroencephalogram
Effusion, pleural, 6-7

Elastic stockings, 9, 62, 63
Eldepryl; see Selegiline
      hydrochloride
Electroencephalogram (EEG),
      neurologic disorders
      and, 205
Electromyography (EMG),
      neurologic disorders
      and, 210
Embolism, arterial, 60-61
Embolus, pulmonary, 7-10
EMG; see Electromyography
Emotional interventions, pain
      control and, 403
Emphysema, 18-20
Endocrine disorders, 212-235
  diabetes mellitus, 217-235
    diabetic ketoacidosis,
        222-231
    hyperosmolar hyperglycemic
        nonketotic syndrome,
        232-233
    hypoglycemia, 233-235
  disorders of pituitary gland,
      212-217
    diabetes insipidus, 212-213
    hypothalamic tumors,
        213-215
    pituitary tumors, 213-215
    syndrome of inappropriate
        antidiuretic hormone,
        215-217
  hyperosmolar hyperglycemic
      nonketotic syndrome,
      232-233
  hypoglycemia, 233-235
Endometrial cancer, 350
Endometriosis, 351-352
End-stage renal disease (ESRD),
      79, 80
Enteral nutrition, electrolyte
      imbalances in, 385-387
Enteral tube and providing
      nutritional support, 381
Environmental control, isolation
      precautions and, 489